the last date stamped

30 MAR 2001

13.5.04

2 9 AUG 2008

- 1 SEP 2008

17.3.09

H-R Wiedemann • J Kunze
Clinical Syndromes
Third Edition

Clinical Syndromes

Third Edition

Professor H-R Wiedemann MD

Kiel

Professor J Kunze MD

Berlin

with contributions from Dr F-R Grosse

Osterholz-Scharmbeck

Fourth, fully revised, substantially enlarged German edition
Third edition, English translation
With 329 photographic plates

Translation of the German Fourth Edition by
Neil Paget, Dip Trans

Translation of the German Third Edition
by Dr Mary F Passarge

Development Editor: Gina Almond

Project Manager: Jane Tozer

Production: Hamish Adamson

Design and layout: Gisli Thor

Index: Anita Reid

Publisher: Richard Furn

Authorised translation of the fourth German language edition 'Atlas der Klinischen Syndrome' by
H-R Wiedemann, J Kunze 1995
Published in 1997 by Mosby-Wolfe, an imprint of Times Mirror International Publishers Limited
Copyright © Schattauer Verlag GmbH 1995
© 1997 Times Mirror International Publishers Limited
Printed in Italy by Canale
ISBN 0 7234 2950 2

For full details of all Times Mirror International Publishers Limited titles, please write to Times Mirror International Publishers Limited, Lynton House, 7–12 Tavistock Square, London WC1H 9LB, England.

A CIP catalogue record for this book is available from the British Library.

We gratefully dedicate this edition to the following colleagues:

Michael Baraitser, London
J Bruce Beckwith, Loma Linda
Peter Beighton, Cape Town
M Michael Cohen Jr, Halifax
Robert J Gorlin, Minneapolis
Judith G Hall, Vancouver
Pierre Maroteaux, Paris
Victor A McKusick, Baltimore
Giovanni Neri, Rome
John M Opitz, Helena
Jürgen Spranger, Mainz

Preface to the German Fourth Edition

The reviews of the third edition of our Atlas were, it is fair to say, universally favourable about the text, format and illustrations. This applies both to general medical journals and to those from virtually all of the major specialities—from ophthalmology to dermatology, ear, nose and throat surgery, medical genetics, neurology, orthopaedics, radiology and orthodontics. Comments on the latest English edition (1992) were equally positive, for example, in the *Archives of Disease in Childhood* and the *New England Journal of Medicine*. New foreign language editions (Indonesian, Slovak and Czech).are currently in the pipeline by Schattauer.

With this new edition of the Atlas, the senior editor and his valued associate, Professor Jürgen Kunze (Berlin), have undertaken a comprehensive revision of the previous content and substantially enhanced it by adding further 'syndromes', with Professor Kunze, along with numerous helpful colleagues, making a particularly significant contribution.

The introductory comments on the nomenclature of syndromes have been extended and the detailed 'Diagnostic Overview' expanded to reflect the newly incorporated syndromes.

Seven illustrations have been replaced in the section on 'Minor Malformations, Anomalies and Variants in Man' and individual pictures have been substituted or entirely new illustrations inserted in 13 photographic plates for syndromes already included (giving a total of 28 new pictures). Eight previously unillustrated syndromes now have plates (with a total of 47 pictures) and four syndromes have been given additional plates (with 33 new pictures).

Most importantly, the Fourth Edition sees the introduction of 45 'new' syndromes (each accompanied by a photographic plate), which in turn means a further 274 additional pictures.

My long-time associate Mrs Herta Dibbern (Kiel) has meanwhile left the team. I would like to thank her once again for her excellent photographic work, which is amply documented in our Atlas. For their recent photographic services we thank Mrs Hanna Reimers and Mr Claus-Peter Blohm (both based in Kiel) and, especially, Mrs Erika Schäfer (Berlin).

We are particularly indebted also to those colleagues who, quite spontaneously and unselfishly, have supplied us with characteristic data and documents. Special mention should be made here of the contribution made to the previous edition by Professor Folker Hanefeld (formerly of Berlin, then Göttingen), who enriched the Atlas with no fewer than 17 syndromes. For the present edition, the following contributors should be named:

Prof M Becker, Berlin (Alagille syndrome)

Dr P Beyer, Oberhausen (Femoral Hypoplasia—Unusual Facies Syndrome)

Dr M Cohen and Prof S Stengel-Rutkowski, Munich, Dr R J Gibbons, Oxford, and Dr P Meinecke, Hamburg (Alpha-Thalassaemia with Mental Retardation)

Prof F Dressler, Berlin, Dr W Küster, Marburg, and Dr J Woweries, Berlin (Dandy–Walker Syndrome; Tay Syndrome)

Prof W Dudenhausen and Dr C Hofstaetter, Berlin (Pena–Shokeir Phenotype)

Dr U Frank, Braunschweig (Wolf Syndrome)

Dr R Götte and Prof H Versmold, Berlin (Diabetic Embryopathy)

Dr A Groß, Berlin (ABCD syndrome)

Prof G Groß-Selbeck and Dr M Petermöller, Düsseldorf (Kohlschütter Syndrome)

Dr A Grüters-Kieslich and Dr D Schnabel, Berlin (Peutz–Jeghers Syndrome; Vitamin-D dependent Rickets Type II)

Prof R Happle, Marburg (Restrictive Dermopathy)

Dr R C M Hennekam, Amsterdam, and Dr P Meinecke, Hamburg (Peters-Plus Syndrome)

Prof G Henze, Berlin (Chediak–Higashi Syndrome; Kasabach–Merritt Syndrome)

Dr D Hosenfeld, Kiel, Dr A Meindl, Munich *et al* (X-Linked Recessive Chondrodysplasia Punctata)

Dr R Houlston, Oxford, Dr P Meinecke, Hamburg (Floating Harbour Syndrome)

Prof H J Kaufmann, Dr T Riebel, Dr N Sarioglu, Berlin, Prof W Tillmann, Minden (Currarino Triad, Opsismodysplasia, Malignant Osteopetrosis)

Dr R König, Frankfurt a M (Townes–Brocks Syndrome)

Prof U Langenbeck, Frankfurt a M (Fryns Syndrome)

Prof W Lenz†, Münster i W (Cenani–Lenz Syndactyly Syndrome)

P Lorenz, Dresden, and Prof U Stephani, Kiel (CDG Syndrome)

Dr R Maier, Bietigheim (COFS Syndrome)

Dr J Mücke, St Ingbert (Hereditary Early-Onset Lymphoedema; MIDAS Syndrome)

Prof E von Mühlendahl, Osnabrück (Jeune Syndrome)

Dr R Pankau, Kiel (Gordon Syndrome; Kniest Syndrome; Pallister–Killian Syndrome; Williams–Beuren Syndrome)

Dr R Reichenbach and Prof H Theile, Leipzig (Baller–Gerold Syndrome)

Dr J Sperner, Berlin/Lübeck, and Prof G Stoltenburg–Didinger, Berlin (Walker–Warburg Syndrome)

Prof B Stück, Berlin (Adams–Oliver Syndrome)

Prof M Vogel, Berlin (Achondrogenesis Type II; 'Boomerang' Dysplasia)

Dr R-D Wegner, Berlin (Fragile X Syndrome)

For further important assistance during the revision process we extend our thanks to the following individuals (some of whom have already been acknowledged):

Dr K Aeissen, Kiel
Prof G R Burgio, Pavia
Dr G Gillessen-Kaesbach, Essen
Prof W Grote, Kiel
Prof H Helge, Berlin
Prof K Kruse, Lübeck
Dr P Maroteaux, Paris
Dr P Meinecke, Hamburg
Dr L Neumann, Berlin
Dr K Ounap, Tartu
Prof J M Opitz, Helena
H-C Oppermann, Kiel
Dr R Pankau, Kiel

Prof E Passarge, Essen
Prof J Schaub, Kiel
Prof W G Sippell, Kiel
Prof H-L Spohr, Berlin
Prof J Spranger, Mainz
Prof T Voit, Düsseldorf
Prof K Zerres, Bonn

Furthermore, we would like to thank Mrs Yvonne Heitmann (Kiel) and Mrs Monika Schulten (Berlin) for their great commitment. Last but not least, we thank Mr Dieter Bergemann, our publisher, and his experienced staff at Schattauer Publishers for their kind support and excellent work.

On behalf of the authors,   Hans-Rudolf Wiedemann

Preface to the German Third Edition

This *Atlas of Clinical Syndromes* was preceded by *Characteristic Syndromes*, in two editions, five languages, and 15,000 copies distributed around the world. Stimulated by readers and reviewers, the new publication is presented herewith, through the efforts of the editor, his former longtime co-worker Professor Jürgen Kunze, Berlin, and his clinical photographer, Mrs Herta Dibbern.

Compared with its predecessor, the *Atlas of Clinical Syndromes* deals more extensively with the stages of life of adolescence and adulthood, and it includes clinical disorders in which visual signs do not play a prominent role. It presents over 260 disease entities or processes in texts and illustrated plates (with a total of almost 1,700 single pictures) and a further 11 conditions without illustrations. These are preceded by five photographic plates to demonstrate characteristic 'minor anomalies, malformations, and unusual characteristics of man' (69 individual pictures).

In the texts we employ the more recently accepted international nomenclature, although neither rigidly nor exclusively. The nomenclature is briefly presented immediately after the table of contents, before the 'Diagnostic Overview' intended for medical practise. Each section of text has been signed by its author. Literature up to 1989, the year of publication, was taken into consideration. Special attention was devoted to the index.

Warm thanks are due to our numerous colleagues for their energetic and unselfish support of this and, in part, the preceding works. These colleagues include:

M Bauer, Gießen (a.d.L.)
F A Beemer, Amsterdam-Utrecht
G Beluffi, Pavia
C-G Bennholdt-Thomsen†, Cologne
A Blankenagel, Heidelberg
W Blauth, Kiel
G R Burgio, Pavia
O Butenandt, Munich
E Christophers, Kiel
E Dieterich, Kiel-Heide
H Doose, Kiel
C Fauré, Paris
J P Fryns, Leuven
A Fuhrmann-Rieger, Gießen
W Fuhrmann, Gießen
E Gladtke, Cologne
W Grote, Kiel
M Habedank, Aachen
F Hanefeld, Berlin-Göttingen
H-G Hansen, Lübeck
R Happle, Njmwegen
H Hauss, Kiel
P Heintzen, Kiel
H Helge, Berlin
M Hermanussen, Kiel

U Hillig, Marburg
D Hosenfeld, Kiel
E Jiminez, Berlin
H J Kaufmann, Berlin
H Kemperdick, Düsseldorf
C v Klinggräff, Kiel
D Knorr, Munich
K Kruse, Würzburg-Lübeck
T Kushnick, Greenville, USA
B Leiber, Frankfurt a M
W Lenz, Münster i. W.
F Majewski, Düsseldorf
H Manzke, Kiel-Norderney
P Maroteaux, Paris
P Meinecke, Hamburg-Altona
T Michael, Berlin
C Mietens†, Bochum
J Murken, Munich
G Neuhäuser, Gießen
M Obladen, Bochum-Berlin
J W Oorthuys, Amsterdam
H-C Oppermann, Kiel
E Passarge, Essen
W Plenert, Jena
A Proppe, Kiel
H Reich, Münster i W
A Rett, Vienna
A Rütt, Cologne-Würzburg
J Schaub, Kiel
A Schinzel, Zürich
H Schönenberg, Aachen
M Seip, Oslo
W Sippell, Kiel
H-L Spohr, Berlin
J Spranger, Mainz
E Stephan†, Kiel
G Stickler, Rochester, USA
R B Stolowsky, Berlin
B Stück, Berlin
M Vogel, Berlin
R-D Wegner, Berlin
U Wendel, Düsseldorf-Hilden
G G Wendt†, Marburg adL
E Werner, Berlin
K Zerres, Bonn

Furthermore, we would like to thank Mrs Yvonne Heitmann, Kiel and Mrs Erika Schäfer, Berlin, for their efforts. And last but not least we thank Mr Dieter Bergemann, our publisher, and his experienced co-workers from Schattauer Publishers for their kind criticism and fine work.

In the name of all authors, Hans-Rudolf Wiedemann
Kiel

Preface to the German Second Edition

Characteristic Syndromes has met with much interest and approval; the first reprinting was required after two years, and foreign-language editions have appeared. Reviewers have consistently commended the atlas, not only for its basic format and the 'information density' of the texts, but also for the quality of the illustrations. Encouraged by this, and stimulated by frequently expressed wishes that further syndromes be included, we now present a new edition. The basic idea and purpose of this book and its organization have remained unchanged: it is meant for medical practise. (Please refer to the Preface to the first edition.)

In the first edition the photographic material came almost without exception from the archives of the pediatric department of the University of Kiel or from the private files of the first author. In this edition 204, instead of 97, syndromes are illustrated—thus more than doubling the content of the book. This has required 'material help' on the part of kind colleagues. We are grateful for the photographs and clinical data for more than 50 of the newly included malformation complexes and hereditary syndromes. Again, color photographs have been intentionally excluded.

More than 170 acknowledged and generally familiar syndromes are presented here with the goal of 'visual recognition' or tentative diagnosis from appearance.

Additionally about 30 further singular clinical pictures have been included which were apparently previously unknown. These have come almost exclusively from the collected observations of the first author, and for the time being represent special cases or 'personal syndromes'. In our experience the study of this kind of presentation by colleagues frequently leads to their 'recognizing' earlier analogous observations they themselves have made or to helpful associations from other fields—and so to closer definition and classification. Thus, the inclusion of these cases if 'for the good of the cause'. The texts and some of the photographic plates of the first edition have been revised. In addition to a table of contents, a diagnostic overview (which has been expanded to include new groups), and an alphabetical index of the syndromes (including the most important synonyms), the present edition offers a table of particularly noteworthy signs.

In conclusion, clinical genetics has become greatly differentiated and continues to become more so at an increasing rate. As a result, a book such as this contains many, albeit well-deliberated, simplifications. This was unavoidable in order to stay within the prescribed framework.

Finally, we would like to acknowledge the slide collection 'Syndromes' ROCOM/Roche 1982, which supplemented the present edition of the atlas.

Hans-Rudolf Wiedemann
Kiel

Preface to the German First Edition

Was ist das Schwerste von allem? Was dir das Leichteste dünket.
Mit den augen zu sehn, was vor den Augen dir liegt.*

(J.W. v. Goethe, Xenia**, from the literary remains)

'Syndromes' are plentiful in modern medicine. According to G. Fanconi, more than six times as many syndromes can be tabulated now than could be at the beginning of the century. Essentially, this is an effect of advances in research and, therefore, may be viewed positively.

It is important to diagnose syndromes early and to draw the necessary conclusions from the diagnosis. Many syndromes are easy for the physician with a trained eye to recognize. The intention of this book is to aid in this training. Almost one hundred syndromes that can be partially or totally visually comprehended have been presented here, each with an illustrated plate. Most of them represent so-called dysmorphosis syndromes, whereby the manifestations may be present at birth, but also may not be apparent until later. Since this book is meant to be of practical use, the authors have neither followed the strict definition of syndromes nor limited themselves to a sharply delineated category of syndromes.

Blickdiagnosen (diagnoses from appearance) are not to be taken literally to mean 'on sight' or 'instant' diagnoses. To be sure, most of the syndromes presented can be identified by an experienced observer with a physician's eye alone and do not require extensive laboratory tests, which unfortunately and unjustifiably are often given priority by young physicians. But in many cases, a careful history to supplement the impression, and a thorough clinical examination to substantiate the tentative diagnosis, will be required. The text accompanying each of the photographic plates gives the basic guidelines and additional information, concisely formulated.

The frequencies of the syndromes are to be understood within the framework of dysmorphosis syndromes in general. Several stand out, especially Down's syndrome (1 in approx. 650 births), but also neurofibromatosis, Noonan syndrome, Prader–Willi syndrome, Turner syndrome, and several others, perhaps including the newly recognized fetal alcohol syndrome. For the patient at hand and his family it is of no particular consolation that his condition is rare. To him the frequency of his disorder is '100%', and he expects his physician to be well informed about it. Furthermore, 'the rare things in medicine are *not rare*, only observers are rare' (H.R. Clouston, 1939).

Patients with the syndromes presented here will be taken to general practitioners and to colleagues of the most diverse specialities—ophthalmologists and radiologists, dermatologists and psychiatrists, human geneticists and otologists, internists and orthopaedic surgeons, pediatricians and neurologists. This atlas is meant to serve all of them. The diagnostic overview following the table of contents is intended to facilitate locating syndromes that come into question.

Hans-Rudolf Wiedemann
Kiel

*Roughly:
  What is the hardest of all? What you as easiest would deem,
  To see with your eyes, what lies before your eyes.

**Satirical epigrams

Nomenclature of Syndromes

In 1982, a clinical genetics working group (Spranger, Benirschke, J G Hall, Lenz, Opitz, Pinsky, Schwarzacher and D W Smith) published its recommendations for an international nomenclature to describe patients with morphological anomalies. With these recommendations, clinical syndromologists are obliged to orientate their thinking pathogenetically. In addition, classification using the new concepts has important practical significance: it says something about prognosis, recurrent risk and diagnostic measures.

However, the definitions are not to be followed rigidly. Today, no one refers to Marfan 'dysplasia' and even the diagnosis of Potter 'syndrome' is clinically widespread. As a further example, a syndrome-like picture in genetically heterogeneous patients is called Pena–Shokeir phenotype.

The concepts are described below in their strictest sense:

Single morphological defects are divided into malformations, disruptions, deformities, and dysplasias.

A *malformation* is an anomaly resulting when the anlage of an organ, part of an organ or a body region is defective. It arises *ab ovo*. Thus, malformations are of genetic origin.

A *disruption* is a morphological defect resulting from the effects of exogenous factors on an organ with an originally normal anlage and development. Thus, disruptions are of a non-genetic nature.

A *deformity* is an anomaly of form and position of part of the body caused by mechanical factors. It may also arise postnatally. Deformities are likewise of a non-genetic nature and accessible to therapy.

A *dysplasia* is a defect of tissue, whether local or generalized, that leads to morphological anomalies. Generalized dysplasias are genetic in nature.

Multiple morphological defect patterns are defined as follows:

Polytopic field defects are topically differentiable anomalies caused by disturbance of a single embryonal 'developmental field'. Polytopic means: widely separated structures.

A *sequence* is a clinical picture of known pathogenesis but unknown aetiology.

A *syndrome* is a pattern of aetiologically connected anomalies. The pathogenetic mechanism of origin is unknown. If the pathogenesis is defined in part, the clinical picture is designated avoiding the term syndrome (mucopolysaccharidosis).

A *symptom* complex is a recurrent pattern of morphological, functional or both types of changes with unknown or inconsistent pathogenesis and aetiology.

A *disease* is an aetiologically and pathogenetically defined clinical picture.

References:
Spranger J, Benirschke K, Hall J G , Lenz W, Opitz J M, Pinsky , Schwarzacher H G, Smith D W: Errors of morphogenesis: concepts and terms. recommendations of an international working group. *J Pediatr* 1982, 100:160–165.
Spranger J: Krankheit, Syndrom, Sequenz. *Monattssch. Kinderheilkd* 1989, 137:2–7.

Contents

Contents

Contents

Diagnostic Overview

The numbers in bold type are the corresponding syndrome numbers.

Syndromes with prominent anomalies of the cranium, face or both

Syndromes in which tall stature is a (possibly transient) prominent feature

Syndromes with prominent short stature (primordial, postnatal or both; proportionate or disproportionate)

Syndromes with prominent aged appearance

Syndromes with prominent cartilaginous or bony excrescences or bulges of the skeleton or soft tissues

Syndromes with prominent anomalies of the hands or feet

Syndromes with triphalangeal (finger-like) thumbs

Syndromes with hypoplasia or aplasia of the thumbs

Syndromes with shortening of the halluces

Syndromes with marked anomalies of the teeth and/or jaws

Syndromes with haematological signs
See under

Syndromes with muscular hypotonia and neurological signs (apart from seizures, seizure disorders and isolated mental retardation)

Syndromes with obligatory or possible visual involvement

Syndromes with possible hearing impairment or deafness

Syndromes with regular or possible mental retardation and behavioural disorders

Atlas Section

The number in parenthesis and bold type are the corresponding **syndrome numbers**

J.K.

1. Bilateral epicanthus:
In 0.5% of newborns, significant in oriental races. Diminishes markedly with age (formation of the facial features). Common in genetic disorders, e.g. Down syndrome, Williams syndrome, etc.

2. Epicanthus inversus:
Charactistic of blepharophimosis-epicanthus inversus-ptosis syndrome. This is an important sign.

3. Mongoloid slant of the palpebral fissures (up-slanting palpebral fissures):
In 3% of Caucasian newborns, major ethnic variations. Common in oriental races, premature infants and in genetic disorders.

4. Antimongoloid slant of the palpebral fissures (down-slanting palpebral fissures):
In 0.1% of all live-born infants. Frequent in genetic disorders. This is an important sign.

5. Brushfield's spots:
Common in white-skinned individuals, especially in those with fair hair. Characteristic also, for example, in Down syndrome. As pigmentation increases after birth, these white spots on the iris fade.

6. Epibulbar dermoid:
Characteristic of Goldenhar 'syndrome', mandibulofacial dysostosis and Proteus syndrome, associated with epidermal nevus syndrome.

7. Synophrys (eyebrows meeting across the midline):
In 0.2% of newborns, more frequent in coloured and oriental races. More prevalent in genetic disorders, e.g. Cornelia de Lange syndrome.

8. Hypotelorism, coloboma of the iris:
Hypotelorism: familially determined, common in cerebral malformations, e.g. trisomy 13, holoprosencephaly, Opitz trigonocephaly. Coloboma of the iris: rare. Associated with coloboma of the eyelid, optical malformations, Goldenhar 'syndrome', cataract, cleft lip and palate, cerebral malformations. This is an important sign.

9. and 10. Megalocornea:
Principal sign of various retardation syndromes. Not to be confused with keratoconus. Rarely found in isolation within families. This is an important sign.

11. Long eyelashes:
Familial. Otherwise indicative of multicausal mental retardation, e.g. Cornelia de Lange syndrome.

12. Hypertelorism:
In 0.4% of newborns. Isolated within individual families and in association with many genetic syndromes, e.g. Aarskog syndrome, Greig's hypertelorism. This is an important sign.

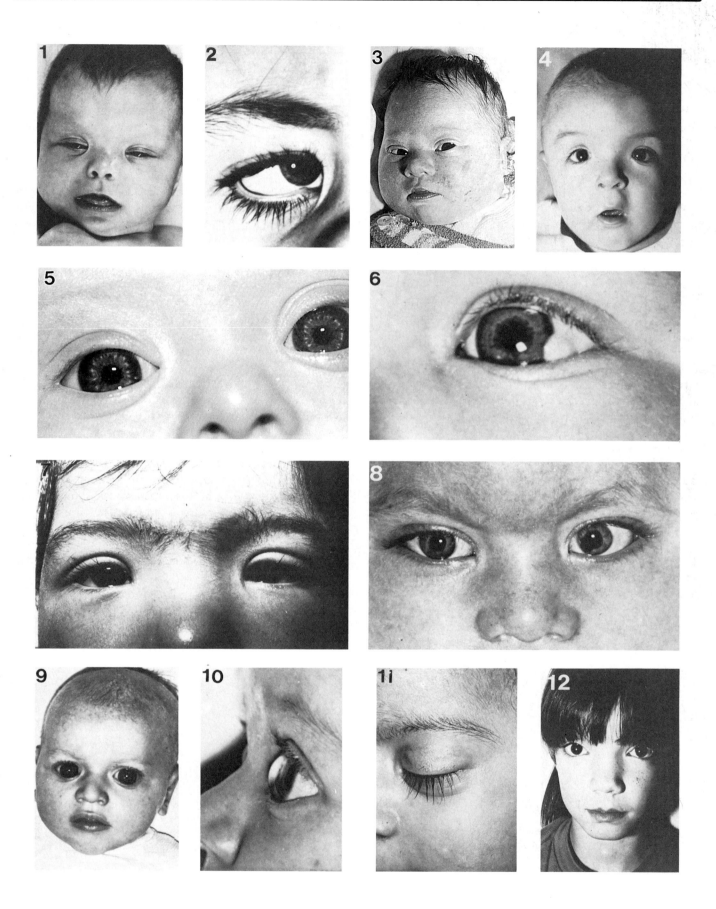

J.K.

1. Naevus flammeus (Bossard spot, frontal; angel's kiss; salmon patch; 'stork mark'):
In over 40% of all newborns. Usually fades in the first year of life. Commonly observed with syndromes, e.g. Wiedemann–Beckwith syndrome.

2. Naevus flammeus = port-wine stain = capillary haemangioma (also 'stork mark'; Unna–Politzer naevus, nuchal):
In over 40% of all newborns; persists in 30% of adults.

3. Depressed nasal bridge:
In over 20% of all newborns; no longer persists with the formation of the facial features after 5 years of age. Simulated in syndromes characterized by a prominent forehead.

4. Pterygium colli, short neck, low nuchal hairline:
In Turner syndrome (XO syndrome), Noonan syndrome, alcoholic embryo-foetopathy, chromosomal disorders, Roberts syndrome, Goldenhar 'syndrome', Klippel–Feil syndrome, etc.

5. Prognathism:
In one out of 25–50 of all newborns, usually familial, e.g. Habsburg prognathism. Associated with many genetic syndromes, e.g. Angelman syndrome.

6. Micrognathia:
In 0.3–0.8% of all newborns, more prevalent in the male sex. Usually becomes less apparent over the first 5 years of life. Widely observed in association with many genetic syndromes, e.g. Pierre Robin syndrome, Franceschetti syndrome, etc.

7. Transverse facial and orbital clefts:
In one out of 100–300 of all facial clefts. Associated with Aperts syndrome, Goldenhar 'syndrome', Franceschetti syndrome.

8. Lisch nodules:
Characteristic of von Recklinghausen's disease (neurofibromatosis), in 90% of all these patients.

9. Vertical median cleft lip:
Characteristic of median cleft face syndrome. Median line syndrome.

10. Interocular blind-ending sinus:
Beware: sinus leading to the base of the brain.

11. Stenosis of the lacrimal ducts:
Secondary synechia following silver nitrate cautery. An isolated, congenital aplasia of the lacrimal canal and/or lacrimal punctum. Symptomatic in LADD syndrome, cyclopia, eyelid malformations. Also observed in families.

12. Conjunctival telangiectasis:
In urticaria pigmentosa syndrome, Coats' disease, Osler's telangiectasis, Rothmund–Thompson syndrome, Louis–Bar syndrome. This is an important sign.

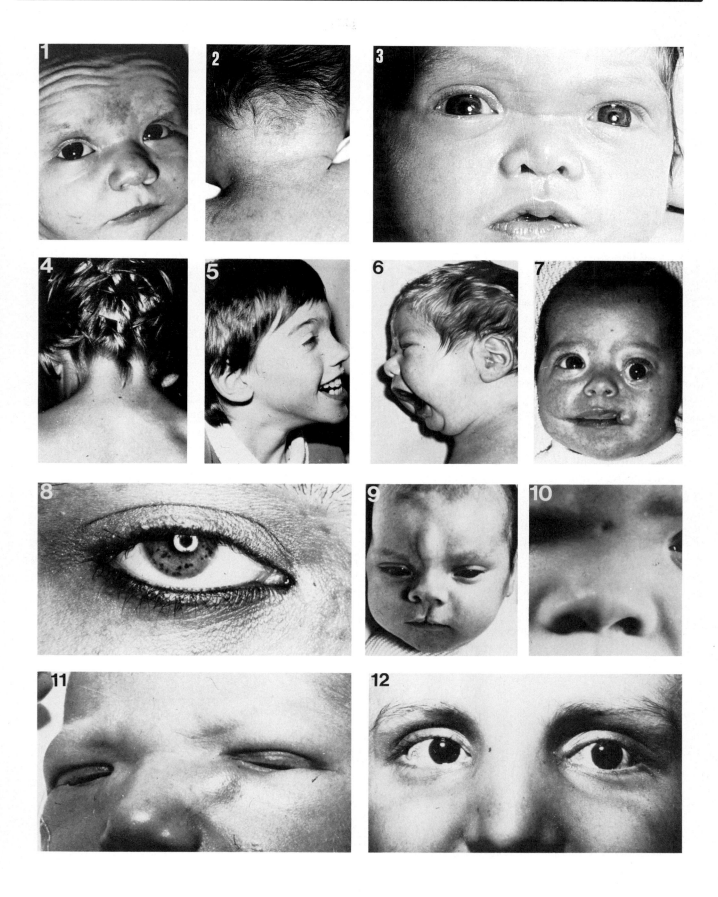

J.K.

1. Protruding ears:
More frequently observed in newborns, often reversible later. In the adult population, encountered in less than 2%. Often harmlessly familial. In the case of reappearance, frequently associated with a functional disorder of the inner ear. Beware: combination with blepharoptosis.

2–4. Auricular tag:
2. Pre-auricular tags, **3. and 4.** 0.2–0.5% of all newborns, usually unilateral, right. Sex ratio 0.6. Sporadic in 90%. Rarely familial. Hearing test should be carried out. Constant sign in Goldenhar 'syndrome', among others. Association with kidney anomalies.

5. Pre-auricular blind-ending sinus or fistulae:
In 0.07–0.2% of Caucasian newborns, common in coloured and oriental races. Usually unilateral, right. Also familial. Sporadic in 50%. Constant sign in cat-eye syndrome, among others. Hearing test should be carried out. Association with kidney anomalies.

6. Auricular tubercle:
In Finland found in over 50% of the population, in Germany 20%, in England 55%. Male:female = 55:45. This is not significant.

7. Inclusion of cystic masses in the helix:
Pathognomic of diastrophic dysplasia.

8. Grooved or notched ear:
In 0.2% of newborns. In 50% of all patients with Wiedemann–Beckwith syndrome.

9. Bipartite tongue:
Determined by a short frenulum which is attached towards the tip of the tongue. Sporadic (pseudofissure of the tongue).

10. Fissured tongue:
Prevalence one out of 12–20 in all age groups. There is a distinct increase with advancing age. Whereas in children a frequency of one out of 100 is observed, in over-40 year olds a frequency of one out of eight can be expected. Male:female = 2.24:1.68. In over 30% of Down syndrome patients. Also familial. Combination with geographic tongue more frequent.

11. Macroglossia:
Rarely familial, postnatally 100% in association with Wiedemann–Beckwith syndrome, also in Down syndrome and hypothyroidism, among others. Later in association with lysosomal thesaurismotic disorders and glycogenoses.

12. Pilonidal sinus:
In 0.1–0.2% of all newborns. Little significance. Look for 'tethered cord'.

13. and 14. Sacral naevus flammeus and sacral skin tag:
Marker for spina bifida occulta, 'tethered cord syndrome', diastematomyelia.

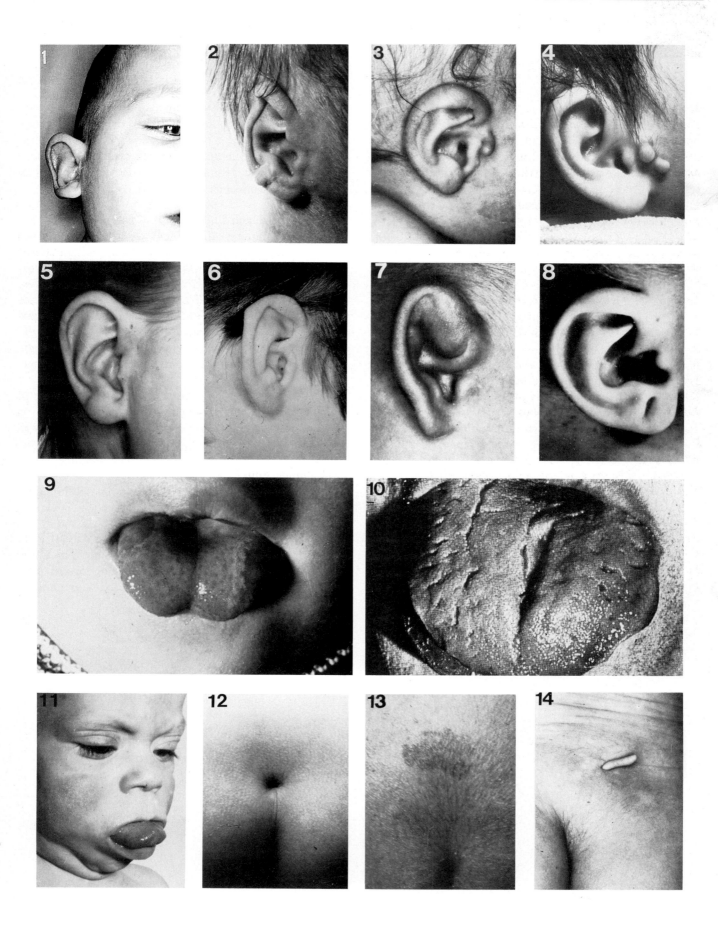

J.K.

1. Café au lait spots:
Found in 3–10% of all newborns. If more than six are observed, larger than 0.5cm in diameter, urgent suspicion of von Recklinghausen's disease (neurofibromatosis). Also in Noonan syndrome, Silver–Russell syndrome.

2. Pigmented naevi with mucous membrane involvement:
Melanocytic naevi in 0.2–0.6% of newborns. Mucocutaneous involvement of the pigmented spots pathognomic of Peutz–Jeghers syndrome.

3. Multiple neurofibromas:
Together with multiple café au lait spots and Lisch nodules, always von Recklinghausen's disease (neurofibromatosis).

4. White spots:
Faint white depigmentations of the skin in the shape of an ash leaf, varying in size and indistinctly defined against normally pigmented skin, always pathognomic of tuberous sclerosis. Not to be confused with chicken-pox scars and neurodermatitis. A sharp definition against healthy skin indicates vitiligo. This is an important sign.

5. Mongolian spot:
In 90% of Asians, 10% of Caucasians, usually sacral. In 97%: regression by 10 years of age. Persistence in 3%. No significance.

6. Accessory nipples:
In 1–2% of all newborns, common in coloured people. Usually sporadic, rarely familial (in 6%), commonly on the left side. In Caucasians, below the normal breast in over 90% of cases; in Japanese, above the normal breast in 88%. Association with kidney anomalies. This is an important sign.

7. Subungual tumour = Koenen tumour:
Pathognomic of tuberous sclerosis.

8. Clinodactyly of the distal phalanges of both fifth fingers:
Up to 1% of all newborns, more prevalent in males. Sex ratio 11:20. Usually sporadic, rarely familial. Harmless anomaly. Common in genetic syndromes, e.g. Down syndrome, Aarskog syndrome, Cornelia de Lange syndrome, Silver–Russell syndrome, etc. DD: Kirner deformity.

9. Simian crease and single crease of the fifth finger:
Simian crease unilaterally in 2–4% of Caucasian newborns; in the oriental population up to 15%. Slight cluster in males (11:20). Bilateral in one out of 1000 newborns. Common in both monogenic and chromosomal disorders, e.g. in 40% of Down syndrome patients. Single crease of the fifth finger: in 0.04–0.08% of newborns. Usually sporadic; radiologically, there is always hypoplasia of the middle phalanx. Empirical experience: simian and single crease of one hand: chromosomal analysis should be performed.

10. Absence of large flexion creases of the fingers:
General signs of arthrogryposis or lack of finger movement during the embryonal and foetal period.

11. Acromial dimple:
Usually bilateral, familial (autosomal dominant). Common in 18p- syndrome, Silver–Russell syndrome.

12. Benign ring-shaped constrictions of the skin:
Usually familial (autosomal dominant), single or multiple. Also in skeletal disorders with shortening of the long bones (dermatomegaly). Not to be confused with amniotic constriction rings.

13. Shawl scrotum:
In 1–2% of all healthy children. Characteristic of patients with Aarskog syndrome and in patients with cryptorchidism.

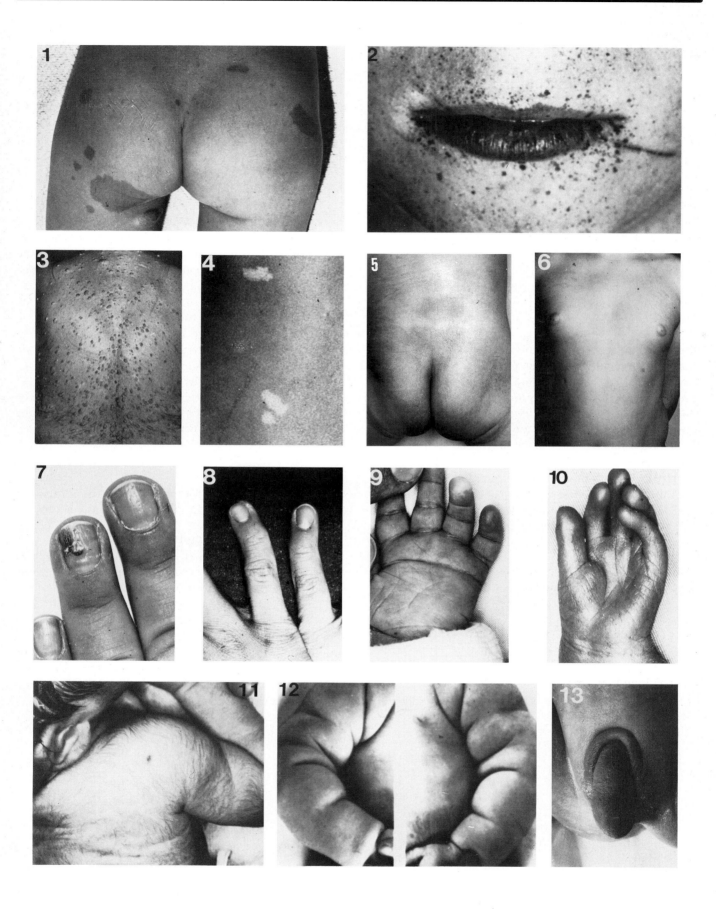

J.K.

1. 'Hitch-hiker thumb':
Pathognomic of Rubinstein–Taybi syndrome, diastrophic dysplasia.

2. Partial cutaneous, interdigital syndactyly:
Cutaneous, partial/total syndactyly is characteristic of many genetic syndromes, e.g. Aarskog syndrome, Greig's cephalopolysyndactyly, etc.

3. Preaxial polydactyly:
Duplication of the fingers on the thumb side, usually unilateral, sporadic. Characteristic, for example, in Greig's cephalopolysyndactyly syndrome, orofaciodigital syndrome type II, trisomy 18, etc.

4. Flexion contractures of the fingers (fifth finger over fourth and second finger over third):
Characteristic, for example, of trisomy 18, Freeman–Sheldon syndrome, distal arthrogryposis type I, Pena–Shokeir phenotype.

5. Partial rudimentary postaxial polydactyly:
Duplication of the fingers on the little-finger side: in Africans, 10 times more frequent than in Caucasians: one out of 100–300 compared with one out of 3300–630, autosomal dominant. Characteristic, for example, of orofaciodigital syndrome type I and II, Greig's cephalopolysyndactyly.

6. Camptodactyly:
In isolated cases, familial, autosomal dominant. Syndromic in trisomy 18, Pena–Shokeir phenotype and other syndromes.

7. Hypoplasia, aplasia of the thumb:
Isolated sign in 20% of all patients with radial defects, two-thirds being unilateral, usually sporadic. Syndromic in Fanconi anaemia, Holt–Oram syndrome, Nager syndrome and others.

8. Triphalangeal thumb:
Either normal position with normal function or inability to oppose with hypoplastic thenar. Sporadic, familial or sign of over-riding genetic syndromes, such as Nager syndrome, tibial aplasia-polydactyly syndrome, Aase syndrome.

9. Reduction of the fourth metatarsal:
Symptomatic of Ullrich–Turner syndrome, pseudo-hypoparathyroidism, spondyloepiphyseal dysplasia tarda, basal-cell naevus syndrome. Also familial as an isolated finding (brachydactyly type E).

10. Hypoplasia of the big toe:
Characteristic of otopalatodigital syndrome I, tibial aplasia syndrome, brachydactyly type D.

11. Partial syndactyly of the second and third toes:
Usually familial, autosomal dominant, zygodactyly. Syndromatic in Dubowitz syndrome, Smith–Lemli–Opitz syndrome and others.

12. 'Sandal gap' (deep crease between hallux and second toe):
0.4% of all newborns. Usually familial. Syndromic in chromosomal disorders, e.g. Down syndrome.

13. Partial postaxial polydactyly of the fifth toe:
Usually familial, autosomal dominant but also a sign of Bardet–Biedl syndrome, Greig's cephalopolysyndactyly syndrome, orofaciodigital syndrome type II.

14. and 15. Parietal foramina and Fenestrae parietales:
Prevalence of around 3% in the Asian population and around 1% in Africans and white people. Transmitted by autosomal dominant inheritance; size (foramina or fenestrae) and location (parietal and frontal) vary within families. They have no clinical significance.

References:
Mehes K: *Informative Morphogenetic Variants in the Newborn Infants.* Budapest: Akademiai Kiado; 1988.
Leppig K A, Werber M M, Cann C I, Cook C A, Holmes J B: Predictive value of minor anomalies. I. Association with major malformations. *J Pediatr* 1987, **110**:530–537.
Little B, Knoll K A, Klein V R, Heller K B: Hereditary cranium bifidum and symmetric parietal foramina are the same entity. *Am J Med Genet* 1990, 35:453–458.

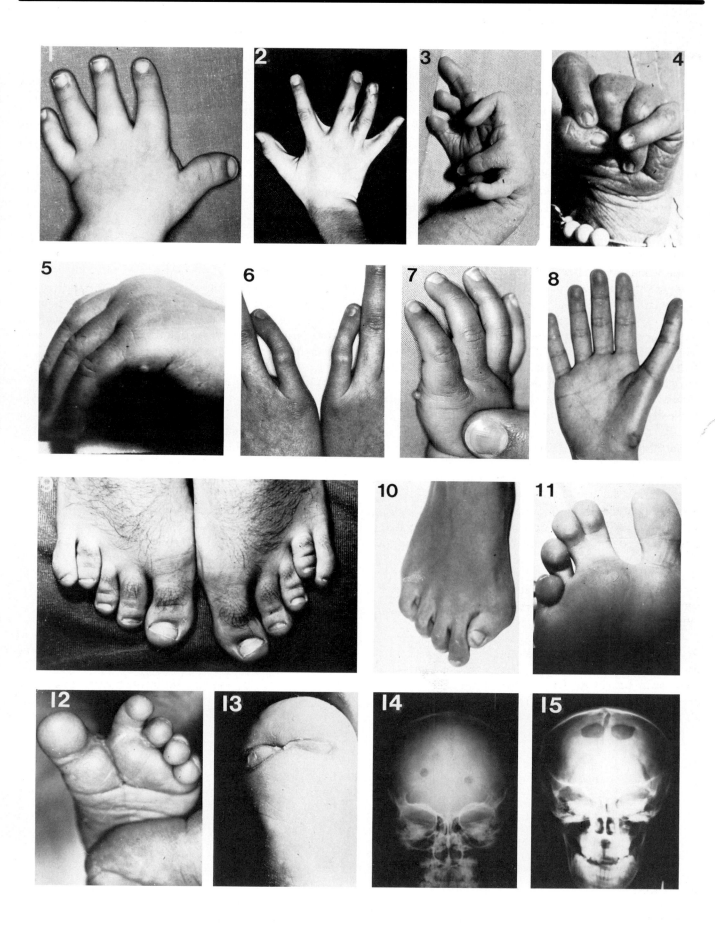

6 Crouzon Syndrome
(Craniofacial Dysostosis)

H.-R.W

A characteristic syndrome with acrocephaly.

Main signs:
- Acrocephaly with a high wide forehead, sometimes with pronounced bulging of the anterior fontanelle region, flat occiput (1–3, 5, 6).
- Exophthalmos (with flat orbits). Slight antimongoloid slant of the palpebral fissures. Convergence of the globes difficult or impossible, divergent strabismus. Possible ptosis (1–6).
- Maxillary hypoplasia with 'parrot-beak' nose, short upper lip, high narrow palate, narrowly spaced teeth; prognathism (2, 3c, 6a, 6c, 7b).

Supplementary findings: Frequently mild to moderate mental retardation. In some cases signs of craniostenosis and optic atrophy with decreased visual acuity. Exceptional is, impaired hearing.

Radiologically, premature craniosynostosis, especially of the coronal and lambdoid sutures; short anterior, deep middle and posterior cranial fossae; often very pronounced digital markings of the skull (7a and 7c).

Manifestation: At birth.

Aetiology: An autosomal dominant hereditary condition with 100% penetrance but variable expression. Increased paternal age; possible significance of germline mosaics. Gene locus on chromosome 10q25-q26.

Frequency: Relatively low but for some time now only a small minority of cases have been published (in 1966 more than 100 published cases were counted). Estimated frequency: one out of 25 000.

Course, prognosis: Mainly dependent on the presence and degree of mental retardation and optic nerve damage.

Differential diagnosis: Above all, Saethre–Chotzen syndrome (7) and Jackson–Weiss syndrome.

Treatment: Symptomatic. Early craniotomy, performed in the first months of life (even in the absence of signs of craniostenosis), depending on the individual's condition and revised at regular intervals. Cosmetic surgery may be indicated eventually to mitigate facial deformity.

Illustrations:
1 A newborn.
2 An infant.
3 and 5 Young preschool children.
4 and 7b A 6-year-old girl.
6 A 10-year-old girl.
7a and c Digital markings of the skull of the child in 4 and 7b at age 10 years.
Some of these children represent definite inherited cases; the others, sporadic cases (interpreted as new mutations).

References:
Vulliamy D G, Normandale P A: Cranio-facial dysostosis in a Dorset family. *Arch Dis Child* 1966, **41**:375.
Kushner J, Alexander E, Davis Jr C H, *et al*: Crouzon's disease (craniofacial dysostosis). Modern diagnosis and treatment. *J Neurosurg* 1972, **37**:434.
Cohen M M Jr: Craniosynostosis… *Birth Defects Orig Art Ser XV* 1979, **5B**:13–63.
Kreiborg S: Crouzon syndrome… *Scand J Plast Reconstr Surg (Suppl)* 1981, **18**.
Marchac D, Renier D: *Craniofacial Surgery for Craniosynostosis*. Boston: Little, Brown and Co; 1982: 211.
Golabi M *et al*: Radiographic abnormalities of Crouzon syndrome. A survey of 23 cases. *Proc Greenwood Genet Ctr* 1984, **3**:102.
Cohen M M Jr: Syndromes with craniosynostosis. In: *Craniosynostosis…* New York: Raven Press; 1986.
Cohen M M Jr: Craniosynostosis update 1987. *Am J Med Genet Suppl* 1988, **4**:99–148.
Rollnick B R: Germinal mosaicism in Crouzon syndrome. *Clin Genet* 1988, **33**:145–150.
Kreiborg S, Cohen M M Jr: Germinal mosaicism in Crouzon syndrome. *Hum Genet* 1990. **84**:487–488.
Navarrete C *et al*: Germinal mosaicism in Crouzon syndrome… *Clin Genet* 1991, **40**:29–34.
Reardon W, van Herwerden L *et al*: Crouzon syndrome is not linked to craniosynostosis loci at 7p and 5qter. *J Med Genet* 1994, **31**:219–221.
Preston R A *et al*: A gene for Crouzon craniofacial dysostosis maps to the long arm of chromosome 10. *Nat Genet* 1994, **7**:149–153.
Li X A, Lewanda A F *et al*: Two craniosynostotic loci, Crouzon…, map to chromosome 10q23-q26. *Genomics* 1994, **22**:418.
Reardon W, Winter R M *et al*: Mutations in the fibroblast growth factor receptor 2 gene cause Crouzon syndrome. *Nat Genet* 1994, **8**:98–103.

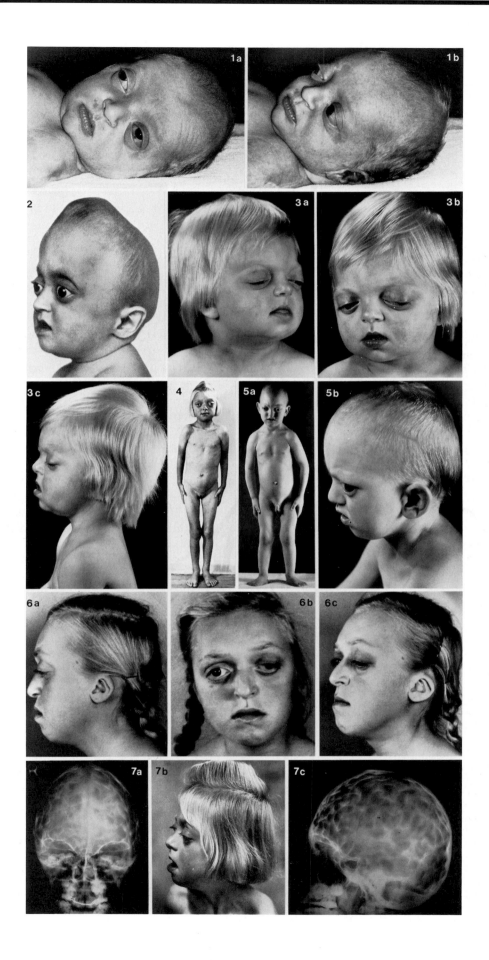

7 Saethre–Chotzen Syndrome

(ACS Type III, Acrocephalosyndactyly Type Chotzen, Chotzen Syndrome)

H.-R.W

A syndrome comprising acrocephaly, relatively characteristic facies, mild to moderate syndactyly of the hands and feet and possible mental retardation.

Main signs:
- Relatively mild acrocephaly with a broad forehead (1–3).
- Face: often markedly asymmetric. Frequently low anterior hairline. Hypertelorism, broad flat nasal bridge, antimongoloid slant of the palpebral fissures, often highly arched eyebrows, possible mild exophthalmos. Ptosis (or blepharochalasis), strabismus. Tear ducts may be narrowed, dystopia canthorum. Beak-like curve of the nose with deviated septum. Possibly low-set ears. Hypoplasia of the maxilla, narrow palate; prognathism (1–3, 4, 6).
- Relatively short stubby fingers (frequently with inturned little finger); exclusively soft-tissue syndactyly between the proximal segments of digits II and III (5) but also of other digits. Normal number of fingers and toes; normal thumbs and big toes. Cutaneous syndactyly of the toes.

Supplementary findings: Frequently, mental retardation, also in combination with neurological or psychological anomalies. Frequently, mild hearing impairment. Small stature.

Possible cryptorchidism.

Radiologically, as a rule premature craniosynostosis of the coronal suture (exceptional is premature synostosis of the metopic suture).

Manifestation: At birth.

Aetiology: Inherited as an autosomal dominant condition. Extremely variable expression; usually complete, occasionally incomplete penetrance. Probable gene locus 7p21 or 7p22.

Frequency: Low but substantially higher than that of Apert syndrome (9).

Course, prognosis: Principally dependent on whether mental retardation is present.

Differential diagnosis: Primarily Crouzon syndrome (6), also Jackson–Weiss syndrome.

Treatment: Early neurosurgical intervention can considerably improve the patient's later appearance.

Illustrations:
1–6 The same boy at ages 4 months and 2 years. Acrocephaly with premature craniosynostosis of the coronal suture. Characteristic facies (including mild ptosis, right convex facial scoliosis, deviated septum and low-set ears). Short stubby fingers with bridge of soft tissue between digits II and III (5), radial deviation of the little fingers; soft-tissue syndactyly between toes III and IV bilaterally. Slight shortness of stature. Psychomotor retardation.

References:

Kreiborg S, Pruzansky S, Pashayan H: The Saethre–Chotzen syndrome. *Teratology* 1972, 6:287.
Pantke A, Cohen Jr M M, Witkop Jr C R: The Saethre–Chotzen syndrome. *Birth Defects Orig Art Ser* 1975, 11:190.
Friedman J M, Hanson J W *et al*: Saethre–Chotzen syndrome... *J Pediatr* 1977, 91:929–933.
Thompson E M, Baraitser M *et al*: Parietal foramina in Saethre–Chotzen syndrome. *J Med Genet* 1984, 21:369–372.
Bianchi E, Arico M *et al*: A family with the Saethre–Chotzen syndrome. *Am J Med Genet* 1985, 2:649–658.
Cohen M M Jr: *Craniosynostosis: Diagnosis, Evaluation and Management.* New York; Raven Press: 1986.
Cohen M M Jr: Craniosynostosis update 1987. *Am J Med Genet, Suppl. 4,* 1988 27:95–148.
Legius E, Fryns JP *et al*: Auralcephalosyndactyly: a... variant of the Saethre–Chotzen syndrome? *J Med Genet* 1989, 26:522–524.
Marini R, Temple K *et al*: Pitfalls in counseling the craniosynostoses. *J Med Genet* 1991, 28:117–121.
Cristofori G, Filippi G: Saethre–Chotzen syndrome with trigonocephaly. *Am J Med Genet* 1992, 44:611–614.
Brueton L A *et al*: The mapping of a gene... evidence for linkage of the Saethre–Chotzen syndrome to distal chromosome 7p. *J Med Genet* 1992, 29:181–185.
Fehlow P, Fröhlich B *et al*: Neuropsychiatrische Begleitsymptome bei Saethre–Chotzen-Syndrom. *Fortschr Neurol Psychiatr* 1992, 60:66–73.
Reardon W, McManus S P *et al*: Cytogenetic evidence that the Saethre–Chotzen gene maps to 7p21.2. *Am J Med Genet* 1993, 47:633–636.
Adès L C *et al*: Jackson–Weiss syndrome... *Am J Med Genet* 1994, 51:121–130.
Rose C S P, King A A J *et al*: Localization of the genetic locus for Saethre–Chotzen syndrome to a 6cM region of chromsome 7... *Hum Molec Genet* 1944, 3:1405–1409.
Reardon W, Winter R M: Saethre–Chotzen syndrome. *J Med Genet* 1994, 31:393–396.

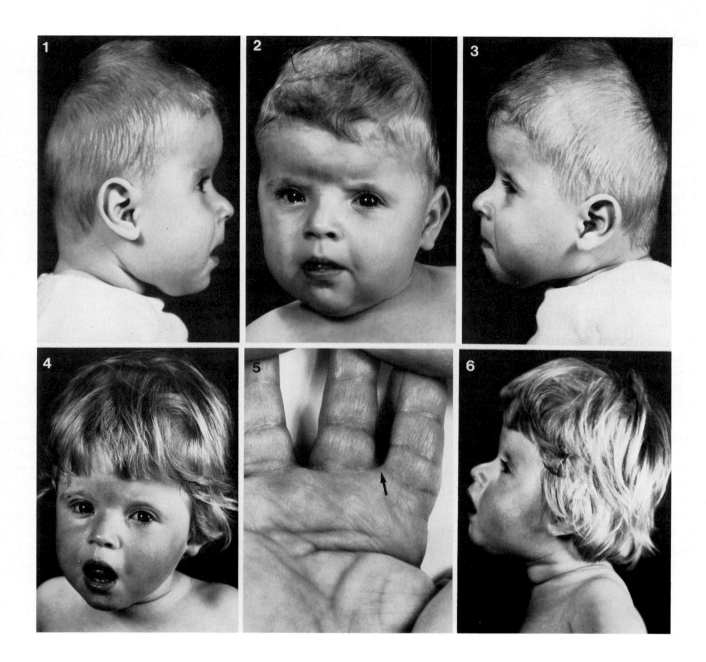

8 Pfeiffer Syndrome

(ACS Type V, Acrocephalosyndactyly Type Pfeiffer)

A syndrome comprising acrocephaly, facial dysmorphism, broad stubby thumbs and halluces and mild to moderate syndactyly.

Main signs:
- Acrobrachycephaly (**1–3**).
- Face: broad with a flat profile, hypertelorism, broad low nasal bridge, antimongoloid slant of the palpebral fissures, high-arched palate and small upper and, in some cases, lower jaw (**1 and 2**).
- Halluces (**4**) and thumbs stubby, broad and short and usually deviated. Various degrees of soft-tissue syndactyly, usually between digits II and III.

Supplementary findings: Possible small stature.

On radiograph, the anterior fontanelle may be enlarged (**3**), with premature closure especially of the coronal suture; various malformations, especially of the first rays of the hands and feet, e.g. trapezoidal first phalanges of the halluces.

Manifestation: At birth.

Aetiology: Inherited as an autosomal dominant condition; markedly variable expression, with complete penetrance. Possible occurrence of germline mosaics. Gene loci on chromosome 8.

Frequency: Low.

Course, prognosis: On the whole, favourable.

Differential diagnosis: Other acrocephalosyndactyly syndromes. It has been discussed whether Pfeiffer syndrome and Saethre–Chotzen syndrome or Apert syndrome (**7** *and* **9**, respectively) represent different grades of severity of a single hereditary defect. Cohen makes a distinction between the the 'classic' Pfeiffer syndrome presented here and two subtypes (previously observed only in sporadic cases), one of which is characterized by the presence of a cloverleaf skull (*12*), the other by severe proptosis oculorum (without a cloverleaf skull); both are prognostically far less favourable.

Treatment: Corrective surgical measures for the cranium and/or hands may be indicated.

Illustrations:
1–5 The same 2-month-old girl. Acrobrachycephaly with flat occiput; distinct interparietal bone; wide open anterior fontanelle with premature ossification of the coronal suture and part of the sagittal suture (**3**). Hypertelorism, antimongoloid slant of the palpebral fissures, strabismus. Broad, stubby thumbs and halluces with mild cutaneous syndactyly.
Normal female karyotype. The mental development of this girl, who underwent early cranial surgery and whose progress has been followed for years, is within normal limits.

References:
Naveh S, Friedman A: Pfeiffer syndrome: report of a family and review of the literature. *J Med Genet* 1976, **13**:277.
Bull M J, Escobar V, Bixler D *et al*: Phenotype definition and occurrence risk in the acrocephalosyndactyly syndromes. *Birth Defects Orig Art Ser* 1797, **15/5B**:65.
Sanchez J M, de Negrotti T C: Variable expression in Pfeiffer syndrome. *J Med Genet* 1981, **18**:73.
Vanek J, Losan Fr: Pfeiffer's type of acrocephalosyndactyly in two families. *J Med Genet* 1982, **19**:289–292.
Kroczek R A *et al*: Cloverleaf skull associated with Pfeiffer syndrome: pathology and management. *Eur J Pediatr* 1986, **145**:442–445.
Rasmussen S A, Frias J L: Mild expression of the Pfeiffer syndrome. *Clin Genet* 1988, **33**:5–10.
Hall J G: Mild expression of the Pfeiffer syndrome. *Clin Genet* 1988, **34**:144.
Muenke M, Epstein C J *et al*: Cytogenetic and molecular genetic studies in patients with Pfeiffer syndrome. *David W. Smith workshop on malformations...*, 1991, Lake Arrowhead, Calif, Sept. 27–Oct. 1.
Stone P, Trevenen C L *et al*: Congenital tracheal stenosis in Pfeiffer syndrome. *Clin Genet* 1990, **38**:145–148.
Cohen M M Jr: Pfeiffer syndrome update, clinical subtypes and guidelines for differential diagnosis. *Am J Med Genet* 1993, **45**:300–307.
Muenke M, Schell U *et al*: A common mutation in the fibroblast growth factor receptor 1 gene in Pfeiffer syndrome. *Nat Genet* 1994, **8**:269–274.

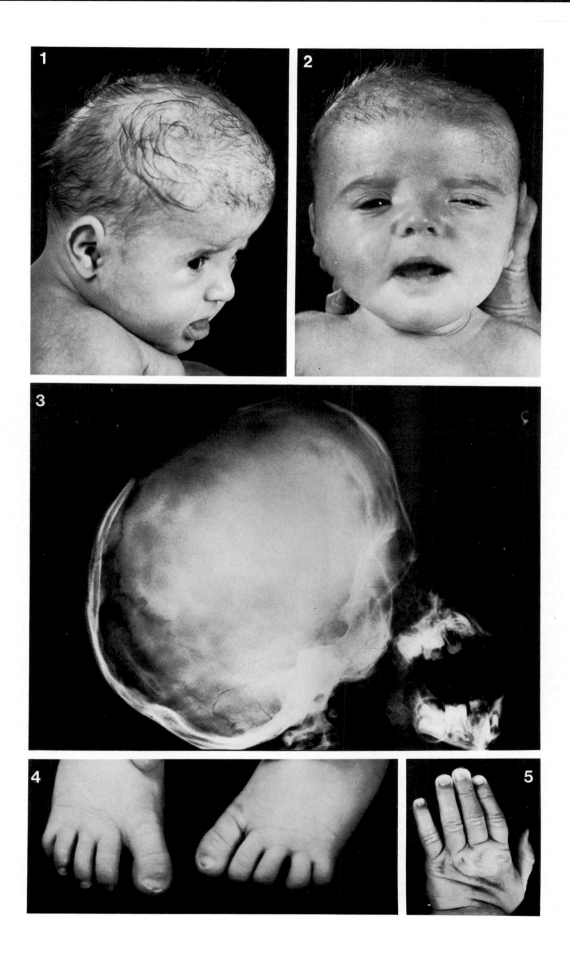

9

Apert Syndrome
(ACS Type 1, Acrocephalosyndactyly Type 1)

H.-R.W

A characteristic syndrome comprising acrocephaly, facial dysmorphism and extensive symmetrical syndactyly of the fingers (including osseus) and toes.

Main signs:

- Acrocephaly with high prominent forehead, flat occiput (**1, 2, 4, 6**).
- Flattish face with a horizontal supra-orbital groove, hypertelorism, flat orbits with exophthalmos, strabismus, slight antimongoloid slant of the palpebral fissures and often a small, up-turned (sometimes beak-like) nose and low-set ears. Maxillary hypoplasia, narrow palate (sometimes cleft); narrowly spaced teeth (**1, 2, 4, 6**).
- Extensive syndactyly to almost complete spoon-like deformity of the hands (**4–7**), generally with bony fusion of the second to fourth fingers (**10**), which often share a common nail (**5**). Fingers often short (**4**), ends of thumbs frequently broad and distorted (**7**). Soft-tissue syndactyly of many or all toes; big toe stubby and deformed (**8, 9, 11, 12**).
- 16% of newborns weigh more than 4000g.

Supplementary findings: Abnormally short upper extremities (**4**), impaired mobility of the elbow and shoulder joints, anomalies of the shoulder girdle. Short stature.

Frequently, mental retardation, which may be severe. However, in about 80% of the patients an IQ of 50–70 can be expected.

Radiologically, irregular premature craniosynostosis, especially of the coronal and often of the lambdoid sutures; short anterior and deepened middle and posterior cranial fossae; maxillary hypoplasia; possible digital markings of the skull (**3**). Sometimes anomalies of the cervical vertebral column; epiphyseal dysplasias.

Numerous other possibly associated malformations (cardiac, urinary, gastrointestinal or respiratory tracts; also various cerebral anomalies: megalencephaly, corpus-callosum malformations, gyration anomalies, white-matter hypoplasia).

Manifestation: At birth. Pronounced short stature from infancy.

Aetiology: An autosomal dominant hereditary condition. However, the vast majority of cases are sporadic and represent new mutations (such as occur more frequently with increased paternal age); significance of germline mosaics still inadequately explained.

Frequency: Low (in 1960, 150 published cases were counted); approximately one out of 100000 live births.

Course, prognosis: Essentially dependent on the severity of the typical malformations, the presence or development of mental impairment and the possible manifestations and consequences of additional defects in other organ systems. Relatively high mortality in the first years of life. Sonography and CT of the skull immediately after birth are recommended. In preschool children, height falls from the fiftieth to the fifth percentile, the process being exacerbated during the school years with rhizomelic reduction of the lower extremities. Puberty at the normal time.

Treatment: Symptomatic. Early neurosurgical intervention for acrocephaly (in the first months of life), even in the absence of signs and symptoms of craniostenosis. Corrective surgery of the extremities should be undertaken sufficiently early, at a time determined in consultation with the hand surgeon.

Pyschological guidance and all necessary handicap aids.

Illustrations:

1, 2, 6 newborns. **4** A 5-year-old child. **12** A 3-year-old boy. **2, 5, 9** The first child of a 33-year-old father. Premature craniosynostosis of the coronal suture, bifid uvula; suspected cardiac defect; only mild mental retardation at follow-up. **3, 7, 8, 10, 11** X-rays and close-ups of the child in **4**.

References:

Spranger J W, Langer Jr L O, Wiedemann H-R: *Bone Dysplasias. An Atlas of Constitutional Disorders of Skeletal Development.* Stuttgart and Philadephia: G Fischer and W B Saunders; 1974.

Stewart R E, Bixon G, Cohen A: The pathogenesis of premature craniosynostosis in acrocephalosyndactyly (Apert's syndrome). *Plast Reconstr Surg* 1977, **59**:699.

Beligere N, Harris V, Pruzansky S: Progressive bone dysplasia in Apert syndrome. *Radiology* 1981, **139**:593.

Allanson J E: Germinal mosaicism in Apert syndrome. *Clin Genet* 1986, **29**:429–433.

Kim H, Uppal V et al: Apert syndrome and fetal hydrocephaly. *Hum Genet* 1986, **73**:93–95.

Patton M A, Goodship J *et al*: Intellectual development in Apert's syndrome... *J Med Genet* 1988, **25**:164–167.

Rollnick B R: Male transmission of Apert syndrome. *Clin Genet* 1988, **33**:87–90.

Gorlin R: Apert syndrome with polysyndactyly of the feet. *Am J Med Genet* 1989, **32**:557.

Cohen M M Jr, Kreiborg S: The central nervous system in the Apert syndrome. *Am J Med Genet* 1990, **35**:36–45.

Cohen M M Jr *et al*: Birth prevalence study of the Apert syndrome. *Am J Med Genet* 1992, **42**:655–659.

Kreiborg S *et al*: Cervical spine in the Apert syndrome. *Am J Genet* 1992, **43**:704–708.

Cohen M M Jr *et al*: Upper and lower airway compromise in the Apert syndrome. *Am J Med Genet* 1992, **44**:90–93.

Czeizel A E *et al*: Birth prevalence study of the Apert syndrome. *Am J Med Genet* 1993, **45**:392.

Cohen M M Jr, Kreiborg S: 1. An updated pediatric perspective on the Apert syndrome. *Am J Dis Child* 1993, **147**:989–993. 2. Growth pattern in the Apert syndrome. *Am J Med Genet* 1993, **47**:617–623. 3. Skeletal anomalies in the Apert syndrome. *Am J Med Genet* 1993, **47**:624–632.

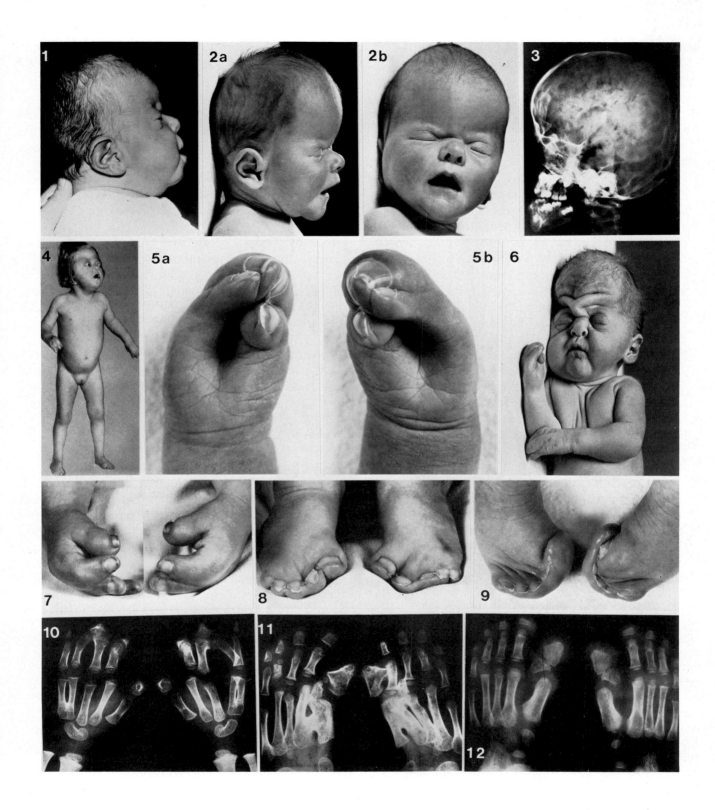

10

Opitz Trigonocephaly Syndrome

(C Syndrome [after the initial of the family name of the first cases described])

H.-R.W

A genetic syndrome with characteristic facies, peculiar conformation of the palate, short neck, cutis laxa, joint disorders, microcephalic mental retardation and, in some cases, polysyndactyly.

Main signs:
- A somewhat triangular-shaped cranium, narrowing at the top (trigonocephaly) as a result of craniosynostosis, with the forehead showing a prominent median ridge and in some cases bitemporal depressions (1 and 4). In some cases, naevus flammeus of the glabella, hypertrichosis of the forehead. Hypotelorism. Mongoloid slant of the palpebral fissures, strabismus, epicanthic folds (1 and 2) and other eye anomalies; broad short nasal bridge and pug nose, long philtrum and diverse anomalies of the external ears (low-set or rotated ears, soft pinnae due to paucity of cartilage and others). High palate, very narrow especially anteriorly, between abnormally wide alveolar ridges (sometimes with frenulae between the latter and the buccal mucous membrane). Macrostomia, micrognathia.
- Loose skin, especially of the neck. Widely spaced nipples. Hyperextensibility, dislocation or contractures of the large joints.
- Failure to thrive in most cases. Hypotonia. Increasing tendency to microcephaly with corresponding psychomotor retardation. In isolated cases, agenesis of the corpus callosum or other cerebral anomalies.
- In some cases short hands and/or fingers (possible aplasia of phalanges of the fingers and/or toes), club feet; postaxial, less frequently pre-axial, polydactyly, clinodactyly and cutaneous syndactyly (9 and 10).

Supplementary findings: Possible cardiovascular defects; lung, kidney or other internal malformations. Also deformities of the thorax, exomphalos, genital anomalies, short extremities, short stature.

Manifestation: At birth.

Aetiology: This syndrome, which is in most cases observed sporadically and is phenotypically very variable, appears in most cases to be the expression of an autosomal recessive gene but may possibly also be the result of anomalies on chromosome 3. Careful, sometimes repeated, chromosomal analysis is indicated, especially in the light of the great difference in recurrence risks.

Frequency: Only 35 cases have been described to date. However, the syndrome is probably not extremely rare.

Course, prognosis: After initial, usually severe failure to thrive, frequently death in early infancy. Surviving children are usually severely retarded.

Differential diagnosis: The Meckel–Gruber syndrome (45) and the Smith–Lemli–Opitz syndrome (281) should be considered in some cases, as well as a number of chromosomal aberrations that may be accompanied by trigonocephaly.

Treatment: Conservative, symptomatic.

Illustrations:
1–8 A 5-month-old boy. Microdolichotrigonocephaly (1–4). Bilateral buphthalmos. Pug nose. Long philtrum. Macrostomia (1 and 2); high narrow palate; pre-auricular pits (5). Short neck, deformation of the thorax; ventricular septal defect; cryptorchidism. Laxity of the skin and musculature. Short hands with bilateral fifth-finger clinodactyly and simian crease (6 and 7); club feet with hypoplasia of rays III–V. A repeated chromosomal analysis (after an initial 'normal' result) showed a pericentric inversion of chromosome 3.
9 and 10 The hand of a 9-month-old, typically affected (normal karyotype) boy with precentral hexadactyly, brachydactyly and fifth-finger clinodactyly.

References:
Oberklaid F, Danks M: The Opitz trigonocephaly syndrome. Am J Dis Child 1975, 129:1348.
Antley R M, Sung Hwang D, Theopold W, Gorlin R J, Steeper T, Pitt D, Danks M, McPherson E, Bartels H, Wiedemann H-R, Opitz J M: Further delineation of the C (trigonocephaly) syndrome. Am J Med Genet 1981, 9:147–163.
Flatz S D, Schinzel A, Doehring E: Opitz trigonocephaly syndrome: report of two cases. Eur J Pediatr 1984, 141:183–185.
Fryns J P, Snoeck L, Kleczkowska A et al: Opitz trigonocephaly syndrome and terminal transverse limb reduction defects. Helv Paed Acta 1985, 40:485–488.
Sargent C, Burn J, Baraitser M et al: Trigonocephaly and the Opitz C syndrome. J Med Genet 1985, 22:39–45.
Reynolds J F, Johnston K M et al: Nosology of the C syndrome. Abstracts of the 10. anniversary David W. Smith workshop on malformations and morphogenesis. May 1989: Madrid; 34.
Lalatta F et al: 'C' Trigonocephaly syndrome... Am J Med Genet 1990, 37:451–456.
De Koster J et al: Opitz C syndrome... Am J Med Genet 1990, 37:457:459.
Stratton R F et al: C syndrome with apparently normal development. Am J Med Genet 1990, 37:460–462.
Camera G et al: 'C' trigonocephaly syndrome... Am J Med Genet 1990, 37:463–464.
Haaf Th et al: Opitz trigonocephaly syndrome. Am J Med Genet 1991, 40:444–446.
Cabral de Almeida J C et al: C syndrome and omphalocele... Am J Med Genet 1992, 43:385.
Cleper R et al: Varadi syndrome... or Opitz trigonocephaly syndrome... Am J Med Genet 1993, 47:451–455.

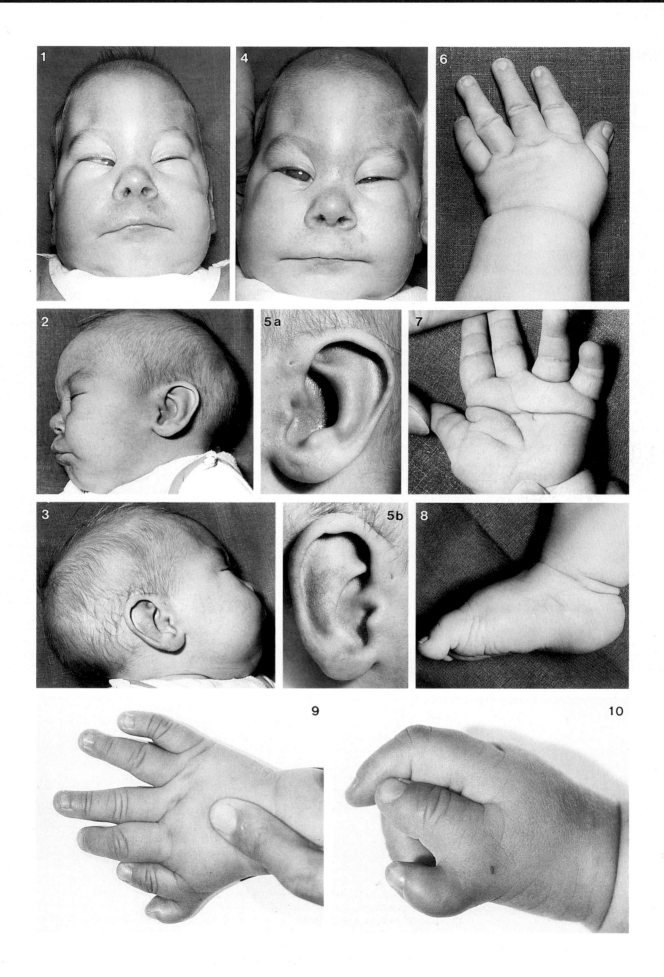

11 Carpenter Syndrome
(ACPS Type II, Acrocephalosyndactyly Type Carpenter)

H.-R.W

A syndrome comprising acrocephaly, facial dysmorphism, brachysyndactyly of the hands and polysyndactyly of the feet.

Main signs:
- Oxy- and acrobrachycephaly with bulging fontanelle (1). In some cases marked bulging of the temporal areas, symmetrically or asymmetrically (1 and 3), with resemblance to or actual formation of a cloverleaf skull (12).
- Face broad and flat with exophthalmos, dystopia canthorum, possible mongoloid or antimongoloid slant of the palpebral fissures and epicanthic folds, low-set and posteriorly rotated ears, high-arched palate and micrognathia (1 and 2). Short thick neck.
- Short hands; brachy-, campto- and clinodactyly; broad thumbs; cutaneous syndactyly between the middle and ring fingers, in some cases more fingers are involved (1 and 2). Short and very wide halluces, may appear bifid, with various degrees of syndactyly of the toes.

Supplementary findings: Frequently, cardiac defects, mild mental retardation, anomalies of the cornea, truncal obesity, short stature, urogenital anomalies.

Coxa valga, genu valgum, lateral dislocation of the patella, pes varus.

Radiologically, characteristic configuration, deviation and duplication in the region of the thumbs and big toes (4 and 5). Brachy- or amesophalangia of the fingers and toes.

Manifestation: At birth.

Aetiology: An autosomal recessive hereditary condition; variable expression.

Frequency: Low (40 cases reported up to 1987).

Course, prognosis: Essentially dependent on the presence and degree of primary mental retardation and on early surgical treatment of the cranium and, in some cases, the heart.

Diagnosis, differential diagnosis: Greig's cephalopolysyndactyly syndrome (236) can be easily ruled out by the less severe cranial deformity; in addition, it is transmitted by autosomal dominant inheritance.

Bardet–Biedl syndrome (159), suggested by the obesity, hypogenitalism, mental retardation and polydactyly, can be excluded by the shape of the skull, the facies, the duplication of the halluces and syndactyly of the Carpenter syndrome and by the absence of tapetoretinal degeneration. The ACPS observations of Goodman *et al* and Summit *et al* probably fall within the domain of the Carpenter syndrome.

Treatment: Surgical measures, as required, on the cranium, the extremities and the heart.

Illustrations:
1–5 A female infant with the Carpenter syndrome. Cutaneous syndactyly of the third and fourth fingers and of the first to third toes bilaterally; broad, stubby thumbs and halluces. Radiologically, deviation of the hypoplastic proximal phalanx of the thumb and hypo- and aplasia of various middle phalanges or, alternatively, coarse broadening of the first ray of both feet, with duplication of the proximal and distal phalanges of the halluces.

References:
Pfeiffer R A, Seemann K B, Tünte W *et al*: Akrozephalopolysyndaktylie. *Klin Pädiat* 1977, **189**:120.
Verdy M, Dussault R G *et al*: Carpenter's syndrome... *Acta Endocrinol* 1983, **104**:6–9.
Robinson L K, James H E *et al*: Carpenter syndrome: natural history and clinical spectrum. *Am J Med Genet* 1985, **20**:461–469.
Cohen D M, Green J G *et al*: Acrocephalopolysyndactyly type II - Carpenter syndrome... *Am J Med Genet* 1987, **28**:311–324.
Gershoni-Baruch R: Carpenter syndrome: marked variability of expression to include the Summitt and Goodman syndromes. *Am J Med Genet* 1990, **35**:236–240.

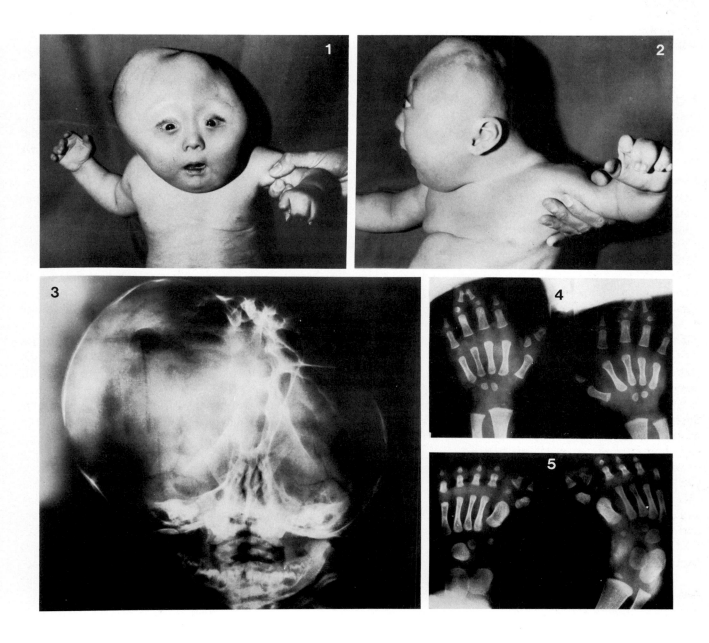

12 Cloverleaf Skull
(Crâne en Trèfle)

A cloverleaf-like deformity of the skull resulting from premature closure of the cranial sutures, occurring both alone and as part of a number of fairly extensive and well-defined clinical syndromes.

Main signs:
Marked bubble-like outpouching of the cranium upwards and bilaterally outwards at the temporal areas, with downward displacement of the ears to an almost horizontal position, depressed nasal bridge and exophthalmos (**1 and 2**). Hydrocephalus (**3**).

Supplementary findings: Increased intracranial pressure, muscle wasting, impaired psychomotor development.

Manifestation: At birth.

Aetiology: Aetiologically and pathogenetically heterogeneous. Cloverleaf skull can occur in the Apert (*9*), Carpenter (*11*), Crouzon (*6*), Saethre–Chotzen (*7*) and Pfeiffer (*8*) syndromes; with camptomelic dysplasia (*129*), thanatophoric dysplasias type II (*119*) and some other skeletal dysplasias; with certain chromosomal aberrations and other disorders; in combination with impaired mobility of the large joints (especially frequently the elbows) and as an apparently isolated finding.

Frequency: Low (more than 150 case reports in the literature).

Course, prognosis: Unfavourable; as a rule, early death.

Treatment: Symptomatic neurosurgical measures may be indicated.

Illustrations:
1 and 2 A 2-month-old infant with cloverleaf skull as an isolated finding. Normally proportioned trunk and extremities. No externally recognizable anomalies apart from the cranial. No joint disorders. The pneumoencephalogram shows markedly dilated lateral ventricles in the protruding temporal areas. (Child died at age 5 months.)

References:
Holtermüller K, Wiedemann H-R: Kleeblattschädel-Syndrom. *Med Mschr* 1960, **14**:439.
Wiedemann H-R, Ostertag B: Kleeblattschädel und allgemeine Mikromelie. *Klin Pädiatr* 1974, **186**:261.
Aksu F, Mietens C: Kleeblattschädel-Syndrom. *Klin Pädiatr* 1979, **191**:418.
Cohen M M Jr: Craniosynostosis… *Birth Defects Orig Ar. Ser XV* 1979 **5B**:13–63.
Banna M, Omaloja M F *et al*: The cloverleaf skull. *Br J Radiol* 1980, **53**:730–732.
Turner P T, Reynolds A F: Generous craniectomy for Kleeblattschädel anomaly. *Neurosurg* 1980, 6:555–558.
Kremens B, Kemperdick H *et al*: Thanatophoric dysplasia with cloverleaf-skull. *Eur J Pediatr* 1982, **139**:298–303.
Zuleta A, Basauri L: Cloverleaf skull syndrome. *Child's Brain* 1984, 11:418–427.
Kozlowski K, Warren P S *et al*: Cloverleaf skull with generalized bone dysplasia. *Pediatr Radiol* 1985, 15:412–414.
Gathmann H A, Vitzthum H, Aksu F: Zur Klinik und Pathogenese der 'Kleeblattschädel-Anomalie'. In: *Entwicklungsstörungen des Zentralnervensystems.* G Neuhäuser (ed) Stuttgart: Kohlhammer, 1986; 90–98.
Kroczek R A, Mühlbauer W *et al*: Cloverleaf skull associated with Pfeiffer syndrome… *Eur J Pediatr* 1986, 145:442–445.
Benallègue A, Lacette F *et al*: Crâne en trèfle… *Ann Génét* 1987, **30**:113–117.
Dambrain R, Fround M *et al*: Considerations about the cloverleaf skull. *J Craniofac Genet Dev Biol* 1987, 7:387–401.
Say B, Poznanski A K: Cloverleaf skull… *Pediatr Radiol* 1987, 17:93–96.
Cohen M M Jr: Cloverleaf syndrome update. *Proc Greenwood Genet Ctr* 1987, 6:186–187.
Cohen M M Jr: Craniosynostosis update 1987: *Am J Med Genet Suppl* 1988, 4:99–148.
Clark R D, Eteson D: Kleeblattschädel association with Saethre–Chotzen syndrome. *Third Manchester Birth Defects Conference*, Manchester, 25-28. October 1988.

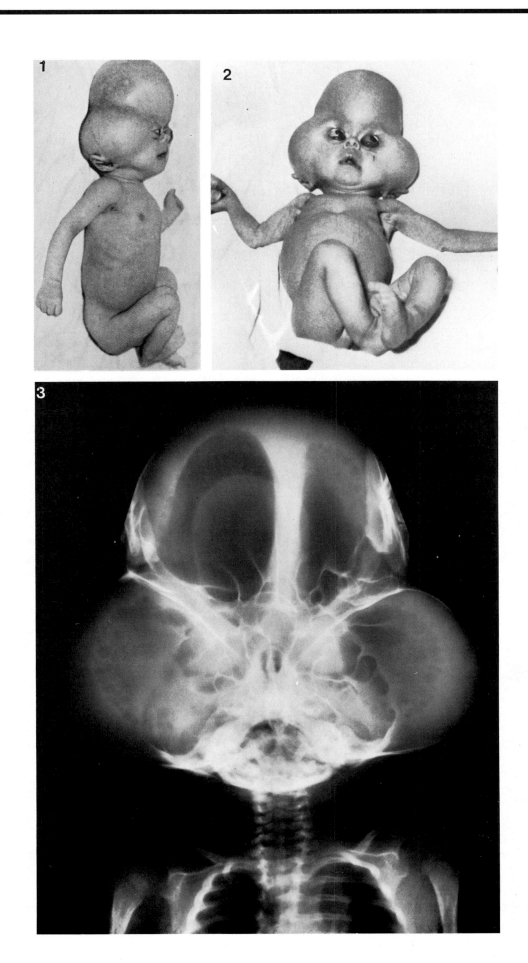

13 Antley–Bixler Syndrome

J.K.

A craniostenosis syndrome with severe midface hypoplasia, proptosis, humeroradial synostoses and choanal atresia.

Main signs:
- Craniofacial signs: brachycephaly, prominent forehead, proptosis, midface hypoplasia, dysplastic ears, deep nasal bridge, choanal atresia/stenosis, craniosynostosis.
- Extremities: camptodactyly, long hands and fingers, multiple joint contractures, impaired extension/flexion of the elbow, supination possible in some cases.
- Skeletal radiology: humeroradial synostoses, bowed femora, femoral fractures, carpal fusion. Shortened skull base. Premature closure of the cranial sutures.

Supplementary findings: Stenoses of the external auditory canal, conductive hearing and inner ear disorders. Respiratory impairment due to choanal stenosis. Flat thorax, flat pelvis. 'Rocking-chair feet'. Partial cutaneous syndactyly. Hypoplastic labia, fused labia minora, large clitoris. Renal duplication, hydronephrosis, utero-obstruction.

Manifestation: Intra-uterine (humeroradial synostoses) and at birth.

Aetiology: Fourteen cases observed to date, of which 12 in females and two in males, three sets of siblings. Possibly autosomal recessive inheritance.

Pathogenesis: Unknown.

Frequency: Fourteen case reports.

Course, prognosis: Eighty per cent of the children die shortly after birth as a result of respiratory disorders with choanal atresia and stenosis. Development of premature craniostenoses. Mental retardation possibly as a result of the craniostenoses. One 10-year-old girl is mentally normal. Orthopaedic problems as a result of the joint contractures. Tendency to fractures.

Differential diagnosis: Acrocephalosyndactyly (7–9, 11).

Treatment: Surgical repair of the choanal stenosis. Physiotherapy of the ankylosis. Neurosurgical intervention in the case of craniostenoses. Correction of urological malformations. Prenatal diagnosis of humeroradial synostoses.

Illustrations:
1a–c 13 days old, acrocephaly, prominent forehead, brachycephalic, midface hypoplasia, dysplastic ears, low broad nasal bridge, bilateral choanal stenosis; **d and e** Impaired extension/flexion of the elbow joint bilaterally, deep dimples; **f–i** Humeroradial synostoses, long hands; **j** Clitoral hypertrophy; **k** Long fingers; **l and m** Contractures of the knee joints, no bowed femora.

References:
Schinzel A, Salvodelly G et al: Antley–Bixler syndrome in sisters: a term newborn and prenatally diagnosed fetus. *Am J Med Genet* 1983, 14:139–147.
Escobar L F, Bixler D, Sadove M, Bull M J: Antley–Bixler syndrome from a prognostic perspective: report of a case and review of the literature. *Am J Med Genet* 1988, 29:829–836.
Dawn DeLozier-Blanchet C: Antley–Bixler syndrome from a prognostic perspective. *Am J Med Genet* 1989, 32:262–263.
Hassell S, Butler G: Antley–Bixler syndrome: report of a patient and review of literature. *Clin Genet* 1994, 46:372–376.

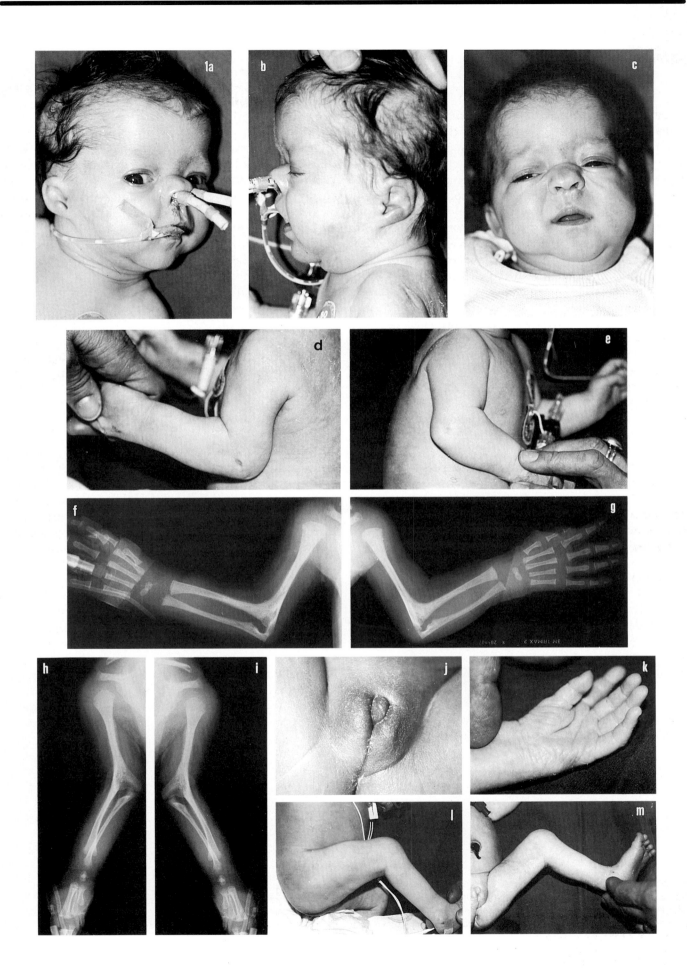

14 Oto-palato-digital Syndrome Type 1

J.K / H.-R.W

A malformation syndrome with typical facial dysmorphism, signs of bone dysplasia, particularly in the form of 'frog hands' and 'frog feet', cleft palate and impaired hearing.

Main signs:
- Characteristic facies with broad prominent forehead, hypertelorism, antimongoloid slant of the palpebral fissures, marked supra-orbital bulging, broad nasal bridge, flat midface and microstomia with down-turned corners of the mouth (3, 4, 11, 12). Prominent occiput. Low-set ears. Micrognathia and cleft palate.
- Broad and short distal phalanges of the hands and feet, particularly of the first ray, the shortness of which is due mainly to hypoplasia of the metacarpal or first metatarsal and the proximal phalanx. Frequently clinodactyly of the little finger. Partial syndactyly. All in all, reminiscent of a 'frog hand' or 'frog foot' (5–8). Enlargement and limited mobility of the large joints.
- Frequently, moderate conductive-hearing impairment. Tendency to otitis, sinusitis and mastoiditis. Frequently, mild mental retardation.

Supplementary findings: Slight shortness of stature. Dental anomalies.
Fusion and deformity of the metacarpals and metatarsals with additional ossification centres and ossicles. Incomplete fusion of the neural arches, generally involving several vertebrae. Vertical clivus.

Manifestation: At birth.

Aetiology: Hereditary disorder, with mode of inheritance not yet definitely established. X-linked recessive is probably the predominant type but X-linked dominant and autosomal dominant with sex-limited expression have also been suggested. Females are usually much less severely affected. Gene locus Xq26-28.

Frequency: Including the children shown here, 69 cases in males and 34 in females were known up to 1981.

Course, prognosis: Normal life expectancy.

Diagnosis, differential diagnosis: Other syndromes with broad, short halluces and thumbs, such as Münchmeyer (252) or the Rubinstein–Taybi syndrome (87), etc, can easily be excluded by the total picture. The same should be true for the Larsen syndrome (230), with its flat facies and joint deformities.
An X-ray of the feet is especially valuable in confirming a tentative clinical diagnosis of oto-palato-digital syndrome.

Comment: A further X-linked disorder, which has similar facial dysmorphism, has been designated oto-palato-digital syndrome type II (229). This is distinguished by more extensive skeletal changes (narrowed thorax, marked bowing of the long bones of the extremities, absence of the fibulae, etc.), a hearing defect as a constant feature and a much less favourable prognosis.

Treatment: Symptomatic.

Illustrations:
1–6 The index case at age 7 years. Birth measurements and present size within normal limits. Condition after total correction of tetralogy of Fallot. Bifid uvula, slightly impaired hearing, frequent otitis. Intellect in the low, normal range. Limited movement of the large joints, thenar hypoplasia. Malformations in the carpal and tarsal regions with synostoses in the latter. Wide defect of the neural arches from the lower thoracic to the sacral vertebrae.
7–12 The brother of the index patient at age 12 years. Birth measurements and present size within normal limits. Essentially the same somatic findings, however, complete median cleft of the soft palate (surgically corrected), no cardiac defect; no X-ray of the vertebral column.
13 and 14 The sister of the two brothers at age 13 years. On the basis of the similar facial features, she may be regarded as a gene carrier. Except for slightly limited movement at her wrists, she has no further anomalies.

References:
Fitch N, Jequier S *et al*: The oto-palatodigital syndrome, proposed type II. *Am J Med Genet* 1983, **15**:655–664.
Kaplan J, Maroteaux P: Syndrome oto-palato-digital de type II. *Ann Génét* 1984, **27**:79–82.
Brewster Th G, Lachmann R S *et al*: Oto-palato-digital syndrome, type II... *Am J Med Genet* 1985, **20**:249–254.
Pazzaglia U E, Beluffi G: Oto-palato-digital syndrome in four generation... *Clin Genet* 1986, **30**:338–344.
Marec B le, Odent S *et al*: Syndrome oto-palato-digital de type I... *Ann Génét* 1988, **31**:155–161.
Hoar D J, Field L L, Beards F, Hoganson G, Rollnick B, Hoo J J: Tentative assignment of gene for oto-palato-digital syndrome to distal Xq (q26-q28). *Am J Med Genet* 1992, **42**:170–172.

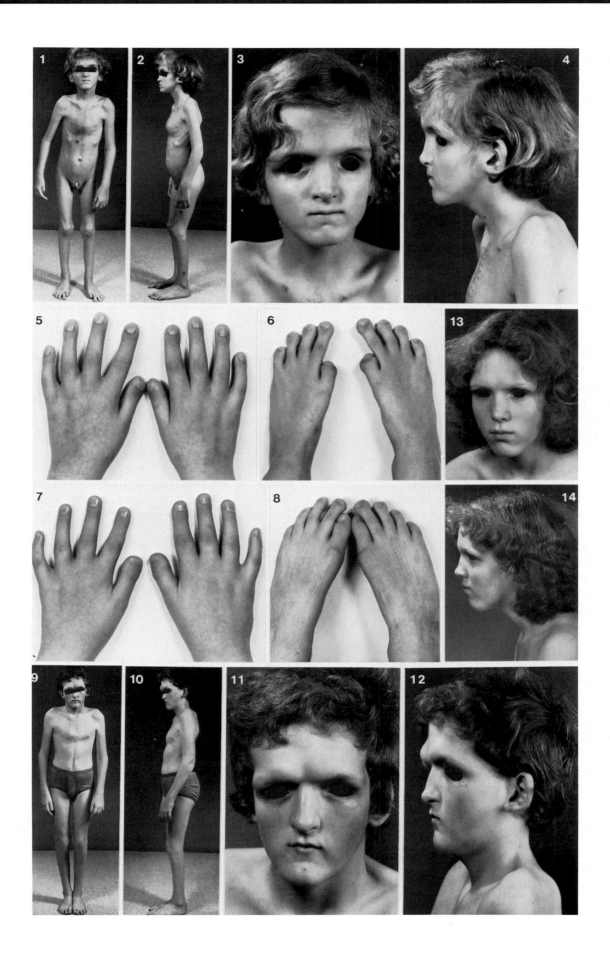

H.-R.W

A syndrome comprising unusual coarse facies, mental retardation, small stature, generalized hypotonia and characteristic hands; males far more severely affected than females.

Main signs:

- Narrow, rectangular protruding forehead appearing bitemporally compressed. Coarse, straggly scalp hair, prominent supra-orbital ridges, hypertelosim, antimongoloid slant of the palpebral fissures, pronounced eyebrows, thick upper eyelids, sometimes ptotis; broad nasal bridge and short, broad pug nose with a thick septum and alae; pouting lower lip, prognathism, mouth usually open, hypodontia, dysodontiasis and large, fleshy ears (2, 4–7).
- Mental retardation, considerable (IQ usually below 50) in males, substantially less severe in females. Frequently, hearing defect. Also increased susceptibility to seizures.
- Small stature, of varying degrees, height possibly below the third percentile.
- 'Full' forearms. Plumpish, lax, soft hands with tapered, hyperextensible fingers (8). Short halluces.

Supplementary findings: Hypotonia of the joints and ligaments. Cutis laxa and poor muscle performance (1). Frequently kyphoscoliosis (3), pectus carinatum or excavatum and pes valgus. Clumsy, wide-based gait. (These findings are all especially pronounced in males.)

Radiologically, distal phalanges of the fingers short and distally distended ('tufted'); dysplastic middle phalanges, short rays of the halluces, coxa valga, thick ossa frontalia and other signs.

Manifestation: At birth or later (increasing coarseness of the facial features; increasingly apparent short stature).

Aetiology: Possibly a systemic connective tissue disorder. Anomalies of proteoglycan metabolism in cultured fibroblasts and other abnormalities have been described. The syndrome is X-linked (no male-to-male transmission), with diminished expression in females. The gene appears to be located on the short arm of the X chromosome (Xp22.2-22.1). Female 'carriers' can be recognized mainly by facial characteristics or peculiarities of the hands and fingers (see above).

Frequency: Low; to date, 80 reported cases.

Course, prognosis: The signs become more marked with age.

Differential diagnosis: Other forms of mental retardation and short stature with coarse facies, especially fragile X syndrome (55), Sotos syndrome (74), Williams–Beuren syndrome (276).

Treatment: Symptomatic. Test early for impaired hearing. All handicap aids. Genetic counselling for the parents.

Illustrations:
1–8 The same proband with typical signs of the syndrome.

References:
Tentamy S A, Miller D, Hussels-Maumenee I: The Coffin–Lowry syndrome: an inherited faciodigital mental retardation syndrome. *J Ped* 1975, **86**:724.
Fryns J P, Vinken L, van den Berghe H: The Coffin syndrome. *Hum Genet* 1977, **36**:271.
Wilson W G, Kelly Th E: Early recognition of the Coffin–Lowry syndrome. *Am J Med Genet* 1981, **8**:215–220.
Hunter A G W, Partington M W *et al*: The Coffin–Lowry syndrome… *Clin Genet* 1982, **21**:321–335.
Beck M, Glössl J *et al*: Abnormal proteodermatan sulfate in three patients with Coffin–Lowry syndrome. *Ped Res* 1983, **17**:926–927.
Vine D T *et al*: Etiology of the weakness in Coffin–Lowry syndrome. *Am J Hum Genet* 1986, **39**:A 85.
Machin G A, Walther G L *et al*: Autopsy findings in two adult siblings with Coffin–Lowry syndrome. *Am J Med Genet Suppl* 1987, **3**:303–309.
Gilgenkrantz S, Mujica P *et al*: Coffin–Lowry syndrome: a multicenter study. *Clin Genet* 1988, **34**:230–245.
Hanauer A, Alembik Y *et al*: Probable localisation of the Coffin–Lowry locus… *Am J Med Genet* 1988, **30**:523–530.
Young I D: The Coffin–Lowry syndrome. *J Med Genet* 1988, **25**:344–348.
Miyazaki *et al*: Calcified ligamenta flava in a patient with Coffin–Lowry syndrome: biochemical analysis of glycosaminoglycans. *Jpn J Hum Genet* 1992, **35**:215–221.
Biancalana *et al*: Confirmation and refinement of the genetic localization of the Coffin–Lowry syndrome locus in Xp22.1-22.2. *Am J Hum Genet* 1992, **50**:981–987.
Hartsfield J K *et al*: Pleiotropy in Coffin–Lowry syndrome: sensorineural hearing deficit… *Am J Med Genet* 1993, **45**:552–557.
Biancalana V, Trivier E *et al*: Construction of a high-resolution linkage map for Xp22.1-p.22.2 and refinement of the genetic localization of the Coffin–Lowry syndrome gene. *Genomics* 1994, **22**:617–630.

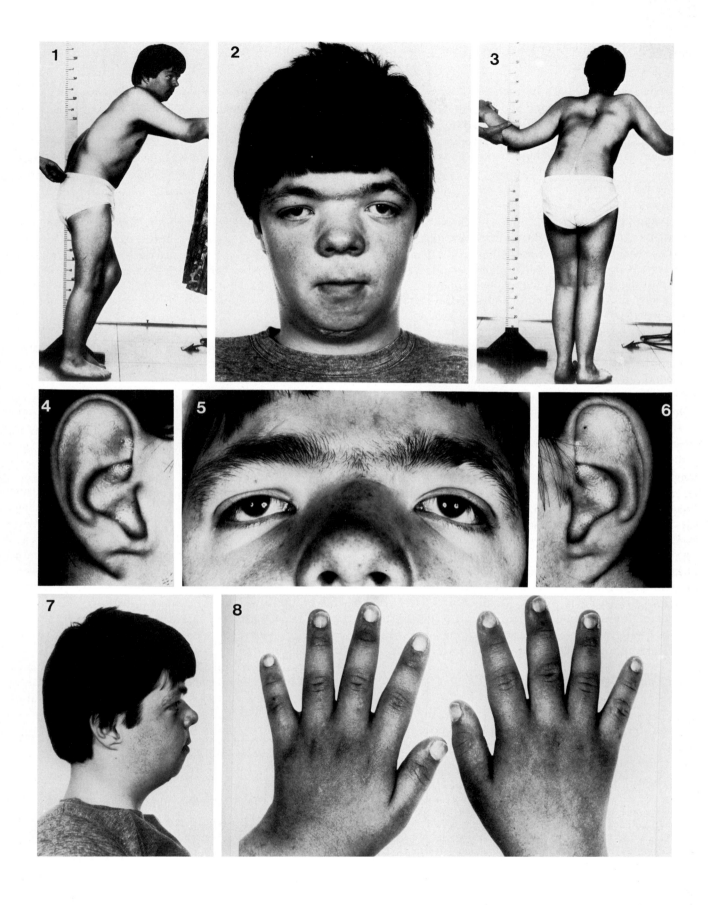

16 Kabuki Syndrome
(Kabuki Make-up Syndrome, Niikawa–Kuroki Syndrome)

J.K

A variable syndrome with characteristic facies, moderate mental retardation, postnatal shortness of stature, skeletal anomalies and persistent foetal fingertip pads.

Main signs: The name 'Kabuki make-up' syndrome was derived from the characteristic make-up technique of the Kabuki performers, a traditional Japanese theatrical profession.
- Unremarkable pregnancy, term birth, practically no prenatal growth retardation, neonatal hyperbilirubinaemia and hypoglycemic tendency.
- Characteristic 'Kabuki' facies: ectropion in the lateral third of the lower eyelid, long palpebral fissures, epicanthus medialis, arched eyebrows, sparse in the lateral third, blue sclerae (33%), depressed nasal tip, short nasal septum, cleft lip, cleft palate, bifid uvula, large protruding ears with dysplastic antihelices, pre-auricular fistulae, abnormal dentition, low occipital hairline, micrognathia.
- Mental retardation: IQ approximately 80.
- Neurological anomalies: neonatal hypotonia, feeding problems, microcephaly (in 30–50%), seizures (33%), strabismus.
- Skeletal anomalies: hyperextensible joints, short fifth finger (shortened middle phalanx of the fifth finger), scoliosis (50%), hip dysplasia (30%).

Supplementary findings: Fingertip pads in nearly 100% of all patients, increased ulnar loops, absence of the digital triradius c or d, increase in loops on the hypothenar eminence.

Congenital cardiac defects: aortic abnormalities such as coarctation of the aorta, bicuspid aortic valves. Urogenital anomalies. Premature breast development. Precocious puberty. Undescended testes, small penis. Hirsutism. Malrotation of the colon, anal atresia, rectovaginal fistula. Microcephaly, deafness. Increased susceptibility to infection, recurrent otitis media. Hypodontia, lower-lip pits.

Manifestation: Soon after birth.

Aetiology: Unknown. No observations in siblings. Chromosomal disorders of the X or Y chromosomes were found in three children. No increased consanguinity.

Occasional indications of familial similarities. One family with autosomal dominant inheritance.

Pathogenesis: The persistence of the fingerpads, regression of which generally begins after the tenth to twelfth week of pregnancy, indicates disturbed embryonal development.

Frequency: More than 100 patients reported: 62 from Japan, 45 in caucasians. Incidence in Japan is one out of 32000 newborns.

Course, prognosis: Three-quarters of patients exhibited retarded growth. Short stature from the first year of life. Increased risk of infection. Mild to moderate mental retardation.

Differential diagnosis: Robinow syndrome (*113*), Langer–Giedion syndrome (*232*), van der Woude syndrome (*35*), Coffin–Lowry syndrome (*15*).

Treatment: Symptomatic. Orthopaedic measures in the case of scoliosis. Protection against infections in the case of otitis and pneumonia.

Illustrations:

1 A girl from age 4 months to 9 years with mongoloid slant of the palpebral fissures, a short philtrum, large protruding ears (additionally, cleft palate, short stature, brachydactyly, delayed development and otitis).

2 A girl, age 1 year, circumference of the head 44cm (tenth percentile), width of the palpebral fissures 27mm, corresponding to the 97th percentile ('big eyes'), discrete eversion of the lower eyelids, arched eyebrows, flat nasal bridge, broad nasal tip, large dysplastic ears.

3 Boy, age 3 years, short stature, microcephaly, characteristic facies, retardation, cutis laxa.

4 8 years and 6 months, boy, short stature, microcephaly, ptosis, convergent strabismus, wide palpebral fissures, large ears (after plastic surgery, as previously protruding); also brachydactyly, hyperextensible joints, cleft palate.

1 from: Schrander-Stumpel *et al*. The Kabuki (Niikawa-Kuroki) syndrome: further delineation of the phenotype in 29 non-Japanese patients. *Eur J Pediatr* 1994 ,153:438–445 ().

References:

Niikawa N, Matsuura N, Fukushima Y *et al*: Kabuki make-up syndrome: a syndrome of mental retardation, unusual facies, large and protruding ears and postnatal growth deficiency. *J Pediatr* 1981, 99:565–569.

Meinecke P, Rodewald A: Kabuki make-up syndrome in a caucasian. *Dysmorphology Clin Genet* 1989, 3:103–107.

Kuroki Y, Suzuki Y *et al*: A new malformation syndrome of long palpebral fissures, large ears, depressed nasal tip, and skeletal anomalies associated with postnatal dwarfism and mental retardation. *J Pediatr* 1991, 99:570–573.

Niikawa N, Kuroki Y *et al*: Kabuki make-up (Niikawa–Kuroki) syndrome: a study of 62 patients. *Am J Med Genet* 1988, **31**:565–589.

Halal F, Gledhill R, Dudkiewicz A: Autosomal dominant inheritance of the Kabuki make-up (Niikawa–Kuroki) syn. *Am J Med Genet* 1989, **33**:376–381.

Philip N, Meinecke P *et al*: Kabuki make-up (Niikawa–Kuroki) syndrome: a study of 16 non-Japanese cases. *Clin Dysmorphology* 1992, 1:63–77.

Francescini P, Vardeu M P *et al*: Lower lip pits and complete idiopathic precocious puberty in a patient with Kabuki make-up (Niikawa–Kuroki) syndrome. *Am J Med Genet* 1993, **47**:423–425.

Schrander-Stumpel C, Meinecke P *et al*: The Kabuki (Niikawa–Kuroki) syndrome: further delineation of the phenotype in 20 non-Japanese patients. *Eur J Pediatr* 1994, 153:438–445.

Hughes H E, Davies S J: Coarctation of the aorta in Kabuki syndrome. *Arch Dis Child* 1994, 70:512–514.

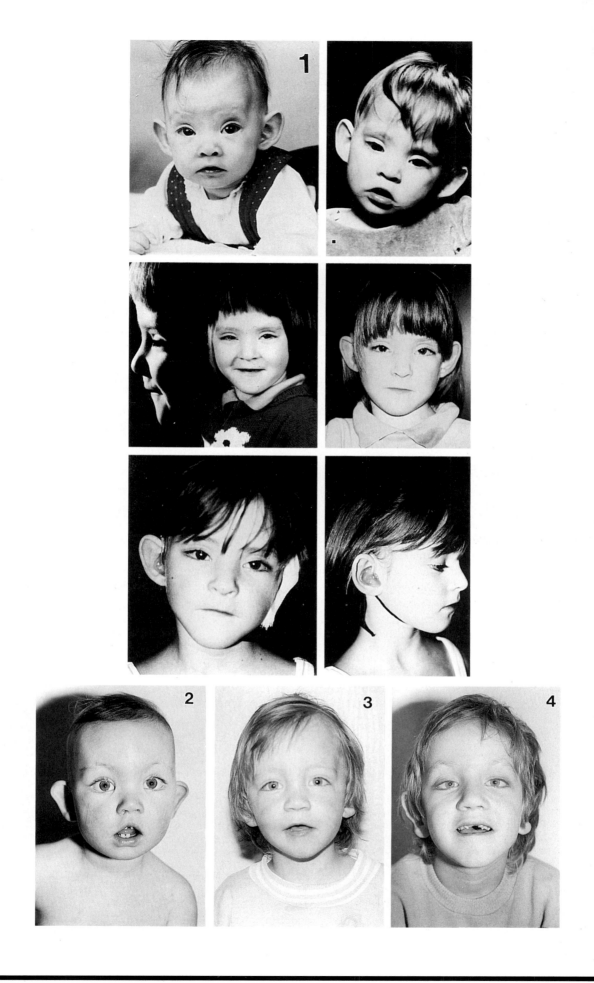

17 Megalocornea-Mental Retardation Syndromes
(MMR Syndromes, Neuhäuser Syndrome)

J.K.

A group of different retardation syndromes with megalocornea and neurological disorders.

Main signs:
- Megalocornea (corneal diameter is 13 mm or more). Before 1 year of age, 12.0mm is already suspicious.
- Varying degrees of delayed psychomotor development.

Supplementary findings: Hypoplasia of the iris, iridodonesis, myopia, micro- and macrocephaly. Convulsive disorder. Craniofacial characteristics: prominent forehead, broad nasal bridge, antimongoloid slant of the palpebral fissures. Epicanthus medialis, micrognathia. Muscular hypotonia, co-ordination disorders (type 1 = Neuhäuser), abnormal myelination.

Camptodactyly, scoliosis, short stature (type 2 = Frank Temtamy).

Macrocephaly, prominent forehead, broad prominent nasal bridge, antimongoloid slant of the palpebral fissures, malar hypoplasia, retrognathism, narrow thorax, long thin fingers (type 3).

Megaencephaly, adiposity, fleshy ears (type 4 = Frydman).

Unclassifiable forms, for example, with hypothyroidism; with dystrophin-positive muscular dystrophy (own observation).

Manifestation: After unremarkable pregnancy and delivery, delayed psychomotor development. Megalocornea from birth.

Aetiology: Heterogeneous. Autosomal recessive inheritance. Possible variability. Twenty-nine patients known to date.

Pathogenesis: Unknown.

Course, prognosis: Dependent on neurological complications.

Differential diagnosis: Megalocornea as an isolated characteristic can be transmitted by autosomal dominant inheritance and by X-linked recessive inheritance as anterior megalophthalmos. Beware glaucoma and buphthalmus.

Megalocornea is often confused with keratoconus as it occurs in many syndromes: trisomy 21 (49), Marfan syndrome (76), osteogenesis imperfecta (204/205), Ehlers–Danlos syndrome (203), Lowe syndrome (290), Larsen syndrome (230), Weill–Marchesani syndrome, Rothmund–Thompson syndrome (180), Parry–Romberg syndrome, non-ketotic hyperglycinema-adrenomyelodystrophy, Ito syndrome (188), mucolipidosis II (72), SHORT syndrome (321), Walker–Warburg syndrome (314). Frequently associated with disorders of the anterior chamber of the eye.

Treatment: Symptomatic, e.g. seizure control.

Illustrations:

1 Boy age 8 years and 6 months with epilepsy. **2 and 3** Thick fleshy fingers. **4** 'Big eyes': bilateral megalocornea. Diameter 13.9mm. 5 Enlargement from the family album; 9 months old, 'nice big eyes'.

References:

Neuhäuser G, Kaveggia E G, France T D, Opitz J M: Syndrome of mental retardation, seizures, hypotonic cerebral palsy, and megalocornea, recessively inherited. *Z Kinderheilkd* 1975, 120:1–18.
Schmidt R, Rapin I: The syndrome of mental retardation and megalocornea. *Am J Hum Genet* 1981, 33:90A.
Grønbech-Jensen M: Megalocornea and mental retardation syndrome: a new case. *Am J Med Genet* 1989, 32:468–469.
Del Guidice E, Sartorio R, Romano A, Carozzo R, Andria J: Megalocornea and mental retardation syndrome: two new cases. *Am J Med Genet* 1987, 26:417–420.
Frydman M, Berkenstadt M, Raas-Rothschild A, Goodman R M: Megalocornea, macrocephaly, mental retardation and motor retardation (MMMM). *Clin Genet* 1990, 38:149–154.
Kimura M, Kato M, Yoshino K, Ohtani K, Takeshita K: Megalcornea mental retardation syndrome with delayed myelination. *Am J Med Genet* 1991, 38:132–133.
Santolaya J M, Grijalbo A, Delgado A, Erdozain G: Additional case of Neuhäuser megalocornea and mental retardation syndrome with congenital hypotonia. *Am J Med Genet* 1992, 43:609–611.
Verloes A, Journel H, Elmer C, Nisson J P, Le Merrer M, Kaplan J, Van Maldergem L, Deconinck H, Meire F: Heterogeneity versus variability in megalocornea-mental retardation (MMR) syndromes: report of new cases and delineation of 4 probable types. *Am J Med Genet* 1993, 46:132–137.
Antinolo G, Rufo M et al: Megalocornea-mental retardation syndrome: an additional case. *Am J Med Genet* 1994, 52:196–197.

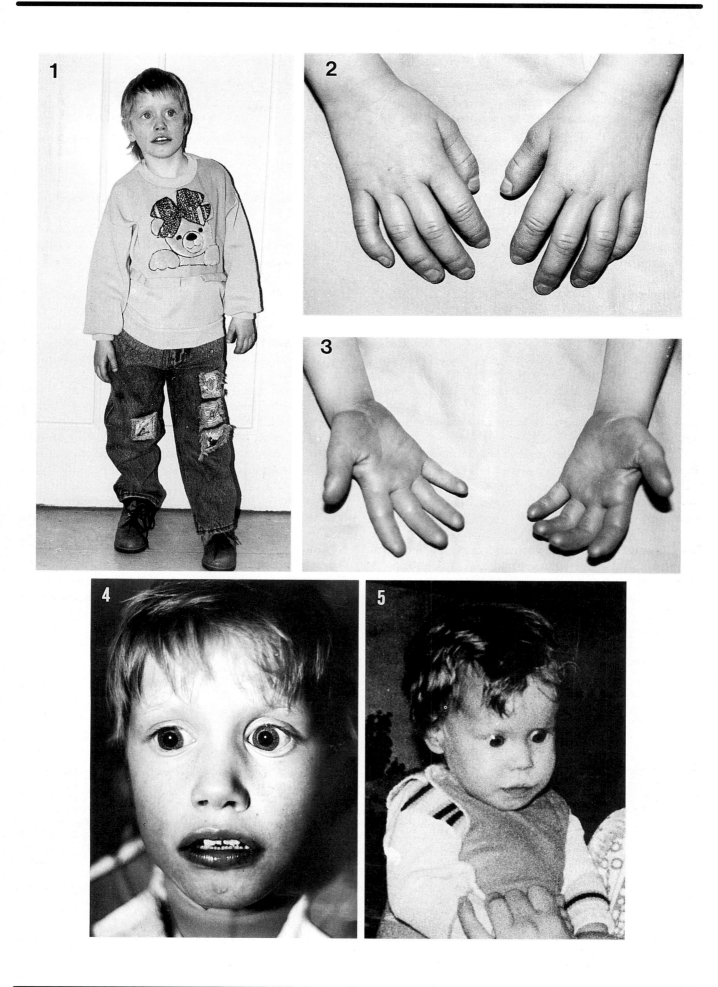

18 Melnick–Needles Syndrome
(Osteodysplasty)

H.-R.W

A highly characteristic syndrome mainly of the skeletal system, the affected having a typical facial appearance.

Main signs:
- Relatively large cranium with high prominent forehead and generally marked delay in closure of the anterior fontanelle. Facial part of the skull small with exophthalmos, hypertelorism, fleshy nose, full cheeks, relatively large ears, micrognathia of the lower jaw, malalignment of the teeth, malocclusion (1).
- Some degree of bowing of the arms and legs with cubitus valgus and genu valgum. Slight shortening of the distal phalanges of the hands and feet, especially of the thumbs.
- Bizarre, characteristic radiological changes (especially cortical irregularities and narrowing of the diaphyses) of the long bones (2), the ribs (4), clavicles, shoulder blades and the pelvis (5) with severe coxa valga; other areas also affected in this generalized skeletal dysplasia.

Supplementary findings: Narrow thorax with possible impairment of respiration. Frequently, dorsal kyphosis and/or scoliosis and hip dysplasia; club feet may be present. Hyperextensibility of the joints and skin, diastasis recti abdominis, hernias. Mental development not affected. Look out for a possible hearing defect and anomalies of the urinary tract.

Manifestation: Pre- and postnatally. Apart from the abnormal facies and delayed closure of the anterior fontanelle, the patients usually attract attention because of an abnormal gait and 'bowed' limbs.

Aetiology: Monogenic hereditary disease, autosomal dominant or X-linked dominant, associated with lethality in males and survival in females.

Frequency: Very low (about 45 observations have been reported in the literature).

Course, prognosis: Not infrequently initial failure to thrive and increased susceptibility to infections of the upper respiratory tract and the middle ear in the first years of life.

As a rule, normal adult height. Normal life expectancy. Possible difficulties with child bearing due to pelvic deformity. Premature arthrosis.

Diagnosis, differential diagnosis: Prenatal recognition of skeletal changes possible. Some superficial similarities to conditions such as pyknodysostosis (108), craniometaphyseal dysplasia (57), or Engelmann–Camurati syndrome (295), which can be immediately ruled out radiologically.

Partially expressed forms of the syndrome may be recognized only by chance.

Several reports of a 'serpentine fibula–polycystic kidney syndrome', with marked similarities to Melnick–Needles syndrome, appear independently in the literature (Exner, Majewski et al.).

Treatment: Symptomatic. Orthopaedic treatment, as required, especially for the spinal column, the hips and the feet. Dental and orthodontic care.

Illustrations:

1–5 An 8-year-old patient with the fully expressed syndrome. Note in addition the disease-related sclerosis of the base of the skull (3).

References:

Spranger J W, Langer jr L O, Wiedemann H-R: *Bone Dysplasias. An Atlas of Constitutional Disorders of Skeletal Development.* Stuttgart and Philadelphia: G Fischer and W B Saunders; 1974.
Leiber B, Olbrich G, Moelter N et al: Melnick–Needles-Syndrom. *Mschr Kinderheilk* 1975, **123:**178.
Fryns J P, Maertens R, van den Berghe H: Osteodysplastia—a rare skeletal dysplasia. *Acta Paediatr Belg* 1979, **32:**65.
Dereymaeker A M, Christens J et al: Melnick–Needles syndrome (osteodysplasty). Clinical and radiological heterogeneity. *Helv Paediatr Acta* 1986, **41:**339–351.
Donnenfeld A E, Conard K A et al: Melnick–Needles syndrome in males: a lethal multiple congenital anomalies syndrome. *Am J Med Genet* 1987, **27:**159–173.
Krajewska-Walasek M, Winkielman J et al: Melnick–Needles syndrome in males. *Am J Med Genet* 1987, **27:**153–158.
Exner G U: Serpentine fibula—polycystic kidney syndrome... *Eur J Pediatr* 1988, **147:**544–546.
Fryns J P, Schinzel A et al: Hyperlaxity in males with Melnick–Needles syndrome. *Am J Med Genet* 1988, **29:**609–611.
Sauter R, Klemm T et al: Melnick–Needles-Syndrom. *Pädiat Prax* 1988, **37:**173–180.
van der Lely H et al: Melnick–Needles syndrome (osteodysplasty) in an older male... *Br J Radiol* 1991, **64:**852–854.
Eggli K et al: Melnick–Needles syndrome. *Pediatr Radiol* 1992, **22:**257–261.
Majewski F et al: Serpentine fibula—polycystic kidney syndrome and Melnick–Needles syndrome are different disorders. *Eur J Pediatr* 1993, **152:**916–921.

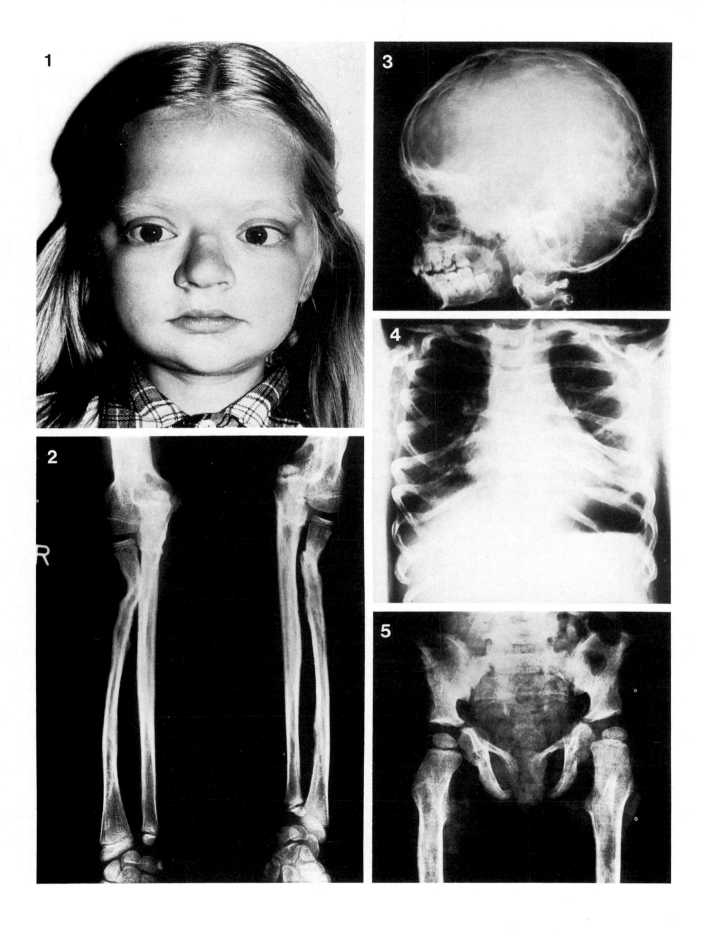

19 Cleidocranial Dysplasia
(Scheuthauer–Marie–Sainton Syndrome)

H.-R.W

A characteristic syndrome especially of the skeleton (cranium, clavicles, pelvis), the affected having a typical physical appearance.

Main signs:
- Large, broad and short cranium with frontal and parietal bossing and a supraglabellar depression (**1 and 3**), persistence of the fontanelles and open sutures for years or for life (**7**); facial part of the cranium relatively small with hypertelorism, broad depressed nasal bridge, in some cases anteverted nares (**2**) and mild exophthalmos (**1**).
- Upper thorax narrow with absent or poorly defined superior and inferior clavicular depressions and drooping, angular shoulders (**2, 4, 5**) with a-, hypo-, or dysplasia of the clavicles (**8**). Hypermobility of the shoulders (**3 and 6**).

Supplementary findings: Narrow pelvis, slender extremities, moderate short stature after infancy. Dysodontiasis (delay of both dentitions, supernumerary teeth) (**9**). Nails may be hypoplastic and brittle (**10**).

Radiologically, delayed maturation with numerous wormian bones in the cranium (**7**), markedly delayed ossification also in the pelvic region, especially the pubic bones. Possible coxa vara (or valga); shortened radii, accessory epiphyses in the metacarpal/metatarsal region, mesobrachyphalangia of the fifth digit, etc.

Manifestation: At birth.

Aetiology: Monogenic hereditary disorder, autosomal dominant, with high penetrance and extremely variable expression. Isolated occurrence of a case in a kindred with no signs of the condition suggests a new mutation. Possible gene locus 8q22. However, the occurrence of an autosomal recessive form has recently also been reported.

Frequency: Not so rare. By 1962, about 700 cases in the literature.

Course, prognosis: Life expectancy normal or slightly reduced. Developmental defects of the teeth and jaws are frequent and may be very troublesome. Tendency to dislocations. Average adult height 156.5 cm in males, 144.5 cm in females. Narrowness of the pelvis may necessitate Caesarean deliveries.

Differential diagnosis: In newborn and young infants, possible erroneous initial diagnosis of hydrocephalus or osteogenesis imperfecta. Later, possible confusion with the much less frequently occurring pyknodysostosis (*108*) (but with more marked growth deficiency, absence of the supraglabellar depression, clavicular ridges usually normal, no comparable ossification defect of the pelvic bones but above all, osteosclerosis, tendency to fractures, poorly defined submaxillary angle. Autosomal recessive inheritance.) There are also other, rare syndromes with dysplasia of the clavicles.

Treatment: Prompt specialist dental and orthodontic care as needed. Orthopaedic treatment may be indicated.

Illustrations:
Children at ages 30 months (**1**), 42 months and 18 months (**4–6**).

Skull radiograph of a 4-year-old child (**7**): open fontanelles and sutures, markedly widened frontal suture, numerous wormian bones.

Chest radiograph of an 8-year-old child (**8**): aplasia of the clavicles and abnormally positioned scapulae.

Supernumerary incisors in both the upper and lower jaws between persisting deciduous teeth in a 9-year-old child (**9**). Hypoplastic, brittle nails in a 5-year-old child (**10**).

References:
Wiedemann H-R: Gestörte Ossifikation besonders der bindegewebig präformierten Belegknochen: Die Dysostosis cleidocranialis. *Handbuch der Kinderheilkunde,* Vol 6. Heidelberg: Springer; 1967:128ff.
Spranger J W, Langer Jr L O, Wiedemann H-R: *Bone Dysplasias. An Atlas of Constitutional Disorders of Skeletal Development.* Stuttgart and Philadelphia: G Fischer and W B Saunders; 1974.
Goodman R M, Tadmor R, Zaritsky A *et al*: Evidence for an autosomal recessive form of cleidocranial dysostosis. *Clin Genet* 1975, 8:20.
Fleisher-Peters A, Schuch P: Befindlichkeit und Lebensschicksal von Patienten mit Dysostosis cleidocranialis. *der kinderarzt* 1983, **14**:1059–1067.
Yamamoto H *et al*: Cleidocranial dysplasia... *Oral Surg Oral Med Oral Path* 1989, 68:195–200.
Jensen B L: Somatic development in cleidocranial dysplasia. *Am J Med Genet* 1990, 35:69–74.
Chitayat D *et al*: Intrafamilial variability in cleidocranial dysplasia... *Am J Med Genet* 1992, 42:298–303.
Jensen B L *et al*: Development of the skull in infants with cleidocranial dysplasia. *J Craniofac Genet Dev Biol* 1993, 13:89–97.
Jensen B L *et al*: Craniofacial abnormalities in 52 school-age and adult patients with cleidocranial dysplasia. *J Craniofac Genet Dev Biol* 1993, 13:98–108.

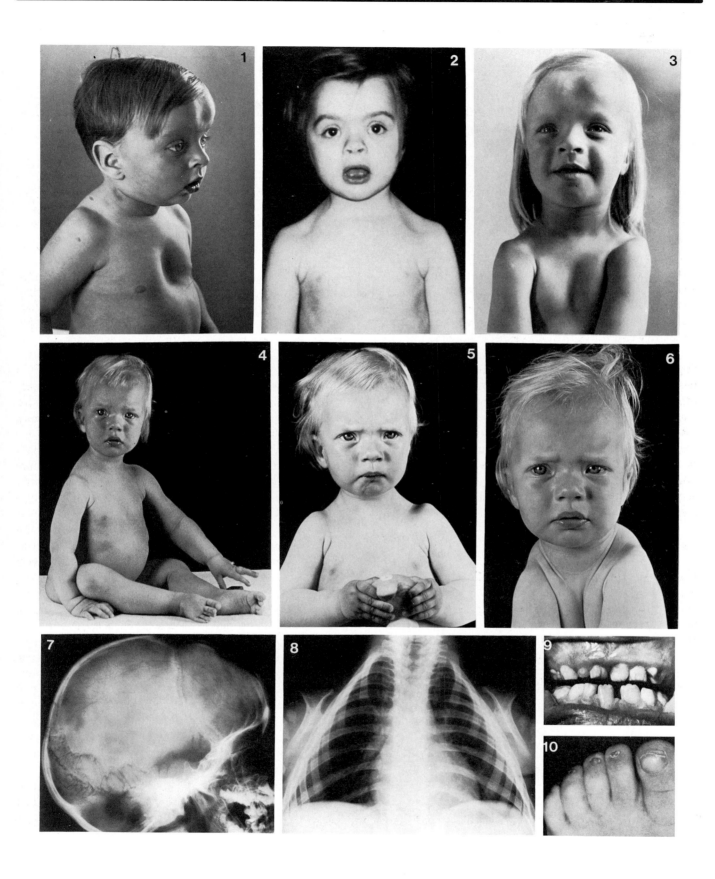

Syndrome of Increasing Macrocephaly with Signs of Cardiac Overload from Intracranial Arterio-venous Shunt

H.-R.W

Progressive macrocephaly (with or without definite hydrocephalus) and signs of cardiac overload (in the absence of congenital heart defect) with intracranial arterio-venous fistula (usually an aneurysm of the great cerebral vein of Galen).

Main signs:
- Abnormal growth of the cranium (**1 and 2**) with development of some degree of dilation of the ventricular system and with minimal to definite signs of increased intracranial pressure.
- Signs of cardiac failure without demonstrable congenital heart disease.
- In most (but not 100% of) patients, a continuous or systolic vascular murmur can be detected over all or part of the cranium; in some patients increased vascularity, pulsations and so on are present. Usually visible are pulsations of the cervical vessels, with thrills and murmurs.

Supplementary findings: Demonstration of an intracranial arterio-venous fistula (arterio-venous aneurysm, generally involving the great vein of Galen) (**3 and 4**).

Manifestation: Macrocephaly apparent congenitally or postnatally. Signs of cardiac overload become manifest sooner or later, depending on the size of the shunt.

Aetiology: Uncertain.

Frequency: Not so rare; many patients probably go undiagnosed.

Course, prognosis: In view of the precarious cerebral and cardiac problems, always dubious.

Diagnosis: Initially, cranial sonography, perhaps computer tomography or subtraction angiography; later, usually angiography of the carotid and vertebral arteries bilaterally.

Differential diagnosis: Intracranial arterio-venous fistula in Osler disease. Family history.

Treatment: The cardiac insufficiency may not respond to medical treatment. Possibly surgery, if necessary, as a last resort, at a time very carefully chosen after consultation between the neurosurgeon and cardiologist.

Comments:
- In any location of the body an extracardiac arterio-venous shunt can, depending on the size, lead to signs of cardiac overload and possibly to life-threatening decompensation.
- Depending on their size, intracranial shunts frequently manifest immediately *post partum* with severe cyanotic cardiac insufficiency. When not manifest until later in infancy or thereafter, developing hydrocephalus and convulsions or subarachnoid haemorrhages and neurological defects may dominate the picture.

The 'craniomegalic' form presented here is one particular, unusual form.

Illustrations:

1, 3 A 5-year-old boy with congenital, progressive macrocephaly (at birth, 39 cm; 11 months, 52.8 cm; 13 months, 54 cm; 4 years, 58 cm). Signs of cardiac overload without evidence of heart defect caused by an extracardial left-to-right shunt. Continuous vascular murmur together with distended veins over the scalp; low voltage electroencephalogram, dilated ventricles and papilledema. Otherwise normal development for age, with no neurological deficit. On angiogram, a large aneurysm of the great vein of Galen; aneurysmal enlargement of the confluence of the sinuses and adjacent vessels caused by arteriovenous shunts to both posterior cerebral arteries; numerous angiomas.

2 The same patient at ages 5, 7 and 8 years. Congenital progressive macrocephaly (at birth, 38 cm; 5 years, 60 cm). Signs of cardiac overload without evidence of heart defect, due to an extracardiac left-to-right shunt. Continuous vascular murmur and prominent veins and pulsations on the scalp; low-voltage electroencephalogram, secondary internal hydrocephalus (Pudenz–Heyer catheter). Otherwise normal development for age, with no noticeable neurological deficit. On angiogram, large aneurysm of the great vein of Galen with some angioma-like enlargement of adjacent vessels caused arterio-venous shunts with both posterior cerebral arteries.

4 Successful operative closure at age 7 years of most of the pathological anastomoses, without neurological sequelae (Professor Yasargil, Zürich).

References:
Gold A P, Ransohoff J, Carter S: Vein of Galen malformation. *Acta Neurol Scand* 1964, 40:(11)1.
Amacher A L, Shillito Jr J: The syndromes and surgical treatment of aneurysms of the great vein of Galen. *J Neurosurg* 1973, 39:89.
Cuncliffe P N: Cerebral arteriovenous aneurysm presenting with heart failure. *Br Heart J* 1974, 36:919.
Kelly Jr J J, Mellinger J F, Sundt Jr T M: Intracranial arteriovenous malformations in childhood. *Ann Neurol* 1978, 314:338.
Benz-Bohm G, Neufang K F R. *et al*: A. v. Missbildung im Bereich der Vena Galeni… *Fortscht. Röntgenstr.* 1985, 142:579–581.

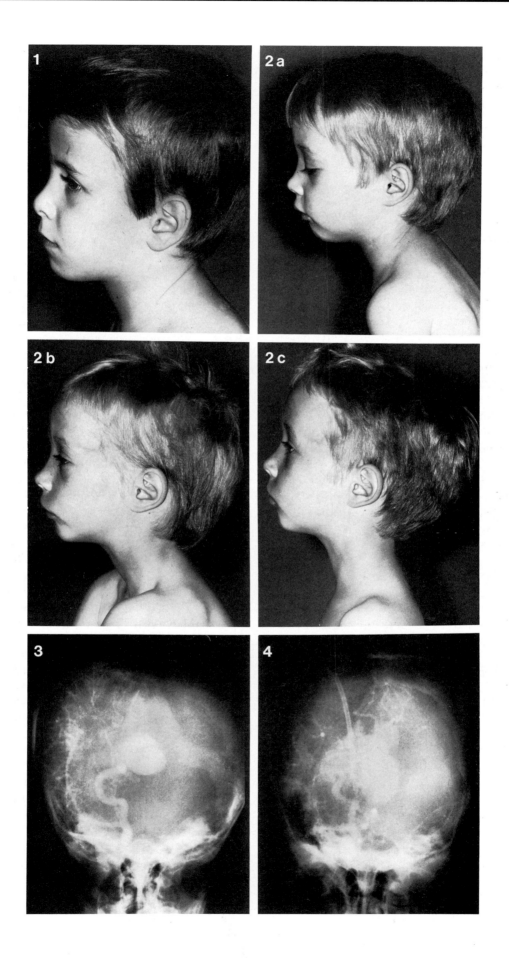

21 Megalencephaly
(Non-neuropathic)

H.-R.W

A condition with primary megalencephaly, occasionally combined with primary developmental retardation, muscular hypotonia, epilepsy or other anomalies, such as cardiac defects.

Main signs:
- Macrodolichocephaly (head circumference increasingly above the 98th percentile, beginning at an early age). Prominent occiput, markedly delayed closure of the anterior fontanelle, which is neither bulging nor tense, prominent forehead. In the children presented here: strikingly deep-set eyes, broad nasal bridge and nose and pointed, receding chin (**1 and 2**).
- In individual patients, primary psychomotor retardation, hypotonia, epilepsy, shortness of stature.

Supplementary findings: In the patients presented here: normal height. Short neck; trunk and extremities somewhat obese and short (**1 and 2**). Heart murmur. Large genitalia (**1a**); testicular volume of the older boy at 20 months, 3–4 ml; at 4 years and 5 months, 5–6 ml.

No evidence of intracranial vascular malformation nor of hydrocephalus. (Unremarkable ventricular system on repeated echo-encephalography; transillumination and bilateral cerebral angiography negative). Ophthalmological examination normal, as were extensive neurological examinations, endocrinological studies, specific tests for storage diseases and other hereditary degenerative diseases and chromosomal analysis.

Skull radiographs: elongated cranium, markedly delayed closure of the fontanelles, somewhat poorly defined and deeply serrated sutures, elongated flat sella turcica, numerous bony lacunae in the lambdoid suture (**3 and 4**).

Further radiographs of the skeleton: discordant bone maturation (areas of distinctly delayed, together with areas of partially accelerated, ossification).

Normal-sized heart with left-sided prominence in both brothers; in the older boy, possible atrial septal defect and idiopathic dilation of the pulmonary artery.

Manifestation: At birth or shortly thereafter.

Aetiology: Autosomal dominant condition with development of signs much more likely in males (up to four times as prevalent).

Course, prognosis: Occasionally complicated by mental retardation (approximately 5–8%) or with epilepsy. No mental deterioration.

Diagnosis, differential diagnosis: Conditions with increased intracranial pressure, the syndrome described on page 40 and other conditions and disease processes associated with macrocephaly must be ruled out. Macrocephaly, without signs of increased intracranial pressure, in a neurologically and developmentally normal child should, especially with familial occurrence, suggest the benign form of megalencephaly shown here and may obviate the use of invasive methods of examination.

Treatment: None or symptomatic.

Illustrations:

1–4 Two siblings, both with psychomotor retardation, the second and third children of young, healthy non-consanguineous parents after a girl and two abortions. Other family members with large heads. The first child is, to a lesser degree, likewise macrodolichocephalic (at 24 weeks, 44 cm; at 4 years and 5 months, 55 cm) and has a cardiac defect (persistent ductus arteriosus, corrected; ventricular septal defect; anomalies of the pulmonary artery), completely normal psychomotor development and slight obesity. Pregnancy and delivery were normal with both brothers. Birth measurements of the older child: 4.3 kg, 59 cm, 38.5 cm. Head circumference of the younger child (**2**) at 13 months, 53 cm (**3**); of the older child at 10 months, 52 cm; 20 months, 57 cm; 30 months, 59 cm; and 32 months (**4**), 61.5 cm. Obesity in the older brother. Resemblance of the brothers increasing.

References:
DeMyer W: Megalencephaly in children. *Neurology* 1972, **22**:634.
Jennings M T *et al*: Endocardial fibroelastosis, neurologic dysfunction and unusual facial appearance in two brothers, coincidentally associated with dominantly inherited macrocephaly. *Am J Med Genet* 1980, **5**:271.
Pettit R E *et al*: Macrocephaly with head growth parallel to normal growth pattern. *Arch Neurol* 1980, **37**:518.
Priestly B L *et al*: Primary megalencephaly. *Z Kinderchirur* 1980, **31**:335.
Lorber J *et al*: Children with large heads... 109 children with megalencephaly. *Dev Med Child Neurol* 1981, **23**:494–504.
Fryns J P *et al*: Mental retardation, macrocephaly, short stature and craniofacial dysmorphism in three sisters. *Clin Genet* 1988, **33**:293–298.
Laubscher B *et al*: Primitive megalencephaly in children... *Eur J Pediatr* 1990, **149**:502–507.
Cole T R P *et al*: Autosomal dominant macrocephaly... *Am J Med Genet* 1991, **41**:115–124.

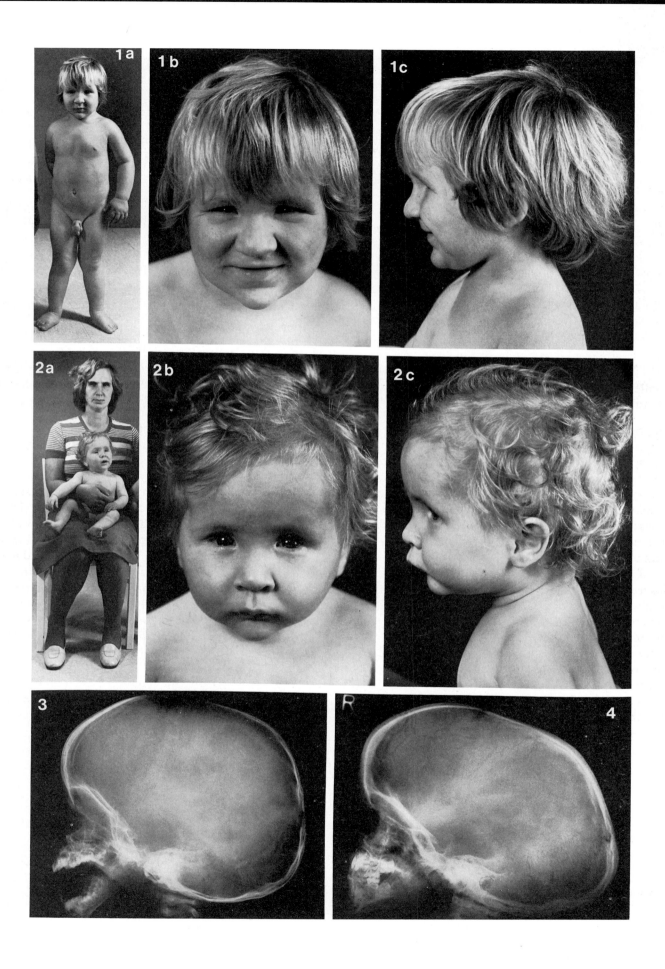

22 Alexander's Disease

J.K.

A progressive, fatal leukodystrophy with megalencephaly, loss of neurological function and mental deterioration.

Main signs:
- Megalencephaly with normal or enlarged ventricles.
- Progressive psychomotor retardation.
- Loss of speech.
- Seizures, spastic tetraparesis, opisthotonus, contractures; pseudobulbar palsy; ataxia.

Supplementary findings: Increasing intracranial pressure; hyperpyrexia, attacks of vomiting. Fluctuating course. A cranial ultrasound scan can be diagnostically helpful.

Histologically, characteristic Rosenthal fibers, progressive fibrinoid degeneration of the fibril-rich astrocytes, demyelinating leukodystrophy, hyaline panmyelopathy.

Manifestation: Three forms with different ages of onset: infantile, juvenile and adult.

Aetiology: Autosomal recessive disorder. To date only one family with three siblings of different sex has been described; otherwise only sporadic cases. Storage disease of the white and grey matter of the central nervous system with subendymal, subpial and perivascular deposition of hyaline and crystalline structures (alpha-B crystals).

Frequency: Very rare. To date, only 20 known patients.

Course, prognosis: Progressive, with fatal outcome, which, with the early form, can occur between the fifth month and the fifth year of life.

Treatment: Symptomatic.

Differential diagnosis: Other megalencephalies. Multiple sclerosis.

Illustrations:
1 Three siblings with progressive macrocephaly (normocephalic at birth; crossing the 97th percentile by the end of the first year of life, then a parallel course above the 97th percentile).
2 The three siblings at ages 14, 15 and 17 years, confined to wheelchairs due to spastic quadriplegia; mental function still well preserved.

References:

Russo L S, Aron A, Anderson P J: Alexanders disease. A report and reappraisal. *Neurology* 1976, **26**:607–614.

Borrett D, Becker L E: Alexander's disease. A disease of astrocytes. *Brain* 1985, **108**:367–385.

Harbord M G, LeQuesne G W: Alexander's disease: cranial ultrasound findings. *Pediatr Radiol* 1988, **18**:227–228.

Iwaki T, Kume-Iwaki A, Leim R K H, Goldman J E: Alpha-B-crystallin is expressed in non-lenticular tissues and accumulates in Alexander's disease brain. *Cell* 1989, **57**:71–78.

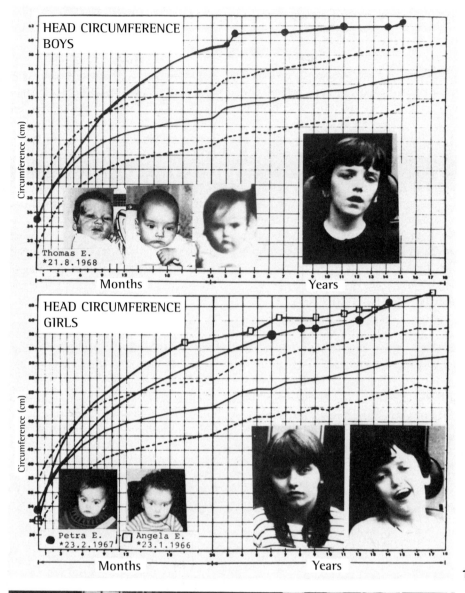

HEAD CIRCUMFERENCE
BOYS

Circumference (cm)

Thomas E.
*21.8.1968

Months   Years

HEAD CIRCUMFERENCE
GIRLS

Circumference (cm)

● Petra E.   □ Angela E.
*23.2.1967   *23.1.1966

Months   Years

1

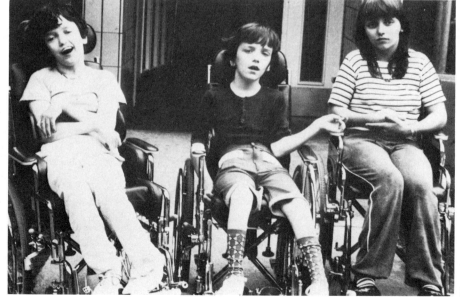

2

23 Frontonasal Dysplasia

(Median Cleft Face Syndrome, Craniofrontonasal Dysplasia; Greig's Hypertelorism)

J.K.

A developmental field defect of heterogeneous aetiology with the signs hypertelorism, brachycephaly, prominent forehead, broad nasal bridge and partial or complete bifid nose.

Main signs:
- Hypertelorism (measure interpupillary distance), prominent forehead with wide bridge of the nose, which may be sagitally grooved or even cleft (then frequently associated with anterior cranium bifidum occultum and/or median cleft of the face), frequently wide open fontanelles with open metopic suture and coronary suture synostosis. Brachycephaly. Facial asymmetry.
- Low nuchal hairline. Widow's peak.
- High palate, widely spaced teeth.

Further signs: Broad neck, possibly pterygium colli; shoulder girdle anomalies with Sprengel's deformity, pseudarthrosis of the clavicles, scoliosis. Longitudinally grooved nails. Pre-axial polydactyly, syndactyly, clinodactyly, abnormalities of the distal phalanges of the fingers and toes, deep crease between hallux and second toe ('sandal-gap'). Agenesis of the corpus callosum, holoprosencephaly, frontal encephalocoeles. Colobomas of the uvea, iris, eyelids, microphthalmia, anophthalmia. Infrequently, small stature and mental retardation.

Manifestation: At birth.

Aetiology: Frontonasal developmental field defect of heterogeneous causes: sporadically occurring, autosomal dominant and autosomal recessive (the latter with severe craniofacial malformations). Females predominate over males 6:1. No transmission has been observed in male lines. Girls are also severely affected. Genetic transmission by an affected woman must be assumed to be 50%.

Frequency: Low. Possibly one out of 250000.

Course, prognosis: Dependent on the degree of severity. As a rule, normal life expectancy.

Differential diagnosis: Frontonasal dysplasia must be phenotypically and genetically differentiated from Greig's hypertelorism syndrome (may be very difficult) and from the familial form of bifid nose occurring as an isolated defect.

Treatment: Symptomatic, plastic surgery may be indicated. Ultrasound and foetoscopic diagnosis in familial cases with female fetuses.

Illustrations:
1–4 Children affected to various degrees.
1 A 1-year-old male with median nasal cleft, broad nasal bridge, median cleft lip and bilateral coloboma of the iris; sister and mother similarly affected.
3 A 3-year-old girl with cranial prominences, colobomas of the alae nasi notches and a severe neurological deficit due to malformation of the brain.

References:

Gollop T R, Kiota M M, Martins R M M *et al*: Frontofacialnasal dysplasia: evidence for autosomal recessive inheritance. *Am J Med Genet* 1984, 19:301–305.
Anyane-Yeboa K, Raifman M A, Berant M *et al*: Dominant inheritance of bifid nose. *Am J Med Genet* 1984, 17:561–563.
Toriello H V, Higgins J V, Walen A *et al*: Familial occurrence of a developmental defect of the medial nasal process. *Am J Med Genet* 1985, 21:131–133.
Bömelburg T, Lenz W, Eusterbrock T: Median cleft face syndrome in association with hydrocephalus, agenesis of the corpus callosum, holoprosencephaly and choanal atresia. *Eur J Pediatr* 1987, 146:301–302.
Morris C A, Palumbos J C, Carey J C: Delineation of the male phenotype in cranio-frontonasal syndrome. *Am J Med Genet* 1987, 27:623–631.
Young I D: Craniofrontonasal dysplasia. *J Med Genet* 1987, 24:193–196.
Meinecke P, Blunck W: Frontonasal dysplasia, congenital heart defect, and short stature... *J Med Genet* 1989, 26:408–409.
Reardon W, Temple I K, Jones B, Baraitser M: Frontonasal dysplasia or craniofrontonasal dysplasia and the Poland anomaly? *Clin Genet* 1990, 38:233–236.
Verloes A, Gillerot Y, Walczak E, van Maldorgem L, Koulischer L: Acromelic frontonasal 'dysplasia': further delineation of a subtype with brain malformation and polydactyly (Toriello syndrome). *Am J Med Genet* 1992, 42:180–183.

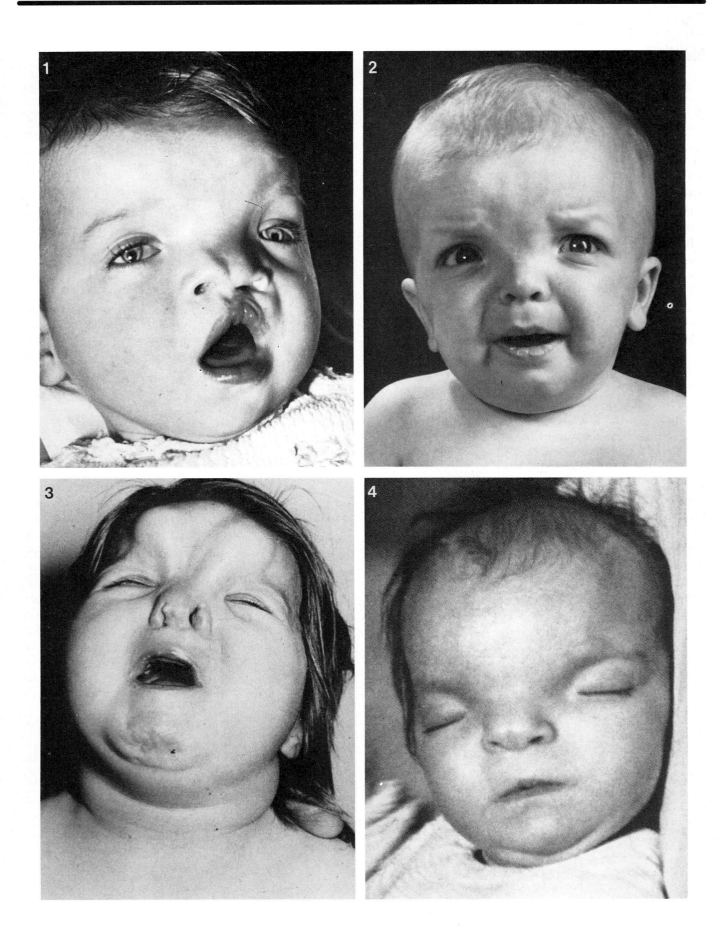

J.K.

A disorder of prechordal development with cyclopia, arhinenecephaly, absent bipolar development of the brain, and facial clefts, of varied aetiology.

Main signs:

- Cyclopia: medial monophthalmia, synophthalmia or anophthalmia. Proboscis (tubular appendage). Nose duplicated, solitary with a single opening or absent (arhinia).
- Ethmocephaly: ocular hypotelorism with or without a proboscis.
- Cebocephaly: ocular hypotelorism with only one nasal opening.
- Premaxillary agenesis: ocular hypotelorism, flat nose, median cleft of the upper lip.
- Minimal facial dysmorphism: variable phenotype with ocular hypotelorism, flat nose, uni- or bilateral cleft lip and coloboma of the iris. Hypertelorism may also occur.
- Alobar, semilobar or lobar holoprosencephaly, mono-ventricular forebrain, rudimentary lobulation of the brain, posterior fissure of the hemispheres.

Supplementary findings: Absence of the ethmoid, mid-section of the sphenoid, vomer, intermaxilla, nasal bones and lacrimal duct system. Hypo- or aplasia of the turbinates. Divided tongue or microglossia, possibly aglossia. Microstomia to astomia. Polydactyly, syndactyly, hypoplastic or absent thumbs, myelomeningocoele, club feet.

Cardiovascular, urogenital and many other internal malformations. Omphalocoele. Anal stenosis.

Manifestation: Primary defect of the prechordal mesoderm. Disturbance before day 21–25 of pregnancy. Ultrasound makes prenatal diagnosis possible. Otherwise diagnosis at birth.

Aetiology: Heterogeneous causes. Different structural chromosomal disorders including trisomies 13 and 18 and triploidy. Recently, several observations of deletions of the long arm of chromosome 7. Rarely familial translocations. As a rule, sporadic occurrence with a 6% recurrence risk. Rarely observations in siblings or transmission with diminished expression over generations. Alcohol embryopathy, diabetic embryopathy. Beware of confusing with Meckel syndrome.

Frequency: Lobar and alobar holoprosencephaly one out of 16 000 live births. With alobar holoprosencephaly female to male 3:1, with lobar form 1:1.

Course, prognosis: Severely affected infants usually do not survive beyond the sixth month of life.

Differential diagnosis: Asymmetric monophthalmus (**4**) and otocephaly (microstomia, agnathia, synotia). Arhinencephaly may also occur in the Kallmann syndrome (*307*) and trisomy 13 (*47*). Greig's hypertelorism or frontonasal dysplasia (*23*), the blepharophimosis-ptosis-epicanthus inversus syndrome (*84*), and the double nose syndrome may have to be ruled out.

Treatment: Symptomatic.

Illustrations:

1 Newborn with intra-uterine growth retardation (46cm, 2 800 g, 28cm head circumference). Convulsions, fluctuating temperature, tachypnoea, dysphagia. Monoventricular prosencephalon, synostoses of the cranial sutures. Death at 24 weeks.

2a and b Prematurely born (31st week of pregnancy) male with cyclopia: centrally located, 1cm orbital cavity with rudimentary eye beneath a 1.8cm long proboscis. Severe microstomia. Distinct medial groove of the flap-like upper lip. Low-set ears, dysplastic pinnae. Low nuchal hairline. Rudimentary tongue. Arhinencephaly, holoprosencephaly. Absence of the cribriform area, only one hemisphere. Double outlet right heart, malrotation I. Partial trisomy for the short arm of one chromosome 3 with balanced parental translocation (3p- 7q+).

3 Newborn with cebocephaly: microphthalmia, ocular hypotelorism, nose with a single opening.

4 Asymmetrical monophthalmia: one healthy eye, one malformed eye with proboscis. Not cyclopia.

References:

Suslak L, Mimms G M, Desposito Fr: Letter to the editor: monozygosity and holoprosencephaly: cleavage disorders of the 'midline field'. *Am J Med Genet* 1987, 28:99–102.

Hattori H, Okuno T, Momoi T *et al*: Brief clinical report: single central maxillary incisor and holoprosencephaly. *Am J Med Genet* 1987, 28:483–487.

Townes Ph L, Reuter L, Rosquete E E *et al*: XK Aprosencephaly and anencephaly in sibs. *Am J Med Genet* 1988, 29:523–528.

Antoniades K, Baraitser M: Proboscis lateralis: a case report. *Teratology* 1989, 40:193–197.

Zwetsloot C P, Brouwer O F, Maaswinkel-Mooy P D: Holoprosencephaly: variation of expression in face and brain in three sibs. *J Med Genet* 1989, 26:274–276.

Corsello G, Buttitta P *et al*: Holoprosencephaly examples of clinical variability and etiologic heterogeneity. *Am J Med Genet* 1990, 37:244–249.

Ronen G M, Andrews W L: Holoprosencephaly as a possible embryonic alcohol effect. *Am J Med Genet* 1991, 40:151–154.

Lurie I W, Wulfsberg E A: 'Holoprosencephaly-polydactyly' (pseudotrisomy 13) syndrome: expansion of the phenotypic spectrum. *Am J Med Genet* 1993, 47:405–409.

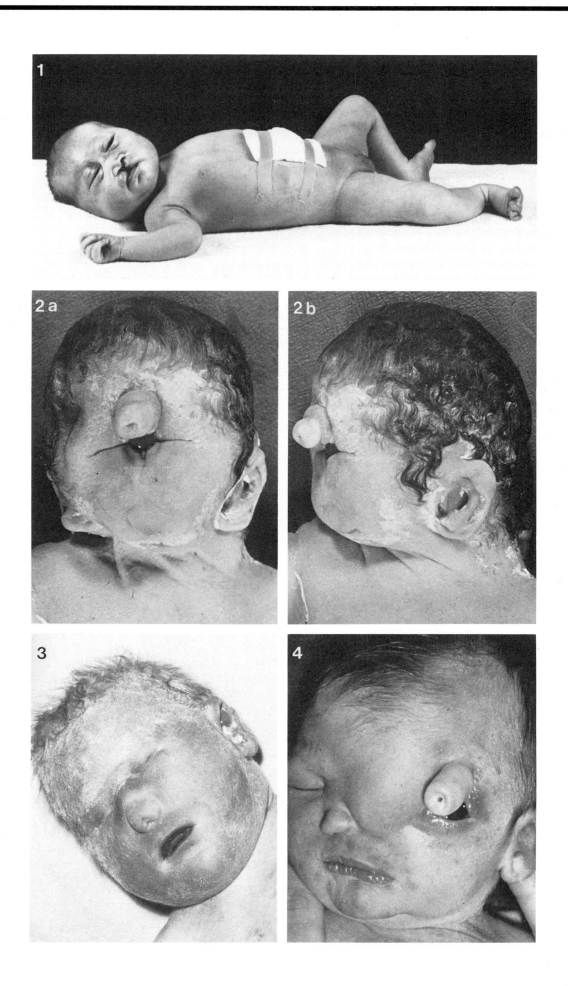

25 Otocephaly

J.K.

A malformation complex comprising agnathia, microstomia and synotia.

Main signs:
- Complete absence of the mandibles (agnathia) or alternatively presence of small fragments.
- Low-set ears and possibly fusion of the lower sections in the region of the absent mandibles. In some cases microtia.
- The oral cavity has a blind ending in the pharynx; the tongue is either absent or small; microstomia.

Supplementary findings: Malformations and fusion of the masticatory muscles; malformations of the auditory ossicles, the temporal palatine bone, the maxilla and the sphenoid. Occasionally, visceral transposition, heart defect.

Manifestation: Prenatally and at birth. To date, 24 cases known, 15 of isolated agnathia, 9 in combination with holoprosencephaly.

Aetiology: Unknown. Prevalence: observed in fewer than one out of 70000 births.

Pathogenesis: Incomplete development of the first pharyngeal arch, midline developmental defect.

Course, prognosis: Lethal malformation complex.

Differential diagnosis: Agnathia–holoprosencephaly (autosomal recessive).

Illustrations:
1 and 2 Thirtieth week of pregnancy, premature female infant, mandibular aplasia, microstomia, fusion of the ears with their lower sections.

References:
Pauli R M, Pettersen J C, Arya S, Gilbert E F: Familial agnathia–holoprosencephaly. *Am J Med Genet* 1983, **14**:677–698.
Leech R W, Bowlby L S, Brumback R A, Schaefer G B Jr: Agnathia, holoprosencephaly, and situs inversus: report of a case. *Am J Med Genet* 1988, **29**:483–490.
Hersh J H, McChane R H, Rosenberg R M, Powers W H Jr, Corrigan C, Pancratz L: Otocephaly-midline malformation association. *Am J Med Genet* 1989, **34**:246–249.
Ades L C, Sillence D O: Agnathia–holoprosencephaly with tetramelia. *Clin Dysmorphology* 1992, **1**:182–184.
Porteous M E M, Wright C *et al*: Agnathia–holoprosencephaly: a new recessive syndrome? *Clin Dysmorphology* 1993, **2**:161–164.

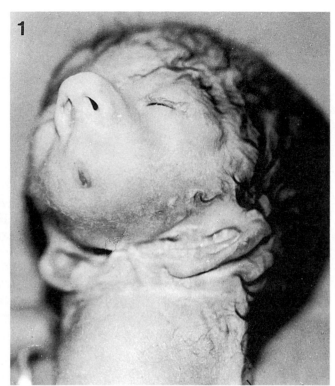

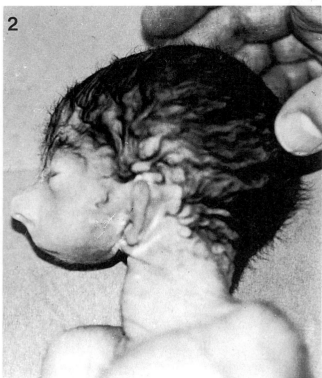

26 An Unknown Malformation Syndrome with Cleft Lip and Cleft Palate

H.-R.W

A syndrome comprising cleft lip and cleft palate, severe psychomotor retardation and internal malformations.

Main signs:
- Bilateral cleft lip; complete cleft maxilla on the left, wide cleft of the palate, incomplete cleft maxilla on the right (1–5). Abnormalities of the skull: acrocephalic cranium with anterior bulging of the right side of the forehead (1–5); delayed closure of the sutures and fontanelles. Low-set ears, dysplastic pinnae (5–8). Complete paralysis of the right facial nerve (2, 3, 5). Abnormal hairline.
- Severe psychomotor retardation.
- Cardiac defect.

Supplementary findings: Short neck with loose nuchal skin. Barrel-shaped chest. Limited motion of the shoulder joints. Retarded bone age.
  Left-sided inguinal hernia. Bilateral cryptorchidism.

Manifestation: At birth.

Aetiology: Undetermined.

Course, prognosis: Early death of the child from renal insufficiency.

Illustrations:
1–8 The above-described child at 31 weeks and 37 weeks. The boy was the second child of healthy young parents (first child healthy); no evidence of parental consanguinity. Child born 6 weeks prematurely (2130 g, 43 cm). Early signs of renal insufficiency; persistent anaemia; no evidence of tubulopathy. Normal male karyotype on chromosome analysis (banding technique). Death at age 18 months. At autopsy, diffuse angiomatosis of the leptomeninges over the frontal lobes of both cerebral hemispheres. No hydrocephalus. Dilation of the pulmonary artery. Right-sided renal aplasia.

Note: Two comparable observations have in the mean time been reported to the author by colleagues.

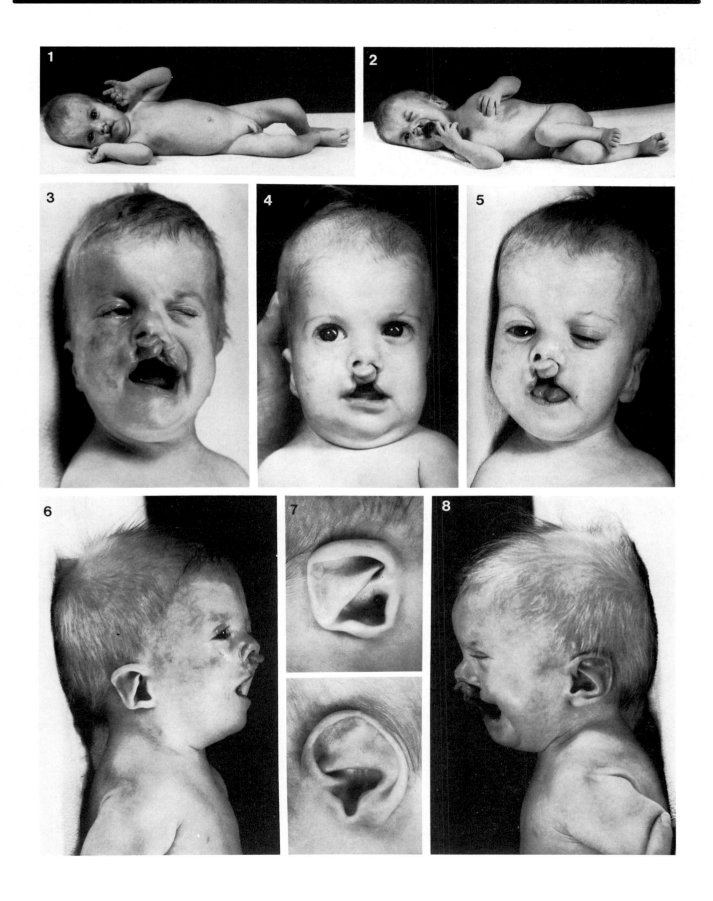

27 Freeman–Sheldon Syndrome

(Craniocarpotarsal Dysplasia; Whistling Face Syndrome)

H.-R.W

A highly characteristic syndrome with mask-like, 'whistling' face, hypoplastic alae nasi, ulnar deviation of the hands, flexion contractures of the fingers and club feet.

Main signs:
- Face: round, full cheeked; mask-like immobility with deep-set, relatively widely spaced eyes, narrow palpebral fissures with slight antimongoloid slant, convergent strabismus; wide, low-set nasal bridge; epicanthus; small nose with hypoplastic alae nasi; long philtrum and small mouth, which is difficult to open, with distinctly pursed lips as though whistling. Paramedian grooves or dimples between the lower lip and the tip of the chin (**1–3**).
- Ulnar deviation of the hands and flexion contractures of the fingers, especially the thumbs (**4**). Therapy-resistant club feet with contractures of the toes.

Supplementary findings: Transverse ridge across the lower forehead or supra-orbital soft-tissue furrow (**3**). Ptosis in some cases, high palate, usually not cleft; occasionally, hearing impairment.

Normal mental development.

Short neck (sometimes with mild pterygium). Usually markedly short stature. Frequently, development of marked scoliosis.

Manifestation: At birth.

Aetiology: Autosomal dominant inheritance. Also, apparent occurrence of an autosomal recessive type in, up to now, six families. X-linked recessive transmission also possible. Heterogeneity.

Frequency: Low. About 100 cases have been described.

Course, prognosis: Life expectancy is not affected.

Diagnosis, differential diagnosis: Exclusion of arthrogryposis (*226–228*) should not cause problems. In children beyond infancy, Schwartz–Jampel syndrome (*288*) may be difficult to rule out. The signs overlap considerably, thus, in 'true' cases of Freeman–Sheldon syndrome extra-facial disturbance of muscle tone may be seen at an early age, frequent contractures of the large joints observed later on, and mild skeletal dysplasias also determined. However, in the Schwartz–Jampel syndrome as a rule no congenital manifestations, demonstrable myotonia (on EMG) and recessive transmission.

Treatment: Surgical treatment of club feet, the fingers, strabismus, the mouth, etc, as needed. Psychological guidance. Genetic counselling of the family.

Illustrations:

1–4 A 1-year-old boy from a healthy family (probable new mutation) with the full clinical picture at birth. Unremarkable psychomotor development. Extreme malpositioning of all fingers (**4**). The left second and right fourth toes are displaced proximally (shortened metatarsals).

References:

Antley R M, Uga N, Burzynski N J *et al*: Diagnostic criteria for the whistling face syndrome. *Birth Defects Orig Art Ser* 1975, **11**:5 61.
Vaitiekaitis A S, Hornstein L, Neale H W: A new surgical procedure for correction of lip deformity in cranio-carpo-tarsal dysplasia (whistling face syndrome). *J Oral Surg* 1979, **37**:699.
Hall J G, Reed S D *et al*: The distal arthrogryposes... *Am J Med Genet* 1982, **11**:185–239.
Kousseff B G, McConnachie P, Hadro T A: Autosomal recessive type of whistling face syndrome. *Pediatr* 1982, **69**:328.
Wang Ts-R, Lin Sh-J: Further evidence for genetic heterogeneity of whistling face or Freeman-Sheldon syndrome... *Am J Med Genet* 1987, **28**:471–475.
Illum N, Reske-Nielsen E *et al*: Lethal autosomal recessive arthrogryposis multiplex congenita with whistling face... *Neuropediatr* 1988, **19**:186–192.
Dallapiccola B, Giannotti A, Lembo A, Sagui L: Autosomal recessive form of whistling face syndrome in sibs. *Am J Med Genet* 1989, **33**:542–544.
Marasovich W A, Mazaheri M *et al*: Otolaryngologic findings in whistling face syndrome. *Arch Otolaryng Head Neck Surg* 1989, **115**:1373–1380.

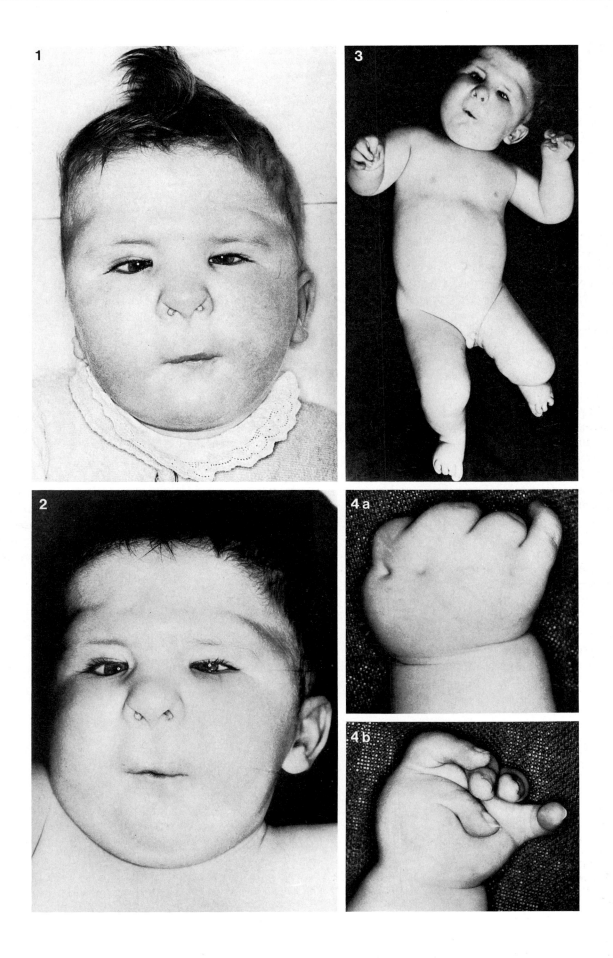

A malformation syndrome with very characteristic facial dysmorphism.

Main signs:
- Antimongoloid slant of the (possibly abnormally short) palpebral fissures with usually distinct coloboma (possibly only indentation) in the lateral half of the lower eyelids (from which the eyelashes may be absent), rarely also of the upper lids (1–4).
- Frontonasal angle often flat (1–3). Possibly aquiline and/or large-looking nose, sometimes with narrow nostrils (1–4).
- Hypoplasia of the zygomata and of the upper and lower jaws with the cheeks appearing sunken (see especially 3a); narrow, receding chin.
- Frequent macrostomia (1b) with high, narrow or cleft palate and dental anomalies.
- Usually considerable malformation of the external ear (microtia; stenosis or atresia of the auditory canal) (1–4). Frequently, defects of the middle and/or inner ear; these are more likely, the more severe the external ear deformity. Possible atrophic areas of skin, blind fistulas or skin tags between the corner of the mouth and the ear (1c)
- (The appearance has been described as fish- or bird-like facies, [1 and 2]).
- Frequent conductive hearing impairment or deafness.

Supplementary findings: Abnormal hair growth from the temples on to the lateral cheeks, towards the corners of the mouth (1a, 3b, 4a).

The facial anomalies can, exceptionally, be asymmetric or even unilateral. Malformations of the eyes such as microphthalmos or coloboma of the iris are unusual.

Choanal atresia in isolated cases.

Diverse extracranial malformations, e.g. cardiac defects may occur. Intelligence normal as a rule (in case of doubt, allow for the patient's psychological handicap and for the possibility of a hearing defect).

Manifestation: At birth; hearing impairment later, if present.

Aetiology: Autosomal dominant inheritance with complete penetrance but variable expression. High proportion of new mutations. Gene locus appears to be on chromosome 5 (5q32-q33.1). Possible existence of a similar autosomal recessive form.

Frequency: Not so rare (in 1964 it was already possible to compare 200 cases from the literature; this number has since more than doubled).

Course, prognosis: Growth of the facial skeleton during childhood may bring some improvement in appearance.

Differential diagnosis: Necessary to rule out the Goldenhar 'syndrome' (30), Nager acrofacial dysostosis (29), postaxial acrofacial dysotosis syndrome (238) and the Wildervanck syndrome (164).

Treatment: Symptomatic. Early evaluation of hearing and prompt application of appropriate aids when needed. Plastic surgery and orthodontic and dental treatment as indicated. Genetic counselling. Prenatal diagnosis possible.

Illustrations:
1 and 3 Two different newborn infants.
2 and 4 Two 3-month-old infants.

The child in 3 represents a hereditary case (father: full clinical picture of the syndrome); the other three children represent probable new mutations. The infants in 1, 2, 4 show bilateral atresia of the auditory canal; the child in 4 does not react at all to noises. Child in 1: cleft palate. Child in 2: bifid uvula, cardiac defect.

References:

Rogers B O: Berry–Treacher Collins syndrome: a review of 200 cases. *Br J Plast Surg* 1964, **17**:109.
Crane J P, Beaver H A: Midtrimester sonographic diagnosis of mandibulofacial dysostosis. *Am J Med Genet* 1986, **25**:251–255.
Dixon M J *et al*: The gene for Treacher Collins syndrome maps to the long arm of chromosome 5. *Am J Hum Genet* 1991, **49**:17–22.
Jabs E *et al*: Chromosomal deletion... in a Treacher Collins syndrome... *Genomics* 1991, **11**:188–192.
Kreiborg Sv *et al*: Cranial base and face in mandibulofacial dysostosis. *Am J Med Genet* 1993, **47**:753–760.
Opitz J M *et al*: Acrofacial dysostoses: review... *Am J Med Genet* 1993, **47**:660–678.
Edery P *et al*: Apparent genetic homogeneity of the Treacher Collins–Franceschetti syndrome. *Am J Med Genet* 1994, **52**:174–177.

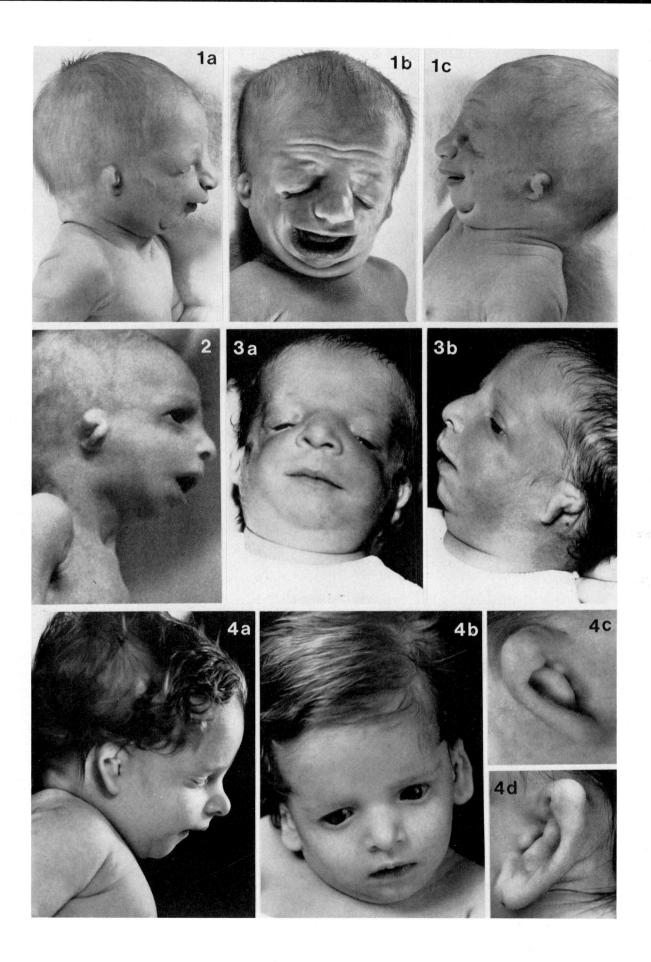

29 Nager Acrofacial Dyostosis

(Nager–de Reynier Type Acrofacial Dystosis; Pre-axial Dysostosis)

H.-R.W
P. Meinecke

A hereditary mandibulofacial dysostosis with hypoplasia of the limbs, especially of the first rays of the upper extremities.

Main signs:

- Facial dysmorphism similar to mandibulofacial dysostosis (28) (**1 and 2**). Frequent cleft palate and conductive hearing defect.
- Anomalies of the thumbs (triphalangism, hypoplasia, aplasia) and in some cases of the neighbouring ray or possibly of the bones of the forearms (hypoplasia of the radius, radio-ulnar synostosis, etc, or even 'phocomelia' involving the shoulder girdle) (**3 and 4**). Varying degrees of hypoplasia may also occur in the lower extremities.

Supplementary findings: Initial difficulties with sucking, swallowing and breathing (as a result of the Robin sequence 39) are not unusual, and may in some cases require tracheostomy or gastrostomy. Small stature appears to be relatively common. Cryptorchidism and dysplastic mamillae may occur, cardiac and/or renal defects are rare.

Possible mild to moderate mental retardation.

Manifestation: At birth; hearing defect later, if present.

Aetiology: Often sporadic occurrence (new mutations? Precise testing of relatives needed). An autosomal recessive gene with variable expression (locus q23?) seems to be predominant but autosomal dominant inheritance also occurs. Heterogeneity. Polytopic field defect acquired during blastogenesis.

Frequency: Low (about 70 case reports to date).

Course, prognosis: Growth of the facial skeleton during childhood may bring about some improvement in appearance.

Differential diagnosis: Acrofacial dysostosis of the mainly postaxial type (238) should not be difficult to rule out because of the different location of the defects. However, there are a substantial number of additional, very rare and in some cases more severe, mandibulo- and acrofacial dysostoses that have not yet been further classified (overview by Opitz et al).

Treatment: Symptomatic. Early hearing tests and immediate special hearing and speech aids when required. Corrective surgery of the hands and corrective orthopaedic, cosmetic, or orthodontic procedures may be indicated. Genetic counselling. Prenatal diagnosis in some cases.

Illustrations:

1–4 A child of healthy nonconsanguineous parents. Bilateral triphalangeal thumb, no radial dysplasia. High palate without cleft; marked mandibular hypoplasia, also on radiograph; hearing apparently not affected. Heart and lower extremities unremarkable.

References:
Burton B K, Nadler H L: Nager acrofacial dysostosis. *J Pediatr* 1977, **91**:84.
Meyerson M D, Jensen K M, Meyers J M *et al*: Nager acrofacial dysostosis: early intervention and long term planning. *Cleft Palate J* 1977 **14/1**:35.
Halal F, Herrmann J *et al*: Differential diagnosis of Nager acrofacial dysostosis syndrome... *Am J Med Genet* 1983, 14:209–224.
Pfeiffer R A, Stoess H: Acrofacial dysostosis (Nager syndrome): synopsis... *Am J Med Genet* 1983, 15:255–260.
Thompson E, Cadbury R *et al*: The Nager acrofacial dysostosis syndrome with the tetralogy of Fallot. *J Med Genet* 1985, **22**:408–410.
Chemke J, Mogilner B M *et al*: Autosomal recessive inheritance of Nager acrofacial dysostosis. *J Med Genet* 1988, 25:230–232.
Le Merrer M *et al*: Acrofacial dysostoses... *Am J Med Genet* 1989, 33:318–322.
Hall Br D: Nager acrofacial dysostosis... *Am J Med Genet* 1989, 33:394–397.
Palomeque A *et al*: Nager anomaly with severe... involvement. *Am J Med Genet* 1990, **36**:356–357.
Aylsworth A S *et al*: Nager acrofacial dysostosis... *Am J Med Genet* 1991, 41:83–88.
Bonthron, D T et al: Nager acrofacial dysostosis: minor familial manifestations... *Clin Genet* 1993, 43:127–131 (1993).
Opitz J M *et al*: Acrofacial dysostoses: review... *Am J Med Genet* 1993, 47:660–678.

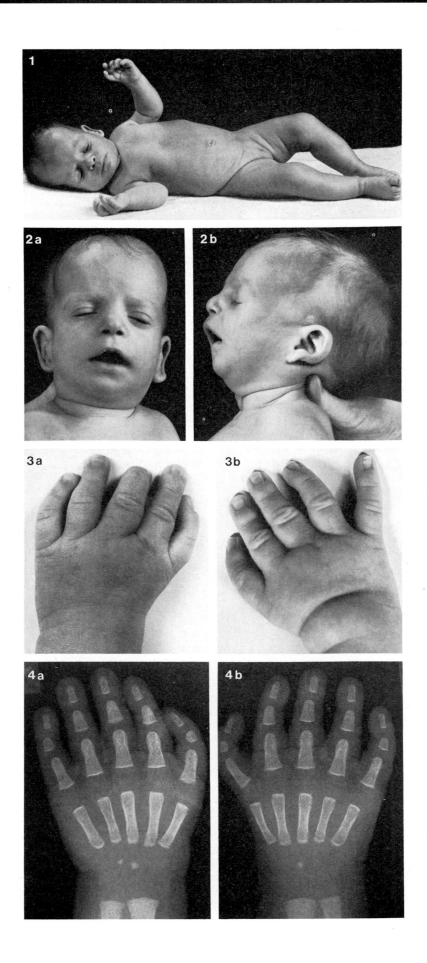

Goldenhar 'Syndrome'

(Goldenhar Anomaly, Goldenhar–Gorlin 'Syndrome', Goldenhar Sequence, Oculoauricular 'Dysplasia', Oculoauriculovertebral 'Dysplasia')

J.K / H.-R.W

A very variable but relatively characteristic malformation complex of eye, ear, malar and, in some cases, vertebral anomalies.

Main signs:

• Often marked facial asymmetry due to unilateral hypoplasia (**2 and 4**); usually, prominent forehead (**1 and 4**), hypoplasia of the zygomatic region and of the mandible, receding chin.

• Epibulbar dermoid or lipodermoid (usually occurring bilaterally on the lateral corneoscleral junction) (**6**); coloboma of the upper lid (usually unilateral). Occurrence also of other ocular anomalies.

• One or more pre-auricular tags, unilateral or bilateral, on a line between the tragus and the corner of the mouth (**1, 3, 4, 7**). Blind fistulas may also be located here. As a rule, microtia or other malformations of the external ear (**7a**).

• Frequent unilateral macrostomia due to a transverse malar cleft (**2 and 4**).

• Usually marked malformations (often hemivertebrae) of the (especially upper) spine, frequently demonstrable only by radiograph (**5**); occasionally scoliosis.

Supplementary findings: Possible cleft lip and/or palate. Frequent dental anomalies.

Possible conductive hearing defect.

Occasionally mental retardation.

Lipomas of the corpus callosum may occur (ultrasound, CT scan).

Cardiac, pulmonary and other anomalies also possible.

Manifestation: At birth; hearing defect later, if present.

Aetiology: A causally heterogeneous and complex developmental field defect in which the manifestations vary markedly in severity. Usually sporadic occurrence (in some cases based on *in-utero* interference of the blood supply). Evidence for autosomal dominant as well as for autosomal recessive inheritance. The majority of affected patients are males. The risk of recurrence after one affected child is about 3%, sibling risk is about 6%.

Frequency: About one out of 3 000–5 000 newborns. Hundreds of cases have been documented.

Course, prognosis: Favourable.

Diagnosis, differential diagnosis: No single sign can be considered obligatory. Differentiation from typical mandibulofacial dysostosis (*28*) should not be particularly difficult, but from hemifacial microsomia (*31*) and from Wildervanck syndrome (*164*) can be practically impossible.

Treatment: Removal of pre-auricular tags and larger dermoids. Closure of malar cleft when present (**6**). Cosmetic surgery may be indicated. Dental care. Early hearing test as a precaution in every case. Hearing aids from early childhood, when needed.

Illustrations:

1–3, 6 An affected infant at 8 and 9 months. Macrocephaly, mild facial asymmetry favouring the left side with distinct hypoplasia of the right mandible. Right lateral epibulbar lipodermoid, right palpebral fissure narrower than the left. One pre-auricular tag on the right, three small tags on the left, one of which lies between the ear and the corner of the mouth. Transverse buccal cleft on the right Capillary angiomas of the midface and occiput. Scoliosis; 13 pairs of ribs. Mental development and hearing apparently unimpaired.

4 and 5 Newborn girl. Facial asymmetry. Three pre-auricular tags on the right; hypoplasia of the zygoma; macrostomia due to small transverse buccal cleft on the right, receding chin; anomalies of the vertebral bodies.

7a and b Newborn girl with left epibulbar dermoid; low-set ears; right microtia with atresia of the auditory canal (left canal abnormally narrow); bilateral pre-auricular tags; macrostomia (without buccal cleft); anomalies of the vertebral bodies (hemi- and block vertebrae); 10 ribs on the right, 11 on the left.

References:

Shokeir M H K: The Goldenhar syndrome: a natural history. *Birth Defects Orig Art Ser* 1977, **13/3C**:67.
Feingold M, Baum J: Goldenhar's syndrome. *Am J Dis Child* 1978, **132**:136.
Setzer E S, Ruiz-Castaneda N *et al*: Etiologic heterogeneity in the oculoauriculovertebral syndrome. *J Pediatr* 1981, **98**:88.
Regenbogen L, Godel V, Goya V *et al*: Further evidence for an autosomal dominant form of oculoauriculovertebral dysplasia. *Clin Genet* 1982, **21**:161.
Boles D J, Bodurtha J *et al*: Goldenhar complex in discordant monozygotic twins... *Am J Med Genet* 1987, **28**:103–109.
Rollnick B R, Kaye C I *et al*: Oculoauriculovertebral dysplasia and variants... *Am J Med Genet* 1987, **26**:361–375.
Beltinger C, Saule H: Imaging of lipoma of the corpus callosum... in the Goldenhar syndrome. *Pediatr Radiol* 1988, **18**:71–73.
Rollnick B R: Oculoauriculovertebral anomaly... *Am J Med Genet Suppl* 1988, **4**:41–53.
Ryan C A, Finer N N *et al*: Discordance of signs in monozygotic twins concordant for the Goldenhar syndrome. *Am J Med Genet* 1988, **29**:755–761.
Kumar A, Friedman J M, Taylor G P, Patterson M W H: Pattern of cardiac malformations in oculoauriculovertebral spectrum. *Am J Med Genet* 1993, **46**:423–426.

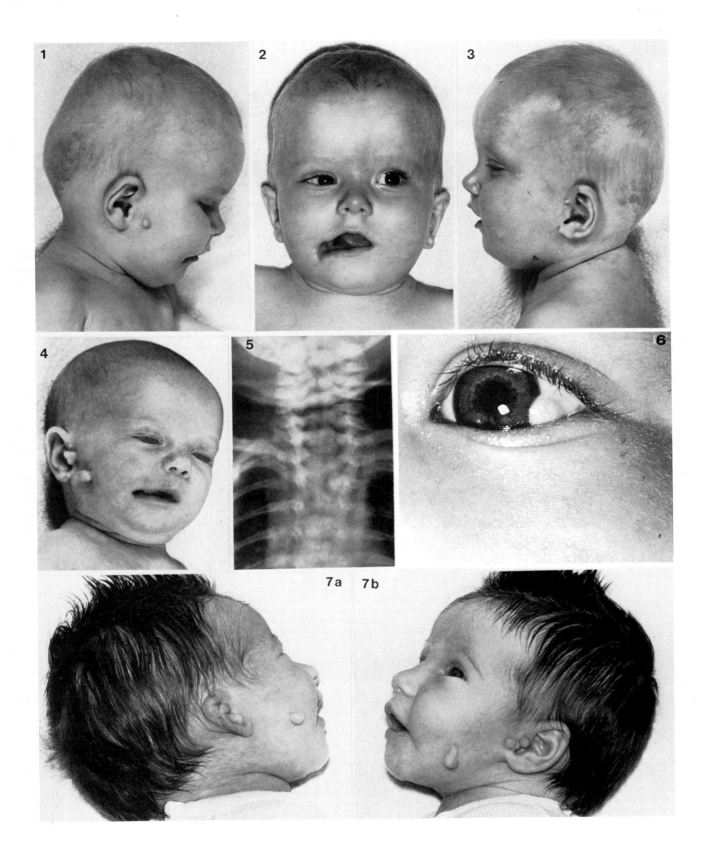

31 | Hemifacial Microsomia

A clinical picture comprising unusual facial asymmetry with unilateral malformation of the ear and ipsilateral hypoplasia, especially of the mandibular ramus and condyle.

Main signs:
- Variable degrees of facial asymmetry caused by unilateral hypoplasia of the jaw and receding chin (1–3).
- Pre-auricular tags or abnormality of the external ear (2). Aplasia in some cases.
- Malocclusion on the affected side.

Supplementary findings: Usually as an exception: anomalies of the eye on the affected side of the face (and usually no dermoid, lipodermoid or coloboma of the upper eyelid).
 Possible hearing impairment.
 Patients with a simultaneous radial anomaly (e.g. triphalangeal thumb) could constitute a separate entity.

Manifestation: At birth or soon after; hearing defect later, if present.

Aetiology: Not uniform; cf. Goldenhar 'syndrome' (30), of which this clinical picture can be considered a favourable variant. Sporadic occurrence as a rule (recurrence risk in first-degree relatives approximately 2–3%).

Frequency: Not so rare (estimates: one out of 3500–5600 live births).

Course, prognosis: Favourable.

Diagnosis, differential diagnosis: Differentiation from mandibulofacial dysostosis (28) is easy; from Goldenhar 'syndrome' (30) is difficult or impossible.
 Hemifacial microsomia has also been observed in association with thalidomide embryopathy (206), diabetic embryopathy (299), foetal primidone syndrome, trisomy 18 (48), cri du chat syndrome (50) and other chromosomal disorders such as Townes–Brockes (313) and branchio-otorenal syndrome, such as the Rokitansky sequence.

Treatment: Corrective cosmetic surgery in some cases. Dental and orthodontic care. An early hearing test is an important precaution. Hearing aids, if indicated, from early childhood onward.

Illustrations:
1–3 A 5 year-old boy from a healthy family. Malformation of the right ear.
2 The patient's appearance after two operations to reconstruct his, now less conspicuous, right ear). Hypoplasia of the right mandible.
Marked, probably combined hearing defect on the right. Normal psychomotor development. Additional abnormalities: limited ability to turn the head to the extreme right, low nuchal hairline, hypoplastic accessory mamilla on the right.

References:
Pashayan H, Pinsky L, Fraser F C: Hemifacial microsomia: oculo-auriculo-vertebral dysplasia: a patient with overlapping features. *J Med Genet* 1970, 7:185.
Stewart R E: Craniofacial malformations. *Pediatr Clin North Am* 1978, 25:500.
Feingold M: Hemifacial microsomia. In Birth defects compendium edn 2. 1979; 511.
Moeschler J, Clarren S K: Familial occurrence of hemifacial microsomia with radial limb defects. *Am J Med Genet* 1982, 12:371–375.
Burck U: Genetic aspects of hemifacial microsomia. *Hum Genet* 1983, 64:291–296.
Rollnick B R, Kaye C I: Hemifacial microsomia and variants. *Am J Med Genet* 1983, 15:233–253.
Connor J M, Fernandez C: Genetic aspects of hemifacial microsomia. *Hum Genet* 1984, 68:349.
Bennum R D *et al*: Microtia: a microform of hemifacial microsomia. *Plast Reconstr Surg* 1985, 76:859–863.
Loevy H T, Shore S W: Dental maturation in hemifacial microsomia. *J Craniofac Genet Dev Biol* 1985, (suppl.1):267–272.
Robinow M *et al*: Hemifacial microsomia... *J Med Genet Suppl* 1986, 2:129–133.
Smakel Z: Craniofacial changes in hemifacial microsomia. *J Craniofac Genet Dev Biol* 1986, 6:151–170.
Farias M, Vargervik K: Dental development in hemifacial microsomia... *Pediatr Dent* 1988, 10:140–143.
Bassila M K, Goldberg R: The association of facial palsy and/or sensorineural hearing loss in patients with hemifacial microsomia. *Am J Med Genet* 1989, 26:287–291.
Kay E D, Kay C N: Dysmorphogenesis of the mandible, zygoma and middle ear ossicles in hemifacial microsomia... *Am J Med Genet* 1989, 32:27–31.
Cousley R R J, Wilson D J: Hemifacial microsomia: developmental consequence of pertubation of the auriculofacial cartilage model?... *Am J Med Genet* 1992, 42:461–466.
Duncan P A, Shapiro L R: Interrelationships of the hemifacial microsomia-VATER, VATER, and sirenomelia phenotypes. *Am J Med Genet* 1993, 47:75–84.

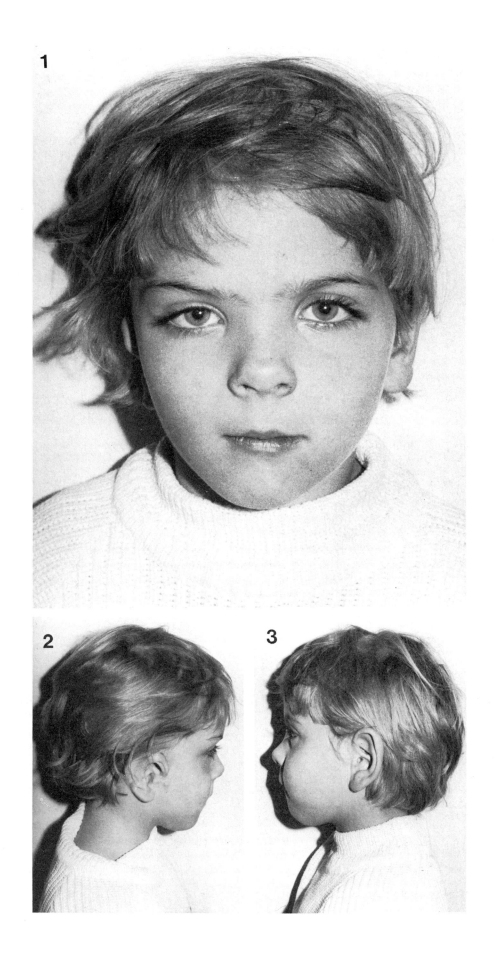

1

2

3

Syndrome of Progressive Hemifacial Atrophy

(Romberg Syndrome, Parry–Romberg Syndrome)

H.-R.W

Localized facial atrophy, possibly associated with focal epilepsy and/or heterochromia iridis complex.

Main signs:
Progressive atrophy of some or all of the tissues on one-half of the face. The whole side of the face may be involved (early stage shown in **1**; further progression since): or patchy or stripe-like areas are affected, such that the changes may resemble a sword wound: 'en coup de sabre' (**2**). The left side of the face is more often affected. In exceptional cases, patients may develop more or less complete hemiatrophy.

Supplementary findings: Frequent pigmentation changes in the affected skin areas; also, discoloration and later loss of hair (eyebrows, eyelashes, and so on). Sensation remains intact on the affected side of the face; motor function barely affected despite muscular involvement.

Involvement of the eye in some cases: sinking in of the eyeball, heterochromia iridis with iridocyclitis; also strabismus, ptosis and other signs.

Headaches or trigeminal neuralgia possible. In some cases contralateral disturbance of neurological function (not infrequently focal epilepsy with contralateral expression); magnetic resonance imaging may then in some cases reveal ipsilateral meningeal and gyral changes as well as ventricular enlargement.

Manifestation: Mainly in the first 2 decades of life.

Aetiology: Uncertain. Uniformity of the syndrome questionable. Occasional familial occurrence suggests that genetic factors at least play a role in these cases.

Frequency: Low.

Course, prognosis: The atrophic process frequently comes to a halt after a course of several years.

Differential diagnosis: Hemifacial microsomia (*31*) and possibly Goldenhar 'syndrome' (*30*).

Treatment: Symptomatic. Cosmetic surgery may be indicated at a later date.

Illustrations:
1 A 27-month-old, normally developed girl from a healthy family. Since the end of her first year of life, increasing 'sinking in' of the whole right side of her face, including soft tissue, bony parts and the eye, with unaltered toddler-like fullness of the left side of the face. Intermittent strabismus on the right. Tongue normal; no depigmentation of the skin; no heterochromia; no neurological findings. Symmetrical development of the remainder of the body, as judged by appearance and measurements.
2 A 7 year and 3-month-old boy, tall and slightly obese, from a healthy family. Underdevelopment of the left side of the face noted since infancy; distinct underdevelopment of the maxillary sinus and teeth on the left compared with the right. On the forehead, two parallel vertical pigmented atrophic areas of skin about 4 cm long and barely a finger-breadth wide, with bony involvement as a localized scleroderma of the 'en coup de sabre' type, the one median, the other 2 cm to the left. Development of these areas in the past few years. Intermittent left-sided headaches. Signs of a mild right-sided spastic hemiparesis with left-sided focal findings in electroencephalogram; no seizure disorder. Mild retardation. Ophthalmological examinations normal to date.

References:
Franceschetti A, Koenig H: L'importance du facteur hérédo-dégénératif dans l'hémiatrophie faciale progressive (Romberg). Études des complications oculaires dans ce syndrome. *J Génét Hum* 1952, 1:27.
Fulmek R: Hemiatrophia progressiva faciei (Romberg Syndrom) mit gleichseitiger Heterochromia complicata (Fuchs-Syndrom). *Klin Mbl Augenheilk* 1974, 164:615.
Muchnik R S, Sherrell J A, Rees T D: Ocular manifestations and treatment of hemifacial atrophy. *Am J Ophthalmol* 1979, 88:889.
Goldhammer Y: Progressive hemifacial atrophy (Parry–Romberg's disease) principally involving bone. *J Laryngol* 1981, 95:643–647.
Asher S W, Berg B O: Progressive hemifacial atrophy. *Arch Neurol* 1982, 39:44.
Lewkonia R M, Lowry R B: Progressive hemifacial atrophy (Parry–Romberg syndrome); report with review of genetics and nosology. *Am J Med Genet* 1983, 14:385–390.
Hall B D *et al*: Progressive hemifacial atrophy (Romberg syndrome) with 'coup de sabre' forehead and scalp lesions... *Proc Greenwood Genet Ctr* 1987, 6:100–101.
Küster W, Kries R V *et al*: Lineare zirkumskripte Sklerodermie unter dem Bilde einer Hemiatrophia faciei. *Pädiatr Prax* 1987/88, 36:131–136.
Menges-Wenzel E M *et al*: Hemiatrophia faciei progressiva (Parry–Romberg-Syndrom). *Mschr Kinderheilk* 1993, 141:922–924.
Terstegge K, Henkes H *et al*: Zerebrale Manifestationen der progressiven fazialen Hemiatrophie... *Radiologe* 1993, 33:585–595.
Terstegge K, Kunath B *et al*: MR of brain involvement in progressive facial hemiatrophy... *AJNR* 1994, 15:145–150.

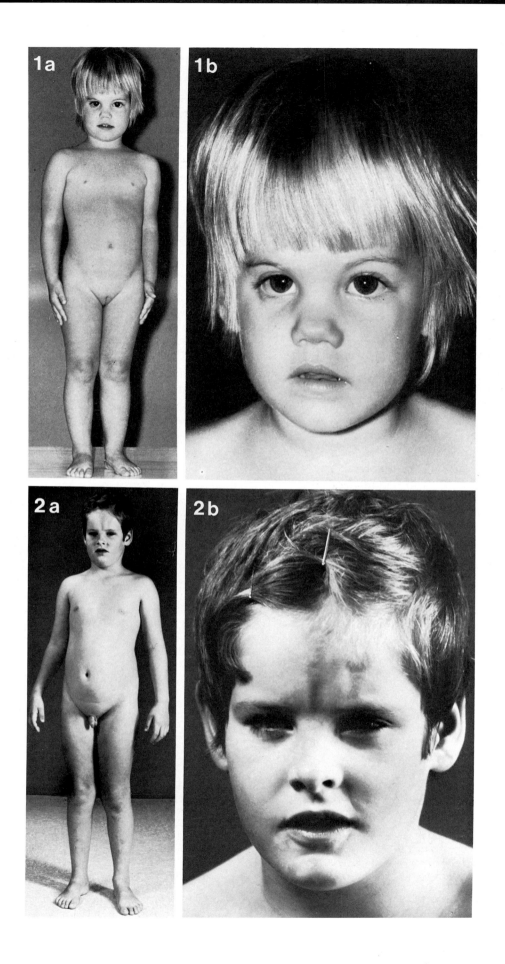

33 Cardiofacial Symptom Complex
(Asymmetric Crying Face Syndrome)

J.K.

Association of cardiac defect and asymmetric crying face.

Main signs:
- Facial asymmetry when crying, unnoticeable when calm.
- Various congenital heart defects.

Supplementary findings: Possible dysplasia of the ear and signs of VATER association: vertebral malformations, renal anomalies, anal atresia, oesophageal atresia, radial peculiarities.

Manifestation: At birth.

Aetiology: Usually sporadic, multifactorial inheritance but occasionally autosomal dominant inheritance.

Pathogenesis: Partial agenesis of the depressor anguli oris muscle. In combination with heart defect: possible developmental field defect.

Course, prognosis: Dependent on the severity of accessory malformations.

Differential diagnosis: Paresis of the facial nerve.
Right-sided asymmetry occurs more frequently with associated malformations than left-sided facial asymmetry.

Illustrations:
1a and b Patient *1* = 5-month-old female infant with distortion of the left-sided labial commissure and absence of the right-sided depressor anguli oris muscle. Auricular dysplasia.
2a and b Patient *2* = 5-month-old female infant with distortion of the left-sided labial commissure and absence of the right-sided depressor anguli oris muscle. Unilateral malformation of the ear.

References:
Nelson K B, Eng P D: Congenital hypoplasia of the depressor anguli oris muscle: differentiation from congenital facial palsy. *J Pediatr* 1972, **81**: 16–20.
Pape K E, Pickering D: Asymmetric crying facies: an index of other congenital anomalies. *J Pediatr* 1972, 81:21–30.
Papadatos C *et al*: Congenital hypoplasia of depressor anguli oris muscle. A genetically determined condition? *Arch Dis Child* 1974, 49:927–931.
Miller M, Hall J G: Familial asymmetric crying facies. *Am J Dis Child* 1979, **133**:743–746.
Monreal F J: Asymmetric crying facies: an alternative interpretation. *Pediatr* 1980, **65**:146–149.
Singhi S, Singhi P, Lall K B: Congenital asymmetric crying facies. *Clin Pediatr* 1980, **19**:673–678.
Lenarsky C, Shewmon D A, Shaw A, Feig S A: Occurrence of neuroblastoma and asymmetric crying facies. Case report and review of the literature. *J Pediatr* 1986, **107**:268–270.

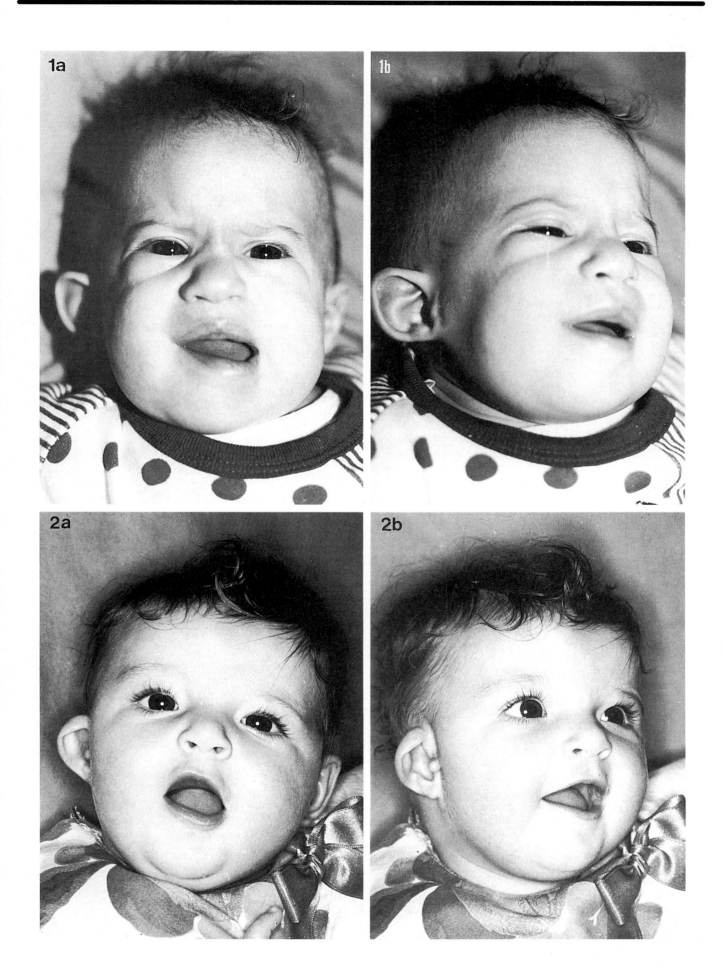

Anomalies in the Mid-anterior Neck Region
(Pterygium Colli Medianum, Rhaphe Mediana Supra-umbilicalis—with or without Vascular Naevi)

H.-R.W

A number of rare anomalies occurring sporadically, alone or in combination, in the anterior mid-line region.

Main Signs:
- Median pterygium colli between the chin and jugular fossa (**1 and 2**). Double origin from the protuberances of the chin (**1b and 2**); variably firm skin folds, which are scar-like in some areas; frequent micrognathia and limited extension of the neck.
- Supra-umbilical cicatricial raphe between the navel and the xiphoid (or extending even further upwards) (**3 and 4**).
- In some cases, a vascular naevus or cavernous haemangioma (the latter not infrequently ulcerating) on the neck and/or face, possibly also in the larynx (**4**).

Supplementary findings: In some cases a median fissure of the throat, characterized by a superficial scar (sometimes up to 1 cm wide) with subcutaneous connective tissue strands between the hyoid or chin (in this case originating from the paramedian tuberosities of the chin) and jugular fossa, where a depression can lead further into a fistula to the superior mediastinum. Infrequently, a median 'cleft' or cleft residue extends deeper or further caudally: cleft of the lower lip, tongue, lower jaw or chin (possibly also just a Pierre Robin sequence); anomalies of the sternum ranging from split sternum to aplasia with respiration-dependent median retraction and billowing of the anterior thorax, in some cases with an extensive ectopia cordis.

Manifestation: At birth and thereafter.

Aetiology: Sporadic occurrence. Developmental field defect of the anterior midline. Practically no risk of recurrence.

Frequency: Rare.

Course, prognosis: Favourable.

Diagnosis: Not difficult. In the newborn the mid-abdominal raphe and the eventual pterygium initially appear as fine, delicate linear scars and only later, with time, become increasingly distinct and firmer. Radiographic examination of the thorax and its organs is imperative. In case of stridor, intralaryngeal haemangiomas must be ruled out.

Treatment: Adequate treatment of progressive haemangiomatosis as required. In addition, cosmetic procedures are generally indicated at the appropriate time.

Illustrations:
1 A 17-year-old girl, otherwise completely normally developed, with median pterygium colli. Laryngopharynx, sternum and the rest of the bony thorax and internal organs normal.
2 A similarly affected 4-year-old boy, otherwise normally developed and without further anomalies.
3 A 21 month old with an upper mid-abdominal raphe, a defect of the manubrium of the sternum and herniation of the lung. Widely spaced nipples.
4 A 3-month-old infant with an upper mid-abdominal raphe, a soft tissue tag in the region of the jugular fossa, widely spaced nipples, facial haemangiomatosis. X-ray of the sternum and the rest of the thorax and thoracic organs normal.

References:

Gotlieb A, Hanukoglu A, Fried D *et al*: Micrognathia associated with asternia and teleangiectatic skin lesion. *Syndrome identification* (March of Dimes Birth Defects Foundation) 1982, 8, 1:10–13.

Leiber B: Angeborene supraumbilikale Mittelbauchrhaphe (SMBR) und kavernöse Gesichtshämangiomatose — ein neues Syndrom? *Mschr Kinderheilk* 1982, 130:84–90.

Gargan T J, McKinnon *et al*: Midline cervical cleft. *Plast Reconstr Surg* 1985, 76:223–229.

Waldschmidt J, Ribbe R, Weineck J: Diagnose und Differentialdiagnose der angeborenen Fisteln und Zysten des Halses. *Z Kinderchi* 1987, 42: 271–278.

Godbersen S, Heckel V, Wiedemann H-R: Pterygium colli medianum and midline cervical cleft: midline anomalies in the sense of a developmental field defect. *Am J Med Genet* 1987, 27:719–723.

Van der Staak F H J, Pruszczynksi M *et al*: The midline cervical cleft. *J Pediatr Surg* 1991, 26:1391–1393.

Maddalozzo J, Frankel A *et al*: Midline cervical cleft. *Pediatr* 1993, 92:286–287.

Gorlin R D *et al*: Midline cervical cleft. *Pediatr* 1993, 92:286–287.

Gorlin R D *et al*: Marked female predilection in some syndromes associated with facial hemangiomas. *Am J Med Genet* 1994, 52:130–135.

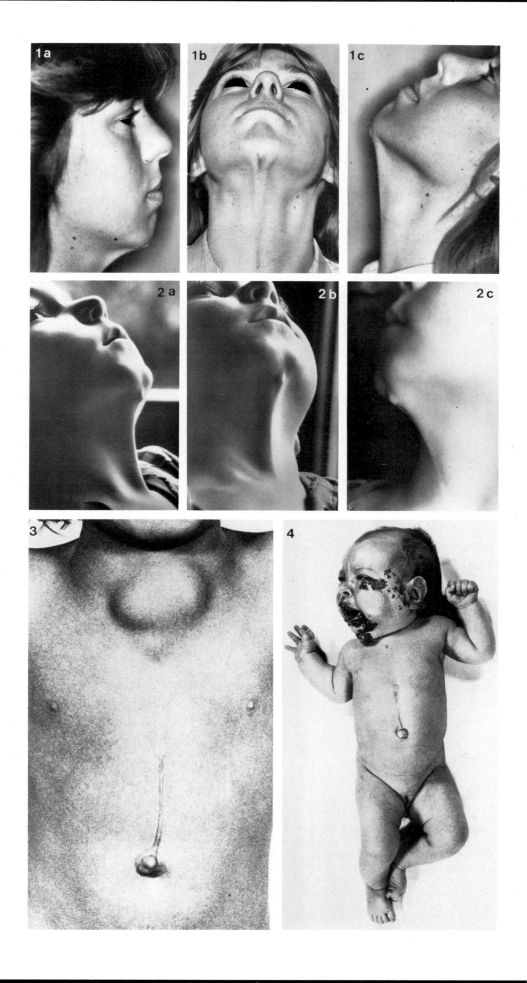

35 Van der Woude Syndrome
(Lower Lip Pits, Cleft Lip and Palate Syndrome)

H.-R.W

A characteristic syndrome comprising pits of the lower lip and cleft lip/palate.

Main signs:
- Generally symmetrical paramedian pits or protuberances of the lower lip ('fistulae labii inferioris') in over 80% of patients (1–4).
- Cleft lip and/or palate (in approximately 60%) (1a).
- Hypodontia (usually, the second incisors and second molars; in approximately 15% of patients).

Manifestation: At birth (dental anomalies later).

Aetiology: Autosomal dominant inheritance with at least 90% penetrance and variable expression. Numerous cases probably represent new mutations. Possible microdeletion in 1q32-41.

Frequency: Relatively high; 1000 or more cases in the literature. Estimation: one out of 40 000 live births.

Course, prognosis: Good.

Diagnosis, differential diagnosis: The occurrence of weak forms should be kept in mind. Differentiation from the OFD syndrome type I (36) and from the popliteal pterygium syndrome, which can also occur with lower lip pits and clefts.

Treatment: Operative correction of the cleft lip and/or palate is foremost.

Illustrations
1–4 Two affected sisters.
1a and b The younger girl at 5 months and at 3 years and 6 months (here, after surgical correction of the cleft lip and palate; before correction of the lower lip).
4 The older sister after cleft palate surgery; before correction of the lower lip. The previous four generations have been similarly affected.

References:
Van der Woude A: Fistula labii inferioris congenita and its association with cleft lip and palate. *Am J Hum Genet* 1954, 6:244–256.
Burdick A B, Bixler D *et al*: Genetic analysis in families with Van der Woude syndrome. *J Craniofac Genet Dev Biol* 1985, 5:181–208.
Schinzel A, Kläuser M: The Van der Woude syndrome... *J Med Genet* 1986, 23:291–294.
Bocian M, Walker A P: Lip pits and deletion 1q32-41. *Am J Med Genet* 1987, 26:437–443.
Wienker T F, Hudek G *et al*: Linkage studies in a pedigree with Van der Woude syndrome. *J Med Genet* 1987, 24:160–162.
Hughes M *et al*: Does van der Woude syndrome map to chromosome 2q34-36? *Proc Greenwood Genet Ctr* 1988, 7:176.
Küster W, Lambrecht J T: Cleft lip and palate, lower lip pits, and limb deficiency defects. *J Med Genet* 1988, 25:565–572.
Murray J C, Nishimura D Y *et al*: Linkage of an autosomal dominant clefting syndrome (Van der Woude) to loci on chromosome 1q. *Am J Hum Genet* 1990, 46:486–491.
Hecht J T, Wang Y *et al*: Van der Woude syndrome and nonsyndromic cleft lip and palate. *Am J Hum Genet* 1992, 51:442–444.
Sander A *et al*: Evidence of a microdeletion in 1q32-41 involving the gene responsible for Van der Woude syndrome. *Hum Mol Genet* 1994, 3:575–578.

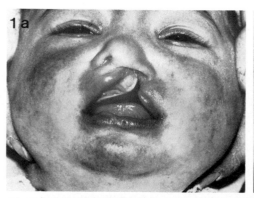

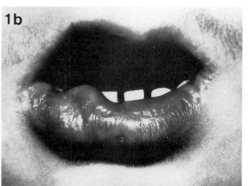

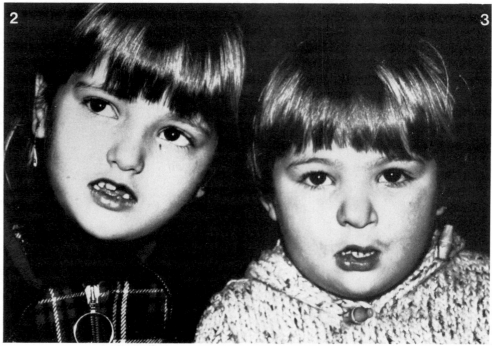

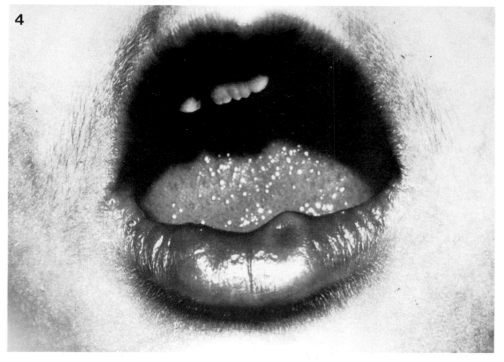

36 Orofaciodigital Syndrome Type 1

(OFD Syndrome 1, Papillon–Léage–Psaume Syndrome)

H.-R.W

A hereditary syndrome in females comprising lobulated tongue, hyperplastic frenula, notched alveolar crests, unusual facies and anomalies of the hands and feet.

Main signs:

- Lobulation of the tongue into two or more lobes (5). Multiple intra-oral hyperplastic frenula, frequently with extensive fixation of the tongue and/or upper lip. Lateral notching of the alveolar ridge of the upper jaw (8); notches are also possible in the anterior alveolar ridge of the lower jaw. High palate or (irregular/asymmetric) cleft palate.
- Unusual facies (1–3): frontal bossing, broad nasal bridge, hypertelorism or telecanthus, hypoplasia of the alae nasi, hypoplasia in the jaw region with dysodontiasis (lower lateral incisors frequently absent), possible median cleft of the upper lip. Milia of the ears and face in infancy, later receding. Dry skin and alopecia of the scalp in some cases.
- Clinodactyly, brachydactyly and syndactyly of the hands and feet (7, 9, 10–12). Exceptional, unilateral or asymmetric polydactyly.

Supplementary findings: About one-half of the patients are mentally retarded (with an average IQ of about 70). Malformations of the brain are not uncommon (e.g. aplasia of the corpus callosum, as with other midline malformation syndromes).

Hamartoma of the tongue in some patients.

Occasionally short stature or deafness. Polycystic kidneys apparently frequent, sometimes with adult-type manifestation.

Manifestation: At birth.

Aetiology: Clinical picture with variable expression, X-linked dominant. As the pleiotropic gene is completely lethal in males, only females are clinically affected (except in Klinefelter syndrome).

Frequency: Low; estimated at one out of 50 000. Two hundred cases published.

Course, prognosis: Life expectancy is probably essentially normal. Dependent on the mental development of the patient.

Differential diagnosis: Orofaciodigital syndrome type II (237) occurs in both sexes (autosomal recessive inheritance); the main differentiating characteristics are bilateral postaxial polydactyly of the hands (less frequently of the feet), hypoplasia of the alae nasi, broad tip of the nose and absence more frequently of the middle than the lateral incisors.

Comment: This sharply outlined syndrome is only one representative of a probably relatively large, still only provisionally classified, heterogeneous and varied group of OFD syndromes (at least eight types); for some of these there are only a few relevant observations.

Treatment: Closure of clefts, removal of hypertrophic frenula, orthodontic and dental care, etc. Surgical correction of the hands and special schooling may be indicated. Genetic counselling is important.

Illustrations:

1–12 A 10-year-old girl with the full syndrome (after operative correction of the inner canthi, upper lip, tongue, palate and hands). Mild mental retardation. Height below the 10th percentile. Flat midface, thin hair.

References:

Melnick M, Shields E D: Orofaciodigital syndrome, Type I: a phenotypic and genetic analysis. *Oral Surg* 1975, **40**:599.
Annerén G, Arvidson B *et al*: Orofaciodigital syndromes I and II... *Clin Genet* 1984, **26**:178–186.
Baraitser M: The orofaciodigital (OFD) syndromes. *J Med Genet* 1986, **23**:116–119.
Connacher A A, Forsyth C C *et al*: Orofaciodigital syndrome type I... *J Med Genet* 1987, **24**:116–122.
Donnai D, Kerzin-Storrar L *et al*: Familial orofaciodigital syndrome type I... *J Med Genet* 1987, **24**:84–87.
Toriello H V: Heterogeneity and variability in the oral-facial-digital syndromes. *Am J Med Genet* 1988, Suppl **4**:149–159.
Goodship J, Platt J *et al*: A male with type I orofaciodigital syndrome. *J Med Genet* 1991, **28**:691–694.
Salinas C F *et al*: Variability of expression of the orofaciodigital syndrome I... *Am J Med Genet* 1991, **38**:574–582.
Gillerot Y, Heimann M *et al*: Oral-facial-digital syndrome I in a newborn male. *Am J Med Genet* 1993, **46**:335–338.

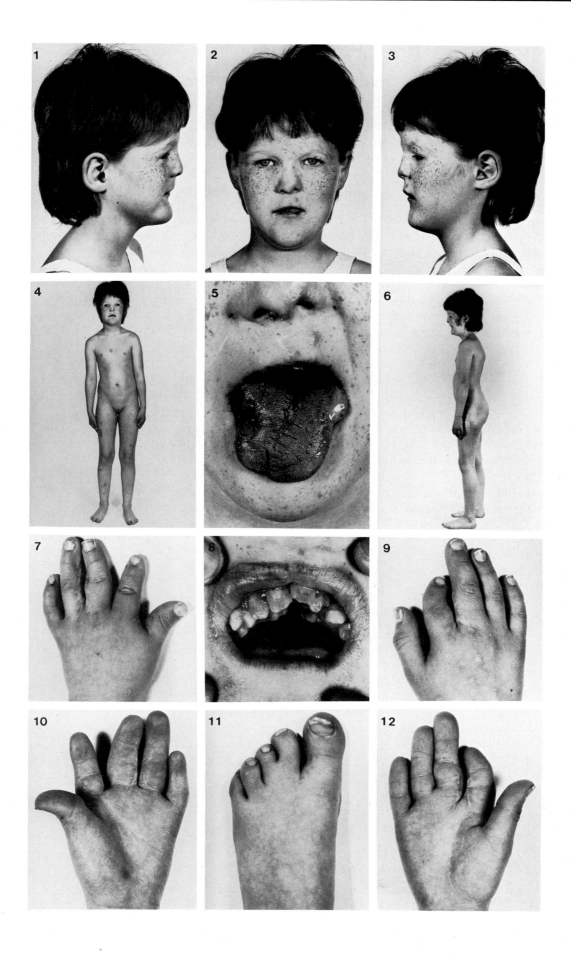

37 Syndrome of Microcephaly and Intra-oral (Fibro-) Lipomatous Hamartomatosis

A syndrome comprising congenital microcephaly, polypoid (fibro-) lipomatous hamartomas of the oral mucous membranes and mild mental retardation.

H.-R.W

Main signs:
- Congenital microcephaly (head circumference of the younger child at birth 33 cm, with birth length of 51 cm; head circumference thereafter always below the third percentile, at 3 years and 6 months it was 45 cm; in her older sibling, 48 cm at 5 years) (1–5). Closure of fontanelles normal for ages.
- Congenital polypoid (fibro-) lipomatous hamartomas of the oral mucosa (multiple tumour-like whitish to yellow–brown growths, rounded to lobular, on the tip, back and edges of the tongue and on the alveolar processes; some removed shortly after birth and some later in infancy; no recurrence). In addition, long tongue, with furrow-like grooving, especially in the younger child (1, 2, 4, 5); residua on the tongue of the older girl (6).
- Slight delay of gross motor development of the older girl (walking unsupported at 18 months), considerable delay in the younger child (walking without support, still somewhat unstable, at 3 years); relatively good mental development of the younger sister and practically normal mental development of the older.

Supplementary findings: Small stature (older girl below the 10th percentile, younger below the third).

In both girls, skin dimples above the knee bilaterally (1). Bluish sclera and hyperextensible joints; muscular hypotonia.

Skin, ocular fundi, neurological examination (in the younger child including computerized tomography scan, echocardiogram, electroencephalogram), alveolar processes, dentition and hands and feet normal. Blood biochemistry, endocrinological examinations (and chromosome analysis in the younger girl) normal.

Manifestation: At birth.

Aetiology: Unknown; genetic basis probable.

Frequency: Unknown.

Course, prognosis: Apparently relatively favourable.

Comment: In the differential diagnosis, an atypical orofaciodigital syndrome type I (36) was especially considered but had to be rejected. It appears to be a 'new syndrome'.

Illustrations:
1–6 The only children to date of young, healthy non-consanguineous parents.

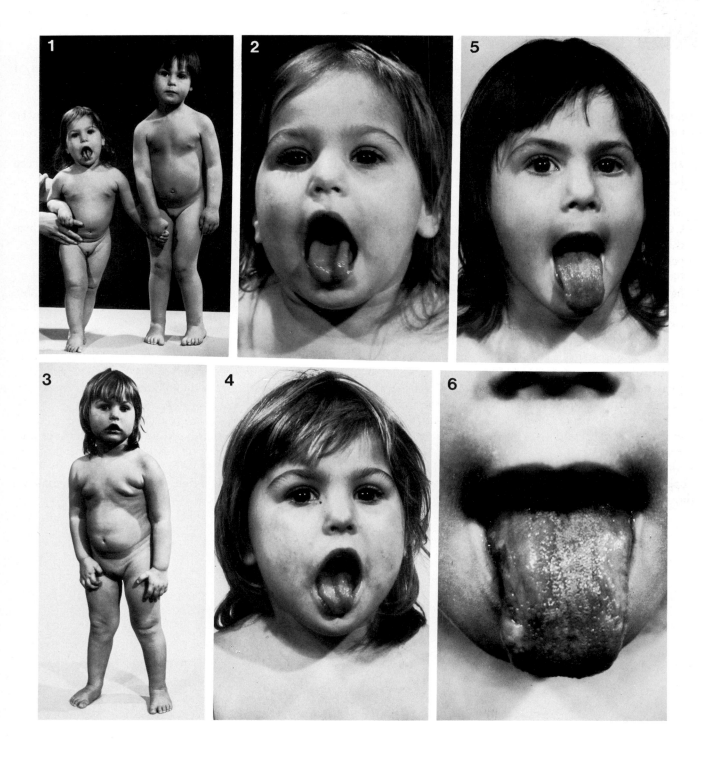

38 Cat-eye Syndrome

(Coloboma–Anal Atresia Syndrome)

H.-R.W / J.K

A syndrome comprising unusual facies, pre-auricular tags and fistulas, coloboma of the iris, anal atresia, other malformations and mental retardation.

Main signs:
- Facies characterized by hypertelorism, antimongoloid slant of the palpebral fissures, low nasal bridge (**1 and 2**). Pre-auricular tags and/or fistulas (**3 and 4**). Generally bilateral coloboma of the iris (retina, choroid) (**2**). Possible microphthalmos, glaucoma, cataract.
- Anal atresia with or without rectovaginal or rectoperineal fistula.
- Mental retardation usual but generally mild.

Supplementary findings: Various malformations of the kidneys and urinary tract. Cardiac defects. Rib anomalies, vertebral malformations, e.g. hemivertebrae, dislocation of the hip, short stature. Mild conductive hearing disorder.

Karyotype shows an extra small chromosome.

Manifestation: At birth.

Aetiology: With in-situ hybridization it could be unequivocally shown that the extra marker chromosome allows the diagnosis of partial trisomy of the long arm of chromosome 22 (22 pter -> q 11 : : q 11 -> 22 pter). Sporadic duplication; rarely the result of a balanced parental translocation.

Frequency: Low. About 60 or more patients have been described.

Prognosis: Dependent on the presence and degree of mental retardation and on the severity of heart and kidney malformations and whether they are correctable.

Differential diagnosis: There is a further 'cat-eye syndrome' with normal chromosomes, positional anomalies of the hands and feet and strikingly long thumbs.

Treatment: Operative correction of the anomalies amenable to surgical treatment and all appropriate handicap aids.

Genetic counselling for the parents.

Illustrations:

1–4 A 5 year and 6-month-old girl after surgery for anal atresia and for partial removal of pre-auricular tags. Duplication of the renal pelves and ureters on pyelography. Development only initially delayed. IQ at 3 years and 6 months: 118.

References:

Schinzel A, Schmid W, Fraccaro M *et al*: The 'Cat Eye-Syndrome':... *Hum Genet* 1981, 57:148.

Duncan A M V, Rosenfeld W *et al*: Re-evaluation of the supernumerary chromosome in an individual with cat eye syndrome. *Am J Med Genet* 1987, 27:225–227.

Kunze J, Tolksdorf M, Wiedemann H-R: Cat-eye-Syndrom. Klinische und cytogenetische Differentialdiagnose. *Humangenetik* 1975, 26:271–289.

Magenis R E, Sheekly R R *et al*: Parental origin of the extra chromosome in the cat eye syndrome: evidence from heteromorphism and in situ hybridization analysis. *Am J Med Genet* 1988, 29:9–19.

Urioste M, Visedo G *et al*: Dynamic mosaicism involving an unstable supernumerary der (22) chromosome in cat eye syndrome. *Am J Med Genet* 1994, 49:77–82.

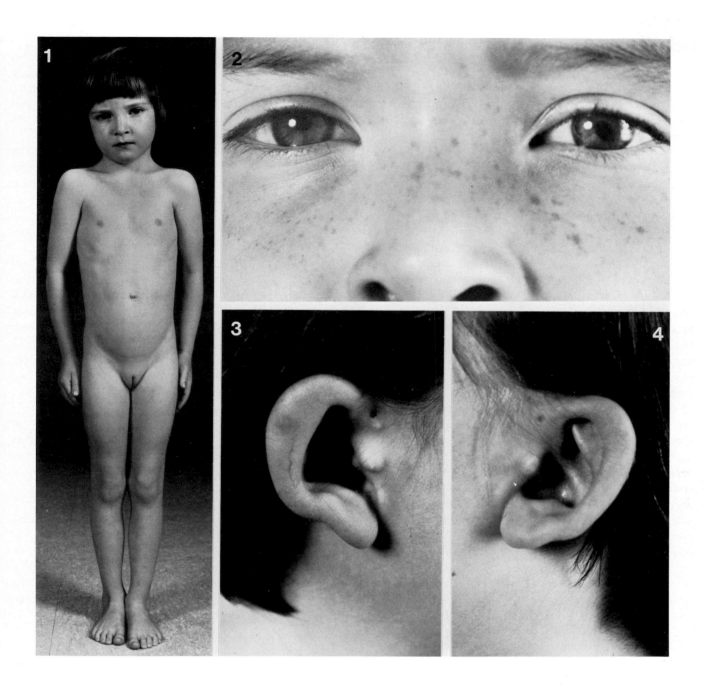

39 Pierre Robin Sequence

(Robin Sequence, Pierre Robin Anomaly, Pierre Robin Complex, Pierre Robin Syndrome, Pierre Robin Triad)

H.-R.W

A characteristic combination of hypoplasia of the lower jaw, glossoptosis and cleft palate.

Main signs:
- Usually marked, sometimes extreme, micrognathia (**1, 2, 4**). As a result, retroglossia, glossoptosis with narrowing of the airway, corresponding stridor and in some cases, signs of hypoxia.
- Cleft palate (**3**), possibly only very high palate or bifid uvula.

Supplementary findings: Bulging of the upper rib cage (**5**) as a result of obstructed respiration. Frequently, mental retardation, whether as a result of hypoxic episodes or other causes (e.g. brain anomalies).

In the literature, the Pierre Robin sequence has been described in association with malformations of a great variety of other organs. Some of these cases can be further classified: e.g. as Nager acrofacial dysostosis (*29*), Catel–Manzke syndrome (*40*), cerebrocostomandibular syndrome (*41*), trisomy 18 syndrome (*48*), oro-acral syndrome (*212*), postaxial acrofacial dysostosis (*238*), Shprintzen syndrome (*278*) - and at least 10 other clinical conditions. However, it has not, up to now, been possible to classify some of them further. For this reason and because of its heterogeneous aetiology, the Pierre Robin triad is considered as a sequence, which can occur alone or as a component of a syndrome. In every newborn with Pierre Robin complex, arthro-ophthalmopathy (Stickler syndrome, *302*) must be ruled out, especially when there is a family history of hereditary myopia, with or without retinal detachment, of cleft palate and of spondyloepiphyseal dysplasia. Examination by a qualified ophthalmologist is indicated.

Manifestation: At birth.

Aetiology: Not genetically uniform. Predominantly sporadic occurrence. No sibling cases among the patients with non-syndromic Pierre Robin sequence. The primary defect is probably the failure of the mandible to attain the proper size during the second embryonal month, so that the tongue is not brought down and forward and closure of the palate is impeded (sequence).

Frequency: Not rare.

Prognosis: For isolated Pierre Robin triad, dependent on the extent of the malformations. Danger of suffocation and of hypoxic brain damage. After survival of the first 2 months of life, prognosis good as a result of development of the mandible (**4 and 5** the same child aged 6 weeks and then 18 months). In a 10-year prospective study of 55 patients, 26% died within the first 3 months of life. Over one-half of the patients presented audiometric anomalies; 13% had delayed speech development.

Treatment: Nurse prone, glossopexy, procedures to extend the lower jaw; tracheostomy should be reserved as a last resort. Tube feeding, possibly gastrostomy.
Surgery for cleft palate.

Illustrations:
1–3 A 4-week-old infant. Frequent asphyxial episodes. Aspiration pneumonia. Treated by nursing prone and tube feeding.
4 and 5 A patient aged 6 weeks and then 18 months. Dyspnoea, stridor, frequent episodes of asphyxia in the first 3 weeks of life. Treatment by nursing prone and tube feeding. Note development of the mandible.

References:

Grimm G, Pfefferkorn A, Taatz H: Die klinische Bedeutung des Pierre–Robin Syndroms und seine Behandlung. *Dtsch Zahn- Mund- und Kieferheilk* 1964, 43:169.
Opitz J M: Familial anomalies in the Pierre–Robin syndrome. *Birth Defects Orig Art Ser* 1969, 5:119.
Cohen M M Jr: The Robin anomaly — its nonspecifity and associated syndromes. *J Oral Surg* 1976, 34:587.
Williams A J, Williams M A, Walker C A *et al*: The Robin anomalad (Pierre Robin syndrome) — a follow up study. *Arch Dis Child* 1981, 56:663.
Carey J C, Fineman R M *et al*: The Robin sequence... *J Pediatr* 1982, 101:858–864.
Heaf D R, Helms P J, Dinwiddie R *et al*: Nasopharyngeal airways in Pierre Robin syndrome. *J Pediatr* 1982, 100:698.
Couly G: Les formes graves néo-natales du syndrome de Pierre Robin. *Arch Fr Pédiatr* 1984, 41:591–594.
Cozzi F, Pierro A: Glossoptosis-apnea syndrome. *Pediatr* 1985, 75:836–843.
Sheffield L J, Reiss J A *et al*: A genetic follow-up study of 64 patients with the Pierre Robin complex. *Am J Med Genet* 1987, 28:25–36.
Couly G, Cheron G *et al*: Le syndrome de Pierre Robin. *Arch Fr Pédiatr* 1988, 45:553–559.
Bull D J, Givan D C, Sadove A *et al*: Improved outcome in Pierre Robin sequence: effect of multidisciplinary evaluation and management. *Pediatr* 1990, 86:294–301.
Chitayat D, Meunier C M, Hodkinson K A, Azouz M E: Robin sequence with facial and digital anomalies in two halfbrothers by the same mother. *Am J Med Genet* 1991, 40:167–172.
Menko F H, Madan K, Baart J A, Beukenhorst H L: Robin sequence and a deficiency of the left forearm in a girl with a deletion of chromosome 4q33-qter. *Am J Med Genet* 1992, 44:696–698.

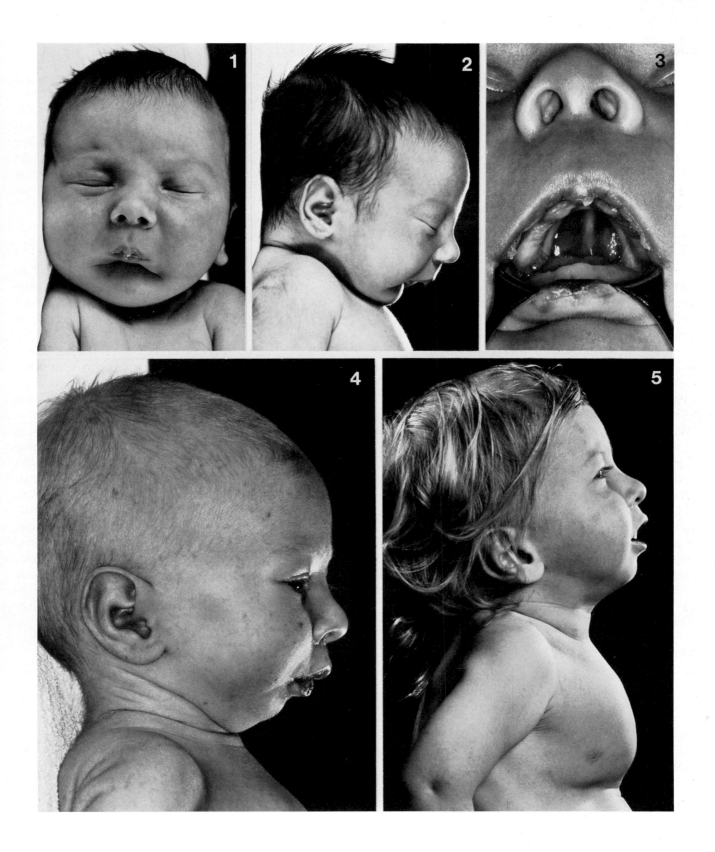

40 Catel–Manzke Syndrome
(Pierre Robin Complex with Accessory Metacarpal of the Index Finger)

H.-R.W

A characteristic combination of the Pierre Robin Complex with a peculiar finger malformation.

Main signs:
- The more or less completely expressed Pierre Robin complex (mandibular hypoplasia, retroglossia, cleft palate); this holds true for all of the patients described to date (18 out of 18) (**1**).
- Positional anomalies of both index fingers, due to a radiologically demonstrable accessory ossicle (rudimentary phalanx, rudimentary metacarpal) between the, sometimes shortened, second metacarpal and the proximal phalanx (16 out of 18 and 17 out of 18, respectively). Usually, radial deviation of the index fingers at the metacarpophalangeal joint and possible ulnar deviation at the first interphalangeal joint (**2–4**).
- Clinodactyly of the little finger (nine out of 18) and in some cases of the other fingers also: possible camptodactyly.
- Congenital cardiac anomalies (eight out of 18; atrial septal defect, ventricular septal defect and others).

Supplementary findings: Possible club feet or other congenital malformations of the feet, small stature, dislocatable knees or other joints.

Manifestation: At birth.

Aetiology: Not established. Sex ratio, to date, 13 male: three female (in two patients the sex was not given). Several sibling cases and striking family histories. Genetic syndrome of very variable expression.

Frequency: To date, 18 patients are known from the literature.

Course, prognosis: Dependent on the severity of the Pierre Robin complex and how prompt and effective its treatment is additionally, on the type, severity and treatment of possible cardiac defects.

Diagnosis: Not difficult in typical patients

Treatment: As in isolated Pierre Robin complex. In addition, care for the cardiac and other anomalies when present. Early consultation with an experienced hand surgeon.

Illustrations:
1 A case of Catel–Manzke syndrome, a boy, at age 6 weeks: hypoplasia of the mandible (with microglossia, glossoptosis and a widely cleft palate); dyspnoea on inspiration and expiration, secondary to the glossoptosis, distended barrel-shaped thorax.
2–4 X-rays of the hands of the proband at 6 weeks, 6 years and 6 months and then 26 years. Accessory bone (metacarpal?) between the second metacarpal and the proximal phalanx of the index finger bilaterally. Eventual fusion of the accessory part with the proximal phalanx and, on the left side, also with the second metacarpal. Radial deviation of both index fingers. Slight brachymesophalangy and clinodactyly of the fifth fingers. No consanguinity of the proband's parents; several cases of mandibular hypoplasia without further abnormalities in the mother's family.

References:

Manzke H: Symmetrische Hyperphalangie des zweiten Fingers durch ein akzessorisches Metacarpale. *Fortschr Röntgenstr* 1966, **105**:425–427.

Sundaram V, Taysi K, Hartmann A F Jr *et al*: Hyperphalangy and clinodactyly of the index finger with Pierre Robin anomaly: Catel–Manzke syndrome... *Clin Genet* 1982, **21**:407–410.

Brude E: Pierre Robin sequence and hyperphalangy — a genetic entity (Catel–Manzke syndrome). *Eur J Pediatr* 1984, **142**:222–223.

Dignan P St J, Martin L W, Zenni E J Jr: Pierre Robin anomaly with an accessory metacarpal of the index fingers. The Catel–Manzke syndrome. *Clin Genet* 1986, **29**:168–173.

Thompson E M, Winter R M, Williams M J H: A male infant with the Catel–Manzke syndrome and dislocatable knees. *J Med Genet* 1986, **23**:271–274.

Skinner S A, Flannery D B *et al*: Catel–Manzke syndrome. *Proc Greenwood Genet Ctr* 1989, 8:60–63.

Bernd L, Martini A K *et al*: Das Catel–Manzke-Syndrom. *Klin Pädiatr* 1990, **202**:60–63.

Wilson G N, King T E *et al*: Index finger hyperphalangy and multiple anomalies: Catel–Manzke syndrome? *Am J Med Genet* 1993, **46**:176–179.

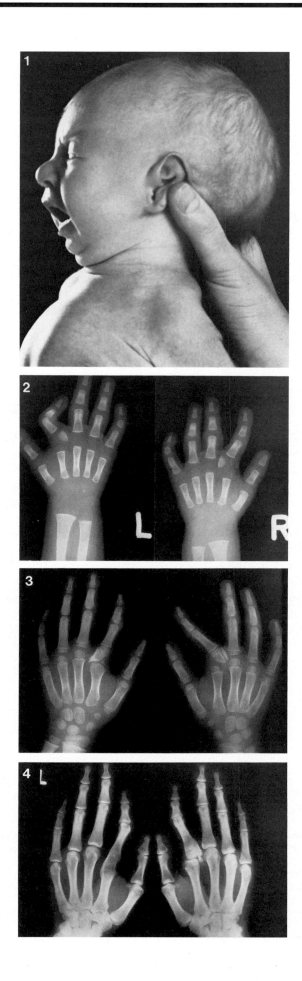

41 (Cerebro-)costo-mandibular Syndrome
(Smith–Theiler–Schachenmann Syndrome; Rib gap Syndrome)

H.-R.W

P. Meinecke

A syndrome of Pierre Robin sequence (micrognathia–glossoptosis–cleft palate), with multiple dorsal rib defects and, occasionally, microcephaly and mental retardation.

Main signs:
- Dorsal rib defects (frequently absence of the 12th rib) and possible vertebral anomalies; the former most frequently of the fifth and sixth ribs and usually symmetrical.
- Pierre Robin sequence, with the mandibular defect being the most constant.
- Microcephaly (or microbrachycephaly) in at least one-third of patients. Mental retardation in approximately one-third of the surviving patients; functional central nervous system disorders also relatively frequent.

Supplementary findings: Hydrocephalus, porencephaly, spina bifida cystica and other anomalies of the central nervous system may occur.

Short neck with nuchal skin fold and Sprengel's deformity in some patients. Possible development of scoliosis.

Occasionally, hearing defects.

Polyhydramnios in some patients.

Manifestation: At birth and subsequently.

Aetiology: A monogenic disorder with variable penetrance and expression can be assumed. As there is evidence for autosomal recessive as well as for autosomal dominant transmission, heterogeneity is likely. (Mild signs of the disorder, including those on chest radiograph, should be sought in members of the proband's immediate family).

Frequency: Low. About 45 patients known to date.

Course, prognosis: Only approximately one-half of the patients observed to date have survived the initial respiratory, feeding and associated problems and, of these, approximately one-half have had diverse central nervous system disorders. The latter can, in some cases, be regarded as resulting from early postnatal hypoxic damage.

Treatment: Initially, that of the Pierre Robin complex (39) or respiratory insufficiency. Later, any appropriate handicap aids.

Genetic counselling. Prenatal diagnosis by ultrasound or radiograph in some cases.

Illustrations:

1–6 A patient, the second child of healthy, young non-consanguineous parents (after a healthy boy).

1 and 2 Microretrognathia with the complete Pierre Robin sequence.

5 The multiple rib defects neonatally.

3 and 4 The bell-shaped deformity of the thorax and the persistent micrognathia of the now 2- and 10-year-old boy, with impaired hearing but completely normal psychomotor development.

6 Marked narrowing of the upper thorax; some of the earlier rib defects have been bridged by bone. At age 10 years, the chest circumference of the proband, who exhibits remarkable physical prowess (at tennis), differs by only 3 cm between maximum inhalation and exhalation (50:47 cm). Nearly all lung-function parameters lie between 45 and 50%. Height (134 cm) and head circumference (52 cm) correspond to approximately -1 SD.

The father of the proband shows mild micrognathia and a high narrow palate.

References:

McNicholl B, Egan-Mitchell B, Murray J P et al: Cerebro-costo-mandibular syndrome... *Arch Dis Child* 1970, **45**:421–424.

Williams H J et al: Cerebro-costo-mandibular syndrome: long term follow-up of a patient and review of the literature. *Am J Roentgenol* 1976, **126**:1223–1228.

Silverman F N et al: Cerebro-costo-mandibular syndrome. *J Pediatr* 1980, **97**:406–416.

Hennekam R C M, Beemer F A, Hujbers P A et al: The cerebro-costo-mandibular syndrome: third report of familial occurence. *Clin Genet* 1985, **28**:118–121.

Smith K G, Sekar K C: Cerebrocostomandibular syndrome. *Clin Pediatr* 1985, **24**:223–225.

Trautman M S, Schelley S L, Stevenson D K et al: Cerebro-costo-mandibular syndrome: a familial case consistent with autosomal recessive inheritance. *J Pediatr* 1985, **107**:990–991.

Meinecke P, Wolff G, Schaefer E: Cerebro-costo-mandibular syndrome ohne cerebrale Beteiligung bei einem 4jährigen Jungen. *Mschr Kinderheilk* 1987, **135**:54–58.

Merlob P, Schonfeld A, Grunebaum M et al: Autosomal dominant cerebro-costo-mandibular syndrome: ultrasonic and clinical findings. *Am J Med Genet* 1987, **26**:195–202.

Drossou-Agakidou V et al: Cerebrocostomandibular syndrome in four sibs, two pairs of twins. *J Med Genet* 1991, **28**:704–707.

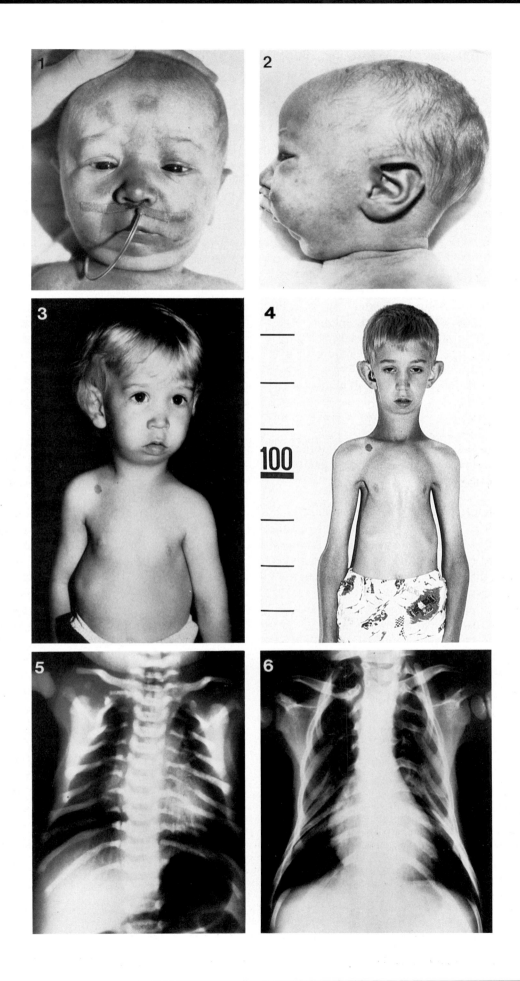

42 Fraser Syndrome
(Cryptophthalmos–Syndactyly Syndrome, Cryptophthalmos Syndrome)

H.-R.W

Syndrome of absence of the palpebral fissure(s), usually with partial or complete absence of eyelids and eyebrows and with defects of the eyes, especially the anterior segment, combined with anomalies of the ears, nose, limbs, urogenital system and other areas.

Main signs:
- Bilateral or unilateral absence of the palpebral fissure (the normal lid structure is replaced by a skin-fold covering that originates from the forehead), with defects of the lids and eyebrows and anomalies of the eyes (defects of the anterior segment; microphthalmia, anophthalmia). Projections of scalp hair extending from the low-lying temples to the lateral eyebrow region (1–4, 6). Cryptophthalmos is not an obligatory feature (10).
- Broad nasal bridge, hypoplasia and notching of alae nasi (1–4, 6, 10).
- Variable dysplasia of the external (possibly also of the inner and middle) ears (2, 3, 6).
- Partial cutaneous syndactyly and more extensive anomalies of the limbs (7–9, 11).
- Bilateral or unilateral agenesis or hypoplasia of the kidneys; genital malformations (hypospadias, vaginal atresia, pseudohermaphroditism) (5).

Supplementary findings: Possible anomalies of the cranial vault, encephalocoele or other malformations of the brain, facial clefts (10), stenosis or atresia in the laryngeal region, anal atresia, malformations of the heart and/or lungs, anomalies of the urinary tract. Frequent occurrence of mental retardation.

Manifestation: At birth.

Aetiology: Autosomal recessive disorder with variable expression; this mode of inheritance can be regarded as certain when ultrasound (or autopsy) shows aplasia or hypoplasia of the kidneys. (Isolated cryptophthalmos does not signify Fraser syndrome and may follow autosomal dominant transmission).

Frequency: Low. Approximately 130 observations in the literature.

Course, prognosis: With cryptophthalmos, dubious to poor with regard to sight. Otherwise dependent on the type and severity of associated defects.

Diagnosis: Cryptophthalmos, anomalies of the ears and nose, syndactyly and urogenital anomalies are the cardinal features; when cryptophthalmos is not present, the spectrum of the other signs should suggest the true diagnosis. It is important to rule out renal anomalies.

Treatment: Rehabilitation and cosmetic surgery if possible. Genetic counselling. Prenatal diagnosis (ultrasound, foetoscopy).

Illustrations:

1, 2, 4–9 A newborn, the third child of healthy parents after two healthy children. The eyeballs are readily palpable bilaterally; median notch of the nose; syndactyly of the hands and feet with hypoplasia of the distal phalanges; ambiguous external genitalia (normal female karyotype); malformations of internal organs.
3 A 10-year-old girl, the second child of consanguineous parents (two healthy siblings). Small eyeball palpable on the left; mixed hearing loss and stenosis of the auditory canal bilaterally; partial cutaneous syndactyly of the hands and feet; vaginal atresia.
10 and 11 A newborn girl who died shortly after birth, the first child of healthy parents. Fraser syndrome without cryptophthalmos.

References:
Burn J, Marwood R P: Fraser syndrome presenting as bilateral renal agenesis in three sibs. *J Med Genet* 1982, 19:360–361.
Lurie J W, Cherstvoy E D: Renal agenesis as a diagnostic feature of the cryptophthalmos–syndactyly syndrome. *Clin Genet* 1984, 25:528–532.
Mortimer G, McEwan H P, Ytes J R W: Fraser syndrome presenting as monozygotic twins with bilateral renal agenesis. *J Med Genet* 1985, 22:76–78.
Koenig R, Spranger J: Crytophthalmos–syndactyly syndrome without cryptophthalmos. *Clin Genet* 1986, 29:413–416.
Thomas I T, Frias J L, Felix V et al: Isolated and syndromic cryptophthalmos. Am. *J Med Genet* 1986, 25:85–98.
Gattuso J, Patton M A, Baraitser M: The clinical spectrum of the Fraser syndrome... *J Med Genet* 1987, 24:549–555.
Bialer M G, Wilson W G: Syndromic cryptophthalmos. *Am J Med Genet* 1988, 30:385–387.
Boyd P A, Keeling J W et al: Fraser syndrome... *Am J Med Genet* 1988, 31:159–168.
Francannet C et al: Fraser syndrome with renal agenesis... *Am J Med Genet* 1990, 36:477–479.
Ramsing M et al: Fraser syndrome... in the fetus and newborn. *Clin Genet* 1990, 37:84–96.
Schauer G et al: Prenatal diagnosis of Fraser syndrome... *Am J Med Genet* 1990, 37:583–591.
Stevens C A, McClanahan C et al: Pulmonary hyperplasia in the Fraser cryptophthalmos syndrome. *Am J Med Genet* 1994, 52:427–431.

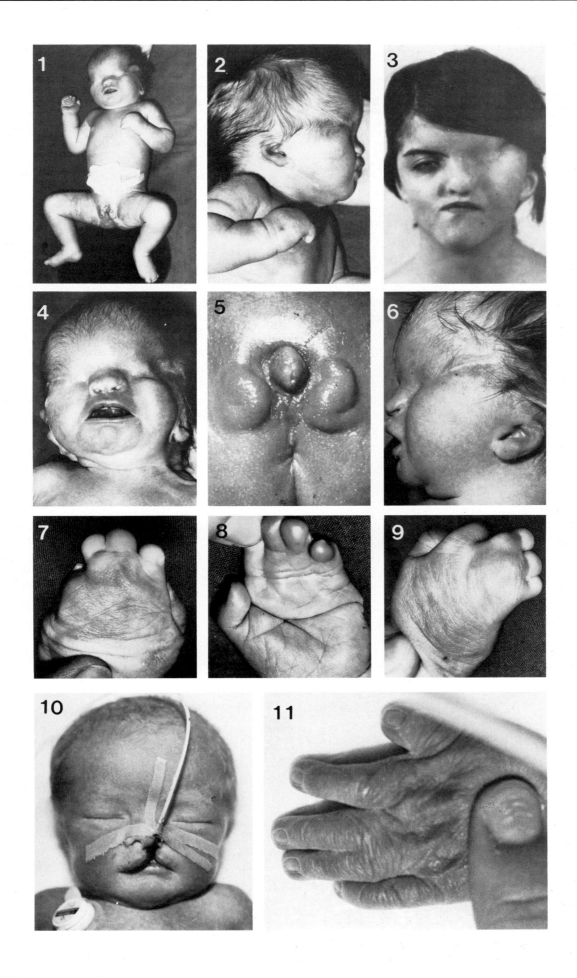

43 'Potter Syndrome'

An aetiologically heterogeneous but clinically, essentially uniform, sequence.

H.-R.W

The term 'Potter syndrome' (oligohydramnios sequence) refers to the effect of prolonged amniotic fluid deficiency on the foetus, with hypoplasia of the lungs, facial dysmorphism and skeletal changes, usually of renal origin. The degree to which the various features are expressed depends mainly on the degree and duration of the oligohydramnios or anhydramnios.

The renal causes include bilateral agenesis of the kidneys and the various different forms of polycystic kidney disease (see table). Also caused by the same pathogenesis: various combinations of renal agenesis; renal dysplasia (polycystic kidneys Potter type II); the end-result of early acting obstructive processes (polycystic kidneys Potter type IV); as a later manifestation, hydronephrosis of different origins.

In a proportion of patients, the kidney changes occur as a part of one of numerous syndromes (e.g. cerebro-oculo-facio-skeletal syndrome (320), Fraser syndrome (42), caudal dysplasia syndrome (168), Meckel syndrome (45), branchio-oto-renal syndrome, prune belly syndrome (165), VATER association (311) and chromosome disorders).

Main signs:
Hypoplasia of the lungs, 'Potter' facies: hypertelorism, prominent skin folds originating from the inner corner of the eye, retrognathia, large dysplastic low-set ears with deficient cartilage formation. Additional malformations in more than 50% of patients: vertebral anomalies, club feet, joint contractures of variable severity, large hands and caudal regression anomalies including sirenomelia.

Supplementary findings: Gonadal dysgenesis, pseudohermaphroditism, anorectal malformations, tracheo-oesophageal malformations (often within the spectrum of the VATER association), cardiovascular malformations.

Manifestation: The Potter phenotype in its various forms is always evident at birth; evidence of the underlying disorder may appear later in the less severe forms.

Frequency: Approximately one out of 3000. The various underlying disorders are much less frequent individually (see table).

Characteristics of the most important forms of polycystic kidney disease which may also lead to Potter phenotype

	Autosomal recessive form (Potter type I)	Autosomal dominant form (Potter type III)	Dysplasia (Potter type II)
Frequency	c. 1:6000 to 1:40 000	c. 1:1000	All forms c. 1:1000
Pathology of the kidneys:			
Shape	Kidney shape retained	Kidney shape retained.	Usually loss of kidney shape.
Size	Enlarged; initially normal size.	Enlarged; initially normal size.	Both enlarged and hypoplastic
Symmetry	Symmetrical	Symmetrical; initially, may be asymmetrical for years.	Often asymmetrical.
Localization of cysts	Collecting tube.	Cysts in all parts of the nephron and collecting tube.	Usually complete loss of the kidney structure; classification often not possible.
Further malformations of the urogenital tract	None.	None.	Additional malformations frequent; usually obstruction.
Liver changes	Congenital fibrosis of the liver a constant feature.	In about one-third of adult cases.	None.
Additional signs	Pancreatic cysts (rare).	Aneurysms of the base of the brain.	Very frequently various malformations.
Main signs	Neonatal period: respiratory insufficiency. With increasing age of survival, renal insufficiency and portal hypertension.	Onset in the third to fifth decades of life, or during childhood; in rare cases in infancy with respiratory problems; renal insufficiency, pain, organomegaly, hypertension, hematuria, urinary tract infections.	Variable: either no signs (unilateral), or Potter sequence. Frequently signs due to additional malformations.
Frequency of the Potter sequence	Low.	Very low.	High.
Inheritance	Autosomal recessive.	Autosomal dominant.	Heterogeneous; multifactorial inheritance; empirical risk of recurrence usually low.

K. Zerres
H.-R.W

Course, prognosis: Fully expressed signs occur when the amniotic fluid deficiency has been marked and prolonged and the prognosis is usually unfavourable. In the less severe forms, the prognosis may occasionally be more favourable, depending on the underlying disorder.

Differential diagnosis: Exclusion of chronic hydrorrhoea gravidarum and diagnosis of the underlying disorder (ultrasound examination of the parents) should be carried out in every case.

Treatment: As a rule, none possible; with less prolonged obstructive processes, operative correction may help preserve (remaining) renal function.

Illustrations:

1 A child with 'classic Potter syndrome': Potter facies, malformations of the hands, genital anomalies.

2a and b Amnion nodosum (plain and enlarged views).

References:

Curry C J R, Jenson K *et al*: The Potter sequence: a clinical analysis of 80 cases. *Am J Med Genet* 1984, **19**:679–702.

Cerebro-oculofacio-skeletal syndrome: Preus M, Kaplan P, Kirkham T H: Renal anomalies and oligohydramnios in the cerebro-oculofacio-skeletal syndrome. *Am J Dis Child* 1977, **131**:62–64.

Meckel syndrome: Fraser F C, Lytwyn A: Spectrum of anomalies in the Meckel syndrome, or: 'maybe there is a malformation syndrome with at least one constant anomaly'. *Am J Med Genet* 1981, **9**:67–73.

Fraser–Cryptophthalmus syndrome: Lurie I W, Cherstvoy E D: Renal agenesis as a diagnostic feature of the cryptophthalmos-syndactyly syndrome. *Clin Genet* 1984, **25**:528–532.

Branchio-oto-renal syndrome: Melnick M, Bixler, D *et al*: Familial branchio-oto-renal dysplasia: a new addition to the branchial arch syndromes. *Clin Genet* 1976, **9**:25–34.

Caudal dysplasia syndrome: Bearn J G: The association of sirenomelia with Potter's syndrome. *Arch Dis Child* 1960, **35**:254–258.

Prune-belly syndrome: Wigger H J, Blanc W A: The prune belly syndrome. *Pathol Ann* 1977, **12**:17–39.

VATER association: Quan L, Smith D W: The VATER association. *J Pediatr* 1973, **82**:104–107.

Zerres K: Genetics of cystic kidney diseases. Criteria for classification and genetic counseling. *Pediatr Nephrol* 1987, **1**:397–404.

Zerres K, Rudnik-Schöneborn S *et al*: Zystennieren im Kindesalter. der kinderarzt 1993, **24**:922–935 (1993).

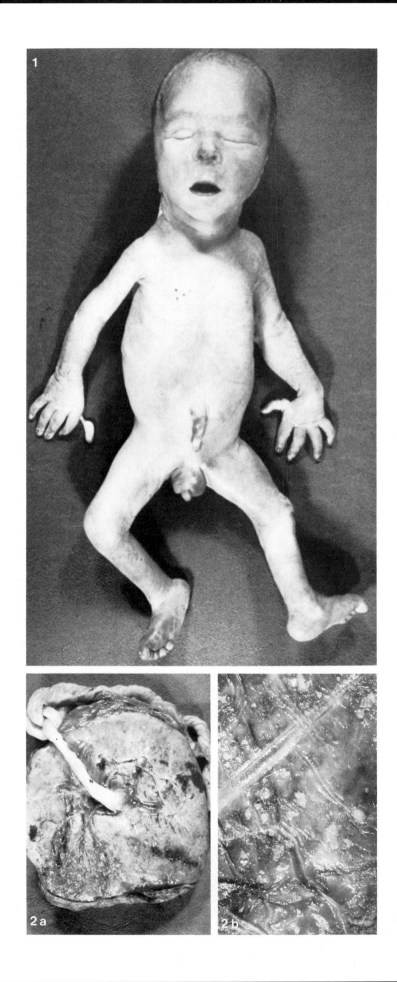

J.K.

A characteristic malformation syndrome (sequence) with fused lower extremities, external and dorsal rotation of these symmelian extremities, dorsally located patellae and ventrally located popliteal fossae, absent external genitalia, anal atresia, renal anomalies and hypoplasia of the lungs.

Main signs:
- Fusion of the lower extremities with absence of one or both feet. The legs and feet are often rotated, with the extensors and flexors reversed in the lower extremities, so that the patellae are dorsal and the popliteal fossae ventral.
- Absence of the external genitalia, imperforate anus, absent rectum.
- Vertebral anomalies, sacral agenesis, pelvic malformations (caudal regression syndrome).
- Renal agenesis (oligohydramnios) or cystic renal dysplasia; horseshoe kidneys; hypoplasia or aplasia of the ureter, urinary bladder and urethra. Asplenia. Single umbilical artery.
- Pulmonary hypoplasia. Cardiac defects, tracheo-oesophageal fistula.
- Potter facies: low-set large dysplastic ears; flattened nose; receding chin; old-appearing, wrinkled face.

Supplementary findings: Intra-uterine growth retardation. External genitalia sometimes represented by small skin tags.
Medial position and malformations of the fibulae. Occasionally, phocomelia of the upper extremities unilaterally or bilaterally. Anomalies of the radius, club hand (talipomanus), absent or extra fingers, syndactyly.

Manifestation: At birth. Should be suspected in pregnancies with oligohydramnios; diagnosis by ultrasound.

Aetiology: Primary defect of the caudal axis skeleton during the third embryonal week. Damage to the primitive streak. Possible exogenous factors. One hundred times more frequent with uniovular twins than with single births. Ratio of males to females is 2.7:1.

Frequency: Low. Approximately one out of 60 000 births. To date, over 300 classic patients reported.

Course, prognosis: Stillbirth or death within a few hours *post partum* (bilateral renal agenesis, pulmonary hypoplasia). In one case, the infant lived for 63 h.

Differential diagnosis: With atypical cases, a smooth transition to VACTERL syndrome (Vertebral anomalies, Anal atresia, Cardiac anomalies, Tracheo-Esophageal fistulas, Radial deformities, Lung hypoplasia) (*312*) of varied aetiology.
Caudal dysplasia syndrome (*168*) and in children of diabetic mothers (*299*), rarely autosomal dominant.

Treatment: No therapeutic efforts known to date can ensure survival. Prenatal diagnosis with ultrasound in women with oligohydramnios and intra-uterine growth retardation.

Illustrations:
1a–d A prematurely born (33rd week) male infant (46 XY) who lived for 2 h: Potter facies, large dysplastic ears lying close to the head, with the upper edge folded in; fused lower extremities in external and dorsal rotation (patellae dorsal, popliteal fossae ventral); dorsolaterally lying dysplastic fibulae with sharp lateral tapering of the bone (1d). Absence of external genitalia in the expected location; para-anal 2 cm-long skin tag corresponded histologically to a primitive penis.
2a–c The first born of male twins (brother free of external malformations); survival for 30 min. Potter facies; fusion of the lower extremities even more extensive than in 1.

References:
Smith D W, Barlett C, Harrah L M: Monozygotic twinning and the Duhamel anomalad (imperforate anus to sirenomelia): a non-random association between two aberrations in morphogenesis. *Birth Defects Orig Art Ser* 1976, Vol XII, 5:53–63.
Temtamy S, McKusick V: The genetics of hand malformations. *Birth Defects Orig Art Ser* 1978, Vol XIV, 3:181–184.
Stevenson R E, Jones K L, Phelan M C: Vascular steal: The pathogenetic mechanism producing sirenomelia and associated defects of the viscera and soft tissues. *Pediatrics* 1986, 78:451–457.
Duncan P A, Shapiro L R: Sirenomelia and VATER association... Dysmorphol. *Clin Genet* 1989, 2:96.
Rodriguez J I, Palacios J, Razquin S: Sirenomalia and anencephaly. *Am J Med Genet* 1991, 39:25–27.

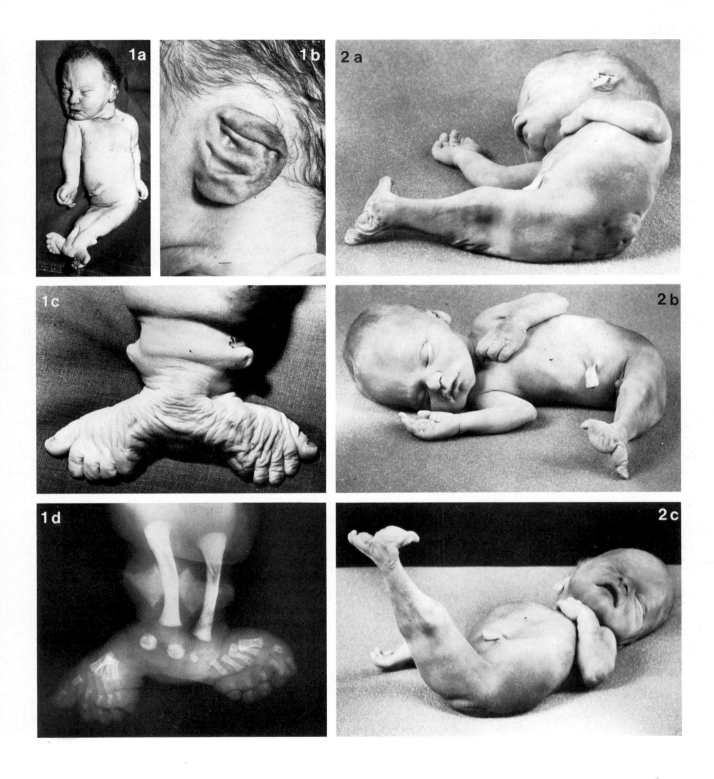

45 Meckel–Gruber Syndrome

(Dysencephalia Splanchnocystica, Gruber Syndrome)

J.K.

An autosomal recessive syndrome with encephalocoele, postaxial hexadactyly and cystic changes of the kidney.

Main signs:
- Encephalocoele; microcephaly, anencephaly.
- Postaxial hexadactyly of the hands and feet.
- Cystic dysplasia of the kidneys and fibrotic and/or cystic changes of the liver.
- Anomalies of the urinary tract (absent renal pelvis, hypoplasia or aplasia of the ureters).
- Oligohydramnios.

Supplementary findings: Facial dysmorphisms; cleft palate, cleft lip; microphthalmia or anophthalmia, hypertelorism; broad, round face with full cheeks, full lips; macrostomia; anomalies of the tongue; narrow chin. Low-set ears. Short neck.

Cardiac defects. Internal and/or external genital anomalies.

Normal pregnancy, oligohydramnios, stillbirth or short survival.

Manifestation: At birth; prenatal diagnosis possible from the 18th week of pregnancy, with modern diagnostic methods (ultrasound). High alpha foetoprotein.

Aetiology: Autosomal recessive defect.

Frequency: Great Britain one out of 140 000; Ashkenazi Jews one out of 50 000; Finland one out of 8500; Massachusetts one out of 13 250; Belgium one out of 3000; Gujarati Indians one out of 1300.

Course, prognosis: Approximately one-third are stillborn; two-thirds of the infants survive for a maximum of 2 h 30 min. Isolated reports of longer survival: 5 months, 8 months, 13 months, 28 months, 3 years, 4 years.

Differential diagnosis: The variability of the Meckel–Gruber syndrome means that the following syndromes should be considered: Potter sequence (43), trisomy 13 (47), hydrolethalus syndrome (323), Smith–Lemli–Opitz syndrome (281).

Treatment: Not relevant; genetic counselling.

Illustrations:
1–4 A newborn male infant: encephalocoele; postaxial hexadactyly of the hands and feet; polycystic kidneys.

References:

Fraser F C, Lytwyn A: Spectrum of anomalies in the Meckel syndrome, or: 'maybe there is a malformation syndrome with at least one constant anomaly'. *Am J Med Genet* 1981, **9**:67–73.
Seller M J: Phenotypic variation in Meckel syndrome. *Clin Genet* 1981, **20**:74–77.
Rehder H, Labbé: Prenatal morphology in Meckel's syndrome. *Prenat Diagn* 1981, **1**:161–172.
Anderson V M: Meckel syndrome: morphologic consideration. *Birth Defects Orig Art Ser*, 1982, Vol **18**, 3B:145–160.
Lowry R B L, Hill R H, Tischler B: Survival and spectrum of anomalies in the Meckel syndrome. *Am J Med Genet* 1983, **14**:417–421.
The Meckel Symposium: *Am J Med Genet* 1984, **18**:559–711.
Young ID, Rickett A B, Clarke D M: High incidence of Meckel syndrome in Gujarati Indians. *J Med Genet* 1985, **22**:301–304.
Shen-Schwarz S, Dave H: Meckel syndrome... review of the literature. *Am J Med Genet* 1988, **31**:349–355.
Pachi A, Giancotti A, Torcia F *et al*: Meckel–Gruber syndrome: ultrasonic diagnosis at 13 weeks... *Prenat Diagn* 1989, **9**:187.
Walpole I R, Goldblatt J, Hockey A, Knowles S: Dandy–Walker malformation (variant), cystic dysplastic kidneys, and hepatic fibrosis: a distinct entity or Meckel syndrome? *Am J Med Genet* 1991, **39**:294–298.

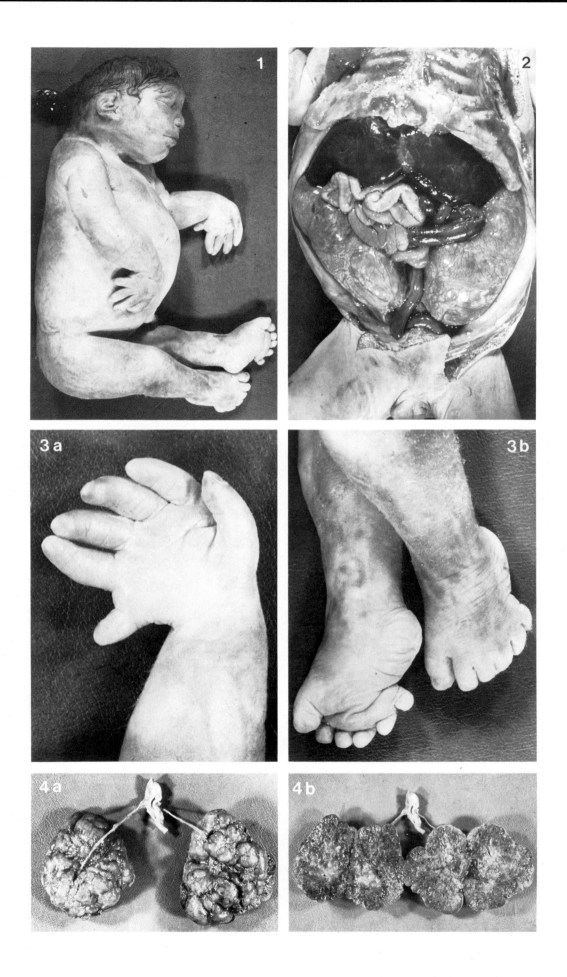

46 Lissencephaly Type 1
(formerly also known as Miller–Dieker Syndrome)

J.K.

A characteristic syndrome with microcephaly, bitemporal depressions, long philtrum and thin upper lip, mild micrognathia, unusual dysplasia of the ears, anteverted nostrils and lissencephaly (agyria).

Main signs:
- Microcephaly, high forehead, prominent occiput.
- Bitemporal depressions of the skull (due to failure of the frontal and temporal lobes to develop properly).
- Long philtrum with thin upper lip.
- Lissencephaly (CT), lissencephaly type I = agyria and/or pachygyria, thick cortex, absent/minimal hydrocephalus. Enlarged ventricles.

Supplementary findings: Polyhydramnios, reduced foetal movements. Low Apgar score, protracted jaundice, small for dates. Mild micrognathia, dysplastic ears, broad nasal bridge, anteverted nostrils, cardiac defects, cryptorchidism, corneal clouding, supernumerary fingers, clino-, camptodactyly, seizures, abnormal muscle tone, severe mental retardation. Postnatal growth retardation.

Manifestation: At birth.

Aetiology: Chromosome 17 disorder in most cases, usually loss of part of the short arm, but ring chromosome 17 and translocation of chromosome 17 also possible. Autosomal recessive inheritance of the Norman–Roberts syndrome (lissencephaly, slanting forehead, hypertelorism, broad prominent nasal bridge, muscular hypertonia, hyper-reflexia, severe mental retardation).

Frequency: Low: up to 20 published cases.

Course, prognosis: Severe mental retardation, seizures, poor growth. Approximately 50% of the children die before 6 months of age, the others in early childhood.

Differential diagnosis: Lissencephaly types I and II are also observed in a few very rare syndromes (Stratton *et al*, Dobyns *et al*), e.g. Walker–Warburg syndrome (*314*), Norman–Roberts syndrome.

Treatment: Symptomatic. Genetic counselling: with de-novo chromosome mutation (high resolution banding) no increased risk of recurrence; with familial translocation, prenatal diagnosis; in the absence of chromosomal abnormality, 25% risk of recurrence.

Illustrations:
1a A 24-day-old girl with bilateral parietal depressions, high forehead, antimongoloid slant of the palpebral fissures, seizures.
1b Micrognathia, long prominent philtrum, anteverted nostrils, dysplastic rotated ears.
2 Cranial computer tomography: lissencephaly (agyria), enlargement of the lateral ventricles.

References:
Jones K L, Gilbert E F, Kaveggia E G *et al*: The Miller–Dieker syndrome. *Pediatrics* 1980, 66:277–281.
Dobyns W B, Stratton R F, Parke J T *et al*: Miller–Dieker syndrome: lissencephaly and monosomy 17p. *J Pediatr* 1983, 102:552–558.
Stratton R F, Dobyns W B, Airhart S D *et al*: New chromosomal syndrome: Miller–Dieker syndrome and monosomy 17p13. *Hum Genet* 1984, 67:193–200.
Dobyns W B, Stratton R F, Greenberg F: Syndrome with lissencephaly. I: Miller–Dieker and Norman–Roberts syndromes and isolated lissencephaly. *Am J Med Genet* 1984, 18:509–526.
Dobyns W B, Kirkpatrick J B, Hittner H M: Syndromes with lissencephaly. II: Walker–Warburg and cerebro-oculo-muscular syndromes and a new syndrome with type II lissencephaly. *Am J Med Genet* 1985, 22:157–195.
Dobyns W B, Gilbert E F, Opitz J M: Further comments on the lissencephaly syndromes. *Am J Med Genet* 1985, 22:197–211.
Kotagal P, Cruse R P, Estes M: Norman–Roberts syndrome. *Am J Med Genet* 1988, 29:681–683.
Mielke R, Lu J H *et al*: Lissencephaly (Letter to the Editor). *Eur J Pediatr* 1988, 147:487.
Warburg M, Prause J K: Reply to the letter. *Eur J Pediatr* 1988, 147:487–488.
Janetti P, Schwartz C E, Dietz-Band J, Light E, Timmermann J, Chessa L: Norman–Roberts syndrome: clinical and molecular studies. *Am J Med Genet* 1993, 47:95–99.

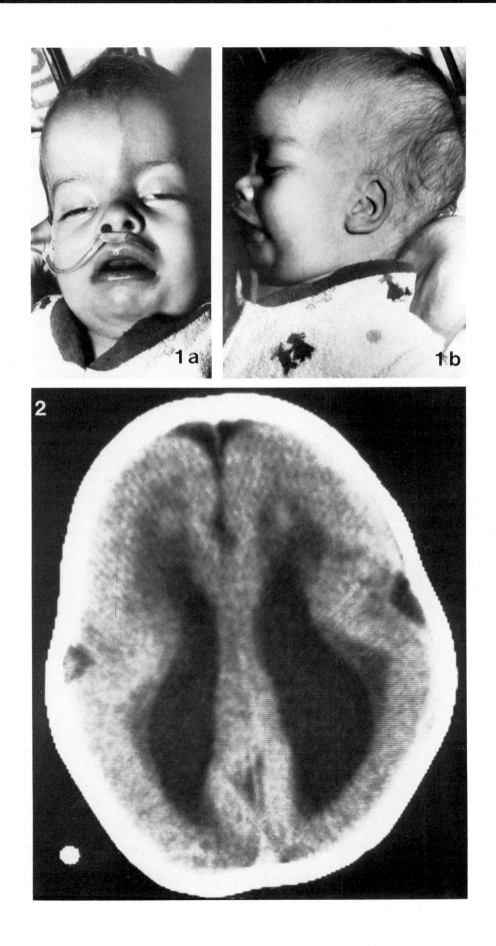

47 Trisomy 13

(D₁-Trisomy Syndrome; Pätau Syndrome; Anglo–American Patau Syndrome)

J.K./ H.-R.W

A malformation syndrome with characteristic facies, polydactyly, primordial growth deficiency, profound psychomotor retardation and multiple other anomalies.

Main signs:
- Intra-uterine growth retardation, birth weight 2600 g.
- Typical facies with slanting forehead, hypo- or hypertelorism, mongoloid slant of the palpebral fissures, microphthalmia or anophthalmia, cleft lip and palate and micrognathia (1, 2, 5, 6).
- Microcephaly, profound psychomotor impairment, seizures; hypotonia, rarely hypertonia.
- Postaxial polydactyly, mainly of the upper extremities, hyperextensible thumbs; narrow, hyperconvex fingernails (3). Simian crease. Protruding calcaneus.
- Localized skin defects in the occipital area (7). Capillary haemangiomas.
- Cryptorchidism, partial fusion of the penis and scrotum, hypospadias.

Supplementary findings: Omphalocoele.
Cardiac defects of various types, especially ventricular septal defect and patent ductus arteriosus.
Polycystic kidneys and anomalies of the urinary tract (horseshoe kidney, single kidney) in 80% of all patients.
Malformations of the brain as with holoprosencephaly (24), anomalies of the cerebellum.

Manifestation: *In utero* and at birth.

Aetiology: Trisomy (in 90%) as a result of meiotic non-disjunction, otherwise due to robertsonian translocations. Genetic imbalance caused by trisomy of chromosome 13 or to a threefold dose of the genetic material located on this chromosome. The extra chromosome almost always exists independently; very rarely, it is attached to another chromosome. Sibling risk: 0.55%. Increased maternal and paternal age (mean ages 31 and 33 years respectively).

Frequency: Approximately one out of 10 000 live births.

Course, prognosis: Severely delayed psychomotor development. Approximately 62% die before reaching 1 year of age. A few survivors can walk with support, understand words, use their own word forms and signs, follow simple commands, recognize and interact, play on their own. Survival rate up to 1 year of age: 45% for girls, 33% for boys; all males and 73% of females die by the fifth year of life; at 10 years of age, less than 10% of girls still alive.

Treatment: Symptomatic. Prenatal diagnosis after birth of an index case, especially in older mothers or in the case of a balanced translocation in one of the parents.

Differential diagnosis: Meckel syndrome (45), where an occipital encephalocoele is usually present (other signs similar); polycystic kidneys. Normal chromosomes.

Illustrations:
1 Patient 1 on the first day of life. Birth measurements: 2230 g, length 48 cm, head circumference 26 cm. Death on the first day of life. Holoprosencephaly, microphthalmia, ventricular septal defect, renal cortical cysts, duplication of the renal pelvis and ureter bilaterally.
2–4 Patient 2 on the first day of life: the ninth child of a 40-year-old woman. Birth measurements within normal limits. Death at age 9 days. Omphalocoele, coloboma of the iris, renal cortical cysts, duplication of the renal pelvis and ureter bilaterally, undescended testes, hypospadias, hypoplasia of the mitral and aortic valves.
5 and 6 Patient 3 at age 7 days. Death on the 19th day of life. Hexadactyly of the hands, microphthalmia, high-arched palate, bifid uvula, persistence of the left superior vena cava, ventricular septal defect, patent ductus arteriosus, horseshoe kidney, bicornate uterus.
7 and 8 Patient 4 at age 3 days. Birth measurements: 2000 g, length 44 cm, head circumference 31 cm. Death at age 2 days. Holoprosencephaly, hexadactyly of both hands, club feet, bilateral cleft lip and palate. Atresia of the pulmonary valve, ventricular septal defect, over-riding aorta, patent ductus arteriosis, bicornate uterus.

References:
Hamerton J L: Human Cytogenetics, 1971, Vol II. Academic Press, New York and London.
Grouchy J de, Turleau C: Atlas des maladies chromosomiques, 2. édit. 1982, Expansion scientifique française, Paris.
Baty B J, Blackburn B L, Carey J C: Natural history of trisomy 18 and trisomy 13: I. Growth, physical assessment, medical histories survival, and recurrence risk. *Am J Med Genet* 1994, 49:175–188.
Baty B J, Jorde L B, Blackburn B L, Carey J C: Natural history of trisomy 18 and trisomy 13: II. Psychomotor development. *Am J Med Genet* 1994, 49:189–194.

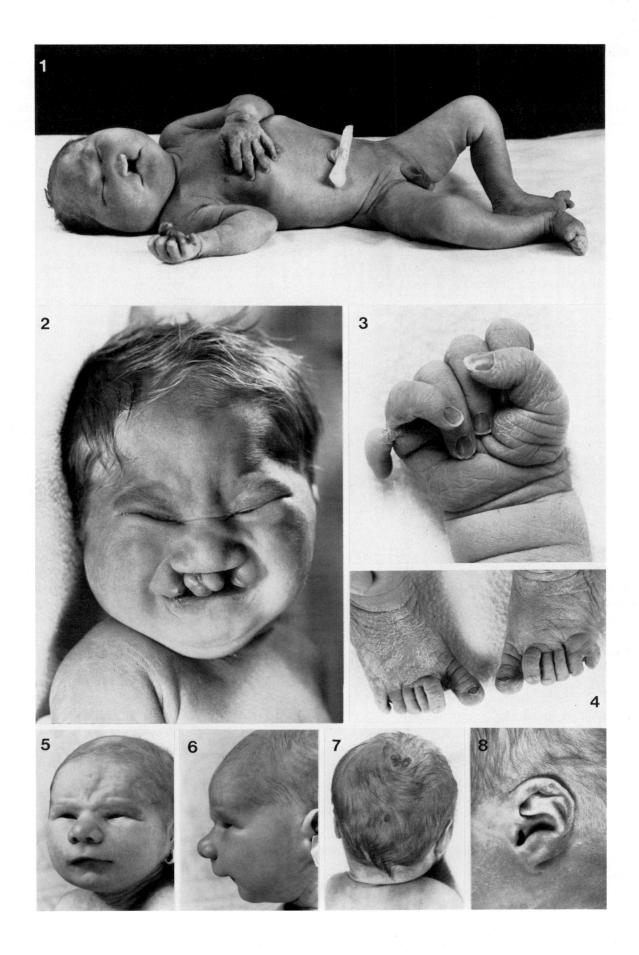

48 Trisomy 18
(Edwards Syndrome)

J.K./ H.-R.W

A syndrome comprising primordial growth deficiency, typical facial dysmorphism, profound psychomotor retardation and multiple other anomalies.

Main signs:
- Intra-uterine growth retardation, birth weight 2200 g.
- Characteristic facies, especially distinguished by protruding forehead, short (sometimes upward-slanting) palpebral fissures, micrognathia, microstomia, short philtrum, not infrequently cleft lip and palate or single components thereof. Narrow, microcephalic skull with prominent occiput, dysplasia of the auricles of the ears (4–8).
- Pronounced prenatal and postnatal growth deficiency.
- Profound psychomotor retardation, seizures; hypertonia after initial hypotonia (1).
- Flexion contractures of the fingers with overlapping of the second and fifth over the third and fourth fingers, respectively (2); hypoplastic nails, especially of the feet; usually partial syndactyly, short dorsi-flexed halluces; protruding calcanei, 'rocker-bottom feet' (3).
- Short sternum; small, relatively widely spaced nipples; umbilical and inguinal hernias; cutis laxa.

Supplementary findings: Aplasia of the radius, polydactyly, syndactyly. Scoliosis.

Anomalies of the central nervous system such as hydrocephalus and myelomeningocoele. Defects of the eyes, blindness.

Cardiac defects, especially ventricular septal defect and patent ductus arteriosus.

Diaphragmatic hernia, omphalocoele.

Hypospadias, cryptorchidism, bifid uterus, ovarian hypoplasia, renal anomalies (hydronephrosis, renal cysts, etc.).

Manifestation: *In utero* and at birth.

Aetiology: Genetic imbalance due to trisomy of chromosome 18 or to a threefold dose of the genetic material located on this chromosome. Almost without exception, the extra chromosome exists as an independent entity (and not translocated onto another chromosome). The maternal chromosome 18 is supernumerary in 75%, the paternal chromosome 18 in 25%.

Frequency: Approximately one out of 8000 births. Predominantly females.

Course, prognosis: At 6 months of age more than 60% of the female trisomy 18 patients are still alive but only 15% of the males. At 1 year of age, 55% of the female patients are still alive but only 10% of the males. At 5 years of age, all of the males have died, whereas 15% of the females are still alive. Risk of recurrence for siblings: 0.55%. In isolated cases, children learn to walk with support, can understand a few words and signs, can react to commands and interact but can rarely play on their own. Trisomy 18 patients can even attain normal intelligence.

Treatment: Symptomatic. Prenatal diagnosis in mothers who have previously borne such a child, especially older mothers, or in the case of a balanced translocation in one of the parents.

Illustrations:
1–3 Patient 1. Birth measurements: 2220 g, length 45 cm, head circumference 31 cm. Death at age 4 weeks. Hypertrophy of the clitoris, stenosis of the aortic isthmus, patent ductus arteriosus, bicuspid pulmonary and aortic valves, ventricular septal defect with over-riding aorta, tandem (fused) kidneys on the left with double renal pelvis.
4 and 5 Patient 2. Birth measurements: 2260 g, length 45 cm, head circumference 32 cm. Death at age 3 days. Partial syndactyly involving all fingers and toes, ventricular septal defect with over-riding aorta, diaphragmatic hernia.
6–8 Patient 3. Birth measurements: 1690 g, length 40 cm, head circumference 31.5 cm. Death at age 8 weeks. Syndactyly, camptodactyly, hypoplastic labia majora, horseshoe kidney, Meckel's diverticulum, diaphragmatic hernia, atrial and ventricular septal defects, bicuspid aortic valve, hypoplasia of the left pulmonary veins.

References:
Hamerton J L: Human Cytogenetics, 1971, Vol II. Academic Press, New York and London.
Schinzel A, Schmid W: Trisomie 18... *Helv Paediat Acta* 1971, **26**:673.
Grouchy J de, Turleau C: Atlas des maladies chromosomiques, 2. édit. 1982, Expansion scientifique française, Paris.
Graham D A, Jewitt M M, Fitzgerald P H: Trisomy 18 mosaicism with complete peripheral lymphocyte trisomy and normal intelligence. *Clin Genet* 1992, **41**:36–38.
Ya-gang X, Robinson W P, Spiegel R, Binkert F, Ruefenacht U, Schinzel A A: Parental origin of the supernumerary chromosome in trisomy 18. *Clin Genet* 1993, **44**:57–61.
Root S, Carey J C: Survival in trisomy 18. *Am J Med Genet* 1994, **49**:170–174.
Baty B J, Blackburn B L, Carey J C: Natural history of trisomy 18 and trisomy 13: I. Growth, physical assessment, medical histories, survival and recurrence risk. *Am J Med Genet* 1994, **49**:175–188.
Baty B J, Jorde L B, Blackburn B L, Carey J C: Natural history of trisomy 18 and trisomy 13: II. Psychomotor development. *Am J Med Genet* 1994, **49**:189–194.
Sarigol S S, Rogers D G: Trisomy 18 mosaicism in a thirteen-year old girl with normal intelligence, delayed pubertal development, and growth failure. *Am J Med Genet* 1994, **49**:94–95.

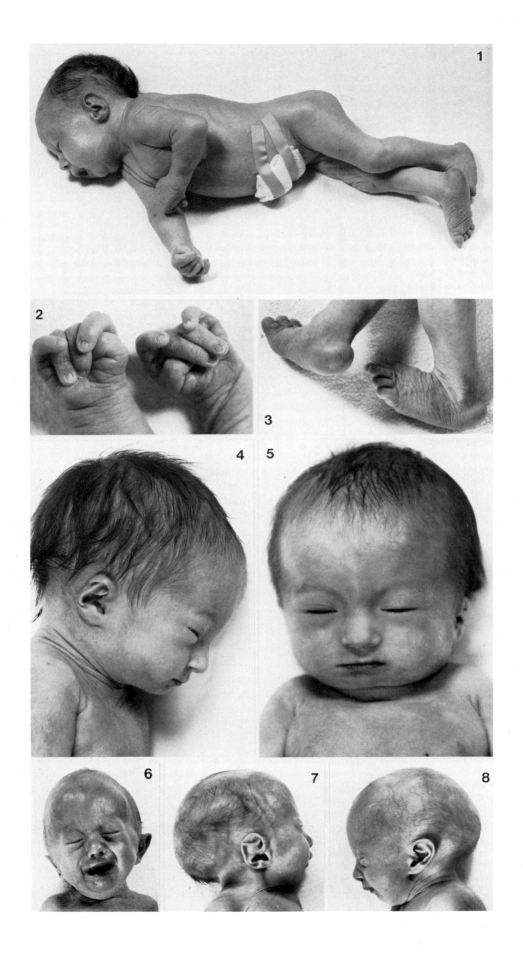

Down Syndrome

(Trisomy 21 Syndrome, Mongolism, Mongoloidism) *J.K./ H.-R.W*

A malformation syndrome comprising mental retardation and very characteristic physical appearance.

Main signs:

- 'Flat face' with mongoloid slant of the palpebral fissures, epicanthus, low nasal bridge, small nose and dysplastic external ears (**1–8, 12–14**) with short cranium and steeply sloping occiput (**14**). Macroglossia (frequently with fissured tongue); dysodontiasis.
- Short-appearing neck with loose skin (more apparent in the young child). Relatively short stature. Short, stubby hands and fingers with frequent clinodactyly of the little fingers and simian crease of the palms (**15**); 'sandal gap' between the first two toes (**13, 16**).
- Muscular hypotonia and generalized hypermobility of the joints with laxity of the ligaments (**9–11**). Atlanto-axial instability in 5–20%.
- Mental retardation, moderate to severe.
- Of all Down patients, 80% develop microcephaly from the sixth month of life (more frequent in females). Twenty per cent of patients are in the lower normal range. In 20–50% there is a reduction of cortical neurons (areas 10, 17, 22), usually in the granular layers. Prenatal retardation of neurogenesis (neuronal migration) and prenatal and postnatal retardation of synaptogenesis.

Supplementary findings: Cardiac defects in almost one-half of the patients (usually septal defects, e.g. arterio-venous canal). Mild exophthalmos; strabismus, nystagmus; small white 'porcelain' (Brushfield) spots in the still pale-coloured iris of the young infant; occasional cataracts, myopia of greater than 5 D in 25%. Duodenal atresia or stenosis in 1–2% of patients.

Hypoplasia of the pelvis with flaring of the ilia and abnormally small angle between the ilium and the roof of the acetabulum on radiograph. Relatively small penis and frequently cryptorchidism (**10**).

Tendency to localized redness of the cheeks and nose (**6**), dryness of the skin, cutis marmorata and constipation; above average frequency of thyroid dysfunction; hearing defects in 78% (of which more than 50% are conductive hearing disorder, 15% labyrinthine deafness, 10% combined hearing defect).

Manifestation: At birth.

Aetiology: Frequently, increased maternal age. The syndrome is the expression of a chromosomal aberration, namely, a trisomy of chromosome 21 or disturbance of the genetic equilibrium caused by a threefold dose of the genetic material located on this chromosome. In over 95% of patients the chromosome exists independently; infrequently (approximately 3%) it is attached to another chromosome (translocation); in 2% mosaics are present. Increased paternal age is not a risk factor for a child with Down syndrome.

Frequency: One case in about 650 births. More than 5% of all mentally retarded children have Down syndrome.

Course, prognosis: Very dependent on the presence and severity of a cardiac defect. Distinctly increased susceptibility to respiratory tract ailments. Increased disposition to acute leukaemia. As infants, rather sluggish and apathetic, but from age 2 or 3 years, hyperactive behaviour. Affected males are infertile. Almost 80% of patients without a cardiac defect reach 30 years of age; 60% of all patients are still alive at age 50 years, 45% at age 60. Height at age 18 years is between 136 and 154 cm for female patients and for males between 140 and 162 cm. From the fourth decade of life, Alzheimer's disease must be expected.

Treatment: Cardiac surgery may be indicated. Physiotherapy and aids for the handicapped. Correction of eye defects (NB: myopia, astigmatism, cataract in 60–85%; strabismus in 43%). For hearing defects, insertion of grommets, hearing aids, speech therapy. Social integration. Genetic counselling for the parents and preventive measures in case of increased risk of recurrence.

Illustrations:

1–8 Facial appearances of two children at ages 4 weeks, 7 months, 10 months and 15 months and ages 21 months, 2 years and 9 months, 6 years 6 months, and 15 years, respectively.

9–11 Hypotonia and hyperextensibility in a child aged 10 months and 18 months, respectively.

12–14 Typical flaccid stance of two children aged 6 years and 6 months and 9 years and 6 months.

15 and 16 Simian crease and 'prehensile' foot with 'sandal gap' in a child aged 6 months and 1 month, respectively.

References:

Hsiang Y-H H, Berkovitz G, Blan Gl L, Migeon C J Warren A C: Gonadal function in patients with Down syndrome. *Am J Med Genet* 1987, **27**:449–459.

Cronk C, Crocker A C, Pueschel S M *et al*: Growth charts for children with Down syndrome: 1 month to 18 years of age. *Pediatrics* 1988, **81**:102–110.

Baird P A, Sadovnick A D: Life tables for Down syndrome. *Hum Genet* 1989, **82**:291–292.

Wisniewski K E: Down syndrome children often have brain with maturation delay, retardation of growth, and cortical dysgenesis. *Am J Med Genet Suppl* 1990, **7**:274–281.

Murken J, Dietrich-Reichart E (eds): Down-Syndrom. R. S. Schulz, Starnberg-Percha 1990.

Antonarakis S E, and the Down Syndrome Collaborative Group: Parental origin of the extra chromosome in trisomy 21 as indicated by analysis of DNA polymorphisms. *N Engl J Med* 1991, **324**:872–876.

Selikowitz M (ed): Down-Syndrom. Akademischer Verlag, Heidelberg, Berlin, New York, 1992.

De Michelena M I, Burstein E, Lama J R, Vasquez J C: Paternal age as a risk factor for Down syndrome. *Am J Med Genet* 1993, **45**:679–682.

Tolksdorf F (ed): Das Down-Syndrom. Ein Leitfaden für Eltern. Stuttgart, Jena, New York: Fischer, 1994.

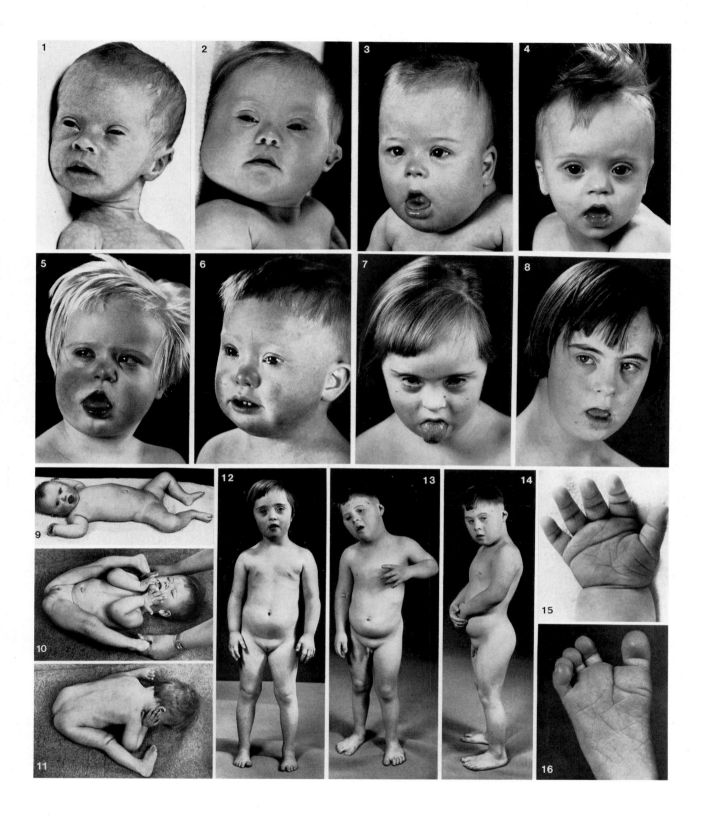

50 Cri Du Chat Syndrome

(Cat Cry Syndrome, Chromosome 5$_p$ Syndrome)

J.K./ H.-R.W

A syndrome comprising typical facial dysmorphism, primordial growth deficiency, psychomotor retardation and cat-like cry in early infancy.

Main signs:
- Face in infancy round and usually flat. Hypertelorism, epicanthic folds, usually antimongoloid slant of the palpebral fissures, strabismus, low broad nasal bridge and micrognathia (1–3).
- Primordial growth deficiency, birth weight under 2600 g.
- Microbrachycephaly and severe psychomotor retardation.
- Cat-like cry (unusually plaintive, high toned, weak) as characteristic feature in early infancy. Abnormal larynx.
- Congenital stridor.

Supplementary findings: Frequently dysplasia or unusual configuration of the external ears (3). Short neck; scoliosis at a later age.

Malocclusion, high palate, bifid uvula.

Partial syndactyly, short metacarpal and metatarsal bones, simian crease.

Muscular hypotonia, inguinal hernia, diastasis recti abdominis.

Manifestation: At birth.

Aetiology: Loss of the tip of the short arm of chromosome 5 (deletion 5p15.2). De-novo deletion in 90%. In 80%, the deletion occurs on a chromosome 5 of paternal origin. As long as neither of the parents has a corresponding translocation, no increased risk of recurrence.

Frequency: Relatively low, approximately one out of 50 000 newborns; up to 1980, about 400 patients had been reported.

Course, prognosis: Marked failure to thrive in infancy. Reduced fertility. Decreased life expectancy. The characteristic cry is lost during the first months of life. Many patients reach adulthood; the oldest patient is 56 years of age.

Differential diagnosis: Wolf syndrome (deletion of the short arm of chromosome 4) (*51*), however, this includes 'fish mouth', cleft lip and palate, coloboma, cardiac defect, hypospadias.

Treatment: Symptomatic. Prenatal diagnosis in cases of increased recurrence risk.

Illustrations:
1, 2, 3 Two affected girls, aged 2 and 6 months.

References:

Niebuhr E: The cri du chat syndrome... *Hum Genet* 1978, 44:227.

Wilkins L E, Brown J A, Wolf B: Psychomotor development in 65 home-reared children with cri-du-chat syndrome. *J Pediatr* 1980, 97:401.

Grouchy J de, Turleau C: Atlas des maladies chromosomiques, 2. édit. Expansion scientifique française, Paris 1982.

Wilkins L E, Brown J A et al: Clinical heterogeneity in 80 home-reared children with cri du chat syndrome. *J Pediatr* 1983, 102:528–533.

Martinez J E, Tuck-Muller C M, Superneau D, Wertelecki W: Fertility and the cri du chat syndrome. *Clin Genet* 1993, 43:212–214.

Overhauser J, Lee-Chen G J, McMahan J, Wasmuth J, Oberlender S, Carlin M E, Niebuhr E: Paternal inheritance of the deleted chromosome 5 in most cri du chat syndrome patients. *Am J Hum Genet (Suppl)* 1988, 45:A 85.

Pettenati M J, Hayworth R, Cox K, Rao P N: Prenatal detection of cri du chat syndrome on uncultured amniocytes using fluorescence in situ hybridization (FISH). *Clin Genet* 1994, 45:17–20.

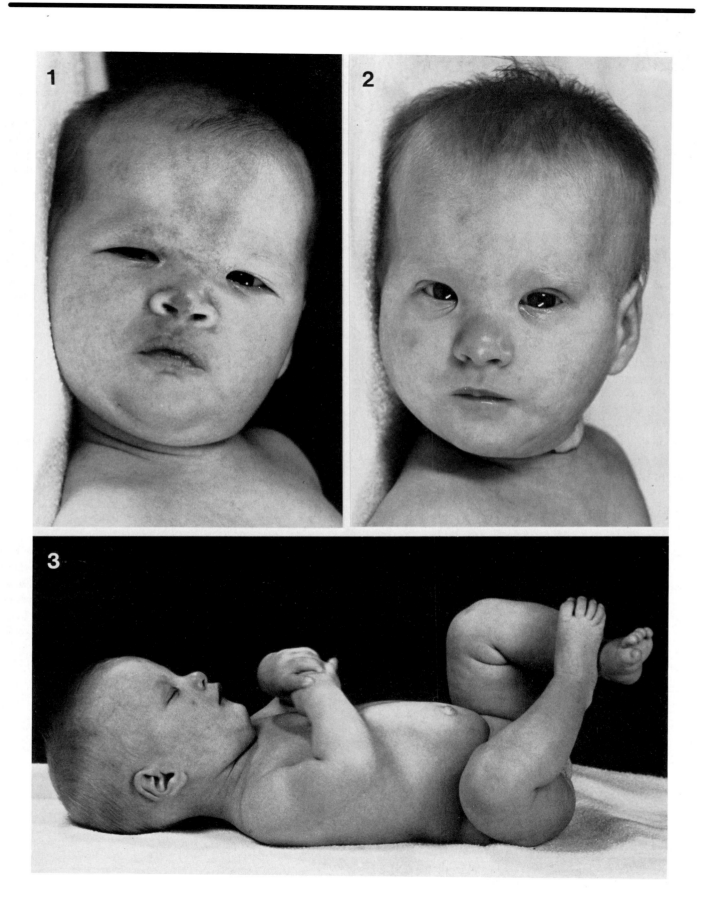

51 Wolf Syndrome
(Chromosome 4p Syndrome, Wolf–Hirschorn Syndrome)

A characteristic chromosome deletion syndrome with microcephaly, abnormally formed cranium, hypertelorism, ptosis, coloboma of the iris, broad hooked nose, dysplasia of the external ears and psychomotor retardation.

Main signs:
- Intra-uterine growth retardation: birth weight around 2000 g with normal period of gestation.
- Microcephaly, cranial asymmetry, haemangiomas of the forehead, prominent glabella, ocular hypertelorism, divergent strabismus, ptosis of the eyelids, antimongoloid slant of the palpebral fissures, coloboma of the iris (30%).
- Narrow external auditory canals, low-set dysplastic ears, pre-auricular tag and pits (50%), broad hooked nose, short philtrum, 'carp mouth', frequent cleft lip or palate, micrognathia.
- Cryptorchidism, hypospadias.

Supplementary findings: Stenosis or atresia of the naso-lacrimal ducts, widely spaced hypoplastic nipples.

Hip dysplasia, club feet, long fingers, hypoplasia or duplication of the thumbs and halluces.

Scalp defects, hernias, diastasis recti.

Cardiac defects, hypoplasia of the cerebellum, agenesis of the corpus callosum, hypoplasia of the olfactory nerve.

Multicystic renal degeneration, hydronephrosis, unilateral renal agenesis, hypoplasia of the uterus, vaginal aplasia.

Manifestation: At birth.

Aetiology: Loss of the tip of the short arm of chromosome 4. Deletion of 4p16. In 24 out of 29 patients examined, this is a deletion of paternal origin. In some of the patients, cytogenic diagnosis is normal. Molecular genetic techniques must be used in diagnosis. Approximately 10% of patients can be explained by a balanced parental translocation. When the parental chromosomes are normal, no increased risk of recurrence.

Frequency: Low; to date over 150 patients described.

Course, prognosis: Increased postnatal mortality (one-third of the patients die in the first year of life). Feeding problems, muscular hypotonia, seizures (80%), increased susceptibility to infections, severe psychomotor retardation, delayed dentition, kyphoscoliosis, delayed or precocious puberty. The oldest patient known, to date, is 24 years old. Two-thirds of the patients have been girls.

Differential diagnosis: Cri du chat syndrome (50).

Treatment: Symptomatic. Prenatal diagnosis in cases of parental translocation.

Illustrations:
1 and 2 Newborn girls.
1 Strabismus, hooked nose, microretrognathia, dysplastic ears.
2 Hypoplastic orbital boundaries, coloboma of the iris on the right, 'carp mouth'.
3a and b Patient 3, aged 3 years: prenatal and postnatal microsomia (weight, length and head circumference far below the third percentile), epilepsy, psychomotor retardation, hypoplasia of the corpus callosum and cerebral medulla, flat nasal bridge, hooked nasal tip, hypertelorism, no development of speech. Cytogenically normal. Molecular genetic deletions of the maternal alleles in the 4p15–16.3 region.

References:
Schinzel A: Catalogue of unbalanced chromosome aberrations in man. De Gruyter, Berlin - New York 1984.
Thies U, Back E, Wolff G, Schroeder–Kurth T, Hager H-D, Schröder K: Clinical, cytogenetic and molecular investigations in three patients with Wolf–Hirschhorn syndrome. *Clin Genet* 1992, **42**:201–205.
Tachdjian G, Fondacci C, Tapia S, Huten Y, Blot P, Nessmann C: The Wolf–Hirschhorn syndrome in fetuses. *Clin Genet* 1992, **42**:281–287.
Dallapiccola B, Mandich P, Bellone E, Selicorni A, Mokin V, Ajmar F, Novelli G: Parental origin of chromosome 4p deletion in Wolf–Hirschhorn syndrome. *Am J Med Genet* 1993, **47**:921–924.
Estabrooks L L, Lamb A N, Aylsworth A S, Callanan N P, Rao K W: Molecular characterisation of chromosome 4p deletions resulting in Wolf–Hirschhorn syndrome. *J Med Genet* 1994, **31**:103–107.

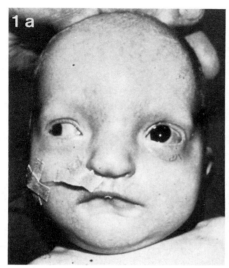
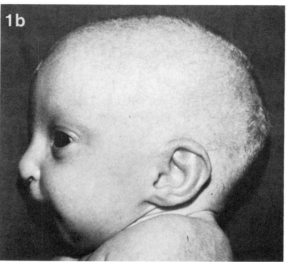
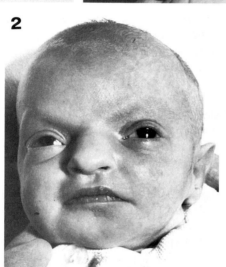
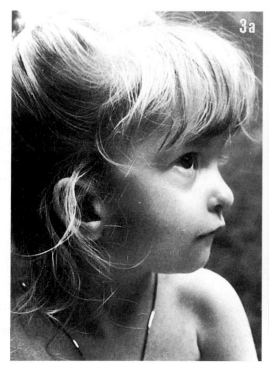
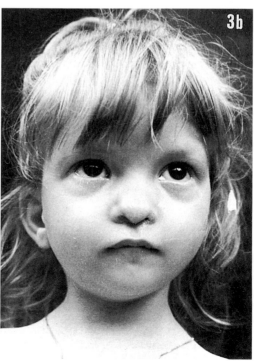

Pallister–Killian Mosaic Syndrome

(Pallister–Killian–Teschler–Nicola Syndrome, Tetrasomy 12p)

J.K.

A chromosomal disorder with the characteristics of severe neonatal muscular hypotonia, little hair growth bitemporally, prominent forehead, coarse face, pigment anomalies, profound mental retardation, seizures, diaphragmatic defects and supernumerary nipples.

Main signs:

- Severe neonatal muscular hypotonia, increase in tendency to premature births, asphyxia, absence of an umbilical artery. Occasionally, 'small for dates' and microcephalic.
- Craniofacial signs: coarseness of facial features, prominent forehead, high hairline; local alopecia, bitemporally pronounced and of the lateral–medial eyebrows and eyelashes; low-set dysplastic ears, hypertelorism, broad flat nasal bridge, exophthalmus, flat upper orbital arches, upward slanting palpebral fissures, epicanthus medialis, small nose, anteverted nostrils, full cheeks, long indistinct philtrum, prominent upper lip, macrostomia, down-slanting labial commissure, high-arched palate, micrognathia (at birth), short neck, frequently nuchal cutis laxa.
- Major malformations: microphthalmia, cataract, keratoconus, aniridia.
- Extremities: disproportionate reduction of the upper and lower extremities, predominantly rhizomelic. Small, broad hands and feet with short fingers and toes. Hypoplasia of the thumbs; occasionally, duplication of the halluces. Tapering fingers. Rarely, atlanto-occipital fusion and only 11 pairs of ribs.
- Cardiac malformations in one-quarter of all patients: ventricular septal defect, coarctation of the aorta, patent ductus arteriosus, atrial septal defect, aortic stenosis. Hypertrophic cardiomyopathy. Pulmonary segmentation disorders, hypoplasia of the lungs (with diaphragmatic defects).
- Abdominal malformations: diaphragmatic defects and hernias, anal atresia and stenosis, ventrally displaced anus.
- Renal malformations: (rare) renal cysts, dysplastic kidneys, ureteral stenosis, hydronephrosis.
- Genital anomalies: cryptorchidism, small scrotum, ambiguous genitalia, large hypoplastic labia, occasional aplasia of the posterior vagina and of the uterus.
- Dermal anomalies: frontotemporal alopecia, sparse eyebrows and eye-lashes; from infancy, patchy, rarely diffuse hyper-, usually, hypopigmentations, predominantly in the upper region of the face and forehead (beware of confusion with Ito syndrome). Accessory nipples.
- Central nervous system anomalies: hydrocephalus (11 out of 46), arhinencephaly (two out of 46).

Supplementary findings: Radio-ulnar synostoses, postaxial polydactyly, absence of the talus, cleft lip and palate, pitted lower lip. Cerebral hypoplasia, cerebral atrophy, laryngomalacia, gastro-oesophageal reflux, impaired hearing.

Manifestation: At birth.

Aetiology: Mosaic tetrasomy 12p in lymphocyte cultures in up to 2% of patients; in fibroblasts in 50–100%; in amniotic and bone-marrow cells in 100%. Higher rate of chromosomal abnormalities from abnormal cutaneous areas. Always sporadic isochromosome of the short arm of chromosome 12.

Pathogenesis: Unknown.

Frequency: Approximately 50 patients have been described.

Course, prognosis: 50% die prenatally, perinatally or postnatally, however, many reach 10–15 years of age. The oldest patient is 45 years of age. The phenotypic changes with increasing age are thick lips, macroglossia, protrusion of the tongue, prominent mandibles. Joint contractures, kyphoscoliosis. Seizures from childhood. Confinement to bed, no development of speech. A few of the survivors attend special schools.

Differential diagnosis: Ito syndrome (*188*), Fryns syndrome (*318*).

Treatment: Symptomatic.

Illustrations: 1a–c 21 months old, retarded, female, frontal bossing, thin scalp hair, broad nasal bridge, long philtrum with narrow upper lip, hypertelorism, sparse eyebrows, depigmentation above the left eyebrow (weight, length and circumference of head around the tenth percentile). **d** Sacral pits. **e and f** Pre-axial hexadactyly.

References:

Reynolds J F, Daniel A et al: Isochromosome 12p mosaicism (Pallister mosaic aneuploidy of Pallister–Killian syndrome): report of 11 cases. *Am J Med Genet* 1987, **27**:257–274.

Warburton, D, Anyane-Yeboa, K, Francke, U: Mosaic tetrasomy 12p: four new cases, and confirmation of the chromosomal origin of the supernumerary chromosome in one of the original Pallister-mosaic syndrome cases. *Am J Med Genet* 1987, **27**:275–283.

Peltomäki P, Knuutila S et al: Pallister–Killian syndrome: cytogenetic and molecular studies. *Clin Genet* 1987, **31**:399–405.

Quarrell O W J, Hamill M A, Hughes H E: Pallister–Killian mosaic syndrome with emphasis on the adult phenotype. *Am J Med Genet* 1988, **31**:841–844.

Soukup S, Neidich K: Prenatal diagnosis of Pallister–Killian syndrome. *Am J Med Genet* 1990, **35**:526–528.

Schinzel A: Tetrasomy 12p (Pallister–Killian syndrome). *J Med Genet* 1991, **28**:122–125.

McLean S, Stanley W et al: Prenatal diagnosis of Pallister–Killian syndrome: resolution of cytogenetic ambiguity by use of fluorescent in situ hybridization. *Prenat Diagn* 1992, **12**:985–991.

Bernert J, Bartels I et al: Prenatal diagnosis of the Pallister–Killian mosaic aneuploidy syndrome by CVS. *Am J Med Genet* 1992, **42**:747–750.

Pankau R, Diebold U, Jenderny J, Kautza M, Dörner K: Killian–Teschler–Nicola-Syndrom. *Monatsschr Kinderheilkd* 1992, **140**:340–342.

McPherson E W, Ketterer D M, Salsburey D J: Pallister–Killian and Fryns syndromes: nosology. *Am J Med Genet* 1993, **47**:241–245.

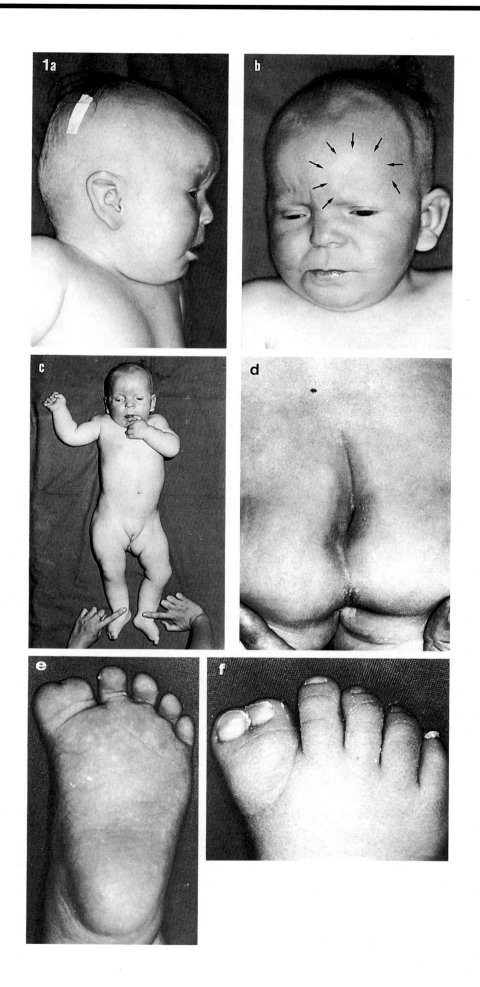

53 Happy Puppet Syndrome
(Angelman Syndrome)

J.K.

Mental retardation, microcephaly, unusual facial features, unprovoked laughing spells and ataxic jerky movements of the extremities characterize this syndrome.

Main signs:
- Moderate to severe mental retardation; paroxysms of laughing ('happy'); no development of speech.
- Microbrachycephaly (25% less than third percentile, 98% less than 50th percentile), occipital groove; hypoplasia of the midface, macrostomia, prognathism, protrusion of the tongue when laughing, widely spaced teeth; atrophy of the optic nerve and defective pigmentation of the choroid and iris.
- Stiff gait, ataxic jerky ('puppet') movements of the extremities; muscular hypotonia; occasionally hyperreflexia; characteristically abnormal electroencephalogram with bilateral irregular spike and wave activity (24-h electroencephalogram), frequently (in 80%) unclassifiable clinical seizure disorder.

Supplementary findings: Blue eyes, blond hair, reduced sleep requirement.

Manifestation: Possible prenatal onset. Birth weight 200 g less than healthy siblings. Diagnosis after about 12 months of age. Laughing episodes after the first or second year of life. Onset of epilepsy between the sixth and 42nd months of life. The facial characteristics become more pronounced with time.

Aetiology: Heterogeneous: in 60–80%, there is a loss of maternal alleles as a result of deletion on maternal chromosome 15 (15q11–13) or, alternatively, paternal disomies in approximately 5%. In 2%, there are structural anomalies on chromosome 15. In approximately 20% of patients, no genetic disorders can be detected. These include the familial cases. Imprinting mutations have also been found in 1%.

Frequency: One out of 16 000. Sibling observations rare.

Course, prognosis: No progression of the mental disorder. No development of speech. Decrease of epileptic disorder with age. The oldest known patient to date is 75 years old. Ten per cent of patients never walk without support. Gait disturbance due to scoliosis, joint contractures, hemiplegia, obesity. Feeding difficulties in infancy. Dry during the day in 75% of patients, eating with a spoon in 85%, dressing with assistance in 50%, simple housework in 70%. Normal menarche and menstruation.
Genetic counselling depending on laboratory findings.

Differential diagnosis: Rett syndrome (*54*), ATR-X syndrome (*250*), ataxic cerebral palsy.

Treatment: Symptomatic treatment of epilepsy, if at all indicated.

Illustrations:

1a and b Patient 1, a mentally retarded, microcephalic boy, aged 8 years and 2 months. Hypoplasia of the midface, macrostomia, prognathism, dental prosthesis for severely malpositioned teeth.

2a and b Patient 2, a girl aged 3 years and 9 months. Microcephaly, hypoplasia of the midface, macrostomia, prognathism, widely spaced teeth. Mental retardation.

3a and b Patient 3, a similarly affected girl aged 8 years and 9 months.

References:

Dörries A, Spohr H-L, Kunze J: Angelman ('Happy Puppet') syndrome – 8 new cases with documented cerebral computer tomography: Review of the literature. *Eur J Pediatr* 1988, 148:270–273.

Boyd S G, Harden A et al: The EEG in early diagnosis of the Angelman... syndrome. *Eur J Pediatr* 1988, 147:508–513.

Dittrich B, Robinson W P et al: Molecular diagnosis of the Prader–Willi and Angelman syndromes by detection of parent-of-origin specific DNA methylation in 15q11-13. *Hum Genet* 1992, 90:313–315.

Clayton-Smith J, Webb T et al: Maternal origin of deletion 15q11-13 in 25/25 cases. *Hum Genet* 1992, 88:376–378.

Clayton-Smith J, Pembrey M E: Angelman syndrome. *J Med Genet* 1992, 29:412–415.

Reis A, Kunze J, Ladanyi L, Enders H, Klein-Vogel U, Niemann G: Exclusion of the GABA-receptor β3 subunit gene as the Angelman syndrome gene. *Lancet* 1993, 341:122–123.

Knoll J H M, Wagstaff J, Lalande M: Cytogenetic and molecular studies in the Prader–Willi and Angelman syndromes: an overview. *Am J Med Genet* 1993, 46:2–6.

Clayton-Smith J: Clinical research on Angelman syndrome in the United Kingdom: observations on 82 affected individuals. *Am J Med Genet* 1993, 46:12–15.

Nicholls R D: Genomic imprinting and uniparental disomy in Angelman and Prader–Willi syndromes: a review. *Am J Med Genet* 1993, 46:16–25.

Penner K A, Johnston J, Faircloth B H, Irish P, Williams C A: Communication, cognition, and social interaction in the Angelman syndrome. *Am J Med Genet* 1993, 46:34–39.

Reis A, Dittrich B et al: Imprinting mutations suggested by abnormal DNA methylation patterns in familial Angelman and Prader–Willi syndromes. *Am J Med Genet*, 1994, (in press).

Reis A, Tyler K, Kunze J, Sperling K: Diagnostik des Angelman-Syndroms. *Medizinische Genetik* 1994, 6:22–28.

Greger V, Reis A, Lalande M: The critical region for Angelman syndrome lies between D15S122 and D15S113. *Am J Med Genet* 1994, 53:396–398.

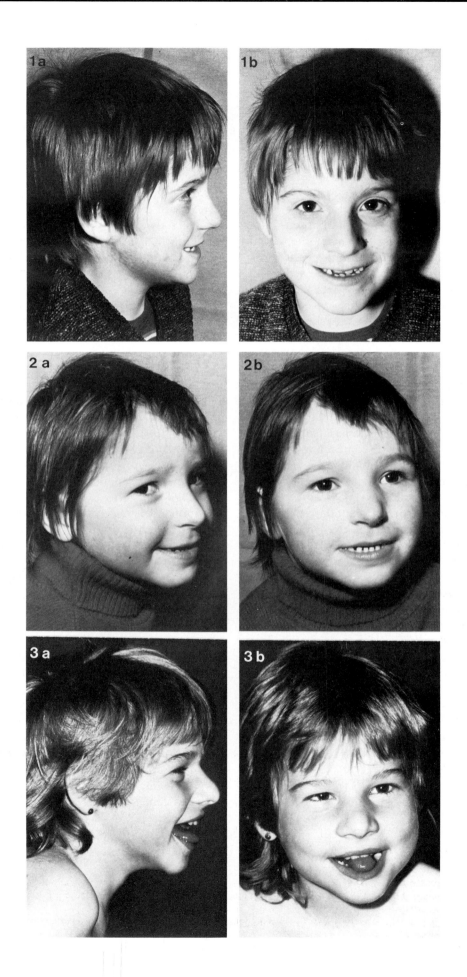

54 Rett Syndrome

J.K.

A progressive syndrome exclusively of females, with cessation of development after the ninth to 18th month of life, rapid mental deterioration with autistic features, stereotyped movements of the hands, tremors of the trunk, ataxia, microcephaly, paraspasm and epilepsy.

Main signs:

- After normal initial development, rapid onset of developmental retardation beginning between the seventh and 18th month of life. Loss of acquired speech, target-specific grasping, purposeful hand movements and interest in the surroundings. Within a year, transition to moderate or severe mental retardation, autism and sleep disorders.
- Cessation of head growth, to microcephaly by the third year of life; ataxia of the trunk and extremities; anxiety, hyperventilation, aerophagia; vasomotor disturbances with sweating, red–blue discoloration of the feet; bizarre patterns of movement ('hand-wringing' in front of the chest or mouth, poor tone, irregular co-ordination), loss of ability to walk, spastic paraparesis, severe progressive kyphoscoliosis, joint contractures, confinement to a wheelchair; constipation. Epilepsy after the fourth year of life; autistic–ataxic dementia.

Supplementary findings: Normal maternal pregnancy, uncomplicated birth at term, no increased abortions, no stillbirths; length and head circumference of the child normal at birth.

No specific laboratory findings: CSF electrophoresis negative as a rule; in some patients decrease or absence of the τ-fraction. Blood ammonia slightly elevated in a few patients. Abnormal electroencephalogram after the third year of life. Nerve conduction velocity normal. Electromyography shows mild signs of denervation; computer tomography of the brain shows mild signs of cerebral atrophy; white matter normal. Non-specific findings on electron microscopy of conjunctival and skin biopsies. Autopsy findings: microencephaly, atrophy of the brain, decreased pigmentation of the substantia nigra, electron-optical increase of neuronal lipofuscin.

Periodic apnoea, intermittent hyperventilation, peripheral vasomotor disturbances.

Manifestation: After the seventh to 18th month of life.

Diagnosis between the third and fifth years of life.

Aetiology: Most likely an X-linked dominant disorder with lethality in male hemizygote embryos. Always new mutations. Seven pairs of monozygotic twins, 11 pairs of discordant twins observed. Eight siblings, one pair of half sisters with the same mother. One case of mother–daughter transmission. Risk of recurrence after first affected daughter: 0.4%. No increase in tendency to abortions in the mothers of daughters affected with Rett syndrome. No patient with Rett syndrome has had children. Isolated observations of 'forme fruste' or atypical forms (Hagberg).

Frequency: Probably underdiagnosed (according to one study, approximately one out of 15 000 girls). To date more than 2000 patients are known worldwide.

Course, prognosis: Progressive course, as described, to spastic quadriparesis, dementia, autism, kyphoscoliosis. Course in four clinical stages: I, early deterioration between the sixth and 18th months of life; II, rapid developmental regression (years 1–4); III, pseudostationary period (years to decades); IV, late motor deterioration (decades) to complete confinement to a wheelchair. Seven per cent reach 40 years of age. Average life expectancy is 28 years. The oldest patient is 68 years of age.

Treatment: No specific therapy known. Trial with dopamine agonists, e.g. bromocriptine. Symptomatic, anticonvulsive treatment in some cases. Physiotherapy. Possibly Ketogenic diet.

Illustrations:

1a Female infant at 3 months, normal psychomotor development, neurologically normal. **1b** The same girl at age 12 years: autistic, ataxic dementia, microcephaly, characteristic 'hand-wringing' movements in front of the chest. **2a and b** A girl aged 2 years and 9 months, with probable normal development in early infancy followed by decrease in performance, on to severe dementia; small cranium, variable muscle tone, constant stereotyped hand-wringing movements, markedly abnormal electoencephalogram.

References:

Hagberg B, Aicardi J, Dias K *et al*: A progressive syndrome of autism, dementia, ataxia and loss of purposeful hand use in girls: Rett's syndrome: Report of 35 cases. *Ann Neurol* 1983, **14**:471–479.
Hagberg B, Goutières F, Hanefeld F *et al*: Rett syndrome: criteria of inclusion and exclusion. *Brain Dev* 1985, 7:372–373.
Hanefeld F: The clinical pattern of Rett syndrome. *Brain Dev* 1985, 7:320–325.
The Rett Syndrome. *Am J Med Genet Suppl* 1. 1986, New York: Liss.
Hagberg B: Rett Syndrome — clinical and biological aspects. 1993, Cambridge University Press.

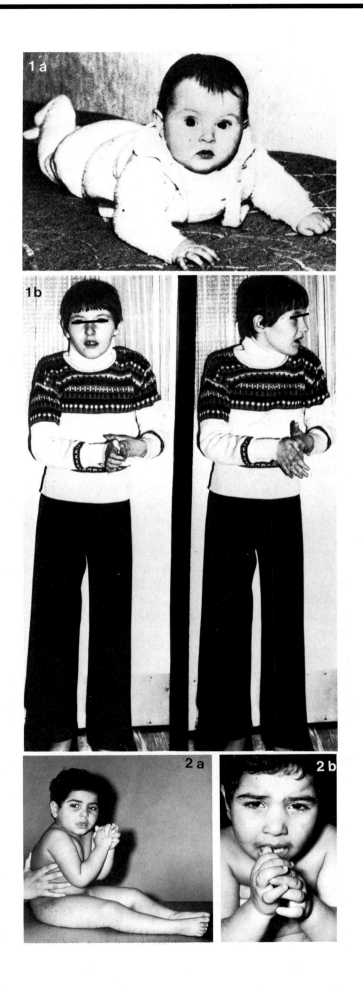

55 Fragile X Syndrome

(Marker X Syndrome; X-linked Mental Retardation; Martin–Bell Syndrome)

The most frequent form of familial mental retardation, mainly in males, with large ears, macro-orchidism and fragile X chromosome.

Main signs:
- Mental retardation of varied severity (IQ below 70 in 25%, 70–84 in 28%).
- Large ears.
- Macro-orchidism (30–75 ml).
- Autism, occasionally.
- Frequency of the fragile X in folic acid-deficient lymphocyte cultures from male probands varies between a few per cent and approximately 50%.

Supplementary findings: Increased weight and head circumference above the 97th percentile at birth. Delayed psychomotor development: muscular hypotonia, thin legs, walking after 18 months, delayed speech (development begins after the third year). Shy as toddlers, with poor social contact. Increasingly hyperactive after age 3–4 years. In adolescence, distinct mental retardation, repetitive speech, echolalia. Occasional seizures. Tall stature, flat feet, hyperextensible joints, prolapse of the aortic and mitral valves, myopia as a result of mesenchymal weakness. The adult male after puberty shows the full clinical picture including typical facial features with long oval face and prognathism. Normal testosterone synthesis, normal testicular histology.

Women and 'fragile X':
- 66% of heterozygous women are normal but approximately 10% of these manifest psychoses.
- 33% of heterozygous women are mentally retarded; of these, 20% become psychotic.
- 50% of heterozygous women do not have cytogenically detectable fragile X.
- 20% of heterozygous women show the same characteristic facial features as affected men.
- Fragile X women show increased fertility (fourfold frequency of twin births).

Manifestation: Delayed psychomotor development after the fifth month of life; delayed speech (development begins after the third year of life); full clinical picture after puberty.

Aetiology: X-linked disorder with anticipation (increasing severity in successive generations): Sherman paradox.

The fragile X marker has been detected (q27.3).

Direct molecular genetic diagnosis is currently possible: detection of triplet expansion (CGG bases) in the fragile X gene with good correlation between the number of repeats and the clinical signs. For a normal person, between six- and 54-fold CGG repeats are found, with 55–200-fold repeats for symptom-free transmitters (e.g. in normal male and female transmitters). In female meiosis, an amplification can occur over 200 repeats, which generally leads to clinical manifestation in male patients. Amplification does not occur in male meiosis.

Frequency: 0.73 fragile X patients out of 1000 schoolboys (Tessa Webb 1986); one fragile X patient out of 1090 men (Opitz 1986); one fragile X patient out of 1500 schoolboys (Gustavson et al 1986); fragile X in up to 7% of mildly mentally retarded schoolgirls with IQs of 55–75 (Turner et al 1980). Prevalence of premutation in the female population is one out of 400.

Course, prognosis: At present there are no life tables. The oldest known patient is 55 years old. Possible decreased life expectancy.

Differential diagnosis: Sotos syndrome (74).

Treatment: No definite results with folic acid therapy. Genetic counselling: In fragile X families, 20% of healthy brothers of fragile X patients have the affected gene. These brothers transmit the gene to their children with no risk of the disorder. However, their daughters will transmit the risk. If the female transmitter is retarded, 50% of her sons will be affected and 30–40% of her daughters. Direct prenatal molecular genetic diagnosis is possible.

Illustrations:
1a–c A characteristically affected 5-year-old boy.
2 A similarly affected 22-year-old man.

References:
Schwinger E, Froster-Iskenius U: Das Marker-X-Syndrom. Klinik und Genetik. Enke, Stuttgart 1984.
X-linked mental retardation 5. 1992, *Am J Med Genet* (Special Issue) Wiley-Liss, A. John Wiley, New York, Chichester, Brisbane, Toronto, Singapore.
Sutherland G R, Gedeon A *et al*: Prenatal diagnosis of fragile X syndrome by direct detection of the unstable DNA sequence. *N Engl J Med* 1991, **325**:1720–1722.
Heitz D, Devys D, Imbert G, Kretz, Mandel J-L: Inheritance of the fragile X premutation is a major determinant of the transition to full mutation. *J Med Genet* 1992, **29**:794–801.
Turner G, Robinson H *et al*: Population screening for fragile X. *Lancet* 1992, 339:1210–1213.
Hull C, Hagerman R J: A study of the physical, behavioral and medical phenotype, including anthropometric measures, of females with fragile X syndrome - *AJDC* 1993, **147**:1236–1241.
Staley L W, Hull C E *et al*: Molecular–clinical correlations in children and adults with fragile X syndrome. *AJDC* 1993, **147**:723–726.
Fahsold R, Pfeiffer R A: Diagnostik und molekulare Grundlagen des fragilen X -(Martin-Bell-) Syndroms. *Pädiat Prax* 1993, **45**:211–216.

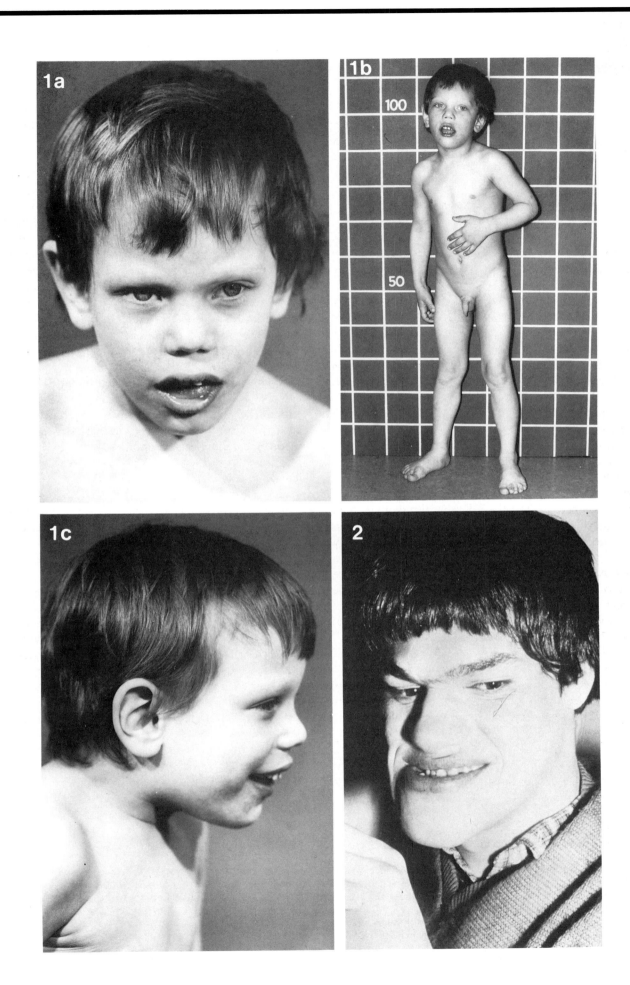

Infantile Cortical Hyperostosis
(Caffey Syndrome; Caffey–Silverman Syndrome)

H.-R.W

A clinical picture occurring chiefly in young infants with firm, frequently asymmetric, soft-tissue swellings, generally of the face or jaw and the extremities, with marked osseous swelling on the X-ray and usually eventual complete recovery.

Main signs:
- Painful, firm, often asymmetric soft-tissue swellings located on the face and/or the extremities and accompanied or heralded by fever and general irritability (1, 3).
- X-rays show periosteal hyperostosis, often severe, usually affecting several areas of the skeleton, preferentially the mandible, clavicles, scapulae, ribs and long bones (2, 4, 5).

Supplementary findings: Occasionally, pseudoparesis of part of an extremity during the acute swelling phase. Leukocytosis, elevated ESR and possible thrombocytosis during the acute phase. Frequently, moderately elevated serum alkaline phosphatase.

Manifestation: Early infancy. (Prenatal onset has also been shown repeatedly on X-ray). The hyperostosis is usually detectable within weeks of the onset of acute external swelling.

Aetiology: Numerous sporadic cases along with increased occurrence in some families, especially in siblings but also in successive generations, for which an autosomal dominant gene with incomplete penetrance and variable expression is thought to be responsible.

Frequency: Relatively low, although approximately 500 patients have been reported.

Course, prognosis: Course occasionally intermittent, with several phases or exacerbations. In isolated cases, a more chronic course may lead to distinct bowing or to overgrowth of the long bones and to marked delay of the gross motor development.

Prognosis as a rule very favourable. Usually complete clinical recovery, followed after several months by radiological recovery.

Differential diagnosis: Trauma (accidental or abusive), inflammatory or toxic conditions and (C or D) vitamin deficiency must be ruled out and perhaps occasionally cherubism (58). Prolonged prostaglandin E_1 treatment can produce an identical radiological picture.

Treatment: Symptomatic. Prevention of contractures. In severe cases, careful administration of corticosteroids may be indicated during the acute phase.

Illustrations:

1 A 9-week-old infant with asymmetric firm soft-tissue swellings on both lower legs and upper extremities.

3 Similarly affected 1-month-old child with anteriorly convex bowing of the tibia.

2 Hyperostosis of the lower edge of the body of the mandible in a 10-month-old infant.

4 and 5 Marked cortical hyperostosis of the tibia and arm bones of the infant in 1.

References:

Spranger J W, Langer L O Jr, Widemann H-R: Bone dysplasias. An atlas of constitutional disorders of skeletal development. Stuttgart and Philadelphia: G Fischer and W B Saunders, 1974.

Finsterbusch A, Rang M: Infantile cortical hyperostosis. Follow-up of 29 cases. *Acta Orthop Scand* 1975, 46:727.

Fried K, Manor A, Pajewski M *et al*: Autosomal dominant inheritance with incomplete penetrance of Caffey disease (infantile cortical hyperostosis). *Clin Genet* 1981, 19:271.

Gentry R R, Rust R S *et al*: Infantile cortical hyperostosis... without mandibular involvement. *Pediatr Radiol* 1983, 13:236–238.

Maclachlan A K, Gerrard J W *et al*: Familial infantile cortical hyperostosis in a large Canadian family. *Can Med Assoc J* 1984, 130:1172–1174.

Langer R, Kaufmann H-J: Pränatale Diagnosestellung bei Caffey'scher Erkrankung... *Klin Pädiat* 1985, 197:473–476.

Tabardel Y, Seghaye M C *et al*: Maladie de Caffey–Silverman néonatale avec thrombocytose... *Arch Fr Pediatr* 1988, 45:263–265.

Töllner U, Alzen G: Das Caffey–Silverman-Syndrom... *pädiat prax* 1988, 37:309–314.

Borochowitz Z, Gozal D *et al*: Familial Caffey's disease and late recurrence in a child. *Clin Genet* 1991, 40:329–335.

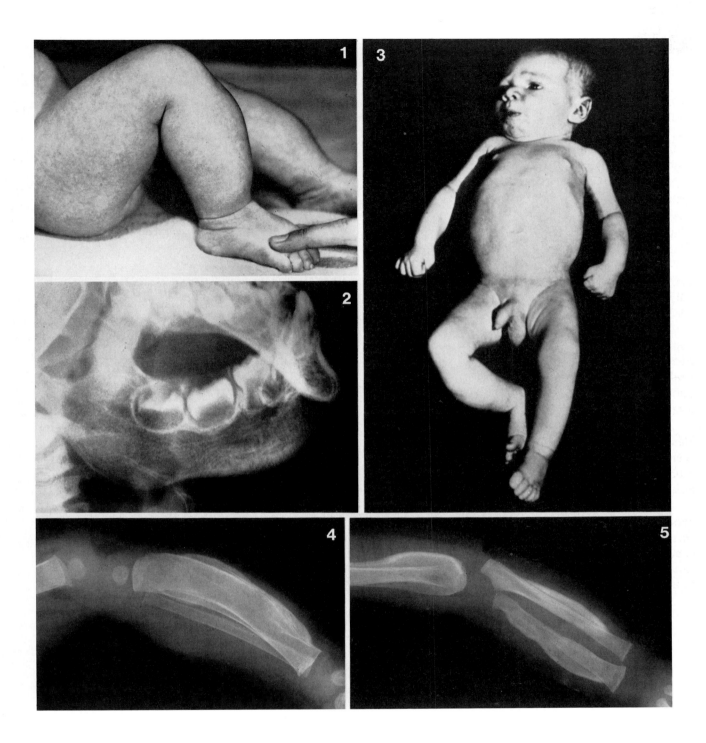

57 Craniometaphyseal Dysplasia

H.-R.W

A hereditary systemic defect of ossification with widening of the metaphyses, thickening of the skull bones and often impaired hearing.

Main signs:
Hypertelorism (2) with paranasal bony ridges (1 and 2) and bulging of the broad nasal bridge and the glabella (3) which, together with a large, occipito-frontally protruding cranium, produce a characteristic appearance. Narrowing of the nostrils with mouth breathing.

Supplementary findings: Compression of the auditory, optic (in some cases to the point of blindness) and facial nerves is usual. Widening of the alveolar crest. Involvement of dentition.

On radiograph, frontal and occipital hyperostosis or sclerosis of the cranium (4); abnormally shaped long bones with club-shaped flaring of the metaphyses (5).

Increased alkaline phosphatase and other biochemical findings possible.

Manifestation: Variable. Possibly from early infancy, more frequently, later in childhood.

Aetiology: Monogenic hereditary disorder with variable expression. Heterogeneity. Autosomal dominant form more frequent than perhaps a more severe autosomal recessive type.

Frequency: Low; approximately 80 patients reported in the literature.

Course, prognosis, treatment: Life expectancy normal as a rule. In mild cases, complete resolution of osseous hyperplasia possible. Good growth. Symptomatic treatment of neural, dental and other complications. Administration of human calcitonin or calcitriol (1,25 $(OH)_2$- vitamin D_3) may have a favourable effect in isolated cases, as shown by recent reports.

Illustrations:
1–3 A 6-year-old boy, normally developed for his age but with defective hearing.
4–6 His radiographs.
6 Typical mild changes.

References:
Spranger J W, Langer L O Jr, Wiedemann H-R: Bone dysplasia. An atlas of constitutional disorders of skeletal development. Stuttgart and Philadelphia: G Fischer and W.B. Saunders, 1974.
Beighton P, Hamersma H, Horan F: Cranio-metaphyseal dysplasia — variability of expression within a large family. *Clin Genet* 1970, 15:252.
Penchaszadeh V B, Gutierrez E R, Figueroa P: Autosomal recessive craniometaphyseal dysplasia. *Am J Med Genet* 1980, 5:43.
Carnevale A, Grether P *et al*: Autosomal dominant craniometaphyseal dysplasia... Clin Genet 1983, 23:17–22.
Cole D E, Cohen M M: A new look at craniometaphyseal dysplasia. *J Pediatr* 1988, 112:577–579.
Key L L, Volberg F *et al*: Treatment of craniometaphyseal dysplasia with calcitriol. *J Pediatr* 1988, 112:583–587.
Fanconi S, Fischer J A *et al*: Craniometaphyseal dysplasia... therapeutic effect of calcitonin. *J Pediatr* 1988, 112:587–591.
Reardon W, Hall C M *et al*: Sibs with... craniometaphyseal dysplasia... *J Med Genet* 1991, 28:622–626.
Gorlin R J: Craniotubular bone disorders. *Pediatr Radiol* 1994, 24:392–406.

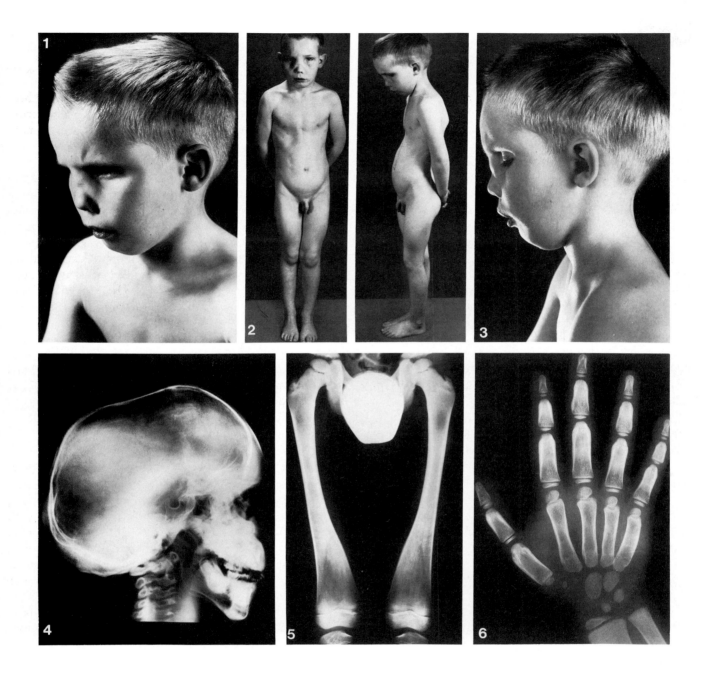

58 Cherubism

H.-R.W

A condition almost exclusively involving the jaw bones, with typical facial dysmorphism.

Main signs:
- Usually bilateral, symmetrical, indolent swelling of the submandibular or malar regions (1–4) due to fibrous replacement of the greater part of the jaw bones (upper and/or lower jaws; lower jaw especially). When the floor of the orbit is involved, the eye is cranially displaced and the sclera is visible below the rim of the iris (1, 3), the 'heavenward' gaze and the 'cherubic' cheeks giving the syndrome its name.
- Hypertelorism almost always present.
- Severely affected primary dentition with many malpositioned or exfoliated teeth (2, 5); hypodontia of the secondary dentition.

Supplementary findings: During the stage of increasing swelling, possible enlargement of the regional lymph nodes and elevation of serum alkaline phosphatase.

Radiograph examination of the rest of the skeleton may show mild cystic translucencies in other areas (e.g. bones of the hands, anterior ends of the ribs).

Manifestation: The first years of life.

Aetiology: Hereditary disorder with autosomal dominant transmission, variable expression and incomplete penetrance in females.

Frequency: Low; apparently, up to 1980, only approximately 100 patients reported.

Course, prognosis: The tumour-like dysplasia affects tooth development, with corresponding results; it may impair nasal breathing and tongue function. After years of progression, the swelling ceases before, during or fairly soon after puberty, then gradually regresses. Thus, it is self-limited and benign. Complete healing but with atrophy of the alveolar processes and reossification of the basal areas of the jaw.

Diagnosis: From appearance, radiographs (5) and, in some cases, histological findings on biopsy (proliferating loose fibrous tissue with spindle cells and multinucleated giant cells; little membranous bone formation).

Treatment: Curettage of tissue hindering nasal breathing or function of the tongue may be indicated. Radiographic therapy contraindicated. Timely application of prostheses. A modelling osteotomy may be indicated after adolescence.

Comment: An autosomal recessive hereditary syndrome comprising cherubism, gingival fibromatosis, hypertrichosis, small stature, mental retardation and epilepsy is called Ramon syndrome.

Illustrations:

1–4 Physically and mentally normal 4-year-old boy with cherubism (mother and sister of the boy similarly affected, the former now in the healing stage). Broad, flat midface with very wide nasal bridge, slight hypertelorism, prominent zygomatic arches, small and flat nose with anteverted nares; eyeball rotated slightly 'heavenwards'. Distension of the lower half of the face. Marked protrusion of the upper dental plates; child unable to close his mouth because of distension of the alveolar processes; severe deficiency of teeth.

5 Vast multicystic distension of the upper and lower jaws with marked thinning of the cortex. Maxillary sinuses cannot be delineated with certainty; zygomatic arches displaced cranially; orbits narrowed; nasal bone almost horizontal; positional anomalies of the tooth buds.

References:
Hoppe W, Spranger J, Hansen H G: Cherubismus. *Arch Kinderheilk* 1966, **174**:310.
Khosla V M, Korobkin M: Cherubism. *Am J Dis Child* 1970, **120**:458.
Peters W J N: Cherubism: a study of twenty cases from one family. *Oral Surg, Oral Med, Oral Path* 1979, **47**:307.
Hoyer P F, Neukam F-W: Cherubismus... *Klin Pädiat* 1982, **194**:128.
Salinas C F, Bradford B F *et al*: Cherubism associated with rib anomalies (Abstract). *Proc Greenwood Genet Ctr* 1983, **2**:129–130.
Pina-Neto J M, Moreno A F C *et al*: Cherubism, gingival fibromatosis, epilepsy and mental deficiency... *Am J Med Genet* 1986, **25**:433–441.

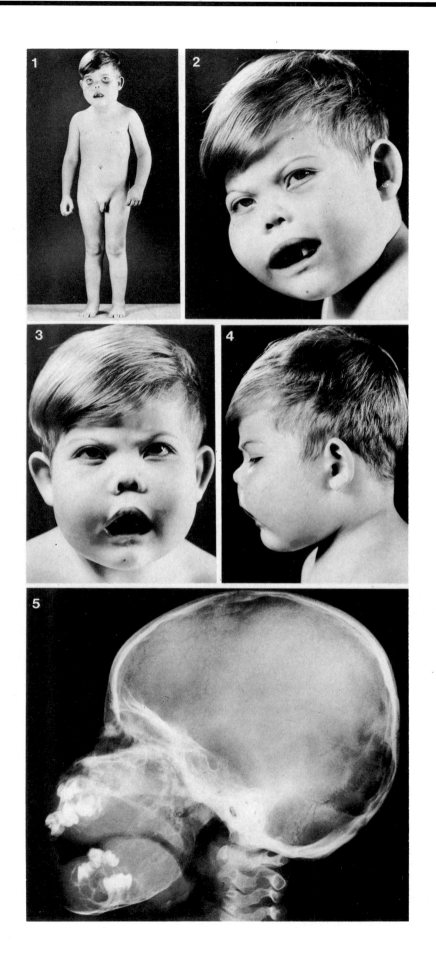

59   Menkes Syndrome

(Kinky Hair Syndrome, Menkes Disease, Steely Hair Syndrome, Trichopoliodystrophy)

H.-R.W

A disease of copper metabolism in boys, with depigmented monilethrix, relatively typical facies, growth retardation, psychomotor retardation, seizures and a poor prognosis.

Main signs:
- Sparse, kinky, short, brittle hair, still pigmented during the first weeks of life, thereafter depigmented. Microscopic twisting in the long axis, varying thickness of the shaft. Sparse eyebrows (**2 and 3**).
- Face puffy; characterized by full cheeks, 'carp mouth', micrognathia, low nasal bridge and short philtrum (**1 and 2**). High palate, broad alveolar ridges. Posteriorly rotated, poorly modelled ears.
- Pale, doughy skin with seborrheic changes (**3**).
- Psychomotor retardation; microcephaly. Seizures. Spasticity alternating with hypotonia.
- Growth deficiency. Metaphyseal flaring, spurs and increased density of the long bones, rosary. Pectus excavatum (**1**), possible club feet.

Supplementary findings: Frequently, small size at birth; early failure to thrive, wasting. Tendency to hypothermia, less frequently, hyperthermia. Increased infections.

Skeleton: wormian bones along the sagittal suture. After the second month of life, flaring of the metaphyses, which gradually regresses during the latter half of infancy (**4 and 5**). Osteoporosis, periosteal bone formation. Vacuolated promyelocytes in the bone marrow. In the fundus oculi, tortuositas vasorum with 'salt and pepper' appearance. On angiography, characteristic corkscrew twisting, elongation and varying calibre of the cerebral, visceral and soft tissue vessels. Subdural haemorrhages. Low levels of copper in serum and some tissues but elevated levels in the mucosa of the small intestine and elsewhere (defective copper distribution). Abnormally elevated copper absorption by cultured fibroblasts.

Manifestation: In the first months of life.

Aetiology: X-linked recessive disorder, thus males affected. Presumed gene locus: Xq13.3. The exact pathogenesis is not clear.

Frequency: Approximately two out of 100 000 live-born males (several hundred patients have been recognized since the first description in 1962).

Course, prognosis: With the onset of seizures in the second to third month of life, arrest of psychomotor development and shortly thereafter loss of acquired abilities, leading to coma, death usually occurs in the second year of life. However, deviations of the clinical course with different variants of the disease occur, including a less severe form with later manifestation and longer survival (into the second decade).

Treatment: Symptomatic. Oral and/or parenteral copper administration has only been shown to alter the course of disease with certainty in individual cases, however, substitution therapy should always be tried initially. Genetic counselling. Prenatal diagnosis, if possible from chorionic villi or cultured amniotic cells (substantially elevated copper level).

Illustrations:

1–5 Photographs and X-rays of an 8-month-old patient. Normal development up to the first seizure at age 10 weeks, then arrest of development and shortly thereafter regression. Frequent infections. Frequent hypothermia. Death at 12 months from meningitis.

References:
Kolb H-J, Guthoff T: Klinische Aspekte des Menkes-Syndroms. *Mschr Kinderheilk* 1987, **135**:827–831.
Menkes J H: Kinky hair disease. In: Neurocutaneous diseases. M. R. Gomez (ed) Boston: Butterworth 1987; 284–292.
Baerlocher K, Nadal D: Das Menkes-Syndrom. *Ergeb Inn Med Kinderheilk* 1988, **57**:77–144.
Gerdes A-M, Tønnesen T *et al*: Variability in clinical expression of Menkes syndrome. *Eur J Pediatr* 1988, **148**:132–135.
Nadal D, Baerlocher K: Menkes' disease... *Eur J Pediatr* **147**:621–625.
Sander C, Niederhoff H *et al*: Life span and Menkes kinky hair syndrome... *Clin Genet* 1988, **33**:228–233.
Westman J A, Richardson D C *et al*: Atypical Menkes steely hair disease. *Am J Med Genet* 1988, **30**:853–858.
Tønnesen T, Gerdes A-M, Damsgaard E *et al*: First trimester diagnosis of Menkes disease... *Prenat Diagn* 1989, **9**:159.
Kreuder J *et al*: Clinical and biochemical consequences of copper-histidine therapy in Menkes disease. *Eur J Pediatr* 1993, **152**:828–832.
Levinson B *et al*: The mottled gene is the mouse homologue of the Menkes disease gene. *Nature Genet* 1994, **6**:369–373.
Mercer J F B *et al*: Mutations in the murine homologue of the Menkes gene... *Nature Genet* 1994, **6**:374–378.
Tümer Z, Tønnesen T *et al*: Detection Sf genetic defects in Menkes disease... *J Inher Metab Dis* 1994, **17**:267–270 +
First trimester prenatal diagnosis of Menkes disease... *J Med Genet* 1994, **31**:615–617.

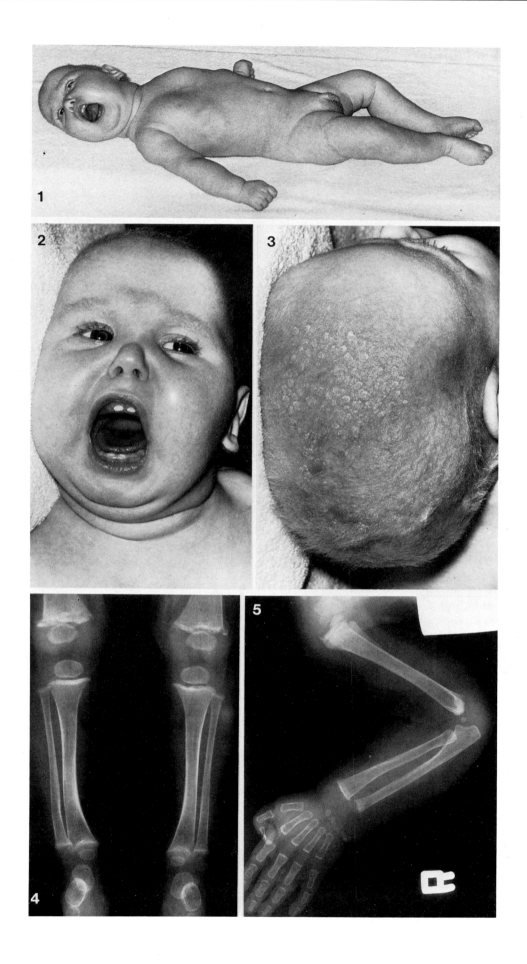

60 Glycogen Storage Disease Type 1
(sometimes also referred to as von Gierke Syndrome)

A hereditary metabolic disease with, when treatment is inadequate or delayed, possible unusual facies, growth failure and markedly protuberant abdomen.

Main signs:
- Unusual facies (best defined as a Rubens or doll face) in some cases (1, 2, 4, 5).
- Very small stature.
- Protuberant abdomen as a result of liver enlargement (3). Hyperlordosis when standing.
- Mental retardation due to hypoglycemia and hypoglycemic seizures.
- Poorly developed hypotonic musculature (3).

Supplementary findings: Acidotic respiration.
Bleeding tendency.
Enlarged kidneys; hepatoma.
Osteoporosis.
Kidney stones, xanthomas, gouty tophi and arthritis.
Fasting hypoglycemia unresponsive to glucagon or adrenaline; elevated lactate, pyruvate, triglycerides, phospholipids, cholesterol and uric acid.

Manifestation: At birth. Growth retardation apparent in late infancy. Xanthomas, gouty tophi and arthritis usually not until adulthood.

Aetiology: Autosomal recessive disease; glucose-6-phosphatase deficiency in the liver, kidneys and mucosa of the small intestines.

Frequency: Low (approximately one out of 400 000).

Diagnosis: By determination of glucose-6-phosphatase activity in a liver biopsy and detection of glycogen deposition in the liver parenchyma.

Course, prognosis: Average life expectancy somewhat reduced because of the metabolic state with lactic acidosis, later by gouty nephritis. Progression of liver enlargement probably limited to childhood.

Treatment: Frequent carbohydrate-rich meals; at night, constant gastric-tube feeding. Alkalization in stress situations during the first years of life; timely antibiotic treatment of bacterial infections; allopurinol to reduce uric acid levels. Liver transplantation has not proved successful.

Illustrations:
1–3 Patient 1 aged 18 months. Delayed development; height deficit 11 cm.
4 and 5 Patient 2 aged 18 months. Height deficit 9 cm. Hypoglycemic seizures up to the sixth year of life. Liver at the level of the umbilicus. Follow-up at age 10 years: no further relative liver enlargement. Height deficit now 13 cm.

References:
Scriver C R, Beaudet A L, Sly W S, Valle D: The metabolic basis of inherited disease. 6. Ed. New York: McGraw-Hill 1989.
Wolfsdorf J I, Crigler J F Jr: Biochemical evidence for the requirement of continuous glucose therapy in young adults with type I glycogen storage disease. *J Inher Metab Dis* 1994, 17:234–242.

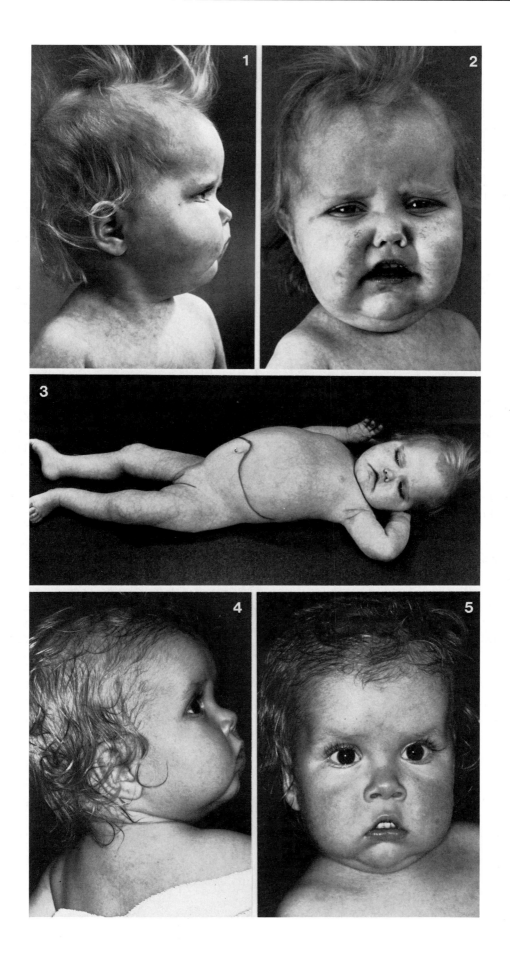

J.K.

An autosomal recessive sphingolipidosis with different clinical forms, characterized by a protruding abdomen due to hepatosplenomegaly, neurological complications of variable severity, cherry-red spot of the retina, thin extremities and growth deficiency.

Main signs:

Type A (acute form with neurological complications): large abdomen as a result of hepatosplenomegaly, feeding difficulties, progressive psychomotor decline within the first to second year of life, thin extremities, yellow–brown discoloration of the skin, cherry-red spot in the macula (50%), corneal clouding, muscular hypotonia. Storage cells in the bone marrow, spleen, adrenal glands and lungs.

Type B (chronic form without neurological complications): enlargement first of the spleen, then of the liver; normal intellect; short stature; dyspnoea; recurrent lung infections.

Type C (chronic form with neurological complications): manifestation after the third year of life; then, regression of speech and intellect, ataxia, grand mal seizures, muscular hypotonia, hyper-reflexia, cholestasis.

Type D (Nova Scotia variant): similar to type C, progressive psychomotor deterioration between the second and fifth years, hepatosplenomegaly, impaired co-ordination, seizures.

Type E (adult form without neurological complications): moderate hepatosplenomegaly (late-onset type C?).

Type F ('sea-blue histiocytosis' is ophthalmoplegic neurolipidosis): hepatosplenomegaly, dementia, ataxia, supranuclear vertical ophthalmoplegia: partial to complete loss of voluntary vertical eye movement, especially downward, as well as vertical optokinetic nystagmus. Analogous horizontal limitations and restricted convergence. Intact: vestibular reflexes, fundus and electroretinogram.

Supplementary findings: *Spleen:* mild haematological sequelae with microcytic anaemia, thrombocytopaenia. *Liver:* slight elevation of SGOT, SGPT and alkaline phosphatase, especially in type B. *Lymph nodes:* enlarged in the mesentery, in the hilum of the spleen, liver and lungs. Thymus and tonsils are infiltrated with storage cells. *Bones:* osteoporosis, coxa valga, dilated medullary spaces in the long bones and metacarpals. *Heart:* endocardial fibro-elastosis. *Lungs:* diffuse reticular and finely nodular infiltrations. *Central nervous system:* atrophy (types A and C up to 50–90% of the normal weight), disorganization of cortical structures, of the basal ganglia, brain stem, spinal cord and spinal ganglia. *Further organs:* special storage cells in the bone marrow: with

May–Grünwald–Giemsa stain numerous large, partly binucleated cells with light, vacuolated cytoplasm and frequently with one or more dark-coloured dense inclusion bodies barely the size of erythrocytes. Less numerous, somewhat smaller storage cells with blue–green cytoplasmic granules ('sea-blue' cytoplasm), which although not specific, suggest type F disease.

Manifestation: Sometimes biochemically diagnosable prenatally, otherwise from birth or after manifestation. *Type A:* organomegaly after the sixth month of life, retardation after 1 year. *Type B:* organomegaly somewhat later than in Type A. *Type C:* neonatal hepatitis with splenomegaly. Hepatomegaly, cholestasia, supranuclear ophthalmoplegia and mental deterioration after the second year. *Type D:* organ and CNS involvement between the second and fourth years. *Type E:* adult form. *Type F:* in the first decade.

Aetiology: Autosomal recessive inheritance. Possible intragenetic and intergenetic heterogeneity. Impaired sphingomyelinase activity in type A (only 10% of normal activity), activity in type B slightly higher than in type A; activity in type C 38–63%, in types D and E normal to elevated. Gene locus for type A: 11p15.4-15.1.

Frequency: Over 100 patients known; of these, 85% type A in Ashkenazi Jews. Type D endemic in Nova Scotia. The opthalmological neurolipidosis has been documented in 39 patients to date.

Course, prognosis: *Type A:* death before the fourth year of life from pneumonia. *Type B:* endangered by pneumonias. *Type C and D:* death between the fifth and 15th years. *Type E:* unknown. *Type F:* death from pneumonia in 12 patients between the fifth and 29th years.

Treatment: No specific therapy. Splenectomy for cosmetic or mechanical indications or in case of hypersplenism. Genetic counselling. Prenatal diagnosis for types A and B only.

Illustrations:

1 A patient, 3 years and 6 months old, with marked hepatosplenomegaly (fundi: 'red spot'). Possibly a mild expression of type A.

2 A younger sibling; **2a** Caput medusae, lipid storage in the skin.

3 A mentally retarded patient, aged 6, with type F. **3a** Paralysis of vertical eye movement.

References:

Boltshauser E, Hanefeld F *et al*: Ophthalmoplegische Neurolipidose. In: Aktuelle Neuropädiatrie 1981, 2:258–270.

Pentchev P G *et al*: A defect of cholesterol esterification in Niemann–Pick disease (type C) patients. *Proc Nat Acad Sci* 1985, **82**:8247–8251.

Kelly D A, Portman B *et al*: Niemann–Pick disease type C: diagnosis and outcome in children, with particular reference to liver disease. *J Pediatr* 1993, **123**:242–247.

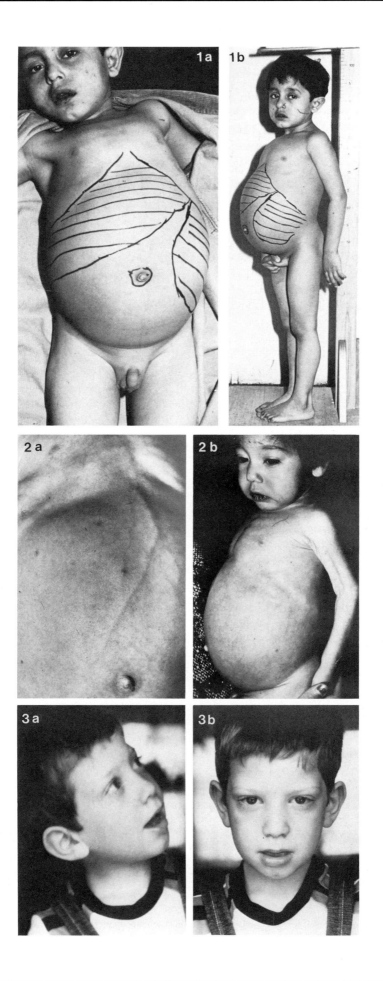

J.K.

Autosomal recessive glucosylceramide lipidoses of the infantile, juvenile and Norrbottnian types.

Main signs:
Type II, Acute Neuropathic Form: Infantile Type. Hepatosplenomegaly, approximately 6 months later neurological complications: cranial nerve and extrapyramidal signs. Trismus, strabismus and retroflexion of the head form the typical triad. Feeding difficulties and problems with secretions due to uncoordinated movements of the oropharynx. Progressive spasticity, hyperreflexia, pathological reflexes. Rarely seizures. Eventual generalized muscular hypotonia and apathy. Recurrent pneumonias.
Type III, Subacute Neuropathic Form: Juvenile Type. Hepatosplenomegaly, then spasticity, ophthalmoplegia, ataxia, retardation, seizures.
Norrbottnian Type. Clinical course in five stages. Growth retardation after the first year of life (-1 to -5 SD), thoracic kyphosis, hip pain, fractures of the neck of the femur, other fractures of the bones, moderate to excessive splenomegaly, abdominal pain with episodes of unexplained fever, hepatomegaly, hyperplasia of the lymph nodes, dyspnoea (due to enlarged spleen), irregular pigmentation of the areas of skin exposed to sun, intellectual retardation after the first year of life, disorder of fine and coarse movements, spastic paraparesis, seizures, oculomotor apraxia, mild hearing defect.

Supplementary findings: Foam cells with cytoplasm of 'wrinkled paper' appearance and eccentric nuclei of varied size, demonstrable in all organs: in the reticuloendothelial system, in the red splenic pulp, in the sinusoids of the liver and lymph nodes, in alveolar capillaries, in bone marrow, in the adventitia of arterioles, in veins and lymph vessels and capillaries; also in the pancreas, the thyroid and the adrenalglands.
Norrbottnian Type: radiologically, decrease of the cortex and Erlenmeyer flask deformity of the distal femur, vertebral compression, acute cystic necrosis of the head of the femur, also of the trochanter. Shortly before death, fine granular pulmonary markings. Microcytic normochromic anaemia, leukopaenia, thrombocytopaenia, epistaxis, petechiae, decreased factors V, VII–XII. Gaucher cells in bone marrow. Abnormal electroencephalogram.

Manifestation: *Type II:* third to 18th month; *Type III:* late infancy to adulthood; *Norrbottnian Type:* birth to 14th year of life.

Aetiology: The most frequent autosomal recessive storage disease of glycolipid metabolism due to subnormal activities of glucocerebrosidase. Intragenetic heterogeneity. Interestingly, the Norrbottnian Type may run different courses within the same family. Molecular genetic and therefore prenatal diagnosis of all types is possible.

Frequency: *Type I (167):* one out of 2500 births among the Ashkenazi Jews; *Type II:* less frequent than Type I, worldwide; *Type III:* less frequent than Type I, worldwide; *Norrbottnian Type:* Northern Sweden, 22 patients to date.

Course, prognosis: *Type II:* death during the first 3 years of life. *Type III:* death between the sixth and 12th years of life. *Norrbottnian Type:* death in the first to third decades, in isolated cases later.
  Cause of death: recurrent infections, pneumonias.

Treatment: See Type I (*167*) but no splenectomy, unless before bone marrow transplantation. Prenatal diagnosis possible.

Illustrations:
1 and 2 Child barely 1 year old with hepatomegaly and Type II. Oculomotor apraxia, amimia.

References:
Dreborg S, Erikson A, Hagberg B: Gaucher disease—Norrbottnian type. I. General clinical description. *Eur J Pediatr* 1980, **133**:107–118.
Blom S, Erikson A: Gaucher disease—Norrbottnian type. Neurodevelopmental, neurological and neurophysiological aspects. *Eur J Pediatr* 1983, **140**:316–322.
Rappaport J M, Ginns E I: Bone-marrow transplantation in severe Gaucher's disease. *N Engl J Med* 1985, **311**:84–88.
Zlotogora J *et al*: Genetic heterogeneity in Gaucher disease. *J Med Genet* 1986, **23**:319–322.
Erikson E: Gaucher disease—Norrbottnian type (III). *Acta Paediatr Scand Suppl* 1986, **326**:1–42.
Beaudet A L: Gaucher's disease. *N Engl J Med* 1987, **316**:619–621.
Hobbs J R, Hugh Jones K, Shaw P J *et al*: Beneficial effect of pre-transplant splenectomy on displacement bone marrow transplantation for Gaucher's disease. *Lancet* 1987, I:1111–1115.
Tsuji S, Choudary P V, Martin B M *et al*: A mutation in the human glucocerebrosidase gene in neuronopathic Gaucher's disease. *N Engl J Med* 1987, **316**:570–575.
Lewis B D, Nelson P V, Robertson E F, Morris C P: Mutation analysis of 28 Gaucher disease patients: the Australian experience. *Am J Med Genet* 1994, **49**:218–223.

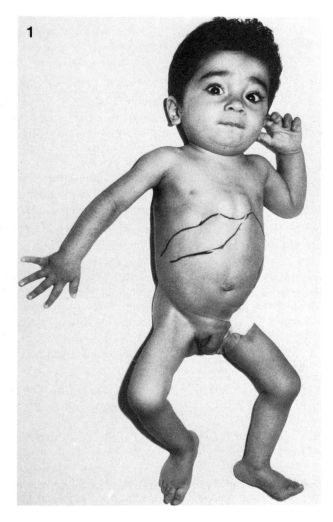

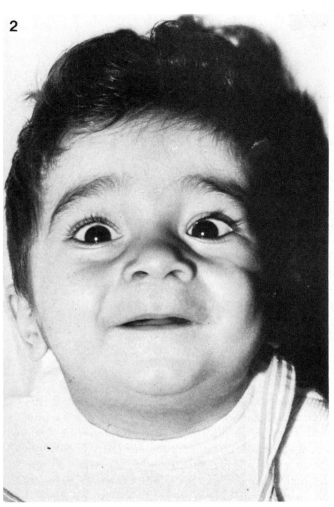

63 GM₂ Gangliosidoses: Tay–Sachs Disease and Sandhoff's Disease

J.K.

Tay–Sachs disease and Sandhoff's disease are autosomal recessive GM₂ gangliosidoses with hexosaminidase defects, rapid psychomotor deterioration, hypotonia to generalized paralysis and eventual spasticity, deafness, blindness, seizures and cherry-red spot of the macula.

Main signs:

- Increasing muscular weakness after the third month of life, startle reflex in response to noise, progressive psychomotor decline, loss of sitting and standing reflexes.
- After 18 months of age in Tay–Sachs patients, or earlier in Sandhoff's patients, progressive deafness, blindness, seizures, pareses, spasticity.
- Doll-like face with pale translucent skin, long eyelashes, fine hair and unusual pink facial colouring.
- Cherry-red spot in the macular region in over 95% of patients.
- Mild hepatosplenomegaly in Sandhoff's disease patients.

Supplementary findings: Vomiting, starting in early infancy and increasing; recurrent pneumonias; progressive macrocephaly after the 16th month of life, as a result of cerebral gliosis (probably less as a result of ventricular enlargement). Lipidosis of the cortical, autonomic and rectal mucosa neurons with ballooning of the cytoplasm and peripherally displaced nucleus. Central demyelinization, cortical gliosis. No pathological changes of the visceral organs in Tay–Sachs disease, slight hepatosplenomegaly in Sandhoff's disease.

Manifestation: Biochemically, after birth. Clinically, earliest signs between the third and sixth months of life.

Aetiology: Tay–Sachs disease is an autosomal recessive disorder caused by hexosaminidase A deficiency. Hexosaminidase A consists of two non-identical subunits, the alpha chain, coded by a locus on chromosome 15 and the beta chain, coded by a locus on chromosome 5. Mutations of the alpha locus on chromosome 15 lead to Tay–Sachs disease or the juvenile or adult form of GM₂ gangliosidosis. Mutations of the beta locus on chromosome 5 lead to Sandhoff's disease. At present, 11 forms of GM₂ gangliosidosis are known (six hexosaminidase A mutants, three hexosaminidase B mutants and two activator mutants). The gene for Sandhoff's disease is located on the long arm of chromosome 5; for Tay–Sachs disease, on the long arm of chromosome 15 (15q23-24).

Frequency: Tay–Sachs disease: thousands of patients known, especially among Ashkenazi Jews, for whom the heterozygote frequency is one out of 25. Approximately 100 patients with Sandhoff's disease known.

Diagnosis: Demonstration of decreased activity of hexosaminidase A and/or B in serum, leukocytes or fibroblast cultures. Demonstration of heterozygosity possible. Prenatal diagnosis.

Course, prognosis: As a rule, patients die by about the third year of life of recurrent pneumonias.

Treatment: Symptomatic. Genetic counselling, contraception, prenatal diagnosis. Screening programmes to identify heterozygotes especially important for Ashkenazi Jews.

Illustrations:

1 A 16-month-old child with Sandhoff's disease. Exaggerated startle response, especially for acoustic stimuli. Increasing spasticity of the flexors of the upper extremities and extensors of the lower extremities.
2a–c A 1-year-old, severely retarded and hypotonic girl with Tay–Sachs. 'Doll' face; long eyelashes. Hyperacusis. Red spot.

References:

Schulte F J: Clinical course of GM₂ gangliosidoses. A correlative attempt. *Neuropediatrics* 1984, 15:Suppl, 66–70.
Pampiglione G, Harden A: Neurophysiological investigations in GM₁ and GM₂ gangliosioses. *Neuropediatrics* 1984, 15:Suppl 74–84.
Sandhoff K, Conzelmann E: The biochemical basis of gangliosioses. *Neuropediatrics* 1984, 15:Suppl 85–92.
Grebner E E, Jackson L G: Prenatal diagnosis for Tay–Sachs disease using chorionic villus sampling. *Prenat Diagn* 1985, 5:305–321.
McKusick K B, Schach S R, Koeslag J H: Social mechanism in the population genetics of Tay–Sachs and other lethal autosomal recessive disease: a computer simulation model. *Am J Med Genet* 1990, 36:178–182.

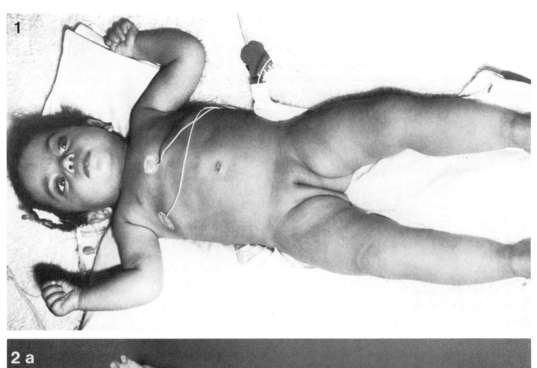

1

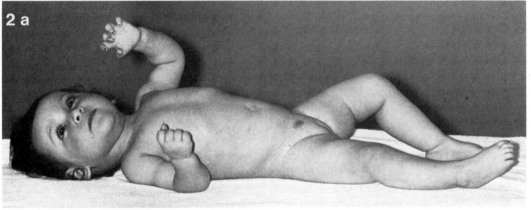

2 a

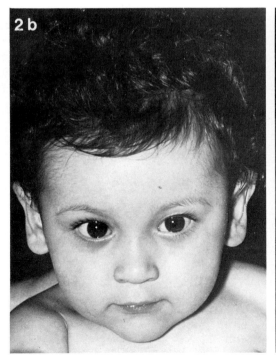

2 b

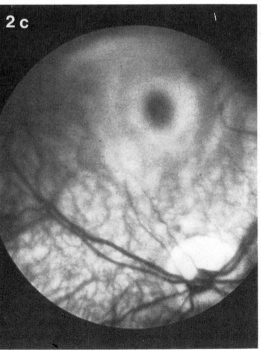

2 c

64 Mucopolysaccharidosis Type I-H
(Hurler Syndrome, Pfaundler–Hurler Disease)

H.-R.W/ J.K.

An autosomal recessive mucopolysaccharide storage disease, which leads to the development of typical facial dysmorphism, short stature, dementia, corneal clouding and hepatosplenomegaly.

Main signs:
- Characteristic facies with low, flat nasal bridge; broad tip of the nose; large nares; hypertelorism; exophthalmos; corneal clouding; thick, pouting lips (**1–4**); large tongue; widely spaced teeth; hypertrophy of the alveolar processes and gums (**8**). Macrocephaly (**6**). Abundant, thick scalp hair (**1 and 2**). Increasing dementia.
- Growth deficiency after initial normal growth in early infancy; short neck; gibbus (**4, 6**).
- Joint contractures (**3**), claw hands (**7**), broad stubby feet. Indurations of the skin and cartilage.
- Protruding abdomen, diastasis recti, hernias.

Supplementary findings: Chronic purulent rhinitis. Abundant lanugo-like body hair.

Heart: valvular defects, enlargement, failure.

Progressive changes of bony structure and form as in dysostosis multiplex: osteoporosis with coarse trabeculations, thickened skull, broad ribs and clavicles, crudely formed scapulae, oval and partly hook-shaped vertebral bodies; broadening and shortening of the long bones (**5**). Dysplasia of the pelvis.

Intracranial pressure frequently increased due to interference with circulation of the cerebrospinal fluid as a result of mucopolysaccharide deposits in the meninges. Increased levels of chondroitin sulphate B and heparan sulphate in the urine; alpha-L-iduronidase in the tissues decreased or not demonstrable.

Manifestation: Biochemically, from birth on; radiologically, the first months of life; clinically, from six months onwards.

Aetiology: Autosomal recessive disease. The above-mentioned mucopolysaccharides are not degraded because of absence of alpha-iduronidase but are stored in various organs, which leads to functional and morphological anomalies of these organs. Gene locus: 4p16.3.

Frequency: Approximately one out of 100 000.

Course, prognosis: Progression until death in the second decade of life (infection, heart failure or aspiration).

Differential diagnosis: The Hunter's syndrome (mucopolysaccaridosis type II) (*65*) affects only males. It is clinically similar but more slowly manifest and milder (however, with relatively early hearing impairment), usually runs a more prolonged course and, as a rule, shows no corneal clouding.

Treatment: Symptomatic. Prevention by means of prenatal diagnosis.

Comment: Alpha-L-iduronidase deficiency can, in addition to the above-described classic Hurler phenotype (mucopolysaccharidosis I-H), also lead to Scheie disease (mucopolysaccharidosis I-S), to Hurler–Scheie variant (mucopolysaccharidosis I-H/S) and to further phenotypes, which are (all?) presumably due to allelic mutations of the same gene. Patients with Scheie disease are of normal height and mental development; they first come to attention in the second decade of life because of joint contractures, impaired vision and corneal clouding. The Hurler–Scheie variant shows an intermediate phenotype.

Illustrations:

1–5 Patient 1 at age 5 years. Height 93 cm (50th percentile for a girl 32 months old), marked dementia, pronounced hepatomegaly.

6 Patient 2 at age 15 months. Height 85 cm (97th percentile), head circumference 52.5 cm (50th percentile for a 10-year-old boy). Hepatomegaly. Bilateral inguinal hernia.

7 and 8 Patient 3. Hand and oral cavity at age 32 months.

References:
Spranger J W, Langer L O Jr, Wiedemann H-R: Bone dysplasias. An atlas of constitutional disorders of skeletal development. Stuttgart and Philadelphia: G Fischer and W B Saunders 1974.
McKusick V A: Heritable disorders of connective tissue. Mosby Saint Louis 1979.
Mueller O T, Shows B et al: Apparent allelism of the Hurler, Scheie and Hurler/Scheie syndromes. *Am J Hum Genet* 1984, **18**:547–556.
Roubicek M, Gehler J et al: The clinical spectrum of alpha-L-iduronidase deficiency. *Am J Hum Genet* 1985, **20**:471–481.
Whitley C B, Gorlin R J et al: A non-pathologic allele (I^W) for low alpha-L-iduronidase enzyme activity vis-a-vis prenatal diagnosis of Hurler syndrome. *Am J Hum Genet* 1987, **28**:233–243.
Spranger J: Mini review: Inborn errors of complex carbohydrate metabolism. *Am J Hum Genet* 1987, **28**:489–499.
Scott H S, Ashton L J et al: Chromosomal localization of the human alpha-L-iduronidase gene (IDUA) to 4p16.3. *Am J Hum Genet* 1990, **47**:802–807.
Beck M, Fang-Kircher S: Mukopolysaccharidosen. Stuttgart, Jena, New York: G Fischer 1993.

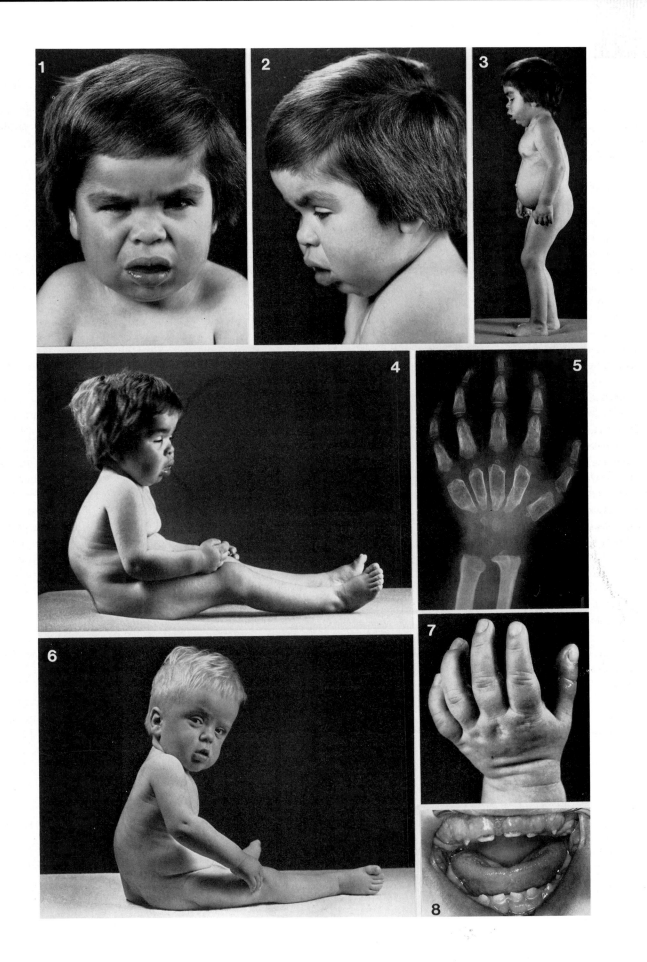

J.K. /H.-R.W

A mucopolysaccharide storage disease exclusively in males and leading to a relatively typical facial dysmorphism, early hearing impairment, hepatosplenomegaly, short stature and generally severe mental retardation.

Main signs:
- Coarse facial features, similar to, but not as pronounced as in Hurler's disease, with broad low nose, hypertelorism, 'full' cheeks, thick lips, large tongue, widely spaced teeth and macrocephaly (**4 and 5**). Impaired hearing beginning in early childhood. NB: usually no corneal clouding. Irritability, mental retardation or dementia (not with type B; see below).
- Short stature after transiently normal growth in the first year or two of life; short neck.
- Joint contractures (**1 and 2**), claw hands (**3**). Induration, usually nodular, of skin and cartilage.
- Pes cavus, hernias (**1 and 2**), diastasis recti. Protuberant abdomen (**2**).

Supplementary findings: Chronic suppurative rhinitis. Hepatosplenomegaly.
Heart: valvular defects, enlargement, cardiac failure.
Changes of bony form and structure as in Hurler syndrome, however, less severe at a given age. Pseudoarthrosis of the femoral head (type B). Increased intracranial pressure from impaired circulation of the cerebrospinal fluid, seldom progressive.
Increased heparan sulphate and chondroitin sulphate B detectable in the urine.

Manifestation: Biochemically, from birth; clinically after the end of the first year of life.

Aetiology: X-linked recessive disease. Gene localized to the long arm of the X chromosome (Xq28). Decreased activity of the enzyme iduronate sulphatase results in storage of mucopolysaccharides in the cells of various organs and thus to anomalies of their functions and morphologies.

Frequency: Approximately one out of 50 000.

Course, prognosis: Slowly progressive in the first years of life. After the fourth or fifth year of life, two forms can be distinguished by their different courses: *Type A*, rapidly progressive with death before the 15th year of life. *Type B*, slowly progressive and with only slight or no noticeable mental impairment and death (usually from cardiac failure) in adulthood. The oldest known patient lived to be 60 years old.

Differential diagnosis: Mucopolysaccharidosis type I-H (*64*).

Treatment: Symptomatic. Genetic counselling. Biochemical identification of the female carriers and prenatal diagnosis possible.

Illustrations:
1–5 Patient (type A) at age 5 years (**1, 2, 4**) and 4 years (**3, 5**). Psychomotor development normal up to 18 months of age; thereafter, developmental standstill. At 111 cm, height still normal. Liver four fingerbreadths below the costal margin. At 5 years and 9 months, a shunt operation for increased intracranial pressure.

References:
Spranger J W, Langer L O Jr, Wiedemann H-R: Bone dyplasias. An atlas of constitutional disorders of skeletal development. Stuttgart and Philadelphia: G Fischer and W B Saunders 1974.
McKusick V A: Heritable disorders of connective tissue. Saint Louis: Mosby 1979.
Young J D, Harper P S *et al*: A clinical and genetic study of Hunter's syndrome. 1. Heterogeneity. *J Med Genet* 1982, 19:401–407.
Archer I M, Young I D *et al*: Carrier detection in Hunter syndrome. *Am J Med Genet* 1983, 16:61–69.
Lykkelund C, Søndergaard F *et al*: Feasibility of first trimester prenatal diagnosis of Hunter syndrome. *Lancet* 1983, II:1147.
Kleijer W J, Diggelen O P van *et al*: First trimester diagnosis of Hunter syndrome... *Lancet* 1984, II:472.
Zlotogora J, Bach G: Heterozygote detection in Hunter syndrome. *Am J Med Genet* 1984, 17:661–665.
Wilson P J, Suthers G K *et al*: Frequent deletions at Xq28 indicate genetic heterogeneity in Hunter syndrome. *Hum Genet* 1991, 86:505–508.
Beck M, Fang-Kircher S: Mukopolysaccharidosen. Stuttgart, Jena, New York: G Fischer 1993.

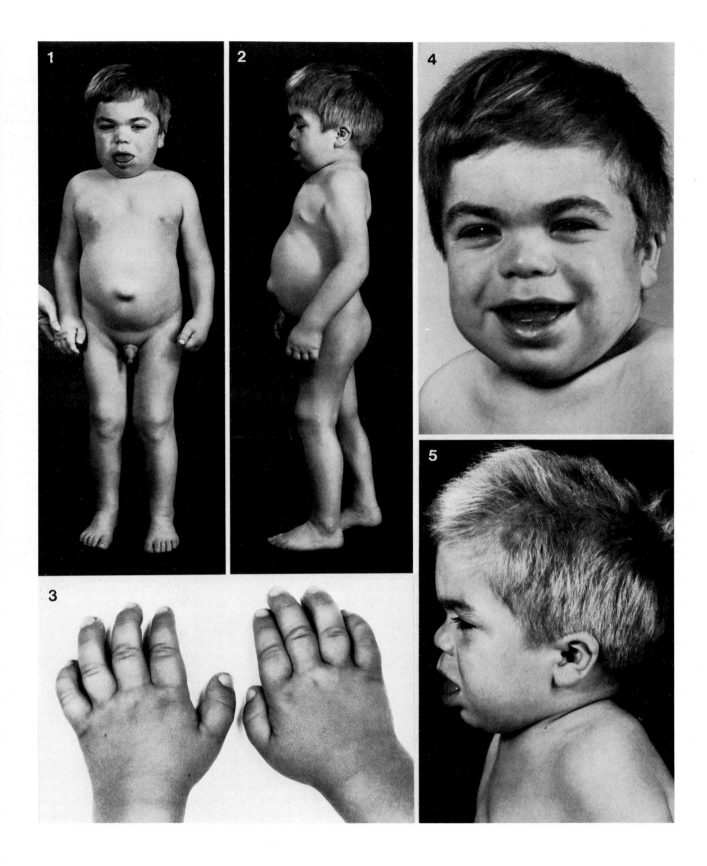

66 Mucopolysaccharidosis Type III
(Sanfilippo Syndrome)

J.K. /H.-R.W

An autosomal recessive mucopolysaccharide storage disease, which leads to a coarsening of the facial features, to behavioural disturbances and dementia and to hepatomegaly.

Main signs:
- Flat nasal bridge; full pouting lips; enlarged tongue; generally coarsened facial features, which in older children are reminiscent of those in Hurler syndrome. Abundant coarse scalp hair; thick bushy eyebrows, sometimes with synophrys (1–5).
- Increasing irritability, aggressiveness, dementia.
- Up to the 10th year of life, above-average height; thereafter, slowing of growth.
- NB: no corneal clouding.

Supplementary findings: Hepatosplenomegaly. Broad dental laminae. Occasionally, umbilical or inguinal hernias, decreased joint mobility. Increased susceptibility to infections. Sleep disorders. Optic atrophy in isolated cases.

Changes of bony structure and form similar to those of mucopolysaccaridosis I-H but much less severe. Increased excretion of the mucopolysaccharide, heparan sulphate in the urine.

Manifestation: Biochemically, from birth; clinically, by behavioural disturbance and mental retardation, usually after the third year and by somatic signs after the fourth or fifth year of life.

Aetiology: Autosomal recessive disease. Heterogeneity. The largely uniform clinical picture is based on the absence of one of the following enzymes: heparan sulphate sulphatase (Sanfilippo syndrome type A), alpha-N-acetylglucosaminidase (type B), acetyl CoA: alpha-glucosaminide-N-acetyltransferase (type C), or N-acetyl-glucosaminide-6-sulphatase (type D). Patients with type A disease are somewhat more severely affected than those with type B (earlier manifestation, more rapid progression); those with type C appear to take an intermediate course. Gene locus type III D: 12q14.

Frequency: Approximately one out of 30 000.

Course, prognosis: Characterized by rapid loss of mental and motor abilities, so that meaningful communication becomes impossible by 6–10 years of age. Spastic tetraplegia with dysphagia in the terminal phase. Death, usually as the result of pneumonia, in the second decade of life.

Treatment: Symptomatic. Genetic counselling. Prenatal diagnosis possible.

Illustrations:
1 and 2 Patient 1, aged 7 years: macrocephaly (head circumference 55.5 cm). Height 138 cm (average height of a 10-year-old girl). IQ 38 (Kramer–Binet). Mild joint contractures.
3–5 Patient 2 aged 3 years. Head circumference, height and psychomotor development still within normal limits. Hepatomegaly. Biochemically type B. Note that the facial features of the younger patient more closely resemble those of Hurler syndrome than do those of patient 1.

References:

Spranger J W, Langer L O Jr, Wiedemann H-R: Bone dyplasias. *An atlas of constitutional disorders of skeletal development.* Stuttgart and Philadelphia: G Fischer and W B Saunders 1974.
McKusick V A: Heritable disorders of connective tissue. Saint Louis: Mosby 1979.
Kleijer W J, Janse H C *et al*: First-trimester diagnosis of mucopolysaccharidosis III A... *N Engl J Med* 1986, **314**:185–186.
Kaplan P, Wolfe L S: Sanfilippo syndrome type D. *J Pediatr* 1987, **110**, 267–271.
Spranger J: Mini review: inborn errors of complex carbohydrate metabolism. *Am J Med Genet* 1987, **28**:489–499.
Toone J R, Applegarth D A: Carrier detection in Sanfilippo A syndrome. *Clin Genet* 1988, **33**:410–403.
Sewell A C, Pontz B F *et al*: Mucopolysaccharidosis type III C (Sanfilippo)... *Clin Genet* 1988, **34**:116–121.
Turki I, Kresse H, Scotto J *et al*: Sanfilippo disease, type C... *Neuropediatrics* 1989, **20**:90–92.
Beck M, Fang-Kirchner S: Mukopolysaccharidosen. Stuttgart, Jena, New York: G Fischer 1993.

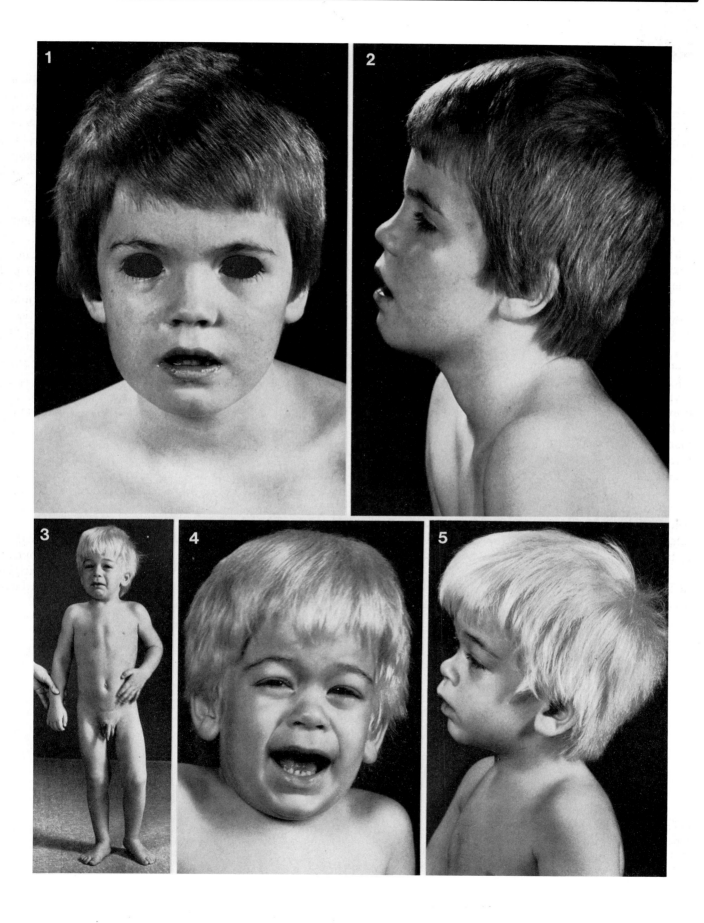

67 Mucopolysaccharidosis Type IV
(Morquio–Brailsford Syndrome, Morquio Syndrome)

J.K. /H.-R.W

A mucopolysaccharide storage disease, which, in its classic form, leads to a relatively typical facial dysmorphism, marked disproportionate short stature, joint dysplasia, corneal clouding and generally to a characteristic clinical picture.

Main signs:
- Moderately coarse facial features with macrostomia, short nose and prominent jaw (**1 and 2**). Corneal clouding, dental caries, grey–blue discoloration of the teeth as a result of enamel hypoplasia.
- Usually severe growth deficiency, especially of the trunk, with a very short neck (**1 and 2**). Head held in dorsiflexion. Pectus carinatum, flaring of the lower rib cage, kyphoscoliosis (gibbus).
- Swelling and limitation of movement at the joints with malpositioning (e.g. ulnar deviation of the hands, pronounced knock-knees), hyperextensibility of the finger joints and instability of the vertebral ligaments. Hands and feet short and stubby.

Supplementary findings: Normal intelligence.
Inguinal hernias. Inelastic, indurated skin. Progressive hearing impairment starting in the first decade of life or thereafter.
Aortic regurgitation.
Changes in bony form and structure similar to those of Hurler syndrome but with more marked changes in the epiphyses and more severe generalized platyspondyly.
Hypoplasia or aplasia of the odontoids.
Increased urinary excretion of the mucopolysaccharides, keratin sulphate and chondroitin-4-sulphate; a tendency to normalization with increasing age in this respect.

Manifestation: Biochemically, from birth; radiologically, in mid-infancy; clinically, from the second to third year of life. Corneal clouding not recognizable without a slit lamp before the age of 10 years.

Aetiology: Autosomal recessive disorder. Heterogeneity. Deficiency of galactosamine-6-sulphate-sulphatase (type A) or beta-galactosidase (type B).

Frequency: Estimated at approximately one out of 100 000.

Course, prognosis: Progression of signs and symptoms. Attainable adult height usually not greater than 1.20 m. Average life expectancy shortened by heart failure and especially as a result of compression of the medulla oblongata and the spinal cord. Life expectancy, which in the past was about 20 years, has been considerably prolonged since the introduction of therapy.

Differential diagnosis: Includes the other mucopolysaccharidoses, especially Hurler syndrome (*64*), which, however, shows mental retardation or dementia, early corneal clouding, a different pattern of mucopolysaccharide excretion in the urine, etc.
Also, differentiation from the skeletal dysplasias especially with severe involvement of the vertebral column [see spondyloepiphyseal dysplasia congenita (*136*); metatrophic dysplasia (*133*); osteodysplasia type Kniest (*138*)].

Treatment: No specific therapy known. Fusion of the upper cervical vertebrae no later than the fifth year of life. Orthopaedic measures. Replacement of the aortic valve may be considered. Hearing aids may be indicated. Psychological care and guidance.

Illustrations:
1 and 2 A 14-year-old patient. Increased excretion of keratan sulphate.

References:
Spranger J W, Langer L O jr, Wiedemann H-R: Bone dyplasias. An atlas of constitutional disorders of skeletal development. Stuttgart and Philadelphia: G Fischer and W B Saunders 1974.
McKusick V A: Heritable disorders of connective tissue. Saint Louis: Mosby, 1979.
Holzgreve W, Gröbe H, v Figura K *et al*: Morquio syndrome: clinical findings in 11 patients with MPS IV A and 2 patients with MPS IV B. *Hum Genet* 1981, 57:360.
Fujimoto A, Horwitz A L: Biochemical efect of non-keratan-sulfate-excreting Morquio syndrome. *Am J Med Genet* 1983, 15:265–273.
Heckt J T, Scott Ch I jr *et al*: Mild manifestations of the Morquio syndrome. *Am J Med Genet* 1984, 18:369–371.
Beck M, Glössl J *et al*: Heterogeneity of Morquio disease. *Clin Genet* 1986, 29:325–331.
Spranger J: Mini review: inborn errors of complex carbohydrate metabolism. *Am J Med Genet* 1987, 28:489–499.
Nelson J *et al*: Clinical findings in 12 patients with MPS IV A... *Clin Genet* 1988, 33:111–130.
Beck M, Fang-Kirchner S: Mukopolysaccharidosen. Stuttgart, Jena, New York: G Fischer 1993.

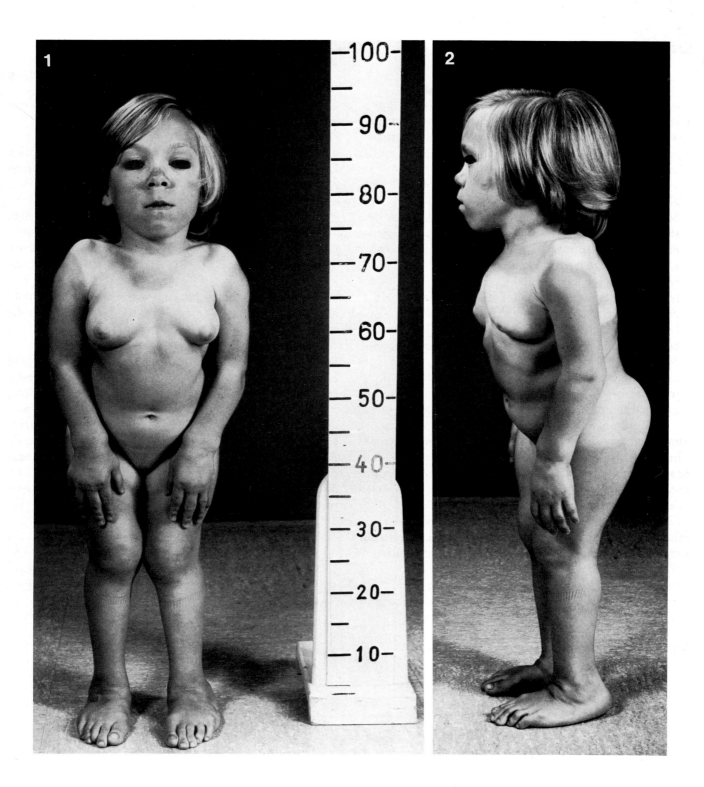

68 Mucopolysaccharidosis Type VI

(Maroteaux–Lamy Syndrome, Polydystrophic Dysplasia)

J.K.

An autosomal recessive mucopolysaccharide storage disease distinguished by characteristic facial changes, corneal clouding, short stature and hearing impairment with normal intelligence.

Main signs:
- Hurler-like facial dysmorphism with large nose; thick lips, low nasal bridge; corneal clouding; macroglossia; widely spaced, late erupting teeth; macrocephaly. Normal intelligence.
- Growth deficiency with increasing curvature of the spine; prominent sternum.
- Mild joint contractures (claw hands).
- Hearing defects of various degrees of severity.
- Large abdomen with hepatosplenomegaly; hernias.

The complete picture resembles that of mucopolysaccharidosis Type I.

Supplementary findings: Recurrent infections of the respiratory tract, diarrhoea, cardiac complications.

Manifestation: The severe form, type A, can be recognized at the end of the first year of life (humpback when sitting). The milder form, type B, is frequently only diagnosed between the sixth and 10th years of life on the basis of growth retardation.

Aetiology: Autosomal recessive disorder with arylsulphatase B deficiency. Intragenetic heterogeneity. Gene localized to the long arm of chromosome 5 (5q13.3).

Frequency: Less than one out of 100 000 births.

Course, prognosis: Patients with the mild form (type B) survive into the third decade of life and longer. They frequently die of cardiac complications. Patients with the more severe form (type A) begin to deteriorate in late infancy and have severe deformities by 3–6 years of age. Exact data on the course after the 10th year of life are poorly documented.

Differential diagnosis: In the late phase, especially mucopolysaccharidosis type I-H (Hurler, 64) but also the other mucopolysaccharidoses (65–67).

Treatment: Symptomatic corrective measures. Treatment of respiratory infections. Prenatal diagnosis and genetic counselling.

Illustrations:
1a and b Patient 1 at age 11 months. Type A clinically diagnosed from the kyphosis apparent when the child was sitting. Facial features not yet remarkable.
2a Patient 2 at age 15 years with hyperlordosis and curvature of the thoracic spine.
2b Hurler-like facies, normal intelligence.
2c Short stature.

References:

Gehler J: Phänotyp bei Heteroglykanosen und Sphingolipidosen. *Monatsschr Kinderheilkd* 1981, **129**:610–620.
Kresse H, Cantz M, von Figura K *et al*: The mucopolysaccharidoses: biochemistry and clinical symptoms. *Klin Wochenschr* 1981, **59**:867–876.
Pilz H, von Figura K, Goebel H H: Deficiency of arylsulfatase B in 2 brothers aged 40 and 38 years (Maroteaux–Lamy syndrome, type B). *Ann Neurol* 1979, **6**:315–325.
Black S H, Pelias M Z *et al*: Maroteaux–Lamy syndrome in a large consanguineous kindred. *Am J Med Genet* 1986, **25**:273–279.
Spranger J: Mini review: inborn errors of complex carbohydrate metabolism. *Am J Med Genet* 1987, **28**:489–499.
Beck M, Fang-Kircher S: Mukopolysaccharidosen. Stuttgart, Jena, New York: G Fischer 1993.

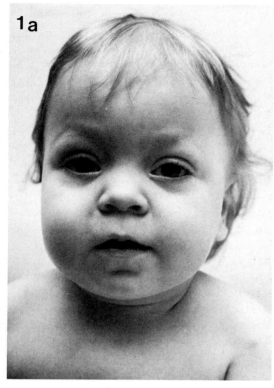

1a

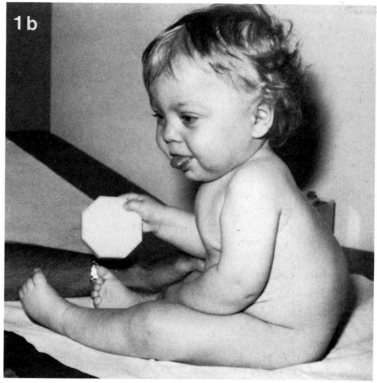

1b

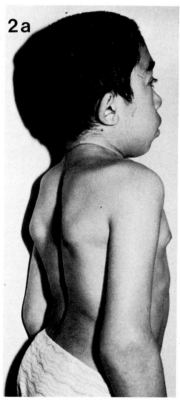

2a

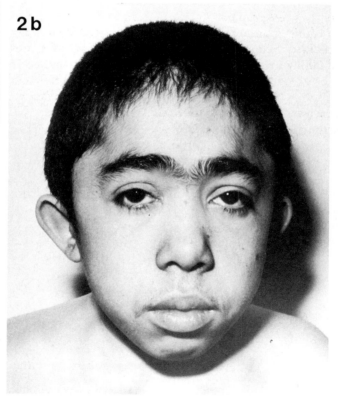

2b

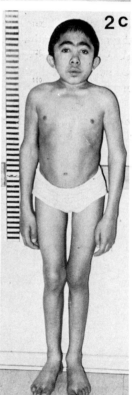

2c

69 Fucosidosis

J.K.

An autosomal recessive oligosaccharidosis with Hurler-like facial dysmorphism, spasticity, hepatomegaly, angiokeratoma corporis diffusum, severe progressive psychomotor retardation and neurological deterioration.

Main signs:
- Macrocephaly, brachycephaly, facial dysmorphism with prominence of the forehead and supra-orbital region, depressed nasal bridge, hypertelorism, exophthalmos, thick growth of scalp hair and eyebrows, thick pouting lips, large tongue, gingival hypertrophy, seizures, spastic tetraplegia. Progressive dementia.
- Short stature, short neck, thoracolumbar gibbus.
- Joint contractures. Claw hands, broad hands and feet with hourglass nails, thick skin, elevated salt content of sweat (type I only), anhydrosis or hypohydrosis, angiokeratoma corporis diffusum over the thorax and inner surfaces of the hands and feet in 50% of all patients.
- Large abdomen, hepatomegaly and cardiomegaly (type I only).

Supplementary findings: Tortuous conjunctival vessels, pigmented retinopathy; mild corneal clouding can occur. Dysfunction of the gall bladder. X-ray: progressive thickening of the diploic spaces, early frontal and supra-orbital synostosis, absent or poorly developed paranasal sinuses. Short odontoid process, cervical platyspondyly, thoracolumbar kyphosis, short sacrum, absent or rudimentary coccyx. Sclerosis and irregularly serrated form and thickening of the roof of the acetabulum, flattening and irregularities of the head of the femur, coxa valga, broadening of the shafts of the long bones.

Manifestation: Biochemically, prenatally and after birth. Clinically: *type I* (infantile type) between the third and 18th months (45% of all patients); *type II* (late infantile–juvenile form) from the first to second year of life; *type III* (adult form) later.

Aetiology: Autosomal recessive disorder. Absence or diminished activity of alpha-L-fucosidase in the liver, lungs, kidneys, brain, skin, lymphocytes and serum. Intragenetic heterogeneity. Further subtypes possible. The gene for fucosidosis has been localized to chromosome 1 (1p34).

Frequency: Approximately 80 patients known; about 45% of them are of the infantile type.

Course, prognosis: *Type I* (infantile type): death around the fifth year of life. *Type II* (juvenile type): death after the 20th year. *Type III* (adult type): too few patients known. Two-thirds of all patients reach the second decade of life.

Differential diagnosis: The phenotype is comparable with that of mucopolysaccharidosis type I-H (Hurler, 64). Angiokeratoma corporis diffusum also occurs with Fabry's disease and aspartyl glucosaminuria, sialidosis, GM_1 gangliosidosis (71), with diseases with unknown primary disorders and also in clinically healthy individuals.

Treatment: Symptomatic. Prevention through prenatal diagnosis.

Illustrations:

1 A 10-year-old fucosidosis patient and his healthy 5-year-old sibling.

2a A 19-year-old patient, brother of the children in 1: thick scalp hair and heavy eyebrows; prominent forehead and supra-orbital ridges; exophthalmos; depressed nasal bridge and broad tip of the nose; thick lips; macroglossia, all in all, coarse facies. Angiokeratoma corporis diffusum on the thorax. Type II fucosidosis.

2b–d Angiokeratoma on the trunk, palms and soles (patient showed broad, somewhat plump feet and broad hourglass nails).

References:

Beaudet A L: Disorders of glycoprotein degradation: mannosidosis, fucosidosis, sialidosis, aspartylglucosaminuria. In: The metabolic basis of inherited disease, 5th edition. Stanbury J B, Wyngaarden J B, Fredrickson D S, Goldstein J L, Brown M S (eds). McGraw-Hill Book company (1983).
Lee F A, Donnell G N, Gwinn J L: Radiographic features of fucosidosis. *Pediatr Radiol* 1977, 5:204–208.
Christomanou H, Beyer D: Absence of alphafucosidase activity in two sisters showing a different phenotype. *Eur J Pediatr* 1983, **140**:27–29.
Jackson K, Dawson G: Molecular defect in processing alpha-fucosidase in fucosidosis. *Biochem Biophys Res Commun* 1985, 133:90–97.
Spranger J: Mini review: inborn errors of complex carbohydrate metabolism. *Am J Med Genet* 1987, 28:489–499.
Fritsch G, Paschke E: Fukosidose. *Pädiat Prax* 1988, 37:469–476.
Willems P J, Garcia C A *et al*: Intrafamilial variability in fucosidosis. *Clin Genet* 1988, 34:7–14.
Willems P J, Gatti R *et al*: Fucosidosis revisited: a review of 77 patients. *Am J Med Genet* 1991, 38:111–131.

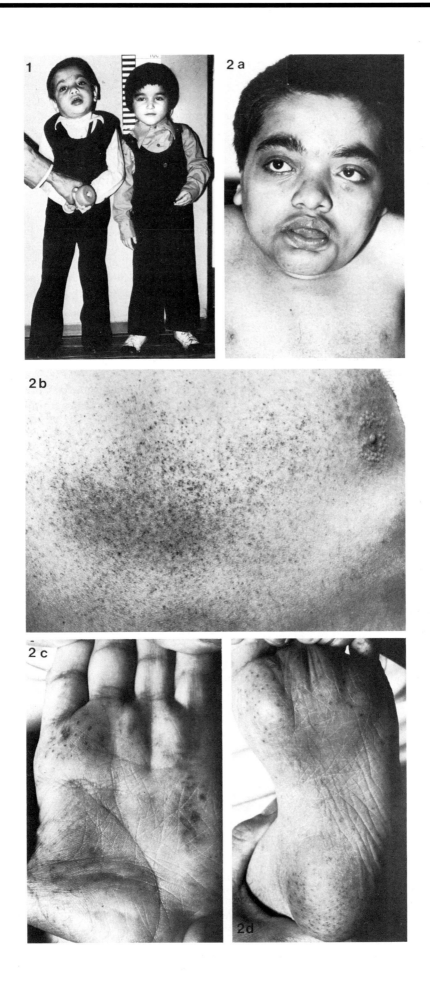

J.K.

An autosomal recessive oligosaccharidosis with an alpha-mannosidase defect, psychomotor retardation or deterioration, macrocephaly, hearing impairment, hepatomegaly and 'dysostosis multiplex'.

Main signs:
- Clinical heterogeneity. *Type I* refers to a severe infantile form and *type II* to a milder, late infantile–juvenile to adult form.
- Psychomotor retardation. Developmental standstill by about the end of the second year of life; coarse facial features; hearing defect.
- Hepatomegaly; hernias.
- Lens opacities and corneal clouding (typical retrolental opacity in the form of a wheel-spoke pattern).
- Thickening of the calvarium; ovoid configuration of the vertebral bodies, which appear flattened and beaked; occasional gibbus.
- Recurrent bacterial infections.

Type I: rapid mental deterioration; marked hepatosplenomegaly; severe dysostosis multiplex; hearing defect.
Type II: mental retardation noted in the school-age child; especially severe hearing impairment; milder skeletal involvement.

Supplementary findings: Vacuolated lymphocytes in most cases; absent mucopolysacchariduria; low IgG level; increased PR interval on electroencephalogram.

Manifestation: Biochemically, from birth. Clinically, *type I*, onset between the third and 12th months; *type II*, onset between the first and fourth years of life.

Aetiology: Autosomal recessive alpha-mannosidase deficiency, intragenetic heterogeneity. Localization of the gene on chromosome 19 (19p13.2-q12). The enzyme activities can be subdivided into two acidic forms, A and B and a neutral form, C. In mannosidosis, types A and B are deficient.

Frequency: Low; about 60 patients have been described up to now.

Course, prognosis: *Type I*: death between the third and 10th years of life from recurrent bacterial infections. *Type II*: survival into adulthood possible.

Differential diagnosis: The clinical picture resembles those of the mild forms of mucopolysaccharidosis. Biochemical assessment.

Treatment: Symptomatic; antibiotics for bacterial infections. Oral zinc therapy unsuccessful. Prenatal diagnosis possible.

Illustrations:
1a–c Patient 1, an 18-month-old girl, type II. Incipient coarsening of facial features, macroglossia, claw hands, 'dysostosis multiplex', retardation.
2a–c Patient 2, likewise type II, 32 months old; coarse facial features with flat profile, depressed nasal bridge, protruding lips; prominent forehead and macrocephaly (above the 97th percentile).
3a–c Patient 3 at 7 years (**a and b**) and 12 (**c**) years; small stature, short neck, coarse facial features, retardation; also type II.

References:
Beaudet A L: Disorders of glycoprotein degradation: mannosidosis, fucosidosis, sialidosis and aspartylglycosaminuria. In: Stanbury J B, Wyngaarden J B, Fredrickson D S, Goldstein J L, Brown M S (eds): The metabolic basis of inherited disease. Fifth edition. McGraw-Hill, New York 1983; 788–802.
Poenaru L *et al*: Antenatal diagnosis in three pregnancies at risk for mannosiosis. *Clin Genet* 1979, **16**:428–432.
Spranger J: Mini review: inborn errors of complex carbohydrate metabolism. *Am J Med Genet* 1987, **28**:489–499.
Wong L T K, Vallance H *et al*: Oral zinc therapy in the treatment of alpha-mannosidosis. *Am J Med Genet* 1993, **46**:410–414.

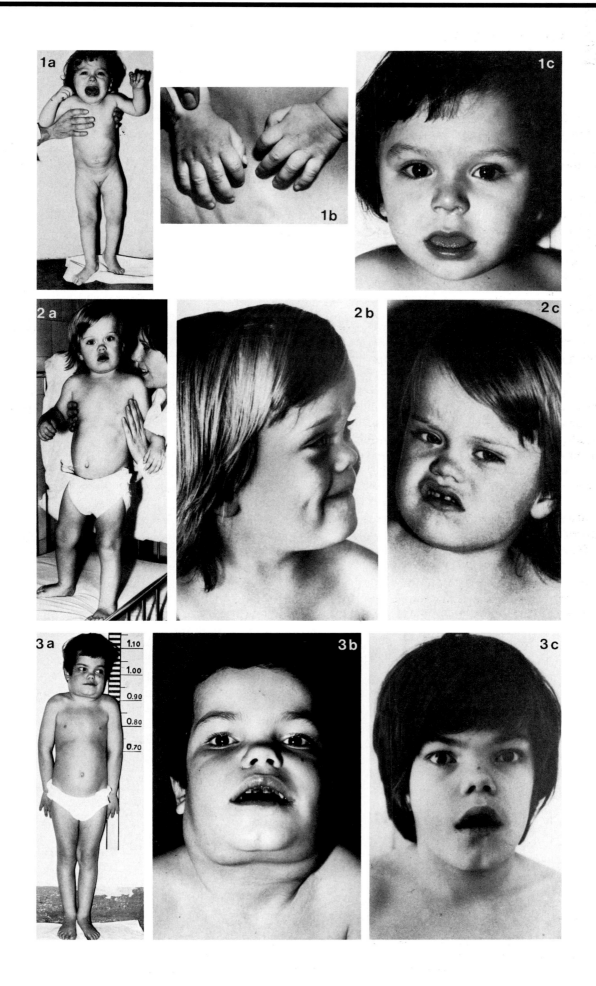

71 GM₁ Gangliosidosis

J.K.

An autosomal recessive storage disease with defective β-galactosidase and very variable phenotype: depending on the form, either an acute infantile onset with rapid neurological deterioration and severe bone deformities or normal intelligence and survival into adulthood.

Main signs:
Infantile form: shortly after birth, generalized oedema of the extremities, poor appetite, vomiting. Subsequently, no sitting or crawling. Mentally dull, irregular respirations, recurrent pneumonias, seizures. Initial muscular hypotonia, followed in the second year by spastic paresis, blindness, deafness.

Prominent forehead, depressed nasal bridge, large low-set ears, coarse facies, gingival hypertrophy, macroglossia, macrocephaly, cherry-red spot on the fundus (50%), dorsolumbar kyphosis.

Juvenile form: later onset. During the first year, normal psychomotor behaviour, good appetite and weight gain. Ataxia after the first year of life as the first sign. Internal strabismus, nystagmus, impaired co-ordination, loss of speech, generalized muscular hypotonia, progressive psychomotor retardation, lethargy, followed by spasticity of the upper and lower extremities. Seizures after the 16th month of life. Recurrent pneumonias. Relatively late development of mild facial dysmorphism.

Adult form: onset in the schoolchild of progressive cerebellar dysarthria, spasticity and ataxia. Mild intellectual decline. Neurological complications ten years after the first symptoms, at about age 20 years.

Supplementary findings: *Infantile form:* deformity of the vertebral bodies with anterior beaking, periosteal new bone formation in the long bones, broadening of the ribs, deformity of the pelvis and bones of the hands and feet. Hepatosplenomegaly.

Juvenile form: eventual blindness, only mild radiological signs.

Adult form: no seizures, no impairment of sight.

Manifestation: Biochemically, from birth; clinically, varied:
Infantile form: shortly after birth, rapidly progressive.
Juvenile form: in the second year of life, slow progression.
Adult form: after the 20th year of life.

Aetiology: Deficiency of ß-galactosidase. The fact that the progression of the different forms is constant within families is explained by intragenetic heterogeneity. Autosomal recessive disorder. Further phenotypic variants are possible. The gene for ß-galactosidase is located on the short arm of chromosome 3.

Frequency: Of the infantile form, presently approximately 100 patients known; of the juvenile form, 20; and of the adult form, more than 25.

Course, prognosis: *Infantile form:* death around the second year as a result of recurrent pneumonias. *Juvenile form:* death between the third and 10th years of life, or shortly after.
Adult form: all known patients have survived to date.

Differential diagnosis: Mucolipidosis type II (I-cell disease) (72).

Treatment: Symptomatic. Genetic counselling. Prenatal diagnosis possible.

Illustrations:
1 and 2 The child in **3** with his brother, who is 6 years and 6 months old. The phenotype of the latter is, in comparison, still normal with some mental deterioration and loss of speech; kyphosis when sitting, awkward gait.
3 An 11-year-old boy with the juvenile form. Macrocephaly, moderately coarse facial features with bushy eyebrows, depressed nasal bridge and macroglossia; short trunk with barrel-shaped thorax and pigeon chest. Impairment of voluntary motor co-ordination; mental deterioration.

References:
Kohlschütter A: Clinical course of GM₁ gangliosidoses. *Neuropediatrics* 1984, **15**:Suppl 71–73.
Pampiglione G, Harden A: Neurophysiological investigations in GM₁ and GM₂ gangliosidoses. Neuropediatrics 1984, **15**:Suppl 74–84.
Sandhoff K, Conzelmann E: The biochemical basis of gangliosidoses. Neuropediatrics 1984, **15**:Suppl 85–92.
Giugliani R, Dutra J C, Pereira M L S *et al*: GM₁ gangliosidosis: clinical and laboratory findings in eight families. *Hum Genet* 1985, 70:347–354.
Spranger J: Mini review: inborn errors of complex carbohydrate metabolism. *Am J Med Genet* 1987, 28:489–499.
O'Brien J S: Beta-galactosidase deficiency. In: Scriver C R *et al*: (eds): The metabolic basis of inherited disease. 6th ed. New York: McGraw-Hill 1989; 1797–1806.

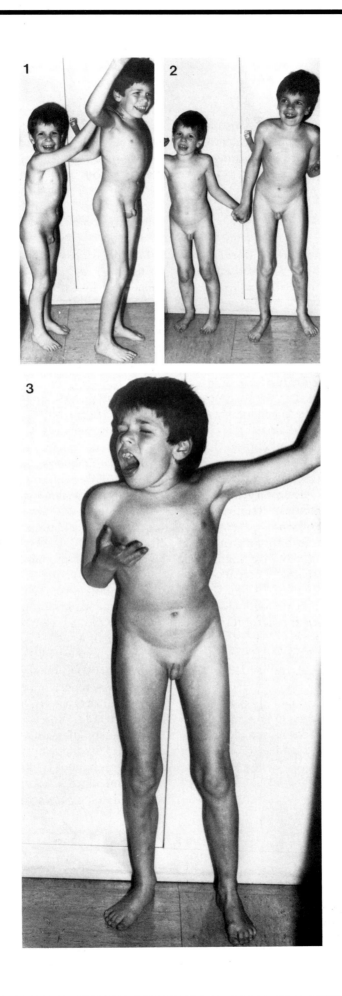

J.K.

An autosomal recessive disorder with elevation of several lysosomal enzymes and Hurler-like signs with variable expression (*type II* = I-cell disease = Leroy Syndrome; *type III* = pseudo-Hurler polydystrophy; *type IV*).

Main signs:

Type II:

- Intra-uterine growth retardation, early coarsening of the facial features, exophthalmos, mouth held open, gingival hyperplasia, thick hair, prominent forehead, scaphocephaly (premature closure of the sagittal suture), depressed nasal bridge.
- Kyphoscoliosis, lumbar gibbus, dislocation of the hip, club feet, joint contractures, hernias. Beaking and wedging of the vertebral bodies, broadening of the ribs, proximal tapering of the metacarpals. Circular periosteal new bone formation, around the shaft of the humerus and other long bones.
- Thick firm skin especially over the finger joints, short fingers, paw-like claw hands.
- Puffy eyelids, corneal clouding, increased corneal diameter.
- Hepatosplenomegaly, cardiomegaly, cardiac defects.
- Disproportionate short stature, severe developmental retardation, recurrent lung infections.

Type III: three different, severe forms;

- Marked limitation of movement in all joints, progressive until puberty. Firm thick skin, paw-like hands, disproportionate short stature, coarsening of the facial features between the sixth and 10th years of life. By the end of the first decade of life, corneal clouding, carpal tunnel syndrome. Intelligence varied: normal to rapidly deteriorating, depending on the form.
- Severe anomalies of the pelvis and spine. Hyperlordosis, hip dysplasia, short neck, final height 130–140 cm.
- No mucopolysacchariduria.

Type IV:

- Slow neurological decline with increased knee and ankle jerks, hypotonia, dystonia, moderate to severe psychomotor deterioration, mild coarsening of facial features.
- Strabismus, corneal clouding.
- No mucopolysacchariduria, no organomegaly, skeleton normal.

Supplementary findings: *Type II:* numerous cytoplasmic inclusion bodies (I-form) in skin fibroblasts. *Type III:* inclusion bodies as in *type II*. *Type IV:* cytoplasmic granular inclusions and lamellar structures in skin cells.

Manifestation: *Type II:* first months of life. *Type III:* age 4–5 years. *Type IV:* in the first decade of life.

Aetiology: Autosomal recessive disorders with decreased intracellular and increased extracellular activities of lysosomal acid hydrolases (10- to 20-fold increase of β-hexosaminidase, iduronate sulphatase, arylsulphatase A in serum). Intragenetic and intergenetic heterogeneity.

Frequency: Low. *Type II:* approximately 50 patients. *Type III:* fewer than 50 patients known. *Type IV:* 20 patients.

Course, prognosis: *Type II:* death before the fifth year of life. *Type III:* the oldest patient is over 50 years old. *Type IV:* the oldest patient is over 32 years old.

Differential diagnosis: *Type II:* Hurler disease (65). *Type III:* mucopolysaccharidosis VI (Maroteaux–Lamy, 68). Classification within type III depends on the diagnostic centre. *Type IV:* mucolipidoses II and III (72). Biochemical elucidation.

Treatment: Symptomatic. Prenatal diagnosis identifies only the homozygotes of type II. Type III can be diagnosed prenatally, likewise Type IV (possibly perform electron microscopic search for inclusion bodies).

Illustrations:

1a and b 7 months old, short stature, coarsening of facial features, thick scalp hair. Prominent forehead, exophthalmos, appears similar to mucopolysaccharidosis (mucolipidosis type II).

2a 16 years old, short stature, lordosis with large protruding abdomen, joint contractures (mucolipidosis type III).

2b Hurler-like appearance, coarsened facies, thick scalp hair, exophthalmos, synophrys, thick lips, depressed nasal bridge. Intelligence normal.

2c and d Joint contractures, short fingers, paw-like claw hands.

References:

Okada S *et al*: I-cell disease: clinical studies of 21 Japanese cases. *Clin Genet* 1985, 28:207–215.
Ornoy A *et al*: Letter to the editor: early prenatal diagnosis of mucolipidosis IV. *Am J Med Genet* 1987, 27:983–985.
Spranger J: Mini review: inborn errors of complex carbohydrate metabolism. *Am J Med Genet* 1987, 28:489–499.
Pazzaglia U E, Beluffi G *et al*: Study of bone pathology in early mucolipidosis II... *Eur J Pediatr* 1989, 148:553–557.
Nolan C M, Sly W S: I-cell disease and pseudo-Hurler polydystrophy. In: Scriver C R *et al* (eds). The metabolic basis of inherited disease. 6th ed. New York: McGraw-Hill 1989; 1589–1602.
Poenaru L, Mezards C *et al*: Prenatal diagnosis of mucolipidosis type II on first-trimester amniotic fluid. *Prenat Diagn* 1990, 10:231–235.
Chitayat D, Meunier C M *et al*: Mucolipidosis IV: clinical manifestations and natural history. *Am J Med Genet* 1991, 41:313–318.

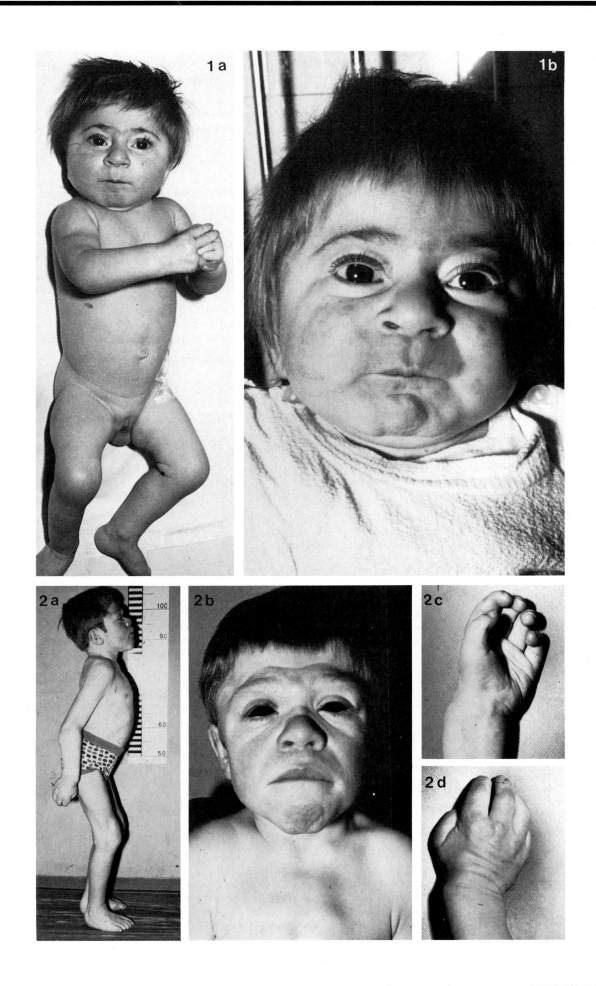

73 Wiedemann–Beckwith Syndrome (WBS)

(Beckwith–Wiedemann Syndrome; Exomphalos–Macroglossia–'Gigantism' Syndrome; EMG Syndrome)

H.-R.W

A congenital, relatively frequent and very characteristic metabolic dysplasia syndrome of practical importance with peculiar facies, 'grooved' ears, congenital and/or postnatal generalized 'gigantism', sometimes with umbilical hernia, muscular macroglossia and other organomegaly in addition to possible severe postnatal hypoglycemia.

Main signs:
- Frequent mild exophthalmos often associated with a relatively small head with protruding occiput and telangiectatic naevi of the upper half of the face in infancy. Hypoplasia of the mid-face, soft-tissue folds under the eyes (see photographic plate opposite). Variously developed slit- or notch-like indentations of the external ears and/or a groove on the dorsal edge of the ear in the great majority of cases (see plate overleaf). Congenital macroglossia, often with macrostomia, prognathism. Omphalocoele (1) or possibly simply development of a large umbilical hernia (2).
- Congenital nephromegaly (ultrasound imperative), hepato-, pancreato- and, in some cases, cardiomegaly.
- Congenital macrosomia and/or postnatal 'gigantism', whereby height, weight, skeletal and dental maturity may be above the norm for years.
- NB: possible severe prolonged therapy-resistant hypoglycemia in the newborn period and infancy.

Supplementary findings: Not infrequently the presence or development of fairly distinct hemihypertrophy (of a lower extremity alone or of the whole half of the body), Infrequent hypertrophy of the clitoris and/or labia or penis.

Substantially increased tendency to neoplasia (especially Wilms tumours and carcinoma of the adrenal cortex), especially in children with distinct hemihypertrophy.

Mental development usually normal (in the absence of severe hypoglycemic damage).

Manifestation: At birth and thereafter (macrosomia)

Aetiology: An autosomal dominant gene with extremely variable expression and incomplete penetrance has been assumed.

In apparently sporadic cases (i.e. thorough investigation for possible carriers negative), new mutation possible, low risk of recurrence. With familial occurrence, transmission normally via the mother; risk of recurrence up to 50%. In atypical cases, chromosome analysis is indicated.

Gene localized on the short arm of chromosome 11 (11p15). Imprinting mechanism.

Frequency: Relatively high, at approximately one out of 12–15 000 newborns; many hundreds of patients have been recognized.

Course, prognosis: After possible postpartum adaptive difficulties (e.g. polycythaemia, hypoglycemia, feeding and respiratory difficulties, and so on), usually good.

Regression of visceromegaly; gradual slowing of growth (often with eventual normal height; normal sexual maturation); tendency to attain normal proportions, including those of facial features and better tongue-to-mouth proportions.

Regular close follow-up examinations, especially of the abdomen for possible tumour development, using ultrasound, are mandatory in the first 6 years of life.

Differential diagnosis: Infant of diabetic mother (but macroglossia, ear grooves, umbilical hernia, etc.).

Hypothyroidism (but accelerated growth and absence of constipation, and so on; blood tests).

Other rare 'overgrowth' syndromes, with signs that in some cases overlap with those of 'WBS', e.g. Perlmans', Simpson–Golabi–Behmel and Marfan syndrome (76).

Treatment: Initially, blood sugar determinations at regular intervals; in some cases appropriate therapy. Repair of omphalocoele, if necessary. Partial glossectomy may be indicated, possibly later in infancy. Orthodontic care.

Orthopaedic treatment for hemihypertrophy.

Genetic counseling. Prenatal diagnosis with ultrasound where indicated.

Illustrations:

1 Premature infant; omphalocoele, macroglossia.

2 A 6-month-old child; typical facies, large umbilical hernia; probably frequent early hypoglycemic seizures; persisting tendency to hypoglycemia.

3, 7, 11 Young children, post–partum surgery for omphalocoele, accelerated growth, mentally normal.

4–6, 8–10, 12–14 Typical facies at various stages of infancy. Subsequent plates: facies during infancy and school age and grooved ears of varying severity and in varying positions.

References:

Wiedemann H-R: Exomphalos-Makroglossie-Gigantismus-Syndrom... *Z Kinderheilk* 1973, **115**:193.

Kosseff A L, Herrmann J, Gilbert E F *et al*: Studies of malformation syndromes of man XXIX: The Wiedemann–Beckwith syndrome. *Eur J Pediatr* 1976, **123**:139.

Sommer A, Cutler E A, Cohen B L *et al*: Familial occurrence of the Wiedemann–Beckwith syndrome... *Am J Med Genet* 1977, **1**:59.

Piussan Ch, Risbourg B, Lenaerts C *et al*: Syndrome de Wiedemann et Beckwith. *J Génét Hum* 1980, **28**:281.

Sotelo-Avila C, Gonzalez-Crussi F, Fowler J W: Complete and incomplete forms of Beckwith–Wiedemann syndrome: their oncogenic potential. *J Pediatr* 1980, **96**:47.

Best L G, Hoekstra R E: Wiedemann–Beckwith syndrome: autosomal-dominant inheritance in a family. *Am J Med Genet* 1981, **9**:291.

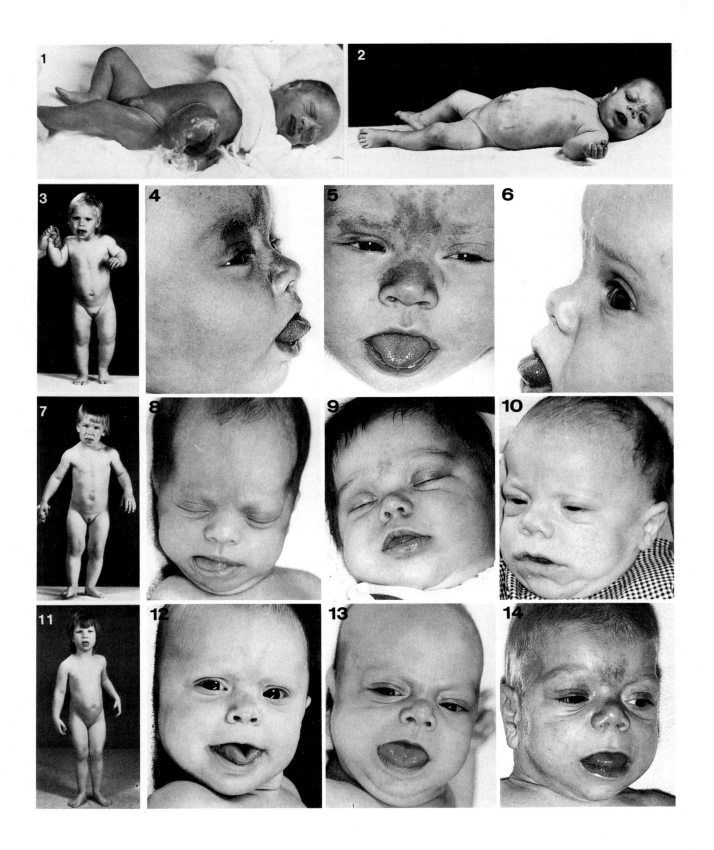

Lemke, J, Meinecke, P. et al: Das Wiedemann-Beckwith-Syndrom. Mschr. Kinderheilk. **134**, 554-557 (1986).

Pettenati, M. J, Haines, J. L. et al: Wiedemann-Beckwith syndrome ... review of the literature. Hum. Genet. **74**, 143-154 (1986).

Engström, W, Lindham, S. et al: Wiedemann-Beckwith syndrome (Review). Eur. J. Pediatr. **147**, 450-457 (1988).

Litz, C. E, Taylor, K. A. et al: Absence of detectable chromosomal and molecular abnormalities in monocygotic twins discordant for the Wiedemann-Beckwith syndrome. Am. J. Med. Genet **30**, 821-833 (1988).

Best, L. G: Familial posterior helical ear pits and Wiedemann-Beckwith syndrome. Am. J. Med. Genet. **40**, 188-195 (1991).

Drut, R. M, Drut, R. at al: Adrenal hyperplastic nodules in Wiedemann-Beckwith syndrome. Birth Defects: Orig. Art. Ser. **29**/1, 367-372 (1993).

Franceschini, P, Guala, A. et al: Monzygotic twinning and Wiedemann-Beckwith syndrome (letter). Am. J. Med. Genet. **46**, 353-354 (1993).

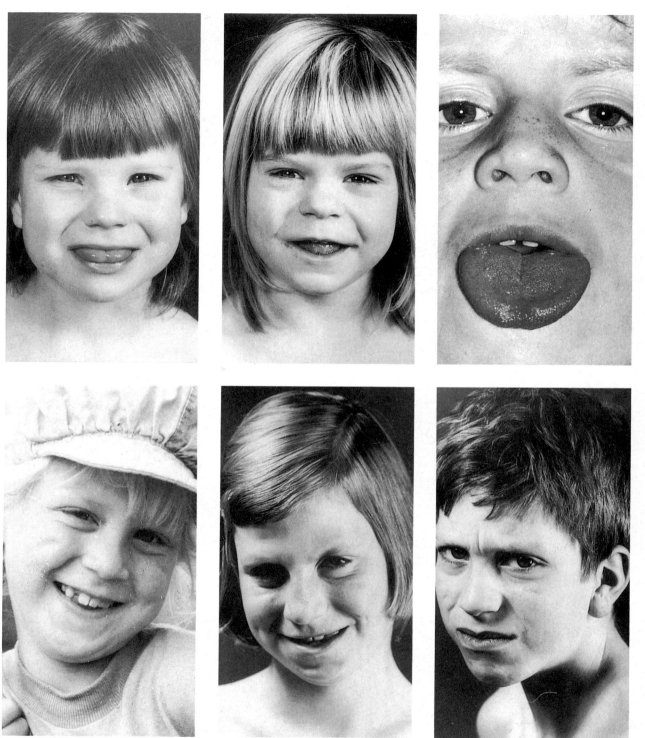

References:

Kunze J, Wiedemann H-R: Das Wiedemann–Beckwith-Syndrom. *Ergeb Inn Med Kinderheilk* 1993, **61**:303–338.

Tommerup N, Brandt C A *et al*: Sex dependent transmission of Beckwith–Wiedemann syndrome... *J Med Genet* 1993, **30**:958–961.

Weksberg R, Teshima I *et al*: Molecular characterization of cytogenetic alterations associated with the Beckwith–Wiedemann syndrome... *Hum Molec Genet* 1993, **2**:549–556.

Cohen M M Jr: Wiedemann–Beckwith syndrome, imprinting IGF2 and H19... (Letter). *Am J Med Genet* 1994, **52**:233–234.

Elliott M, Bayly R *et al*: Clinical features and natural history of Beckwith–Wiedemann syndrome: presentation of 74 new cases. *Clin Genet* 1994, **46**:168–174.

Elliott M, Maher E R: Beckwith–Wiedemann syndrome. *J Med Genet* 1994, **31**:560–564.

Hunter A GW, Allanson J E: Follow-up study of patients with Wiedemann–Beckwith syndrome... *Am J Med Genet* 1994, **51**:102–107.

Mannens M, Hoovers J M N *et al*: Parental imprinting of human chromosome region 11p15.3-pter involved in the Beckwith–Wiedemann syndrome... *Eur J Hum Genet* 1994, **2**:3–23.

Reik, W, Brown, K W *et al*: Allelic methylation of H19 and IGF2 in the Beckwith–Wiedemann syndrome. *Hum Mol Genet* 1994, **3**:1297–1303.

Slatter R E, Elliott M *et al*: Mosaic uniparental disomy in Beckwith–Wiedemann syndrome. *J Med Genet* 1994, **31**:749–753.

Weksberg R: Wiedemann–Beckwith syndrome: genomic imprinting revisited (Letter). *Am J Med Genet* 1994, **52**:235–236.

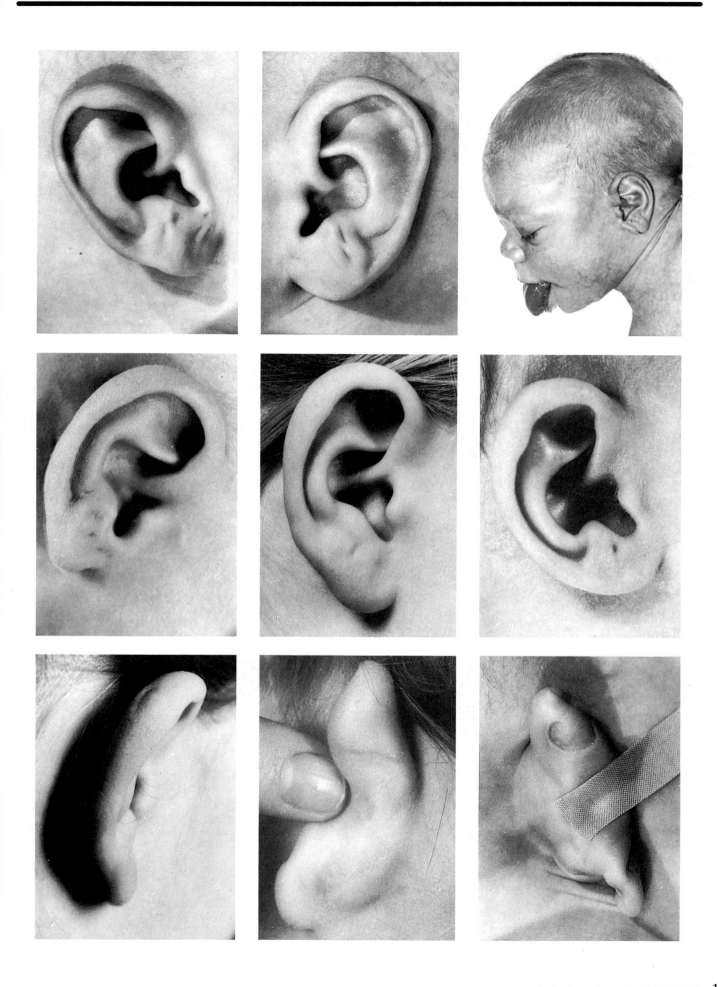

74 Sotos Syndrome
(Sotos Sequence, Cerebral Gigantism Type Sotos)

H.-R.W

An occasional syndrome of childhood 'gigantism', usually with above normal size at birth, unusual facies, acromegalic changes and signs of a (non-progressive) cerebral involvement.

Main signs:
- Congenital macrosomia and/or postnatal somatic 'gigantism' (**3 and 4**) with discordant acceleration of bone age and dentition (phalanges and metacarpals greater than carpals).
- Macrocephaly and abnormally large hands and feet.
- Unusual physiognomy [prominent forehead with high or 'receding' hairline (**1**); hypertelorism; slight antimongoloid slant of the palpebral fissures].
- Congenital non-progressive cerebral impairment with psychomotor retardation, impairment of fine motor activity.

Supplementary findings: Usually dolichocephaly, large ears, prognathism, high palate and unusually long arms. Not infrequently development of kyphoscoliosis. Cranial ultrasound or computerized tomography shows slight to moderate enlargement of the cerebral ventricles, especially the third (no increased intracranial pressure). Electroencephalogram frequently abnormal.

Congenital cardiac defects relatively frequent.

No evidence of a constant endocrinological or biochemical abnormality.

Manifestation: At birth and during infancy.

Aetiology: Genetically determined syndrome. Usually sporadic occurrence. Evidence for dominant as well as possible recessive transmission or gonadal mosaicism. Perhaps heterogeneity.

Frequency: Not particularly rare (several hundred case reports in the literature).

Course, prognosis: Self-limitation of the accelerated growth by the end of the first or at least the beginning of the second decade of life. Onset of puberty at the usual age or somewhat earlier. Adult height within the normal range.

The degree of mental retardation is of considerable importance. Apparently increased tendency to develop malignant tumours.

Differential diagnosis: Other primordial overgrowth syndromes (*73, 75, 76*), including the fragile X syndrome (*55*).

Treatment: Follow-up examinations at regular intervals. All appropriate measures to educate children with developmental or psychomotor retardation. Precautionary measures against or early treatment of scoliosis. Genetic counselling.

Illustrations:

1–4 A child with Sotos syndrome. Length at birth 60 cm. At age 14 months (**1, 3, 4**), average height of a child 32 months old; head circumference corresponding to that of an 8 year old. Hand length of a 5 year old, early eruptions of teeth, bone age 3 years. Prominent forehead with frontal baldness, appearance of a child older than his age; large, somewhat low-set ears; large genitalia; very large feet. Gross motor retardation, clumsy motor performance; clearly enlarged third ventricle. At 28 months, height of a 4 year old; enormous feet. At 3 years and 11 months (**2**), average height of a child 6 years and 3 months old. 'Too old' appearance. Clumsy, restless, mentally subnormal behaviour.

References:

Bale A E, Drum M A *et al*: Familial Sotos syndrome... *Am J Med Genet* 1985, 20:613–624.

Wit J M, Beemer F A *et al*: Cerebral gigantism... *Eur J Pediatr* 1985 144:131–140.

Kaneko H, Tsukahara M *et al*: Congenital heart defects in Sotos sequence. *Am J Med Genet* 1987, 26:569–576.

Verloes A, Sacré J-P *et al*: Sotos syndrome and fragile X chromosomes. *Lancet* 1987, II:329.

Goldstein D J, Ward R E *et al*: Overgrowth, congenital hypotonia, nystagmus, strabismus and mental retardation: variant of dominantly inherited Sotos sequence? *Am J Med Genet* 1988, 29:783–792.

Blackett P R, Coffman M A *et al*: Dominantly inherited childhood gigantism resembling Sotos' syndrome. *Am J Med Sci* 1989, 296:181–185.

Hersh J H, Cole T R P *et al*: Risk of malignancy in Sotos syndrome. *J Pediatr* 1992, **120**:572–574.

Cole T R P, Hughes H E: Sotos Syndrome... *J Med Genet* 1994, 31:20–32.

Maroun Chr, Schmerler S *et al*: Child with Sotos phenotype and a 5:15 translocation. *Am J Med Genet* 1994, 50:291–293.

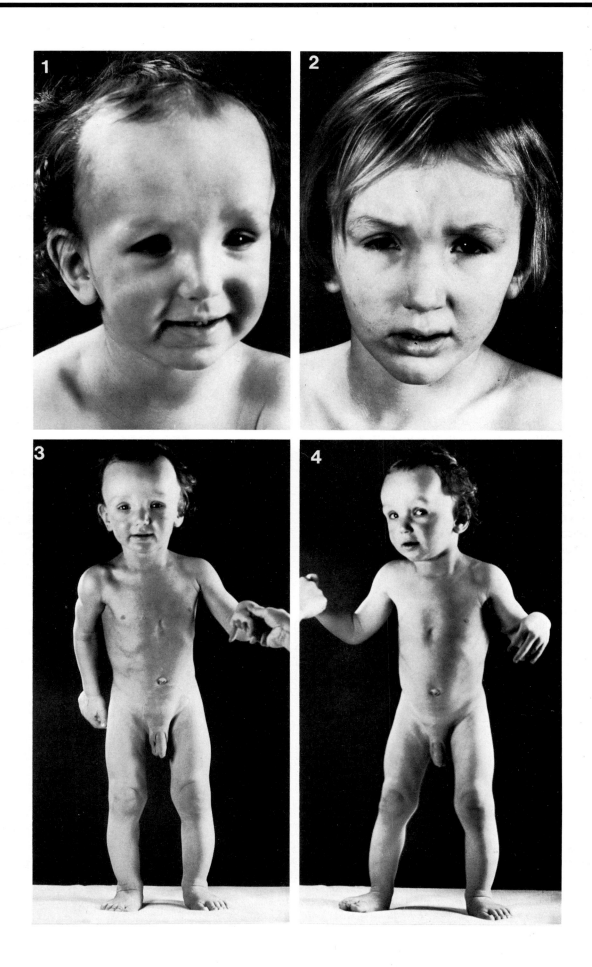

75 Weaver Syndrome

H.-R.W

A further syndrome of childhood 'gigantism', usually with congenital macrosomia, macrocephaly, distinctive facies, psychomotor retardation, unusual voice, increased muscle tone and additional anomalies.

Main signs:

- Congenital macrosomia and/or postnatal somatic 'gigantism' (1).
- Marked macrocephaly (without signs of increased intracranial pressure) with broad, protruding forehead (2).
- Distinctive appearance: marked hypertelorism or telecanthus; broad, low nasal bridge; prominent or long philtrum; receding chin and large ears (1 and 2).
- Developmental retardation a regular feature. Deep, hoarse voice. Muscular hypertonia (less frequently hypotonia).

Supplementary findings: Possible early limitation of movement of the elbows and knees. Club feet. Camptodactyly of the fingers, clinodactyly of the toes, broad thumbs, simian creases in some cases. Thin, deeply inserted nails; prominent fingertip pads.

Loose nuchal skin; inguinal and/or umbilical hernia.

Radiographs: discordant acceleration of bone age (carpals greater than phalanges and metacarpals); low, broad iliac wings; widening of the distal ends of the long bones, especially the femora (3).

Manifestation: At birth and thereafter.

Aetiology: Undetermined. Usually sporadic occurrence. Genetic factors probably play a role, although a definite mode of inheritance has not yet been established.

Frequency: Low (less than 40 patients have been reported since 1974).

Course, prognosis: To date hardly any long-term observations; apparently, final height may be either normal or above/below normal. In each case, mental development is key to the prognosis.

Differential diagnosis: Other primordial 'gigantism' syndromes (73, 74, 76).

Treatment: Symptomatic. Any measures to promote psychomotor development. Early measures should be taken to prevent obesity.

Illustrations:

1–3 A 15-month-old boy, the first child of healthy, young, nonconsanguineous parents. Birth at term after a normal pregnancy: 57 cm, 4970 g and head circumference 36 cm; club feet. At 15 months, 93 cm (like a child 30 months old), about 17 kg and head circumference 52 cm (both those of a 4 year old).

References:

Weaver D D, Graham C B, Thomas I T *et al*: A new overgrowth syndrome with accelerated skeletal maturation, unusual facies and camptodactyly. *J Pediatr* 1974, 84:547.

Fitch N: The syndromes of Marshall and Weaver. *J Med Genet* 1980, 17:174.

Majewski F, Ranke M, Kemperdick H *et al*: The Weaver syndrome: a rare type of primordial overgrowth. *Eur J Pediatr* 1981, **137**:277.

Meinecke P, Schaefer E *et al*: The Weaver syndrome in a girl. *Eur J Pediatr* 1983, 141:58–59.

Farrell S A, Hughes H E: Weaver syndrome with pes cavus. *Am J Med Genet* 1985, 21:737–739.

Ardinger H H, Hanson J W *et al*: Further delineation of Weaver syndrome. *J Pediatr* 1986, 108:228–235.

Thompson E M, Hill S *et al*: A girl with Weaver syndrome. *J Med Genet* 1987l, 24:232–234.

Greenberg F, Wasiewski W *et al*: Weaver syndrome... *Am J Med Genet* 1989, **33**:127–129.

Teebi A S, Sundareshan T S *et al*: A new... disorder resembling Weaver syndrome. *Am J Med Genet* 1989,33:479–482.

Ramos-Arroyo M A, Weaver D *et al*: Weaver syndrome... review... *Pediatrics* 1991, 88:1106–1111.

Cole T R P, Dennis N R *et al*: Weaver syndrome. *J Med Genet* 1992, 29:332–337.

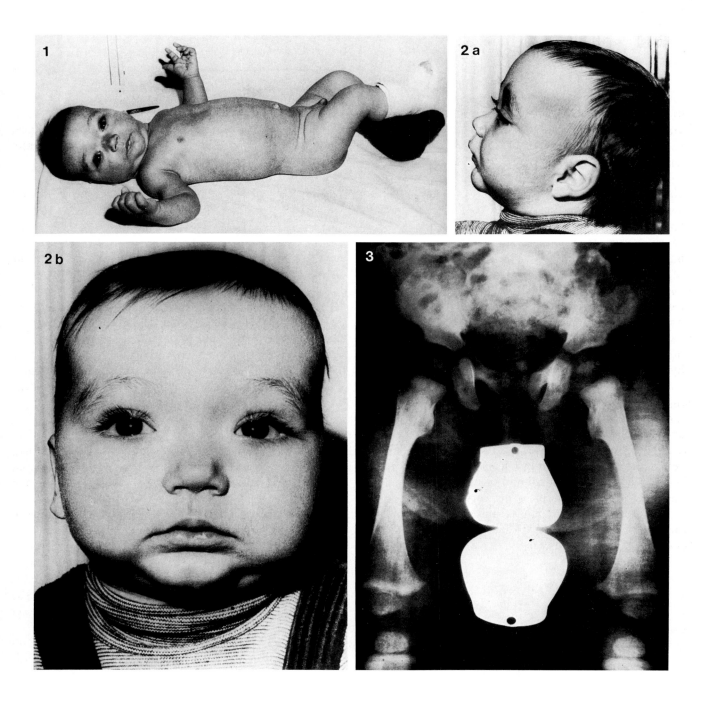

76 Marfan Syndrome
(Arachnodactyly)

H.-R.W

A characteristic hereditary disorder with disproportionate tall stature, defects of the eyes and tendency to develop aortic aneurysms.

Main signs:
- Tall stature, mainly due to excessively long extremities, particularly the distal portions, resulting in eunuchoid body proportions and arachnodactyly (**1, 2, 8**)
- Marked deficit of fatty tissue. Muscular hypoplasia and hypotonia (**1, 4, 6**).
- Long, narrow face with high palate (**1, 4**) and narrowly spaced teeth; dolichocephaly.
- Signs of connective tissue weakness; hernias, hyperextensible joints, dislocation of the joints, kyphoscoliosis, pes planus, striae and others; pectus carinatum or excavatum (**1, 4, 7**).

Supplementary findings: Dislocation of the lenses in about 75% of patients, usually upwards; when less pronounced, recognizable on slit-lamp examination; danger of glaucoma. Usually marked myopia. Retinal detachment. Round lenses. Blue sclera.

General dilation of the aorta (aortic valve incompetence), dissecting aneurysm. Less frequently similar involvement of the pulmonary artery or the mitral and tricuspid valves (prolapse of the mitral valve).

Manifestation: In infancy. However, usually not diagnosed until childhood or later.

Aetiology: Autosomal dominant disorder with variable expression; new mutations may be assumed for about 15% of patients, often associated with increased paternal age. Fibrillin-1 defect. Gene locus on 15q21.1 (a second gene locus assumed on 3p24.2-p25).

Frequency: Varied estimates between one out of 10 000 and one out of 50 000 of the general population.

Course, prognosis: Death as a result of cardiovascular complications possible at any age, especially after puberty. On average, patients attain 30–50 years. If valvular endocarditis develops, the prognosis is very poor. Danger of going blind.

Differential diagnosis: Homocystinuria (79) must be ruled out in every case because it is basically amenable to therapy. Stickler syndrome (302). Contractural arachnodactyly (78). Klinefelter syndrome (308). Certain forms of Ehlers–Danlos syndrome (203). See also neonatal Marfan syndrome (77).

Treatment: Limitation of growth by means of hormone therapy at the appropriate time, also as an attempt to prevent severe scoliosis. Propranolol seems to slow the development of aneurysms. Vascular or cardiac surgery may be indicated. Avoidance of marked physical exertion. Genetic counselling.

Illustrations:

1–3 Patient 1 at age 14 years: height 174 cm, weight 48 kg (normal weight of a girl 159 cm tall). Both second toes shortened operatively, as they were 1.5 cm longer than the halluces. No evidence of cardiac defect at present. Myopia.

4 Patient 2 at age 9 years. No definite evidence of a cardiac defect. Myopia on the right, astigmatism on the left, round lenses. No dislocation of the lenses. Height at 13 years, 196.5 cm.

5 and 6 Patient 3 (sister of **4**) at age 6 years. Suspected to have ballooning of the mitral valve. Round lenses, no dislocation. Normal amino acid chromatogram. Height at age 10 years, 174.5 cm.

7 The Marfan thumb sign (the thumb folded across the palm distinctly extends beyond the ulnar edge of the hand).

8 Positive (Murdoch) wrist sign in a 19-year-old patient: the first and second fingers clearly encircle the wrist.

References:

Pyeritz R R, McKusick V A: The Marfan syndrome: diagnosis and management. *N Engl J Med* 1979, 772.

Donaldson R M, Emanuel E W, Olsen E G J *et al*: Management of cardiovascular complications in Marfan syndrome. *Lancet* 1980, II:1178.

Chemke J, Nisani R, Feigl A *et al*: Homozygosity for autosomal dominant Marfan syndrome. *J Med Genet* 1984, 21:173–177.

Burgio R G, Martin A *et al*: Asymmetric Marfan syndrome. Am. J. Med. Genet. 30, 905-909 (1988); see also *Am J Hum Genet* 1990, 46:661–671.

Kainulainen K, Pulkkinen L *et al*: Location on chromosome 15 of the gene defect causing Marfan syndrome. *N Engl J Med* 1990, 323:935–939.

Viljoen D, Beighton P: Marfan syndrome: a diagnostic dilemma. *Clin Genet* 1990, 37:417–422.

Kainulainen K, Karttunen L *et al*: Mutations in the fibrillin gene... *Nature Genet* 1994, 6:64–69.

Pereira L, Levran O *et al*: A molecular approach to the stratification of cardiovascular risk in families with Marfan's syndrome. *N Engl J Med* 1994, 331:148–153.

Collod G, Babron M-C *et al*: A second locus for Marfan syndrome maps to chromosome 3p24.2-p25. *Nature Genet* 1994, 8:264–268.

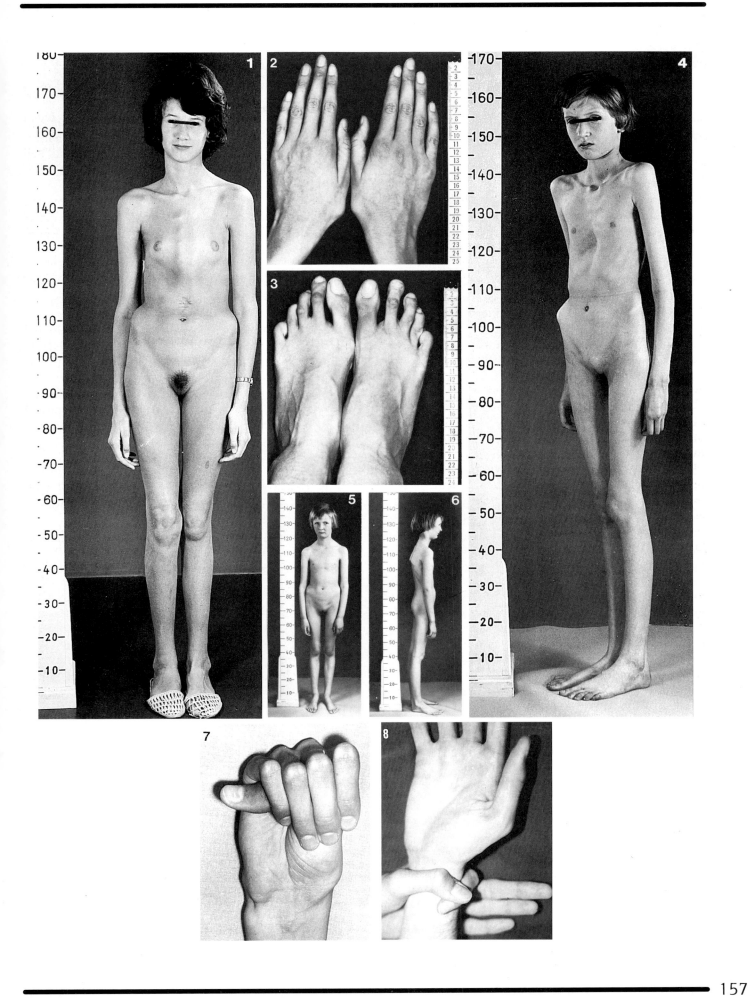

77 Neonatal Marfan Syndrome
(Infantile Marfan Syndrome)

J.K.

A very severe, frequently lethal form of the Marfan Syndrome.

Main signs:

Skeletal symptoms

- (in reverse order of frequency): especially noticeable arachnodactyly; hyperextensible joints of the fingers, hands and feet; pectus carinatum, excavatum; dolichocephaly; unusual facies: broad nasal bridge, bluish sclerae, antimongoloid slant of the palpebral fissures, low-set ears, large and flaccid; high-arched palate, partial cleft palate; micrognathia; scoliosis; malar hypoplasia. Prominent forehead. 'Old man' appearance.

Symptoms of the eye:

- Ectopia lentis (upwards), iridodonesis, myopia, keratoconus. Large, deep-set eyes (enopthalmos), increasing axial eyeball length, flat cornea.

Cardiac peculiarities:

- Dilation of the aortic root, mitral valve prolapse, heart murmurs, tricuspid valve prolapse, ventricular enlargement, ventricular hypertrophy, open Botallo's duct, patent foramen ovale, septal defects, rupture of the aorta, dissecting aneurysm of other vascular regions.

Supplementary findings: Measurement of birth dimensions, age of parents, duration of pregnancy and data about family history do not help to identify high-risk pregnancies or newborns with Marfan syndrome.

Manifestation: At birth, up until the third month of life.

Aetiology: Only 10 out of 54 newborns with Marfan syndrome had a positive family history. Thus, it is usually a case of dominant new mutations. The familial cases evidently run a milder course.

Pathogenesis: Hypotheses: possible defects of the microfibrillar protein fibrillin. Possible combined defect of the fibrillin and decorin. Possible defect of mitochondrial complex I.

Course, prognosis: Increased lethality in the first year of life: aortic dissection, cardiopulmonary insufficiency.

Differential diagnosis: Homocystinuria (79); familial mitral valve prolapse; contractural arachnodactyly (Beals–Hecht, 78); Stickler's arthrophthalmopathy (302).

Treatment: Use of beta blockers delays dilation of the aorta.
  Careful monitoring in the case of existing dilations of the aorta, in order to ensure correct timing of surgical prosthetic care (Bentall operation).

Illustrations:

1 6-month-old female infant, large, old appearance with deep-set eyes (compared with a healthy 6-month-old infant).

2 and 3 Particularly noticeable arachnodactyly (compared with a healthy infant of the same age).

4 Newborn with Marfan syndrome (mother 206 cm, Marfan patient). Distinct arachnodactyly.

References:

Gross D M, Robinson L K, Smith L T, Glass N, Rosenberg H, Duvic M: Severe perinatal Marfan syndrome. *Pediatr* 1989, 84:83–89.

Morse R P, Rockenmacher S, Pyeritz R E, Sanders S P, Bieber R R, Lin A, MacLeod P, Hall B, Graham J M jr: Diagnosis and management of infantile Marfan syndrome. *Pediatr* 1990, 86:888–895.

Buntinx I M, Willems P J, Spitaels S E, Van Reempst P, De Paepe A, Duman J E: Neonatal Marfan syndrome with congenital arachnodactyly, flexion contractures and severe cardiac valve insufficiency. *J Med Genet* 1991, 28:267–273.

Superti-Furga A, Raghunath M, Willems P J: Deficiencies of fibrillin and decorin in fibroblast cultures of a patient with neonatal Marfan syndrome. *J Med Genet* 1992, 29:875–878.

Raghunath M, Superti-Furga A, Godfrey M, Steinmann B: Decreased extracellular deposition of fibrillin and decorin in neonatal Marfan syndrome fibroblasts. *Hum Genet* 1993, 90:511–515.

Christodoulou J, Petrova-Benedict R, Robinson B H, Jay V, Clarke J T R: An unusual patient with the neonatal Marfan phenotype and mitochondrial complex I deficiency. *Eur J Pediatr* 1993, 152:428–432.

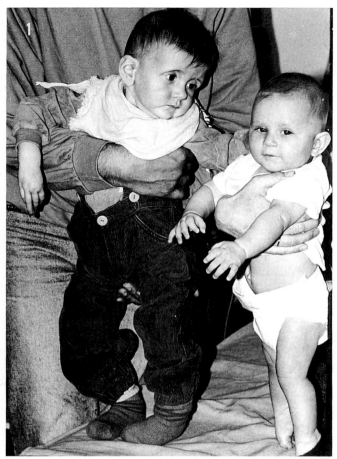

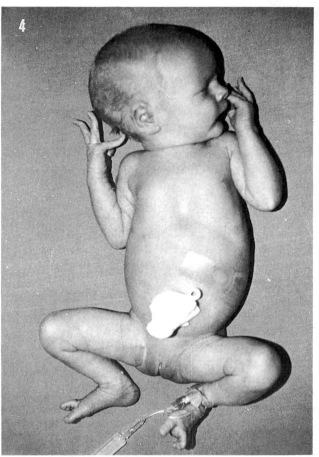

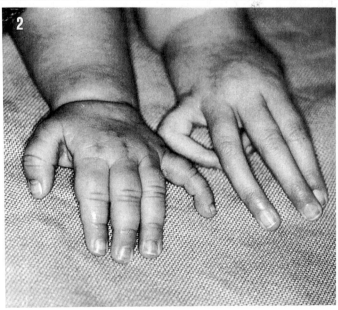

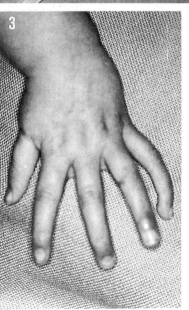

78 Contractural Arachnodactyly
(Beals–Hecht Syndrome, CCA Syndrome)

H.-R.W

A syndrome of arachnodactyly with multiple congenital contractures of the limbs and characteristic changes of the external ear.

Main signs:
- Multiple, mostly symmetrical, congenital contractures of the finger, knee, ankle, elbow and hip joints (usually only mildly involved). Long, thin extremities, including hands and fingers, feet and toes, the proximal phalanges being especially long. Flexion contractures of the fingers at the proximal interphalangeal joints, often with ulnar deviation; thumbs often adducted; toes may be slightly incurved. Pes equinovarus or calcaneo valgus.
- Height normal or above average. Pectus excavatum or carinatum. Frequent development of kyphoscoliosis. Asthenic, Marfanoid habitus. Hypotonia.
- Eyes somewhat deep-set in some cases; external ears may be posteriorly rotated with anomalies of the helix or antihelix and concha, giving the appearance of crumpled ears; high palate, retrognathia. Short neck.

Supplementary findings: No dislocation of the lens or iridodonesis as seen in Marfan syndrome (76) and homocystinuria (79), however, ocular anomalies may occur.

Cardiovascular disorders (as in Marfan syndrome) are much less frequent but may occur, e.g. prolapse of the mitral valve.

Strict differentiation from Marfan syndrome questionable.

Manifestation: At birth.

Aetiology: Autosomal dominant disorder with variable expression. Fibrillin-2 defect. Gene locus: 5q23-31.

Frequency: Low (to date few more than 100 patients in the literature).

Course, prognosis: Initially, motor retardation possible, especially as a result of knee and ankle contractures.

Normal life expectancy (unless, as an exception, a serious cardiac defect is present). The contractures tend to improve, whereas the kyphoscoliosis, when present, tends to progress.

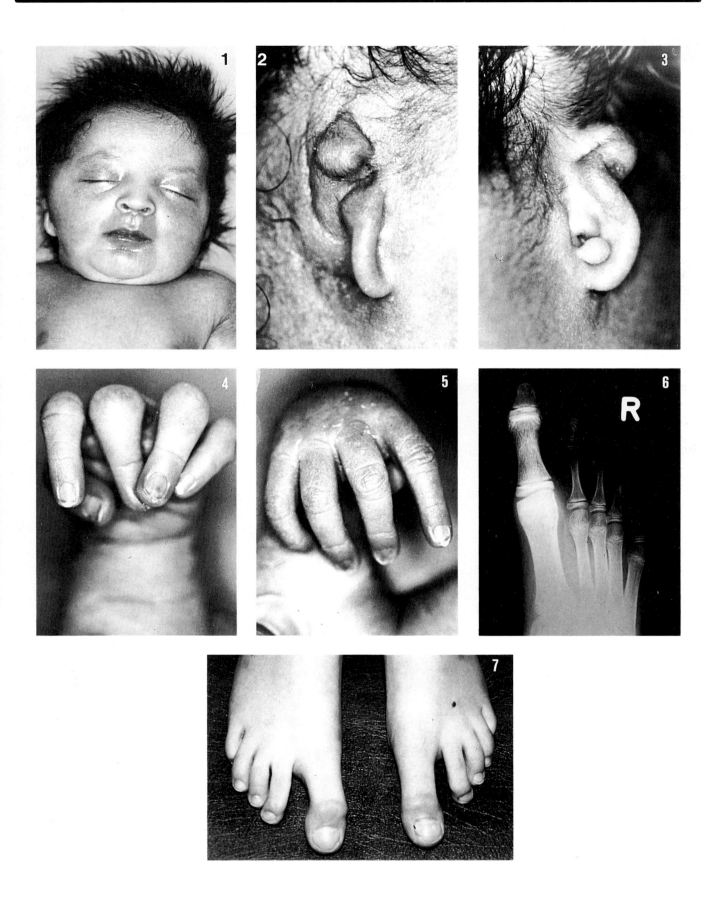

Differential diagnosis: Arthrogryposis (226); differentiation possible from the complete clinical picture.

In the rare case of mental subnormality and rib and vertebral anomalies (supernumerary), a chromosomal aberration (trisomy 8) must be ruled out.

Treatment: Symptomatic, with intensive physiotherapy; surgical correction of malpositioned fingers, if necessary. Genetic counselling.

Illustrations:

1–5 (previous page) An 8-day-old male infant: partial helical aplasia ('crumpled ears'), stenosis of the auditory canal, arachnodactyly with congenital digital contractures.

6 and 7 Characteristic extension of the first ray in a 12-year-old patient.

1–3 (opposite) A mentally normal boy at age 3 years and 6 months, the second child of healthy parents, after the birth of a healthy girl. Birth length 57 cm; subsequent height measurements above the 97th percentile. Congenital flexion contractures of the fingers and bilateral clinodactyly of the fifth finger; long narrow feet, initially in slight club-foot position (later, valgus deformity and pes planus). Large cranium; hypertelorism; high, narrow palate with bifid uvula, slight micrognathia; large ears, posteriorly rotated on the right. Bluish sclera; eyes otherwise negative at repeat follow-up examinations. Winged scapulae; 'pigeon chest' deformity of the thorax; pronounced muscular hypotonia; inguinal hernias. Kidneys normal. Chromosome analysis with banding negative. Low excretion of 5-hydroxyproline.

Persistent ductus arteriosis (ligation at age 3 years). Persistence of the left superior vena cava; surgical repair of severe aortic dilatation and aortic valve replacement at age 5 years. Death caused by heart failure at 5 years and 8 months.

References:

Beals R K, Hecht F: Congenital contractural arachnodactyly. *J Bone Jt Surg* 1971, **53-A**:987.

Bjerkreim I, Skogland L B, Trygstad O: Congenital contractural arachnodactyly. *Acta Orthop scand* 1976, **47**:250.

Meinecke P, Schaefer E *et al*: Congenitale kontrakturelle Arachnodaktylie... *Klin Pädiatr* 1983, **185**:64–70.

Anderson R A. Koch S *et al*: Cardiovascular findings in congenital contractural arachnodactyly... *Am J.Med Genet*.1984, **18**:265–271.

Arroyo M A R, Weaver D D *et al*: Congenital contractural arachnodactyly... review... *Clin Genet* 1985, **27**:570–581.

Tamminga R, Jennekens F G J *et al*: An infant with Marfanoid phenotype and congenital contractures... *Eur J Pediatr* 1985, **143**:228–231.

Currarino G, Friedman J M: A severe form of congenital contractural arachnodactyly... *Am J.Med Genet* 1986, **25**:763–773.

Huggon I C, Burke J P *et al*: Contractural arachnodactyly with mitral regurgitation and iridodonesis. *Arch Dis Child* 1990, **65**:317–319.

Lee B, Godfrey M *et al*: Linkage of Marfan syndrome and a phenotypically related disorder to two different fibrillin genes. *Nature* 1991, **352**:330–334.

Viljoen D, Ramesar R *et al*: Beals syndrome: clinical and molecular investigations... *Clin Genet* 1991, **39**:181–188.

Bawle R, Quigg M H: Actopia lentis and aortic root dilatation in congenital contractural arachnodactyly. *Am J.Med Genet* 1992, **42**:19–21.

Viljoen D: Congenital contractural arachnodactyly (Beals syndrome). *J Med Genet* 1994, **31**:640–643.

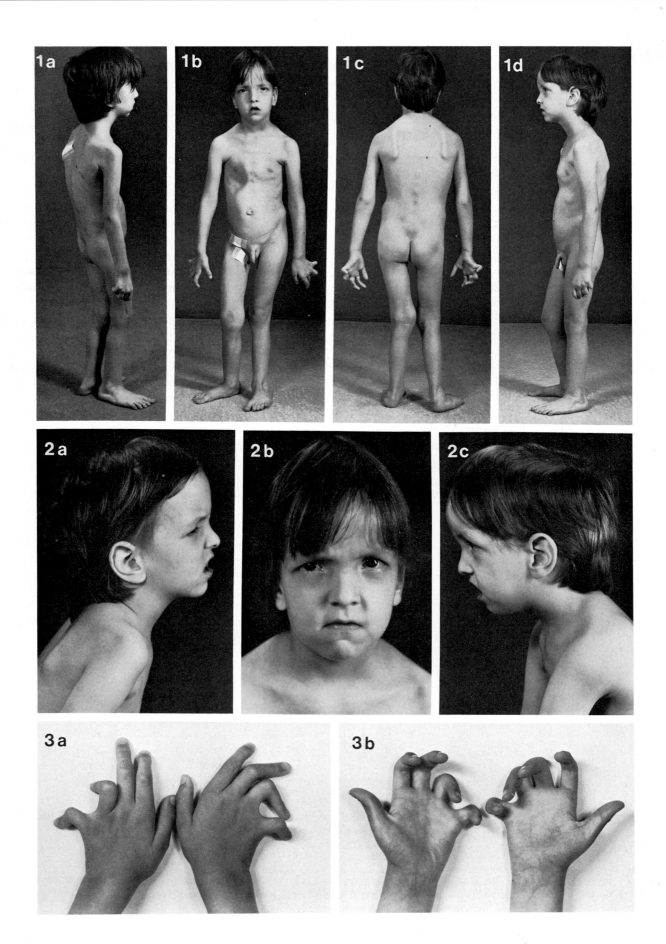

163

79 Homocystinuria

A metabolic disorder leading to tall stature, visual disorders and frequently also mental retardation.

Main signs:
- A clinical picture similar to Marfan syndrome, with age-dependent progressive changes: tall stature with often eunuchoid body proportions, conspicuous in childhood and increasing until puberty; arachnodactyly; deficient subcutaneous fat. Long, narrow face (especially **1–3**); high palate.
- Pectus carinatum or excavatum (**2 and 6**), scoliosis or kyphoscoliosis, knock-knees (**2**), hernias (**2**, postoperative), ankylosis, 'waddling' gait.
- Thin, sparse, dry blond hair; strikingly reddened cheeks, translucent skin. Tendency to eczema.
- In one-half to two-thirds of all patients, mental retardation of various grades of severity. Behavioural disturbances with decreased ability to concentrate, irritability, limited social contact, etc. Possible mild microcephaly.

Supplementary findings: Dislocation of the lens, usually inferiorly, occurring no later than the second decade of life; myopia; possible cataracts, secondary glaucoma, retinal detachment.

Tendency to form thrombo-emboli, even in early childhood and in every region of the body; severe premature arteriosclerosis due to homocystinemic damage to the endothelium.

Seizures in some cases.

Hepatomegaly.

Osteoporosis, punctate calcifications of the distal radial and ulnar epiphyses; shortened metacarpal IV in some patients.

Homocystine in the urine, hypermethioninemia, or enzyme defects in fibroblasts demonstrable.

Manifestation: Biochemically, in the first weeks of life; clinically, in childhood or later.

Aetiology: Autosomal recessive disorder with absence of the enzyme cystathionine synthetase (gene located on the long arm of chromosome 21 (21q22.3). Subdivided into type A and type B according to whether responsive or unresponsive to vitamin B_6 therapy.

In addition, there are further biochemically defined types of homocystinuria which, however, do not show the clinical picture described here (genetic heterogeneity).

Frequency: Approximately one out of 50 000–150 000 of the population.

Course, prognosis: Life expectancy of untreated patients substantially shortened because of thrombo-embolic complications.

Diagnosis: Initially by means of special urinary tests and subsequent quantitative determination of homocystine in the blood plasma and urine. With thrombo-embolism of unknown origin in childhood, homocystinuria must always be considered.

Differential diagnosis: Marfan syndrome (76), in which, however, dislocation of the lens is usually congenital and upwards, cheeks are not flushed, hair is normal, joints are hyperextensible. Furthermore, no mental retardation, no analogous tendency to thrombo-embolism, no progression of signs and usually a family history of similarly affected persons.

Treatment: Approximately 50% of patients respond to high doses of vitamin B_6 (with simultaneous folic acid substitution), type A. Life-long treatment is required. Type B can be favourably influenced by a methionine-deficient and L-cystine-enriched diet on a long-term basis.

Great restraint is needed with operative procedures, especially all avoidable procedures involving the vascular system (venepuncture, etc.) because of the danger of triggering thrombo-embolism. Genetic counselling. In some cases, use of prenatal diagnostic possibilities.

Illustrations:

1–4 Patient 1 at age 5 years 6 months. Height 129 cm (average height of a 7-year-old boy). Moderate mental retardation. Blond hair, reddened cheeks. Dislocation of the lenses and myopia diagnosed at age 2 years.

5–7 Patient 2 aged 3 years 9 months. Height 109 cm (average height of a 5 year old). No mental retardation. Blond hair. Flushed cheeks, eczema. At age 2 years and 6 months slight myopia. No osteoporosis. Neither patient responded to treatment with pharmacological doses of vitamin B_6.

References:

Fowler B, Børresen A L: Prenatal diagnosis of homocystinuria. *Lancet* 1982, II:875.

Munnich A, Saudubray J-M *et al*: Diet-responsive proconvertin (factor VII) deficiency in homocystinuria. *J Pediatr* 1983, 102:730–734.

Wilcken D E L, Wilcken B *et al*: Homocystinuria—the effects of betaine... *N Engl J Med* 1983, 309:448–453.

Boers G H J, Fowler B *et al*: Improved identification of heterozygotes for homocystinuria... *Hum Genet* 1985, 69:164–169.

Skovby Fl: Homocystinuria. *Acta Pediatr Scand Suppl* 1985, 321.

Amram S, Palcoux J B *et al*: Homocystinurie pyridoxino-résistante. *Arch Fr Pédiatr* 1986, **43**:715–717.

Abbott M H, Folstein S E *et al*: Psychiatric manifestations of homocystinuria... *Am J Med.Genet* 1987, 26:959–969.

Gu Z *et al*: Identification of a molecular genetic defect in homocystinuria... (Abstract). *Am J Hum Genet* 1991, 49:406.

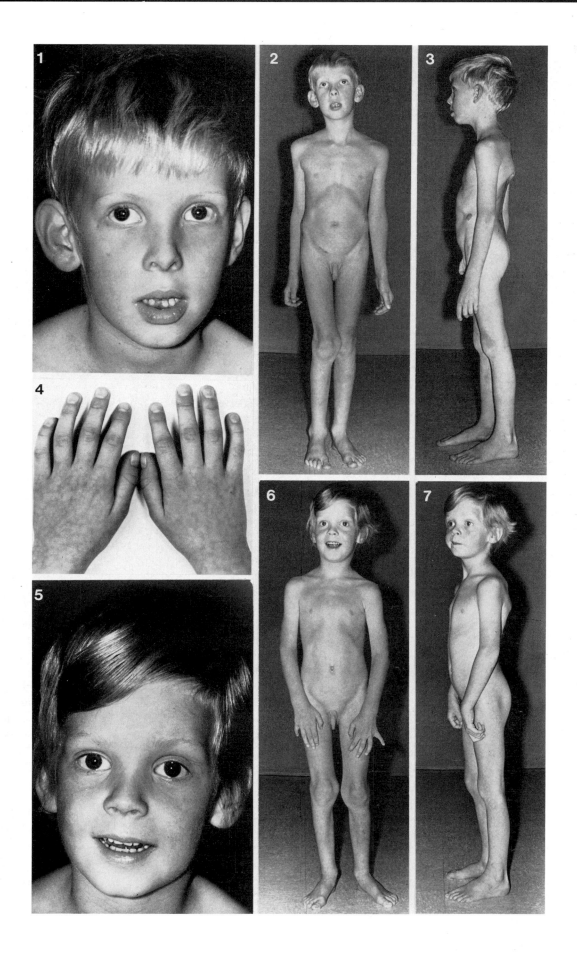

80 XYY Syndrome

H.-R.W/ J.K.

A tall-stature syndrome in males, with frequent behavioural disorders and an extra Y chromosome.

Main signs:
- Tall stature (greater than 180 cm).
- Behavioural disorders in 50%.
- Delayed speech development.

Supplementary findings: Average intelligence. Psyche frequently labile; patients may be unstable, easily led astray and have a history of deviant behaviour.

Increased occurrence of minor anomalies: relatively large head, asymmetrical cranium, dysplastic ears, epicanthus, strabismus, micrognathia; radioulnar synostostes, clinodactyly, single-crease fifth finger, simian crease; pectus carinatum, inguinal hernias.

Tendency to acne and early varicosities of the lower leg and leg ulcers. Double 'Y-chromosomal sex chromatin' demonstrable in a simple screening test; confirmation of the abnormal sex chromosome constitution by chromosome analysis.

Manifestation: Tall stature beginning in puberty, severe acne.

Aetiology: The syndrome, expressing the chromosomal aberration of a supernumerary Y chromosome, is caused by faulty separation of the chromosomes during spermatogenesis.

Frequency: Approximately one out of 1000 newborn boys.

Course, prognosis: Average final height of about 1.85 m; occasionally, patients may be much taller. Extreme tallness is a marked psychological handicap, impairing the patient's ability to cope. Possible infertility (cryptorchidism, hypospadias, small testes, reduced spermatogenesis, Sertoli-cell-only configuration).

Differential diagnosis: Other tall-stature syndromes, especially Marfan syndrome (76), XXY syndrome (308).

Treatment: Hormonal therapy, if excessive growth is anticipated. Psychological guidance; psychotherapy may be indicated.

Illustrations:

1 and 2 The same patient at age 14 years (1.82 m) and 18 years (2.02 m).

References:
Any comprehensive paediatric or internal-medicine textbook.
Robinson A, Lubs H A *et al*: Summary of clinical findings: profiles of children with... 47, XYY *karyotypes Birth Defects Orig Art Ser,* 1979, Vol. XV, Nr 1:261–266.
Grass F, McCombs J *et al*: Reproduction in XYY males ... implications for genetic counseling. *Am J Med Genet* 1984, **19**:553–560.
Netley C T: Summary overview of behavioural development in individuals with neonatally identified X and Y aneuploidy. *Birth Defects Orig Art Ser,* 1986, Vol. XXII, Nr. 3:293–306.
Robinson A, Bender G B, Linden M G: Summary of clinical findings in children and young adults with sex chromosome anomalies. *Birth Defects Orig Art Ser,* 1991, Vol. 26, Nr 4:225–228.

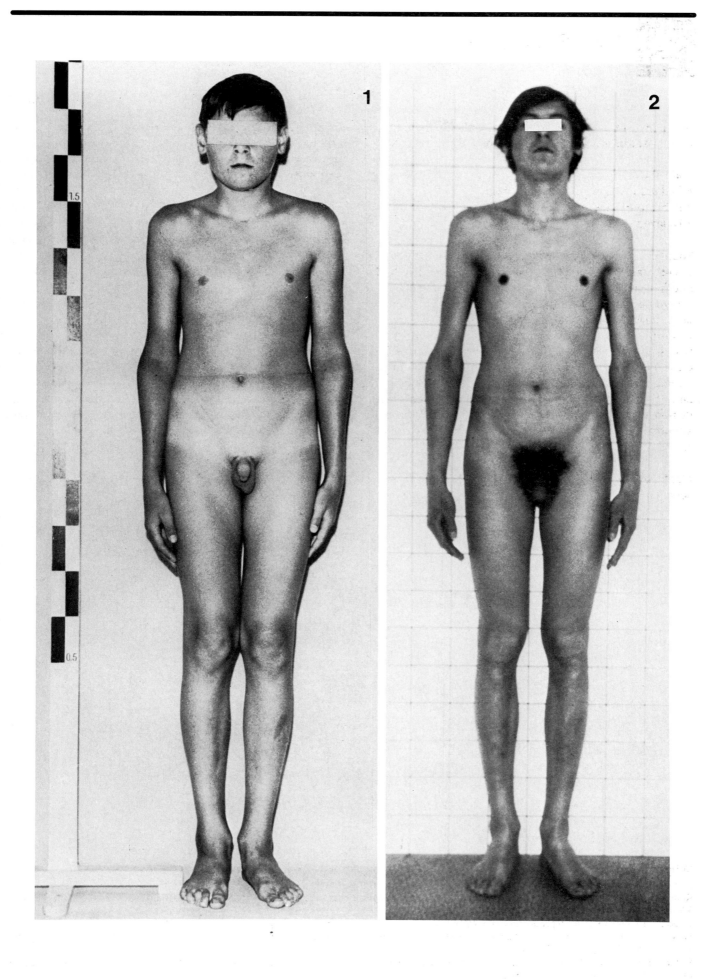

81 Malformation–Retardation Syndrome Caused by Incomplete Triploidy

J.K./H.-R.W

A syndrome of primary subnormality, frequent asymmetry, genital anomalies and psychomotor retardation with mosaic triploidy.

Main signs:
- Prenatal and postnatal growth deficiency with relatively large, elongated cranium, micrognathia and sometimes low-set poorly formed ears (**1**).
- Frequent asymmetry of the body because of underdevelopment of one-half of the face or one extremity (**2a, 2b, 3a**).
- Hypogenitalism in males (micropenis, cryptorchidism, sometimes hypospadias or intersex features) (**2a, 3a**).
- Mental retardation; possible seizure disorder.
- Chromosomally: mosaic triploidy (2N/3N).

Supplementary findings: Average birth weight approximately 2200 g. Diverse anomalies of the hands and feet: club foot, syndactyly, camptodactyly, clinodactyly and others (**3b and 3c**). Pigmentation anomalies in some patients.

Manifestation: At birth.

Aetiology: The presence of (in the case of the patient in 1–3, 4%) triploid cells (in the given case, 69 XXY) as a mosaic (2N/3N).

Frequency: Low; to date only 20 patients reported.

Course, prognosis: Not infrequently, initial failure to thrive. Otherwise the prognosis is mainly dependent on the degree of psychomotor or mental retardation.

Diagnosis, differential diagnosis: The initial assumption has repeatedly been Silver–Russell syndrome (*82*), however, psychomotor retardation and comparatively good body weight should facilitate clinical differentiation. In case of doubt, chromosomal analysis of cultured skin fibroblasts.

Treatment: Symptomatic. Appropriate handicap aids.

Illustrations:
1–3 The same patient, the second child of healthy, young, non-consanguineous parents, after a healthy brother.
1 Somewhat small neonate (47 cm; 2400 g; head circumference 34 cm) with relatively large cranium, micrognathia, radial abduction of both hands.
2 The patient at 3 years.
3 At 4 years and 6 months. Hypoplasia of the left side of the face and the left upper extremity. At both ages, height corresponded to the 10th percentile, head circumference 50–75th percentile. Genu valgus. Micropenis and bilateral undescended testes. Obvious mental retardation.
3b and 3c Proximally displaced thumbs; cutaneous syndactyly of fingers III/IV, of toes II–IV; clinocamptodactyly of both fifth fingers bilaterally, hypoplasia of the fifth toes; 'sandal gap' between the first two toes.
For a long time, the patient was assumed to suffer from the Silver–Russell syndrome. Internal organs: horseshoe kidneys.

References:
Graham J M, Hoehn H, Lin M S et al: Diploid-triploid mixoploidy: clinical and cytogenetic aspects. *Pediatrics* 1981, **68**:23–28.
Tharapel A T, Wilroy R S, Martens P R et al: Diploid-triploid mosaicism: delineation of the syndrome. *Ann Génét* 1983, **26**:229–233.
Meinecke P, Engelbrecht R: Fehlbildungs-Retardierungssyndrom infolge inkompletter Triploidie. *Mschr Kinderheilk* 1988, **136**:206–208.
Küster W, Beckmann H, Gebauer H J et al: Triploidie bei neugeborenen. *Mschr Kinderheilk* 1988, **136**:210–213.
McFadden D E, Kalousek D K: Two different phenotypes of fetuses with chromosomal triploidy: correlation with parental origin of the extra haploid set. *Am J Med Genet* 1991, **38**:35–538.
Järvelä I E, Salo M K, Santavuori P, Salonen R K: 46, XX/69, XXX diploid-triploid mixoploidy with hypothyroidism and precocious puberty. *J Med Genet* 1993, **30**:966–967.
Niemann-Seyde S C, Rehder H, Zoll B: A case of full triploidy (69, XXX) of paternal origin with unusually long survival time. *Clin Genet* 1993, **43**:79–82.

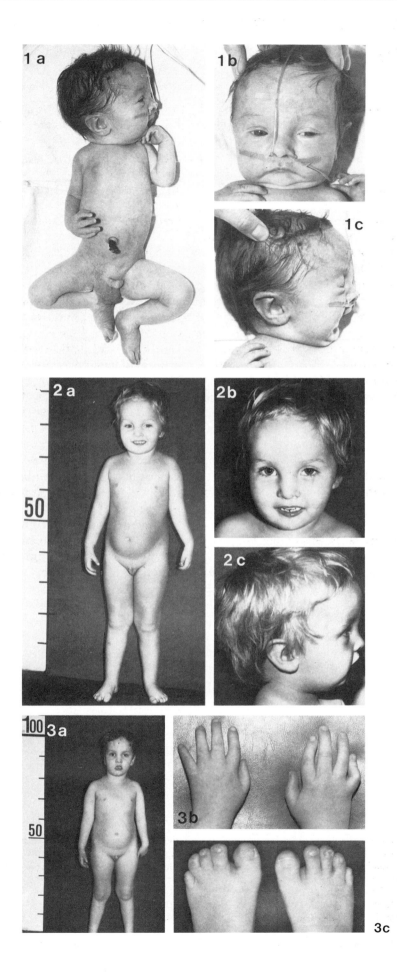

82 Silver–Russell Syndrome
(Russell–Silver Syndrome)

H.-R.W/J.K.

A syndrome comprising marked prenatal and postnatal slenderness, growth retardation, a relatively very large cranium with correspondingly small triangular face and micrognathia, fairly marked asymmetry of the body and clinobrachydactyly of the little fingers.

Main signs:
- Congenital small size (length and weight) with birth at term. Disproportionately large cranium (**1**) with prominent forehead, high hair line and frequently very late closure of the anterior fontanelle, however, normal head circumference at birth and normal further development: 'pseudohydrocephalus'. Small triangular face, often with fine, small nose, short philtrum and large thin-lipped mouth with down-turned corners. Micrognathia (**3**).
- Postnatal continuation of slow growth in height and especially weight (under or at the third percentile; final height approximately 150 cm). Not infrequently, distinct asymmetry because of underdevelopment of one side of the body or a part thereof. The upper extremities may be relatively short (**2a**) and the lower extremities long. Very slender build, also with narrow thorax and insufficiently developed musculature (**2**).
- Clinodactyly or clinobrachydactyly of the little fingers. Delayed bone age (**4**).

Supplementary findings: High squeaky voice persisting for years. Marked tendency to sweat heavily.

Café au lait spots of the skin; hip or other skeletal dysplasias; malformations of the urogenital system. With marked asymmetry of the lower extremities, tilting of the pelvis and secondary scoliosis.

Possible signs of dissociated precocious puberty; most frequently, early elevation of gonadotropin in the urine.

Gross motor development may be delayed. Exceptionally, mental retardation (approximately 15% of patients).

Manifestation: Prenatally and postnatally.

Aetiology: Insufficiently explained. Usually sporadic occurrence. Patients with sex-linked dominant, autosomal dominant or autosomal recessive inheritance are the exception.

A gene locus on the long arm of chromosome 17 was suspected (17q25).

The syndrome shows considerable phenotypic variability.

Frequency: Moderately low but over 200 publications:

Course, prognosis: Usually relatively favourable (apart from the small adult height); in individual patients, dependent on the degree of expression of the clinical picture and on the significance of possible additional malformations and handicaps.

Differential diagnosis: A wide spectrum of clinical pictures with congenital growth retardation need to be considered, including Floating Harbor (*83*), Rubinstein–Taybi (*87*), and Dubowitz (*95*) syndromes. SHORT syndrome (*321*).

Treatment: Physiotherapy and possibly orthopaedic care or alternatively nephro-urological or psychological care may be needed. Growth hormone deficiency and response to high doses of HGH may occur.

Illustrations:
1-3 A 2-year-old girl of normal psychomotor development (birth at term, 1800 g and 49 cm). Height age, 18 months (i.e. below the 10th percentile); weight age, 9 months (i.e. below the third percentile). Congenital hemiatrophy of the whole right side of the body, including the ear and nose (osseous atrophy shown in **3a**); secondary tilting of the pelvis and mild secondary scoliosis. Relatively large but normal-for-age cranium (46.5 cm). Prominent, slightly bulging forehead. Small face; microretrognathia. Clinobrachydactyly of the fifth fingers; syndactyly on the right. Rather unusually tall lumbar vertebral bodies. Ectopic ureterocoele with megaureter and hydronephrosis on the left and with left quiescent accessory kidney and ureter. Markedly elevated gonadotropins in the urine.

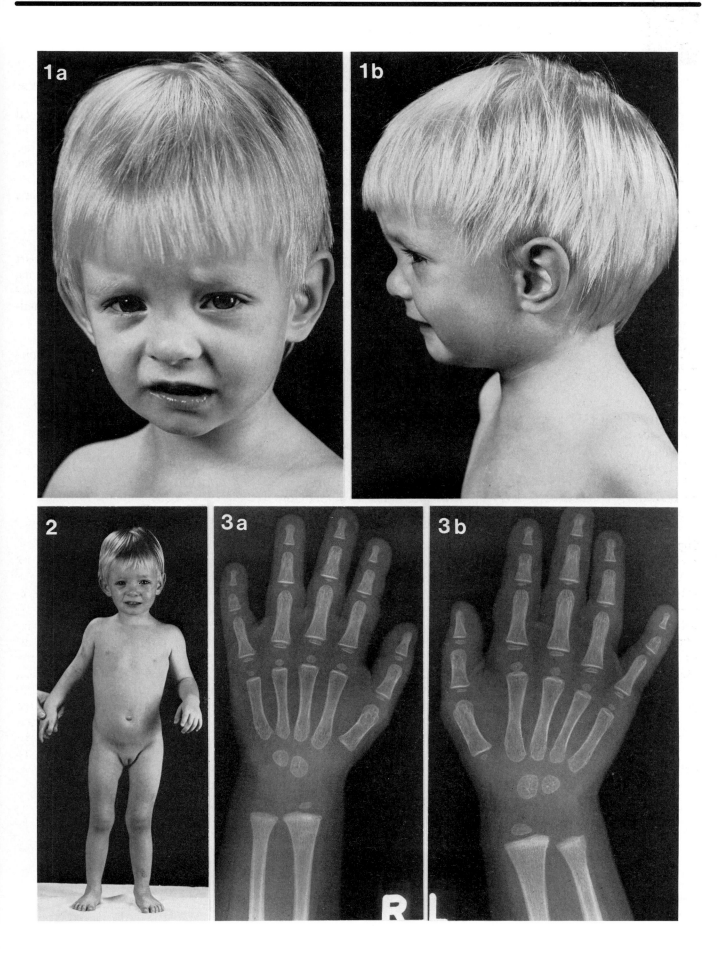

H.-R.W

Illustrations:

1–5 A child born at term with birth weight 1750 g; mental development within normal limits. Shown at 4 years and 6 months (52 cm, 3220 g), at 3 years and 4 months (75 cm, 5500 g) and 12 years and 5 months (126.5 cm, 14.8 kg) (in each case, far below the third percentile). Extremely slender build. Dolichocephaly with large protruding forehead and high and initially thin hairline, head circumference normal for age. Right half of the face somewhat fuller than the left. Slightly low-set ears. Congenital ptosis of the left upper eyelid. Relatively large, thin-lipped mouth with slightly down-turned corners. Microretrognathia. Overbite, narrowly spaced teeth, especially in the lower jaw; caries. Squeaky voice.

Short upper extremities. Slight clinobrachydactyly of the little fingers; bilateral zygodactyly with a double nail on the left second toe.

Extremely narrow, slim hand with markedly delayed bone age. Pseudo-epiphyses of metacarpals I and II proximally and hypoplastic middle phalanx of fifth finger.

Possible ventricular septal defect. Slightly dilated right renal pelvis on pyelography; hypospadias.

Profuse sweating.

References:

Silver H K, Kiyasu W, George J *et al*: Syndrome of congenital hemihypertrophy, shortness of stature and elevated urinary gonadotropins. *Pediatrics* 1953, **12**:368–375.
Russell A: A syndrome of 'intra-uterine' dwarfism recognizable at birth with cranio-facial dysostosis, disproportionately short arms and other anomalies (5 examples). *Proc Roy Soc Med* 1954, **47**:1040.
Tanner J M, Lejarraga H, Cameron N: The natural history of the Silver–Russell syndrome: a longitudinal study of thirty-nine cases. *Pediatr Res* 1975, **9**:611–623.
Angehrn V, Zachmann M, Prader A: Silver–Russell syndrome. Observations in 20 patients. *Helv Paed Acta* 1979, **34**:297–308.
Saal H M, Ragon R A, Pepin M G: Reevaluation of Russell–Silver syndrome. *J Pediatr* 1985, **107**:733–737.
Partsch C J, Hermanussen M, Sippell W G: Treatment of Silver–Russell type dwardism with human growth hormone... *Acta Endocrinol Suppl* 1986, **279**:139–146.
Davies P S, Valley R, Preece M A: Adolescent growth and pubertal progression in the Silver–Russell syndrome. *Arch Dis Child* 1988, **63**:130–135.
Patton M A: Russell–Silver syndrome. *J Med Genet* 1988, **25**:557–560.
Chitayat D, Friedman J M *et al*: Hepatocellular carcinoma in a child with familial Russell–Silver syndrome. *Am J Med Genet* 1988, **31**:909–914.
Donnai D, Thompson E, Allanson J, Baraitser M: Severe Silver–Russell syndrome. *J Med Genet* 1989, **26**:447–451.
Duncan P A, Hall J G, Shapiro R, Vibert B.K: Three-generation dominant transmission of the Silver–Russell syndrome. *Am J Med Genet* 1990, **35**:245–250.
Samm M, Lewis K, Blumberg Br: Monozygotic twins discordant for the Russell–Silver syndrome. *Am J Med Genet* 1990, **37**:543–545.
Lai K Y C, Skuse D *et al*: Cognitive abilities associated with the Silver–Russell syndrome. *Arch Dis Child* 1994, **71**:490–496.

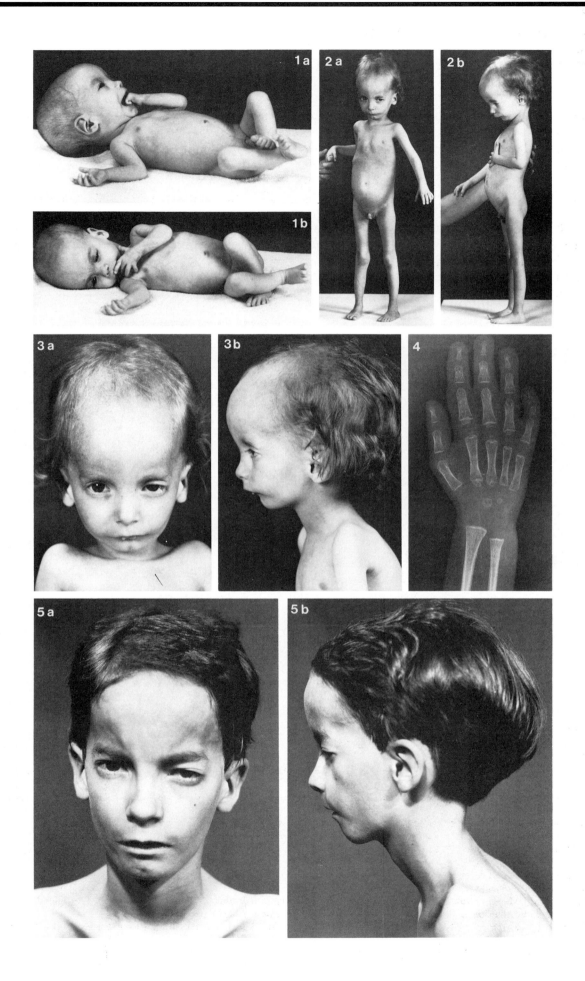

83 Floating Harbor Syndrome

J.K.

A short-stature syndrome with delayed speech development and unusual facial features.

Main signs:
- Primordial growth deficiency, postnatally persistent short stature, birth weight below the third percentile, delayed bone maturation.
- Delayed speech development, mild mental retardation, normal motor development in two-thirds of the patients observed.
- Craniofacial dysmorphism: bulbous nose, short philtrum, thin lips, large mouth, malocclusion, deep-set eyes, long eyelashes, dorsally rotated ears, triangular-shaped face.

Supplementary findings: Low occipital hairline, hirsutism, short neck, clinodactyly, brachydactyly, broad thumbs, hyperextensible joints, distended abdomen (coeliac disease).

Manifestation: In early infancy.

Aetiology: To date only sporadic, isolated cases. No increased consanguinity rate.

Pathogenesis: Unknown.

Frequency: Up to 15 isolated reports.

Course, prognosis: Eventual height after puberty between 130 and 140 cm. No growth-hormone deficiency.

Differential diagnosis: Silver–Russell syndrome (*82*), Dubowitz syndrome (*95*), Rubinstein–Taybi syndrome (*87*), 3-M syndrome. SHORT syndrome (*321*).

Treatment: Gluten-free diet in the case of coeliac disease. Speech therapy.

Illustrations:

1 and 2 Age 2 years, pseudohydrocephalus, short palpebral fissures, large nose, broad nasal bridge, broad nasal tip (flared nostrils), short philtrum, micrognathia, hypoplastic ears. Somatotrophic normal.

3–5 Age 4 years, height 90 cm (−3.5 SD), relative macrocephaly. Aloof, retarded.

6 Short metacarpals, especially distally; brachydactyly; delayed bone age.

7 Patient 2, female, age 2 years and 10 months, height 80.4 cm (below third percentile), large nose, broad nasal bridge, mild convergent strabismus, deep-set eyes, long lashes, dorsally rotated dysplastic ears, long philtrum, thin upper lip.

8 and 9 Patient 3, female, age 14 years, 140 cm (below third percentile), circumference of the head 52 cm (below third percentile), mild hirsutism, triangular-shaped face, short philtrum, thin lips, broad nose, deep-set eyes, dorsally rotated ears, incomplete development of the ears.

7–9 from:
R S Houlston, A L Collins, N R Dennis, I K Temple, Further observations on the Floating-Harbor syndrome. *Clin Dysmorphol* 1994, 3:143–149.

References:

Robinson P L, Shohat M *et al*: A unique association of short stature, dysmorphic features, and speech impairment (Floating-Harbor syndrome). *J Pediatr* 1988, **113**:703–706.

Patton M A, Hurst J *et al*: Floating-Harbor syndrome. *J Med Genet* 1991, **28**:201–204.

Majewski F, Lenard H G: The Floating-Harbor syndrome. *Eur J Pediatr* 1991, **150**:250–252.

Chudley A E, Moroz S P: Floating-Harbor syndrome and celiac disease. *Am J Med Genet* 1991, **38**:562–564.

Houlston R S, Collins A L, Dennis N R, Temple I K: Further observations on the Floating-Harbor syndrome. *Clin Dysmorphol* 1994, 3:143–149.

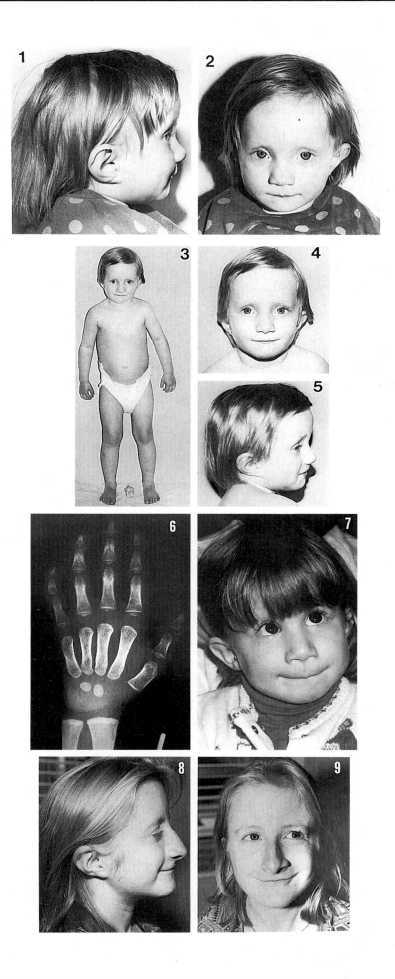

J.K.

A genetically distinct syndrome with epicanthus medialis inversus, lateral displacement of the inner canthi, ptosis and blepharophimosis in addition to female infertility in type I.

Main signs:
- Epicanthus medialis inversus between the upper and lower lids, short palpebral fissure with displacement of the medial angle of the eye (telecanthus). Ptosis, flat nasal bridge, anteverted nares and strabismus.
- Dysplastic ears in some patients.
- Primary hypogonadism with sterility in female type I patients.
- Muscular hypotonia in early infancy.

Supplementary findings: Cardiac defects, occasionally mental retardation. Microphthalmia, anophthalmia, microcornea, hyperopia (hypermetropia), strabismus, nystagmus, amblyopia.

Manifestation: At birth.

Aetiology: Although transmitted as an autosomal dominant condition in type I, infertility affects females only. Penetrance is complete; the sex ratio of corresponding patients in an affected family is therefore shifted to an excess of males. Type II is inherited from both males and females by autosomal dominant transmission with incomplete penetrance. Among the children of affected males, predominantly females are affected and among the children of affected women, predominantly males. The sex ratio of affected individuals within the family is normal. Gene locus: 3q22.3–3q23.

Frequency: Type I is more common than type II. This is significant in genetic counselling of the infertile women.

Course, prognosis: Cardiac defects and mental retardation prevent some patients from living a full life.

Differential diagnosis: Blepharophimosis associated with malformations as part of other syndromes.

Treatment: Ophthalmologic and surgical care. Definition and hormone replacement therapy for ovarian insufficiency.

Illustrations:
1 5-month-old girl.
2 10-month-old girl.
3 14-month-old girl.
All three children have normal psychomotor development, epicanthus inversus, blepharophimosis, ptosis, telecanthus, anteverted nostrils.

References:

Callahan A: Surgical correction of the blepharophimosis syndrome. *Trans Am Acad Ophthalmol Otolaryngol* 1973, 77:687–695.

Pueschel S M, Barsel-Bowers G: A dominantly inherited congenital anomaly syndrome with blepharophimosis. *J Pediatr* 1979, 95:1010–1013.

Zlotogora J, Sagi M, Cohen T: The blepharophimosis, ptosis, and epicanthus inversus syndrome: delineation of two types. *Am J Hum Genet* 1983, 35:1020–1027.

Oley C, Baraitser M: Blepharophimosis, ptosis, epicanthus inversus syndrome (BPES syndrome). Syndrome of the month. *J Med Genet* 1988, 25:47–51.

Jewett T, Rao P N *et al*: Blepharophimosis, ptosis and epicanthus inversus syndrome (BPES) associated with interstitial deletion of band 3q22: review and gene assignment to the interface of band 3q22.3-3q23. *Am J Med Genet* 1993, 47:1147–1150.

Boccone L, Meloni A *et al*: Blepharophimosis, ptosis, epicanthus inversus syndrome, a new case associated with de novo balanced autosomal translocation [46, XY, + (3;7)(q23;q32)]. *Am J Med Genet* 1994, 51:258–259.

Ishikiriyama S, Goto M: Blepharophimosis, ptosis and epicanthus inversus syndrome (BPES) and microcephaly. *Am J Med Genet* 1994, 52:245.

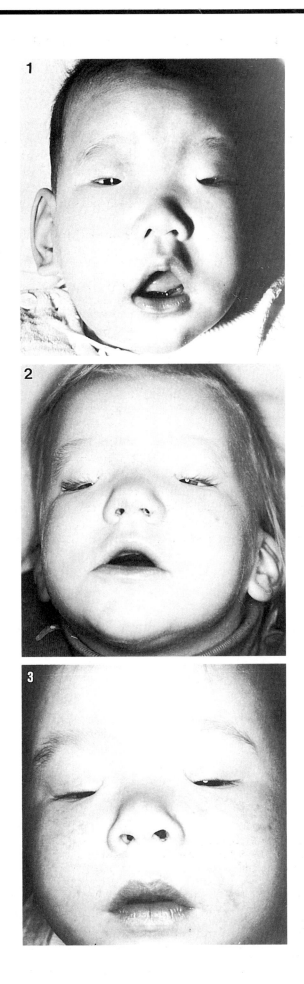

85 Primordial Short Stature with Relative Macrocrania, Peculiar Physiognomy, Further Minor Malformations and Normal Psychomotor Development

H.-R.W

A syndrome of primordial short stature, unusual facies with blepharophimosis, large dolichocephalic cranium and normal mental development.

Main signs:
- Primordial, for the most part proportionate, slender short stature, well under the third percentile. Relative macrocephaly with dolichocephaly (1–3).
- Facies: short, narrow palpebral fissures with slight antimongoloid slant under relatively thick eyebrows. Suggestion of epicanthus bilaterally. Low-set ears. Prominent nose. Small, thin-lipped, narrow mouth, which appears pinched (1, 4). Open bite. Severe caries (secondary to difficulty in caring for the teeth possibly because of the small opening of the mouth).
- Hypogonadism, bilateral cryptorchidism. Simian crease left, suggested on the right; hypoplastic-appearing distal phalanges of the fingers; clinodactyly of the fifth fingers (5).

Supplementary findings: Slumped posture, winged scapulae; dorsal kyphosis, which could be compensated (2 and 3). Psychomotor development normal for age.
Radiographs: dysplasia of the first rib on the left.

Discordant development of the ossification centres on the wrist radiograph and profoundly retarded bone age (by approximately 3 years and 6 months) (5).

Manifestation: At birth.

Aetiology: Undetermined.

Course, prognosis: Apart from short stature, can be expected to be favourable.

Differential diagnosis: Other syndromes with short stature and blepharophimosis.

Treatment: Symptomatic.

Illustrations:
1–5 A 7-year-old boy, the first child of healthy, young nonconsanguineous parents of normal height. A healthy younger brother. Birth of the proband shortly before term with 2250 g and 44 cm. At 7 years and 2 months, 104 cm; head circumference at 6 years and 10 months, 52.3 cm. No abnormality of internal organs; thorough endocrinological examination negative; chromosomal analysis negative.

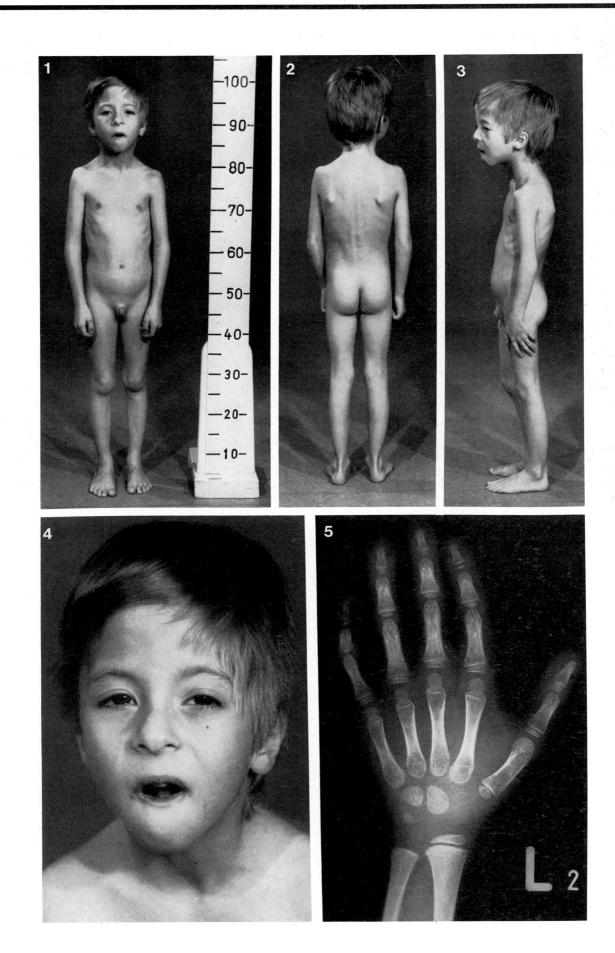

86 Syndrome of Blepharophimosis, Camptodactyly, Short Stature, Mental Retardation and Sensorineural Hearing Impairment

H.-R.W

A syndrome of unusual features of the face, hands and feet, combined with growth disorder, mental retardation and impaired hearing.

Main signs:
- Facies: high forehead, short narrow palpebral fissures, thick eyebrows and mild synophrys; low-set, simple auricles; low nasal bridge and small mouth (with diastema, high palate, bifid uvula) (1–3).
- Camptodactyly of fingers II–V along with clinodactyly of the little fingers (6). Bilateral hallux-valgus deviation and dysplasia of the little toes with rudimentary or absent nails.
- Short stature (below the third percentile at 5 and at 13 years and 6 months) with somewhat short lower extremities (4 and 5).
- Primary mental retardation (IQ 44 at 13 years and 6 months).
- Primary bilateral sensorineural hearing impairment.

Supplementary findings:
Long narrow thorax with mild funnel chest.
Strabismus (operated); ocular fundi normal.
Radiographs: cone-shaped epiphyses of the proximal phalanges of toes II–V bilaterally.

Manifestation: At birth (hearing impairment recognized in late infancy).

Aetiology: Unknown.

Course, prognosis: Affected especially by the severe degree of mental retardation.

Differential diagnosis: Other syndromes associated with short stature and blepharophimosis.

Treatment: Symptomatic.

Illustrations:
1–6 The proband at age 5 years (1, 2, 6) and 13 years and 6 months (3–5). First child of healthy young non-consanguineous parents; premature birth; no serious problems in the first year of life. Several seizures between the third and fifth years of life; neurological examination negative. Electroencephalogram negative, electromyogram normal. Clinical and laboratory examinations negative. Chromosomal analysis negative.

Note: I have since received two comparable reports from colleagues.

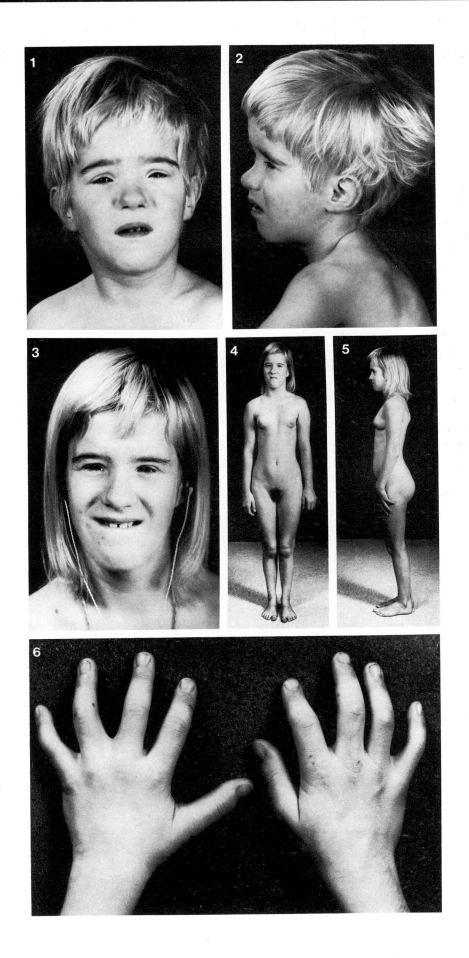

87 Rubinstein–Taybi Syndrome
(Broad Thumb-Broad Hallux Syndrome)

H.-R.W

A syndrome of characteristic facies, microcephalic psychomotor retardation, short stature and anomalies of the hands and feet with broad distal phalanges, especially of the thumbs and halluces.

Main signs:
- Cranium and facies: microcephaly of varied severity, frequently with prominent forehead and large anterior fontanelle. Antimongoloid slant of the palpebral fissures, broad nasal bridge, epicanthic folds, frequent strabismus, prominent eyebrows and eyelids, possible ptosis and mild anomalies of the external ears (1, 2, 6). Beak-shaped nose, aquiline or straight, with anterior prolongation of the nasal septum (2). Microstomia and short upper lip. High palate, slightly receding chin.
- Broad distal phalanges of the thumbs and halluces, also often of other rays (3–7). Thumbs not infrequently radially deviated at the interphalangeal joint ('hitchhiker thumb' 6 and 7). Possible clinodactyly and overlapping toes.
- Psychomotor retardation (IQ usually under 50); frequent electroencephalogram anomalies.
- Short stature (usually about or below the third percentile).

Supplementary findings: Frequently undescended testicles. Frequent hirsutism. Development of kyphoscoliosis. Heart and kidney defects also possible. In some patients, 'soft larynx', causing difficulties with sleeping and anaesthesia; susceptibility to constipation. Increased risk of tumours in the craniocerebral region.

Radiographs may show deformity of the proximal phalanges in patients with abnormal angulation of the thumbs and halluces; sometimes duplication of the hallucal region. Generalized delay of ossification. Possible anomalies of the pelvis, vertebral column or thorax.

Manifestation: At birth and thereafter.

Aetiology: Probably an autosomal dominant new mutation given that occurrence is nearly always sporadic. Frequent concordance in monozygotic twins. Gene locus on chromosome 16 (16p13.3); deletion present in some patients. Practically no increased risk of recurrence in further children of parents with an affected child; 50% risk for the offspring of affected individuals.

Frequency: Among the mentally retarded, up to one out of 500 and higher.

Course, prognosis: For the most part dependent on the degree of mental retardation and the quality of support and education of the child. Average life expectancy probably shortened.

Differential diagnosis: The Saethre–Chotzen (7) and Cornelia de Lange (98) syndromes should not be difficult to exclude.

Treatment: Symptomatic. Any appropriate handicap aids.

Illustrations:
1–5 A girl aged 6 years and 6 months, the second child of healthy non-consanguineous parents after a healthy sibling. Head circumference at birth (with otherwise normal measurements) 32.5 cm; currently 47.6 cm (below the second percentile). Height and weight approximately at the 10th percentile. General developmental retardation. Hirsutism. On radiograph, distinct asymmetry of the facial bones and skull; retarded bone age. Chromosomal analysis negative.
6 and 7 A characteristically affected 4-month-old infant.

References:
Theile U, Draf U, Heldt J P: Das Rubinstein–Taybi–Syndrom. *Dtsch med Wschr* 1978, 1505.
Hennekam R C M, Van den Boogaard M J *et al*: Rubinstein–Taybi syndrome... *Am J Med Genet Suppl* 1990, 6:17–29.
Hennekam R C M, Van Doorne J M: Oral aspects of Rubinstein–Taybi syndrome. *Am J Med Genet Suppl* 1990, 6:42–47.
Hennekam R C M, Stevens C A *et al*: Etiology and recurrence risk in Rubinstein–Taybi syndrome. *Am J Med Genet Suppl* 1990, 6:56–64.
Lowry R B: Overlap between Rubinstein–Taybi and Saethre–Chotzen syndromes... *Am J Med Genet Suppl* 1990, 6:73–76.
Stevens C A, Carey J C *et al*: Rubinstein–Taybi syndrome... *Am J Med Genet Suppl* 1990, 6:30–37.
Imaizumi K, Kuroki Y: Rubinstein–Taybi syndrome... *Am J Med Genet* 1991, 38:636–639.
Tommerup N, van den Hagen C B *et al*: Tentative assignment of a locus for Rubinstein–Taybi syndrome... *Cell Genet* 1991, 58:2002–2003.
Allanson J E: Microcephaly in Rubinstein–Taybi syndrome (Letter). *Am J Med Genet* 1993, 46:244–246.
Marion R W, Garcia D M *et al*: Apparent dominant transmission of the Rubinstein–Taybi syndrome. *Am J Med Genet* 1993, 46:284–287.
Robinson T W, Stewart D L *et al*: Monozygotic twins concordant for Rubinstein–Taybi syndrome and implications for genetic counseling. *Am J Med Genet* 1993, 45:671–673.
Lacombe D: Le syndrome de Rubinstein–Taybi. *Arch Pédiatr* 1994, 681–683.
Masuno M, Imaizumi K *et al*: Submicroscopic deletion... 16p13.3 in... Rubinstein–Taybi syndrome. *Am J Med Genet* 1994, 53:352–354.
Miller R W, Rubinstein J H: Tumors in Rubinstein–Taybi syndrome. *Am J Med Genet* 1995, 56:112–115.

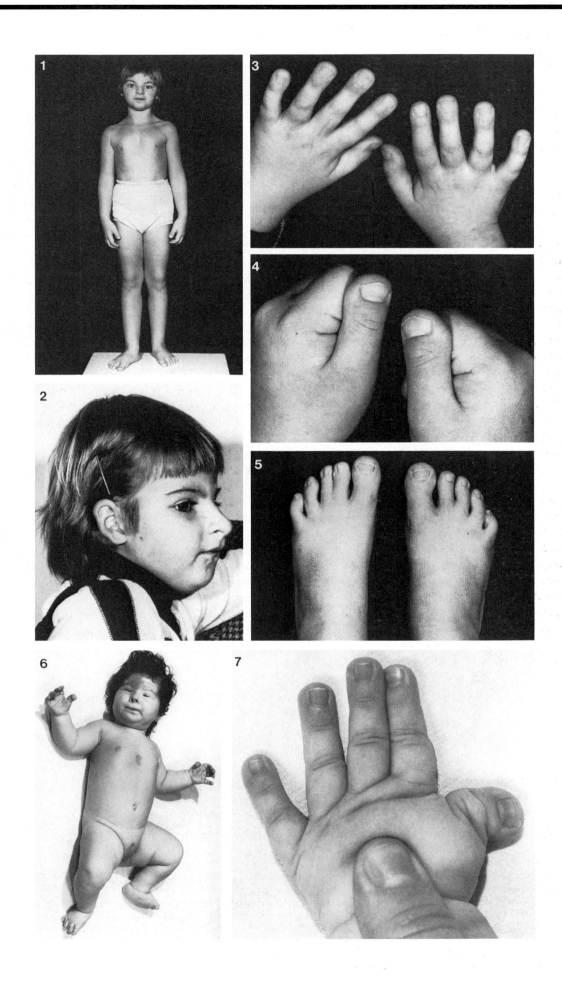

88 Syndrome of Dyscrania or Microcephaly, Psychomotor Retardation and Short Stature with Anomalies of the Hands and Feet

H.-R.W

A familial dyscrania-microcephaly-retardation syndrome with short stature and broad, short thumbs and halluces.

Main signs:
- Dyscrania with high forehead, sloping occiput (1–3); microcephaly.
- Facies: slight antimongoloid slant of the palpebral fissures, low-set ears, slightly receding chin (1-3).
- Psychomotor retardation of variable severity.
- Short stature (can be below the third percentile).
- Short hands and feet with stubby, broad thumbs and halluces (1b–3b, 4, 5).

Supplementary findings: Unilateral undescended testes in both the boys illustrated, as well as inguinal hernias. Micropenis and marked scrotal hypoplasia in the child in 3.

Manifestation: At birth and thereafter.

Aetiology: Genetically determined syndrome; mode of inheritance not yet established.

Treatment: Symptomatic.

Illustrations:

1a and b A 9-month-old infant, the first child of young non-consanguineous parents. Normal birth measurements. Head circumference at 9 months approximately at the second percentile, at 2 years well below the second percentile. Initially, telangiectatic naevi spread over the face. Delayed closure of a very large anterior fontanelle. No psychomotor development (computerized tomography scan: dilated ventricles; electroencephalogram: increased seizure activity). Short stature, on and below the third percentile. Short, stubby thumbs, contracted in the position shown (1b), as are also the halluces. High-arched palate, pectus carinatum, club feet, ventricular septal defect. Optic fundi negative; detailed clinical, laboratory and enzymatic investigations negative. Chromosomal analysis negative.

2a and b, 4 and 5 The 26-year-old mother of the proband: craniofacial dysmorphism, retardation, abnormal thumbs and halluces (also present in the mother's father and her two sisters). Extensive similarities of the mother's and son's palmar ridge patterns.

3a and b The 13-month-old son of one of the sisters of the proband's mother. The first child of young nonconsanguineous parents. Birth 3 weeks before term with 2300 g, 44 cm and 32 cm birth measurements. At 14 months, microcephaly; premature closure of the cranial sutures; computerized tomography scan: partial dilatation of the cerebral ventricles. Psychomotor retardation. Small size (at 14 months, approximately at the third percentile). Plump paw-like hands and plumpish feet, broad thumbs and halluces. Fundi normal. Chromosomes normal (including banded preparations).

Note: A new case that probably corresponds to this syndrome has just been published and a further case has been reported to be by a genetic institute. Both cases also involve boys.

References:
Nevin N C, Stewart F J *et al*: Microcephaly with large anterior fontanelle, generalized convulsions, micropenis and distinct anomalies of the hands and feet. Another example of Wiedemann syndrome? *Clin Genet* 1994, **46**:205–208.

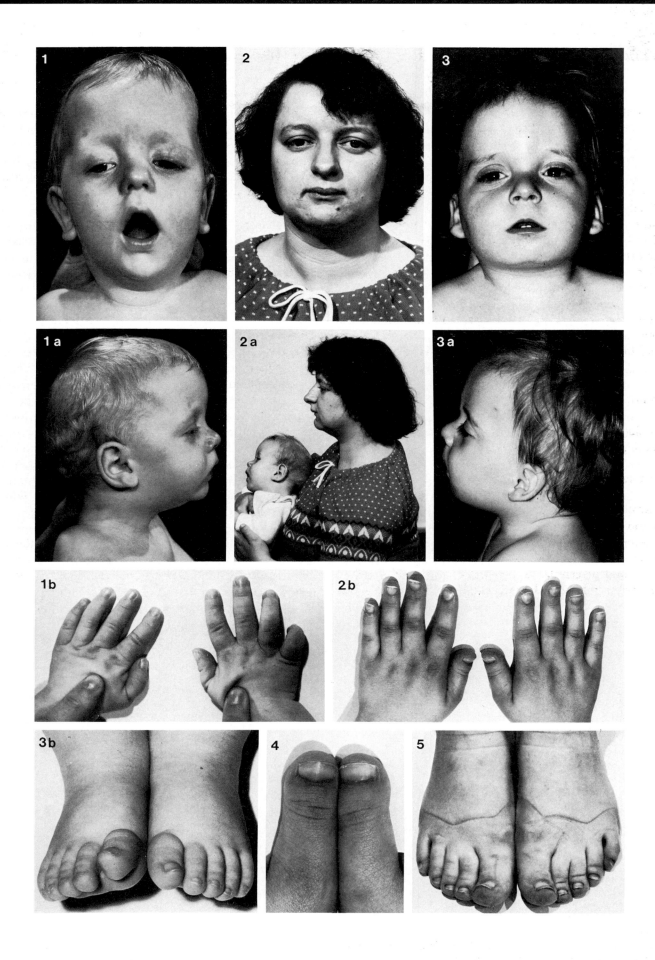

89 Cockayne Syndrome

J.K./H.-R.W

A disorder manifesting, as a rule, from the second year of life onwards and leading to severe dystrophic growth retardation with typical facies, microcephaly, mental retardation, neurological and ocular defects and other anomalies.

Main signs:
- Severe growth deficiency, disproportionate because of the excessive length of the extremities and oversized hands and feet (1).
- Typical facies, narrow, 'sunken' and 'too old', with deep-set eyes, thin nose, prognathism, dental caries (1–3).
- Increasingly apparent microcephaly.
- Progressive neurological defects (ataxia, sometimes tremor; hearing impairment, which may progress to deafness; decreased visual acuity) as well as mental retardation (caused by a special form of orthochromatic leukodystrophy).

Supplementary findings: Development of ocular and visual defects, eventually blindness; retinitis pigmentosa; optic atrophy, cataracts (in approximately one-third of patients); possible corneal clouding.

Hypersensitivity to ultraviolet light with exanthemata and subsequent pigment changes and scarring.

Progressive development of flexion contractures of the large joints and increasing dorsal kyphosis.

Cryptorchidism in some patients; impaired sweating, disorder of water–salt metabolism.

Radiologically, calcifications of the basal ganglia, thickening of the calvaria and other findings.

No evidence of a consistent endocrinological biochemical abnormality.

Manifestation: Starting in the second year of life (after initial normal development for the greater part of the first year of life), however, a congenital form ('type 2') also occurs.

Aetiology: Autosomal recessive disorder. Heterogeneity. Cells are ultraviolet sensitive; defective DNA repair. Gene locus 10q11 (late form).

Frequency: Low; 150 patients have been described to date.

Course, prognosis: Progressive, leading eventually to complete dependence. Substantially decreased life expectancy.

Differential diagnosis: 'Seckel syndrome' (91), Dubowitz syndrome (95), progeria (149), de Barsy syndrome (153), COFS syndrome (320), Bloom syndrome (199) and xeroderma pigmentosum (181) must be excluded.

Treatment: Symptomatic. Avoidance of exposure to sunlight. Cataract operation, hearing aids may be indicated. Genetic counselling of the parents. Prenatal diagnosis.

Illustrations:
1a and b An 8-year-old girl: senile facial appearance, severe psychomotor retardation, pectus carinatum; weight 6 kg, height 95 cm, head circumference 38.5 cm.
2a–c An 18-year-old, the only child of healthy parents. Birth measurements normal, unremarkable development. Starting from the second year of life, marked, progressive, slowing of physical and mental development. Presently, typical senile facial appearance, microcephaly (43.5 cm), short stature (97.5 cm), long extremities with large hands and feet. Ataxia, tremor, mental retardation, photosensitivity. Visual and hearing impairments.
3 The facial appearance of an extremely short 17 year old (mild form).

References:
Soffer D, Grotzky H W, Rapin I et al: Cockayne syndrome: unusual neuropathologic findings and review of the literature. *Ann Neurol* 1979, 6:340.
Houston C St, Zaleski W A et al: Identical male twins and brother with Cockayne syndrome. *Am J Med Genet* 1982, 13:211–223.
Smits M G, Gabreels F J M et al: Peripheral and central myelinopathy in Cockayne's syndrome... *Neuropediatrics* 1982, 13:161–167.
Grunnet M L, Zimmerman A W. et al: Ultrastructure and electrodiagnosis of peripheral neuropathy in Cockayne's syndrome. *Neurology* 1983, 33:1606–1609.
Ohta Sh, Shima A et al: Ultraviolet sensitivity of Cockayne syndrome... *Cong Anom* 1983, 23:399–403.
Lehmann A R, Francis A J et al: Prenatal diagnosis of Cockayne's syndrome. *Lancet* 1985, I:486–488.
Silengo M C, Franceschini P et al: Distinctive skeletal dysplasia in Cockayne syndrome. *Pediatr Radiol* 1986, 16:264–266.
Somer M, Rossi L et al: Cockayne syndrome, early-onset type... *Clin Genet* 1986, 29:473–474.
Sugita K, Suzuki N et al: Cockayne syndrome with delayed recovery of RNA synthesis after ultraviolet irradiation but normal ultraviolet survival. *Pediatr Res* 1986, 21:34–37.
Jaeken J, Klocker H et al: Clinical and biochemical studies in... Cockayne syndrome. *Hum Genet* 1989, 83:339–346.
Patton M A, Giannelli F, Francis A J et al: Early onset Cockayne's syndrome... *J Med Genet* 1989, 26:154 (1989).
Nance M A, Berry S A: Cockayne syndrome: review of 140 cases. *Am J Med Genet* 1992, 42:68–84.
Lehmann A R, Thompson A F et al: Cockayne's syndrome... *J Med Genet* 1993, 30:679–682.
Scott R J, Itin P et al: Xeroderma pigmentosum - Cockayne syndrome... *J Am Acad Dermatol* 1993, 29:883–889.
Miyauchi H, Horio T et al: Cockayne syndrome in two adult siblings. *J Am Acad Dermatol* 1994, 30:329–335.

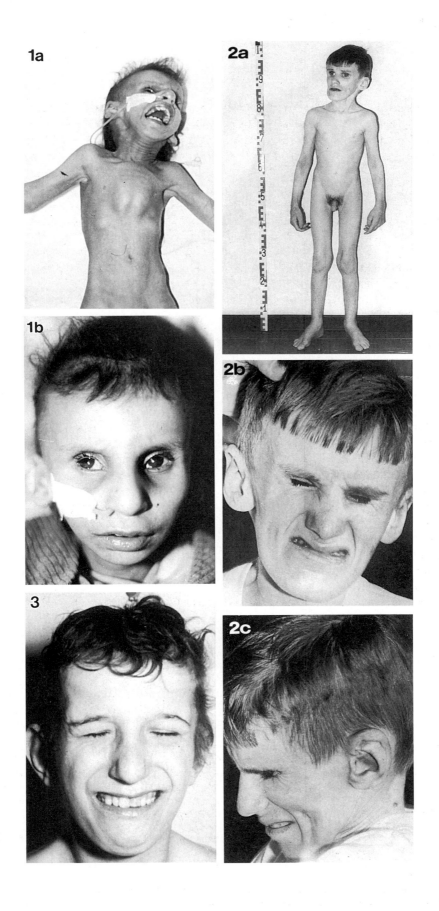

J.K.

Autosomal dominant and autosomal recessive causes with normal or reduced intelligence.

Main signs:
- Circumference of the head below the third percentile.
- Open cranial sutures in early infancy.
- Mental retardation with autosomal recessive and autosomal dominant inheritance reported.

Supplementary findings: Autosomal recessive form with retardation: low, obliquely slanting forehead, flat occiput, frequently severe retardation. In some patients, cataract, short stature, furrowed scalp.

Autosomal recessive form with normal intelligence: receding forehead, normal scalp hair, exopthalmos with laterally slanting palpebral fissures, epicanthus medialis, long straight nose, high nasal bridge, generally widely spaced teeth, malocclusion, micrognathia. Normal intelligence (IQ approximately 100). Autosomal dominant form and average intelligence: no facial dysmorphism. Normal stature. Average school performance. Neurologically and socially normal.

Manifestation: In early infancy. The dominant form is identified after birth.

Aetiology: Autosomal recessive disorder with mental retardation. Frequency: one out of 250 000 newborns. Autosomal recessive inheritance with normal intelligence and facial dysmorphism. Observed 10 times to date. Autosomal dominant inheritance. More than 12 families reported.

Pathogenesis: The autosomal recessive form with mental retardation shows gyral abnormalities and cerebral fissures.

Course, prognosis: Quality of life for the autosomal recessive form with mental retardation depends on the severity of retardation.

Differential diagnosis: Congenital diplegia with microcephaly, premature synostoses, embryopathies with cytomegaly, rubella or toxoplasmosis, microcephaly with choroidoretinopathy, Seckel syndrome (91), X-linked microcephaly with short stature, deafness and genital anomalies, X-linked branchial arch syndrome, syndrome of microcephaly, retardation, skeletal and immune defects, Weaver–Williams syndrome, Nijmegen syndrome, Leung syndrome (microcephaly with lymphoedema of the lower extremities), Nonne–Milroy syndrome (261), syndrome of microcephaly with mental retardation and retinopathy, COFS syndrome (320), syndrome of microcephaly, mental retardation and syndactyly, Filippi type, Norrie's disease.

Treatment: Unknown.

Illustrations:
1 A 10-day-old female newborn with receding forehead and congenital microcephaly.
2 and 3 A 4-day-old female newborn from the 39th week of pregnancy: length 43 cm, head circumference 26.5 cm, receding forehead, long straight nose (autosomal recessive form).
4a–d Autosomal dominant microcephaly and normal intelligence (borderline).

References:
Autosomal dominant microcephaly:
Haslam R H A, Smith D W: Autosomal dominant microcephaly. *J Pediatr* 1979, 95:701–705.
Hecht F, Kelly J V: Little heads: inheritance and early detection. Editorial. *J Pediatr* 1979, 95:731–732.
Burton B K: Dominant inheritance of microcephaly with short stature. *Clin Genet* 1981, 20:25–27.
Ramirez M L, Rivas F, Cantu J M: Silent microcephaly: a distinct autosomal dominant trait. *Clin Genet* 1983, 23:281–286.
Rossi L N, Candini G, Scarlatti G, Rossi G, Prina E, Alberti S: Autosomal dominant microcephaly without mental retardation. *Am J Dis Child* 1987, 141:655–659.
Evans D G R: Dominantly inherited microcephaly, hypotelorism and normal intelligence. *Clin Genet* 1991, 39:178–180.
Autosomal recessive microcephaly:
Cowie V: The genetics and sub-classification of microcephaly. *J Ment Defic Res* 1960, 4:42–47.
Davies H, Kirman B H: Microcephaly. *Arch Dis Child* 1962, 37:623–627.
Kloepfer H W, Platou R V, Hansche W J: Manifestations of a recessive gene for microcephaly in a population isolate. *J Genet Hum* 1964, 13:52–59.
Mikati M A, Najjar S S, Sahli I F, Melhem R E, Mansour S, Der Kaloustian V M: Microcephaly, hypergonadotropic hypogonadism, short stature and minor anomalies: a new syndrome. *Am J Med Genet* 1985, 22:599–608.
Tolmie J L, McNay M, Stephenson J B P, Doyle D, Connor J M: Microcephaly: genetic counseling and antenatal diagnosis after the birth of an affected child. *Am J Med Genet* 1987, 27:583–594.
Teebi A S, Al-Awadi S A, White A G: Autosomal recessive nonsyndromal microcephaly with normal intelligence. *Am J Med Genet* 1987, 26:355–359.

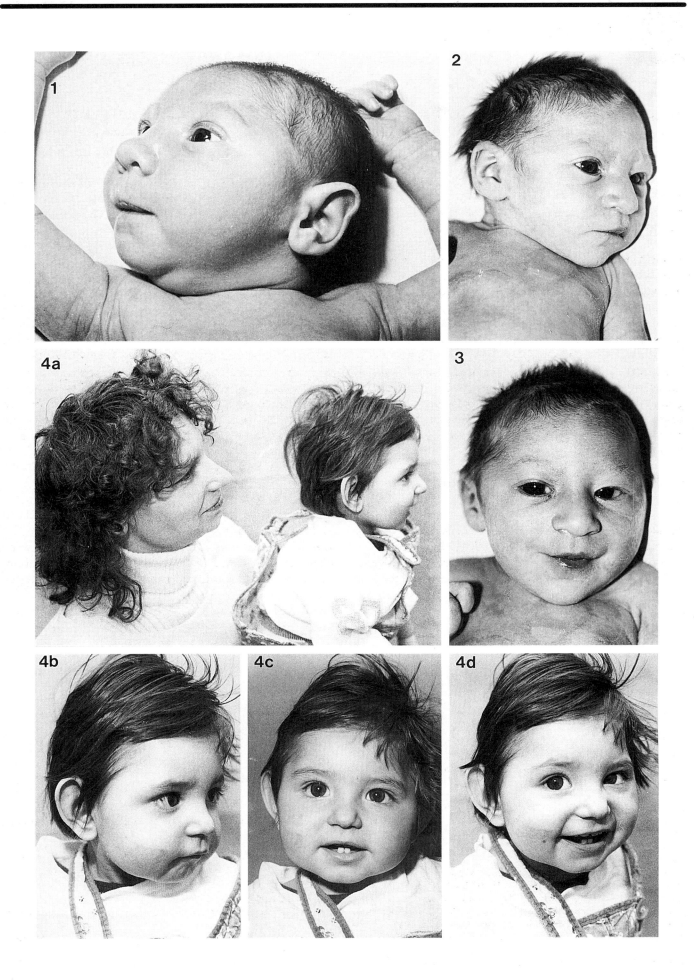

91 Seckel Syndrome

("Bird-headed Dwarfism", Seckel type; Microcephalic Primordial Dwarfism, Seckel Type)

J.K./H.-R.W

A rare, probably heterogeneous, autosomal recessive syndrome with intra-uterine growth retardation, postnatal short stature, mental retardation, microcephaly, prominent nose and micrognathia ('bird-headed' appearance).

Main signs:
- Intra-uterine growth retardation. Birth weight about 1500 g.
- Postnatal continuation of growth deficiency with SD of -5 to -11.
- Microcephaly (-4 to -14 SD), premature closure of the cranial sutures. Mental retardation (IQ below 80).
- Prominent aquiline nose, large eyes, antimongoloid slant of the palpebral fissures, micrognathia, dysplastic ears.

Supplementary findings: High palate, hypoplasia of the dental enamel, retarded bone age, hirsutism, fifth-finger clinodactyly, hip dysplasia, cryptorchidism, clitoral hyperplasia. Further possible malformations of all kinds have been noted.

Manifestation: Prenatally; at birth.

Aetiology: Autosomal recessive disorder.

Frequency: Low; up to 1985, 20 patients were observed.

Course, prognosis: A 13-year-old patient attained a height of 124 cm; the oldest known patient was 104 cm at 22 years of age. One-third of all patients have an IQ below 50; in isolated cases, IQs of 74 and 79 have been recorded.

Differential diagnosis: To be differentiated primarily from osteodysplastic primordial dwarfism types I–III (92). The microcephalic short stature syndrome of Dubowitz (95), alcohol embryopathy (275), the Cornelia de Lange syndrome (98), trisomy 18 (48) and Bloom syndrome (199) can be easily differentiated by phenotype.

Treatment: Symptomatic. Genetic counselling. Ultrasound diagnosis during pregnancy.

Illustrations:
1–3 A characteristically affected newborn.

References:

Majewski F, Goecke R: Studies of microcephalic primordial dwarfism I: approach to a delineation of the Seckel syndrome. *Am J Med Genet* 1982, 12:7–21.

Thompson E, Pembrey M: Seckel syndrome: an overdiagnosed syndrome. *J Med Genet* 1985, 22:192–201.

Butler M G, Hall Br D, Maclean R N et al: Do some patients with Seckel syndrome have hematological problems and/or chromosome breakage? *Am J Med Genet* 1987, 27:645–649.

Stoppoloni G, Stabile M et al: Seckel syndrome... *Ann Genet* 1992, 35:213–216.

Sugio Y, Tsukahara M et al: Two Japanese cases with microcephalic primordial dwarfism: classical Seckel syndrome... *Jpn J Hum Genet* 1993, 38:209–217.

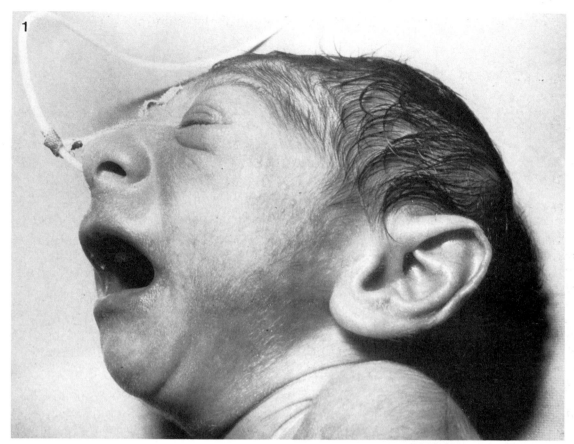

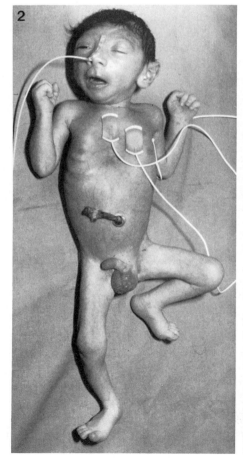

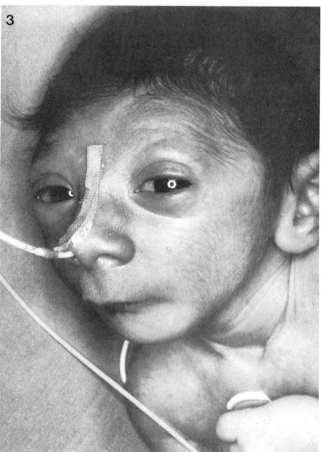

92 Primordial Microcephalic and Osteodysplastic Dwarfism
(Bird-headed Seckel-like Type with Osteodysplasia)

H.-R.W

A clinical picture with very marked prenatal and postnatal growth retardation, microcephaly, prominent nose, receding chin, mental retardation, osteodysplasia and other anomalies.

Main signs:
- Marked intra-uterine growth retardation.
- Postnatal continuation of marked growth deficiency.
- Microcephaly (low and receding forehead; prematurely closed, prominent cranial sutures; prominent occiput); psychomotor retardation.
- 'Bird face' as a result of receding forehead, relatively large eyes, prominent aquiline nose, receding chin.
- Osteodysplasias: S-shaped, long, narrow clavicles; atypical narrowing of the long bones (ventrolateral curving of the femora); abnormally shaped pelvis (ventral prolongation of the iliac crests, absent acetabular angle, elongated pubic and ischial bones, unusually narrow hip-joint space on radiograph) and marked disturbance of metaphyseal growth. Joints very poorly formed, causing an increase of mobility in some and marked limitation in others.

Supplementary findings:
Marked hypotrichosis and dry, finely scaled skin.
Urogenital anomalies.
Fifth finger clinodactyly.

Manifestation: Intra-uterine; at birth.

Aetiology:
Several types of 'Seckel-like' osteodysplastic primordial dwarfism occur, with characteristic skeletal changes. Heterogeneity? Autosomal recessive inheritance seems most likely.

Frequency:
Low. Similarities between the present case and the types 1 and 3 of Majewski *et al.* (it now seems very probable that these types are identical) and especially the observations of Winter *et al.* and Haan *et al.*

Course, prognosis:
Poor with regard to mental development.

Differential diagnosis:
Other types of primordial microcephalic osteodysplastic dwarfism.

Treatment:
Symptomatic. Genetic counselling. Prenatal diagnosis possible by ultrasound in the event of future pregnancies.

Illustrations:
1–9 The second child of young, healthy, non-consanguineous parents after a healthy girl. (1–3, during the newborn period; 4–6 at 6 months; 7–9 at 18 months). Spontaneous birth 9 days after term with birth weight 1200 g, length 36 cm, head circumference 27 cm. Facial asymmetry; strabismus. Hypotrichosis; dry, scaly skin. Hypermobile knees, limitation of movement of the other large joints; rocker-bottom feet. Distally tapering fingers, fifth-finger clinodactyly, bilateral simian crease. Bilateral cryptorchidism. Right-side hydronephrosis with ureteral stenosis. Measurements at 6 months: 3550 g, length 52 cm, head circumference 31 cm. At 3 years and 1 month: length 69 cm, head circumference 34 cm (all measurements well below the second percentile).
Computerized tomography scan: Hydrocephalus *int. et ext. e vacuo;* possible bilateral hypoplasia of the frontal lobes. Severely impaired mental and motor development. Chromosomal analysis of cultured lymphocytes and fibroblasts (including banded preparations) negative.
7–9 Note the extremely delayed osseous development; horizontal acetabular roofs; short, relatively wide femoral necks and narrow joint cavities.

References:
Majewski F, Stoeckenius M, Kemperdick H: Studies of microcephalic primordial dwarfism III: an intra-uterine dwarf with platyspondyly and anomalies of pelvis and clavicles — osteodysplastic primordial dwarfism Type III. *Am J Med Genet* 1982, **12**:37–42.
Winter R M, Wigglesworth J, Harding B N: Osteodysplastic primordial dwarfism: report of a further patient with manifestations similar to those seen in patients with types I and III. *Am J Med Genet* 1985, **21**:569–574.
Verloes A, Lambrechts L *et al*: Microcephalic osteodysplastic dwarfism (type II-like) in siblings. *Clin Genet* 1987, **32**:88–94.
Haan E A *et al*: Osteodysplastic primordial dwarfism... *Am J Med Genet* 1989, **33**:224–227.
Maroteaux P, Badoual J: La chondrodysplasie microcéphalique sublétale. *Arch Fr Pediatr* 1990, **47**:103–106.
Meinecke P, Passarge E: Microcephalic osteodysplastic primordial dwarfism. *J Med Genet* 1991, **28**:785–800.
Shebib S, Hugosson Cl *et al*: Osteodysplastic variant of primordial dwarfism. *Am J Med Genet* 1991, **40**:146–150.
Meinecke P, Passarge E (Letter). *Am J Med Genet* 1992, **43**:628.
Hersh J H, Joyce M R *et al*: Microcephalic osteodysplastic dysplasia. *Am J Med Genet* 1994, **51**:194–199.

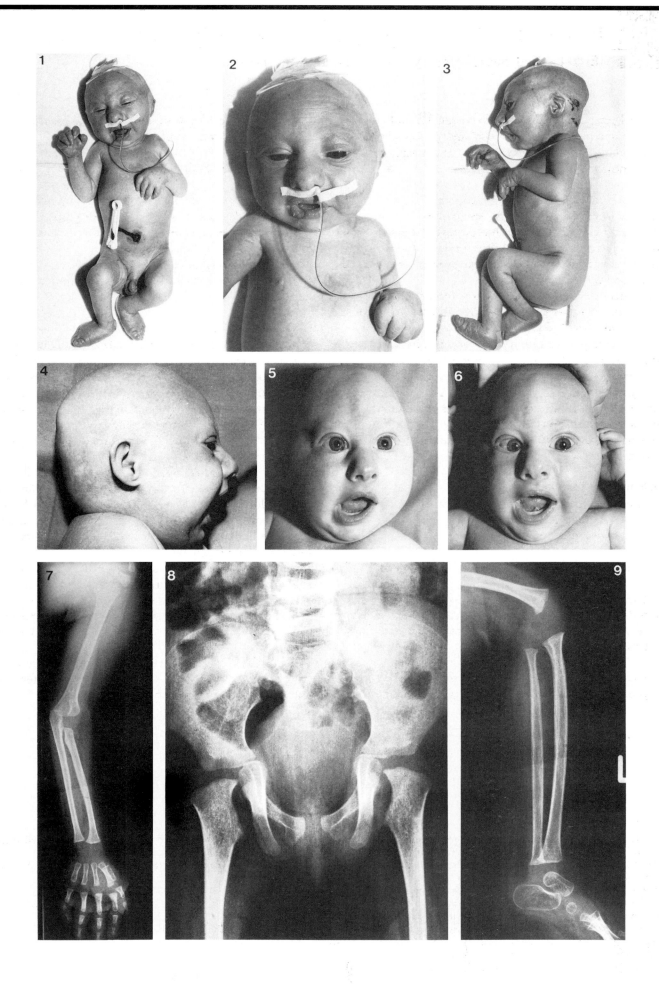

93 A Further Microcephaly-Short Stature-Retardation Syndrome

H.-R.W

An unreported syndrome with unusual facies, microcephaly and mental retardation, short stature, cardiac defects and other anomalies.

Main signs:

- Facies: hypertelorism, blepharophimosis, epicanthic folds, prominent eyebrows, stenosis of the lacrimal duct, convergent strabismus; short, broad nose; gothic palate, retrognathia (**1 and 2**).
- Microcephaly (below the third percentile) with considerable psychomotor retardation.
- Short stature (below the third percentile).
- Ventricular septal defect; persistent ductus arteriosis (operated); patent foramen ovale.
- Complete cutaneous syndactyly of the third and fourth fingers bilaterally (**3**); mild syndactyly of the first and second toes bilaterally.

Supplementary findings: Hypotonia. Hip dysplasia and pes valgus. Unusual cry. Hypoplastic optic papillae, irregular pigmentation of the fundi.

Manifestation: At birth.

Aetiology: Uncertain. Chromosomal analysis normal (high-resolution technique).

Course, prognosis: Poor, in view of the mental retardation.

Diagnosis, differential diagnosis: Other microcephaly-short stature syndromes.

Treatment: Cardiac care, appropriate handicap aids.

Illustrations:

1–3 The second child of healthy parents; sibling healthy. At birth (in the 38th week of pregnancy), obvious intra-uterine growth retardation, with birth weight 1900 g, length 42 cm and head circumference 30.5 cm. Oligohydramnios, small placenta.

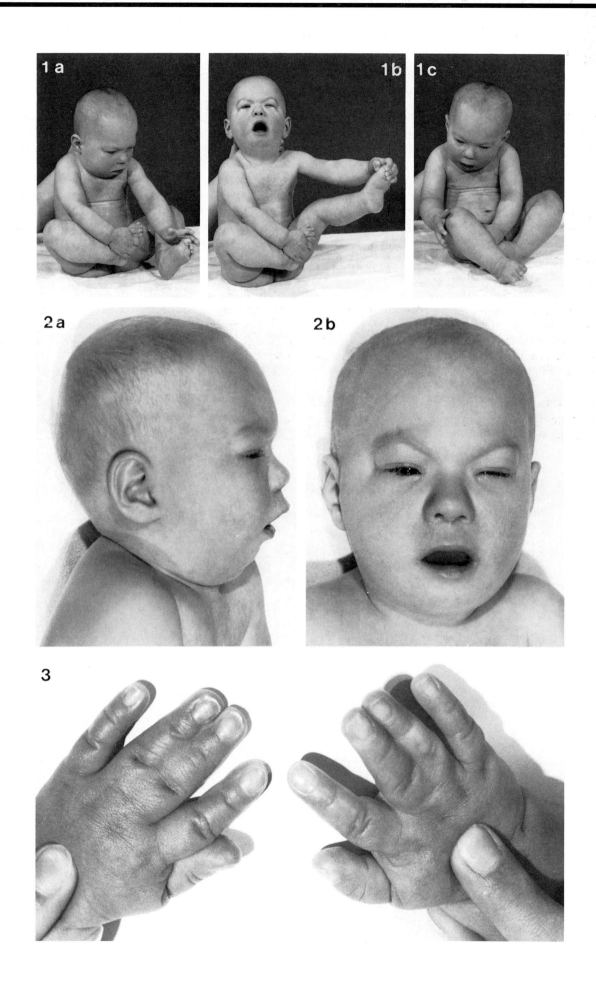

H.-R.W

A characteristic syndrome of growth deficiency, microcephaly, psychomotor retardation, unusual facies, trichosis and aplasia of the terminal phalanges of the fifth fingers and toes.

Main signs:
- Growth retardation of prenatal and postnatal onset with delayed skeletal development. Microbrachycephaly.
- Marked psychomotor retardation. In some patients epilepsy.
- Coarse facies with bushy eyebrows, epicanthus, narrow palpebral fissures, low nasal bridge, broad nose, indistinct philtrum, possible macrostomia, macroglossia and thick lips.
- Sparse growth of scalp hair with hypertrichosis of the face, trunk and proximal extremities.
- Small hands and feet with clinodactyly and aplasia of the distal phalanges of the fifth rays and hypoplasia of further distal phalanges including the nails on the hands and feet.

Supplementary findings:
- Neurological signs in some patients (which may be caused by a variety of cranial malformations). Muscular hypotonia.
- Possibly further skeletal anomalies of the spine, pelvis or other areas.
- Anomalies of the internal genitalia may occur in females. Cardiac abnormalities.
- Normal karyotype.

Manifestation: At birth and thereafter.

Aetiology: Not yet clear. Observations to date for the most part suggest autosomal recessive inheritance but in isolated patients could also indicate autosomal dominant transmission.

Frequency: Low; only approximately 40 relevant patients reported to date.

Course, prognosis: Clouded by a failure to thrive but above all by the mental retardation.

Diagnosis, differential diagnosis: It should be possible to rule out hydantoin embryofoetopathy (255) by the history and trisomy 9p by chromosomal analysis. Brachmann–de Lange syndrome (98) should also be considered.

Treatment: Only symptomatic measures are possible. Appropriate handicap aids.

Illustrations:
1 and 2 A girl aged 5 years and 6 months, normal birth length, microcephalic, mentally retarded, with severe growth retardation (first child of healthy, young, nonconsanguineous parents) with all the characteristic findings. Typical facies, sparse scalp hair, through which the skin of the scalp is visible, and increased facial hair (**1**). Hypoplasia or aplasia of the distal phalanges and nails (**2**). Delayed ossification and hypoplasia or aplasia of the distal phalanx of the fifth ray of the same child at 7 years and 9 months (**3**). The patient showed a hypertonic-hypotonic-ataxic disorder. Normal karyotype.

References:
Coffin G S, Siris E: Mental retardation with absent fifth fingernail and terminal phalanx. *Am J Dis Child* 1970, **119**:433–439.
Haspeslagh M, Fryns J P, van den Berghe H: The Coffin–siris syndrome: report of a family and further delineation. *Clin Genet* 1984, **26**:374–378.
Coffin G S, Siris E: The Coffin–Siris syndrome. *Am J Dis Child* 1985, **139**:12.
Franceschini P, Silengo M C, Bianco R *et al*: The Coffin–Siris syndrome in two siblings. *Pediatr Radiol* 1986, **16**:330–333.
Meinecke P, Engelbrecht R, Schaefer E: Coffin–Siris-Syndrom bei einem 5jährigen Mädchen. *Mschr Kinderheilk* 1986, **134**:692–695.
Bassio W A de: Coffin–Siris syndrome. Chapter 34 in: Neurocutaneous diseases. M. R. Gomez (ed.) 1987:307–310.
Levy P, Baraitser M: Coffin–Siris syndrome. *J Med Genet* 1991, **28**:338–341.
Rabe P, Haverkamp F *et al*: Syndrome of developmental retardation… Coffin–Siris syndrome? *Am J Med Genet* 1991, **41**:350–354.

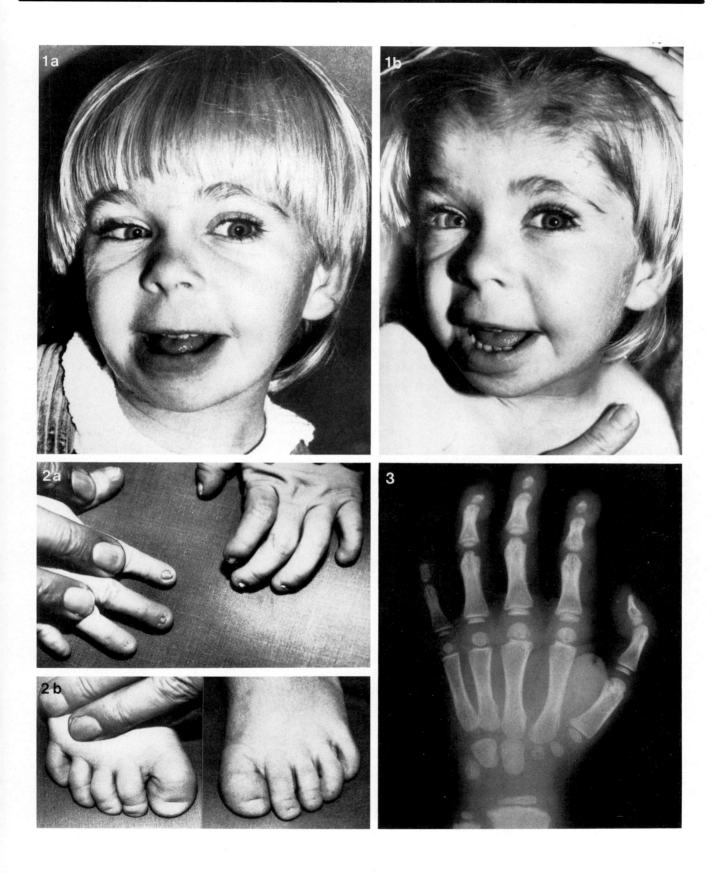

95 Dubowitz Syndrome

H.-R.W

A malformation–retardation syndrome with primordial short stature, unusual facies, marked microcephaly, moderate mental retardation, hyperactivity and eczema.

Main signs:
- Typical facial dysmorphism, especially characterized by upper epicanthic folds, hypertelorism, relatively short palpebral fissures, ptosis, low nasal bridge (most noticeable in the young preschooler). Thin hair, hypoplasia of the lateral eyebrows; dysplasia of the external ears, micrognathia (**1 and 2**)
- Prenatal and postnatal growth retardation. Marked microcephaly with comparatively mild (though not obligatory) mental retardation. Hyperactivity. Muscular hypotonia. High voice.
- Decreased subcutaneous fatty tissue. Eczematous skin changes, especially after exposure to sunlight (**1–4**).

Supplementary findings:
Syndactyly of the second and third toes (**6**).
Pes planus, pes planovalgus. Short, radially deviated fifth fingers (**5**). Tendency to inguinal hernias.
Cryptorchidism.
Vomiting and diarrhoea in infancy.
Immune deficiency. Increased infections. Anaemia.

Manifestation: At birth.

Aetiology: Autosomal recessive disorder. An autosomal dominant form was recently observed for the first time, thus, heterogeneity is likely.

Frequency: Approximately 70 patients have been described since the first description in 1971.

Prognosis: Occasional good catch-up of growth. Improvement of the eczema after the third year of life. Statements about further development are not possible because most of the known patients are still in the early age groups. Apparently there is an increased tendency to aplastic anaemia and the development of malignancies.

Differential diagnosis: Silver–Russell syndrome (*82*). Bloom syndrome (*199*): here, no mental retardation; skin manifestation is not eczema but rather telangiectatic erythema; typical chromosomal abnormalities. Foetal alcohol syndrome (*275*): here, corresponding maternal history, cardiac defect of the child.

Note: The syndrome is not well defined.

Treatment: Symptomatic. Genetic counselling; in case of further pregnancy, prenatal diagnosis by ultrasound.

Illustrations:
1–6 A patient at age 8 years. Birth weight 2750 g. Eczema and vomiting in infancy. IQ 62, hyperactivity. Retractable testes. Measurements at age 8 years: height 106 cm (equivalent to that of a boy aged 4 years and 6 months); weight 12 kg (equivalent to a 21-month-old boy); head circumference 48 cm (equivalent to an 18-month-old boy).

References:
Grosse R Gorlin J, Opitz J M: The Dubowitz–Syndrome. *Z Kinderheilk* 1971, **110**:175.
Majewski F, Michaelis R, Moosmann K, Bierich J R: A rare type of low birthweight dwarfism: the Dubowitz Syndrome. *Z Kinderheilk* 1975, **120**:238.
Orrison W W, Schnitzler E R, Chun R W M: The Dubowitz syndrome: further observations. *Am J Med Genet* 1980, 7:155.
Küster W, Majewski F: The Dubowitz syndrome. *Eur J Pediatr* 1986, 144:574–578.
Shuper A, Merlob P *et al*: The diagnosis of Dubowitz syndrome in the neonatal period... *Eur J Pediatr* 1986, 145:151–152.
Wilhelm O L, Méhes K: Dubowitz syndrome. *Acta Paediatr Hung* 1986, **2**: 67–75.
Winter R M: Dubowitz syndrome. *J Med Genet* 1986, 23:11–13.
Berthold F, Fuhrmann W *et al*: Fatal aplastic anemia in a child with features of Dubowitz syndrome. *Eur J Pediatr* 1987, 146:605–607.
Kondo I, Takeda K *et al*: A Japanese patient with the Dubowitz syndrome. *Clin Genet* 1987, **31**:389–392.
Méhes K: Persönl Mitteilung. 1987.
Belohradsky B H, Egger J *et al*: Das Dubowitz Syndrom. *Erg Inn Med Kinderheilk* 1988, 57:145–184.
Hochreutener H, Schinzel A *et al*: Das Dubowitz Syndrom... *Mschr Kinderheilk* 1990, **138**:689–691.
Ilyina H G, Lurie I W: Dubowitz syndrome... *Am J Med Genet* 1990, 35:561–565.
Thuret I, Michel G *et al*: Chromosomal instability in two siblings with Dubowitz syndrome. *Br J Haemat* 1991, 78:124–125.

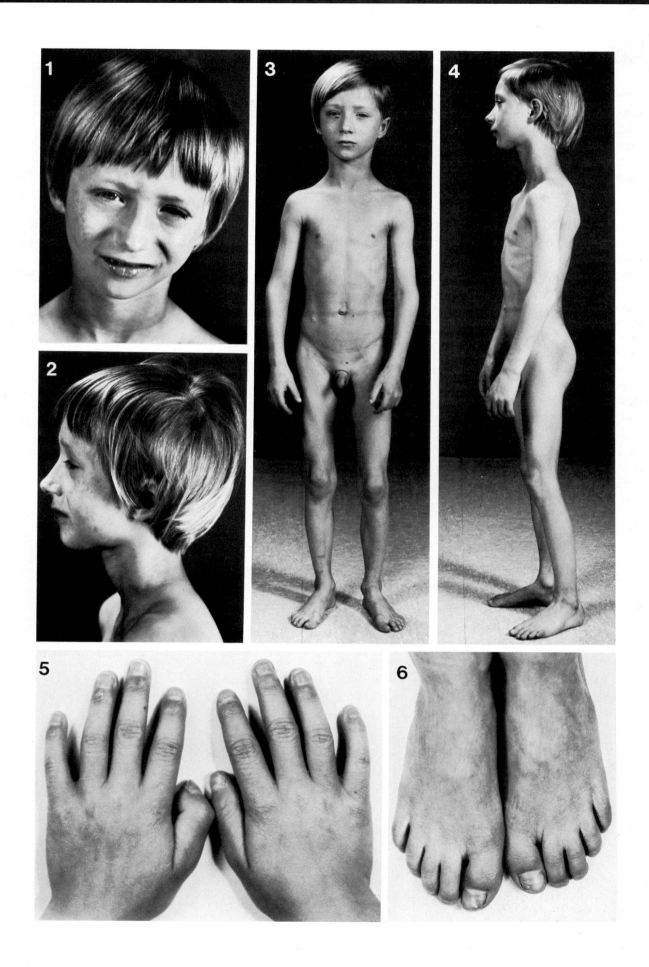

96

A Further Microcephaly-Short Stature-Retardation Syndrome

H.-R.W

An unknown syndrome comprising peculiar facies, microcephaly and mental retardation, short stature anal atresia and other anomalies.

Main signs:
- Facies: antimongoloid slant of the palpebral fissures, bilateral ptosis (left more marked than right; possible third and twelfth cranial nerve paralysis); broad nasal bridge; low-set, prominent, dysplastic ears; thin upper lip and receding chin (1–8).
- Microcephaly (approximately second percentile) with psychomotor retardation.
- Short stature (between the third and 10th percentiles).
- Anal atresia.

Supplementary findings: High palate, dysodontiasis, bifid uvula, patent ductus arteriosus. Synostosis of the first ribs bilaterally; abnormally shaped scapulae and clavicles. Narrow hands; pillar-like legs, lacking contour (6, 9).

Manifestation: At birth.

Aetiology: Unknown.

Course, prognosis: In view of the mental retardation, poor.

Differential diagnosis: Other microcephaly-short stature syndromes.

Treatment: Appropriate handicap aids.

Illustrations:
1–9 The third child of healthy parents; several healthy siblings. Birth measurements 3100 g, 49 cm and 33.5 cm (head circumference). No maternal alcoholism. Chromosomal analysis normal.

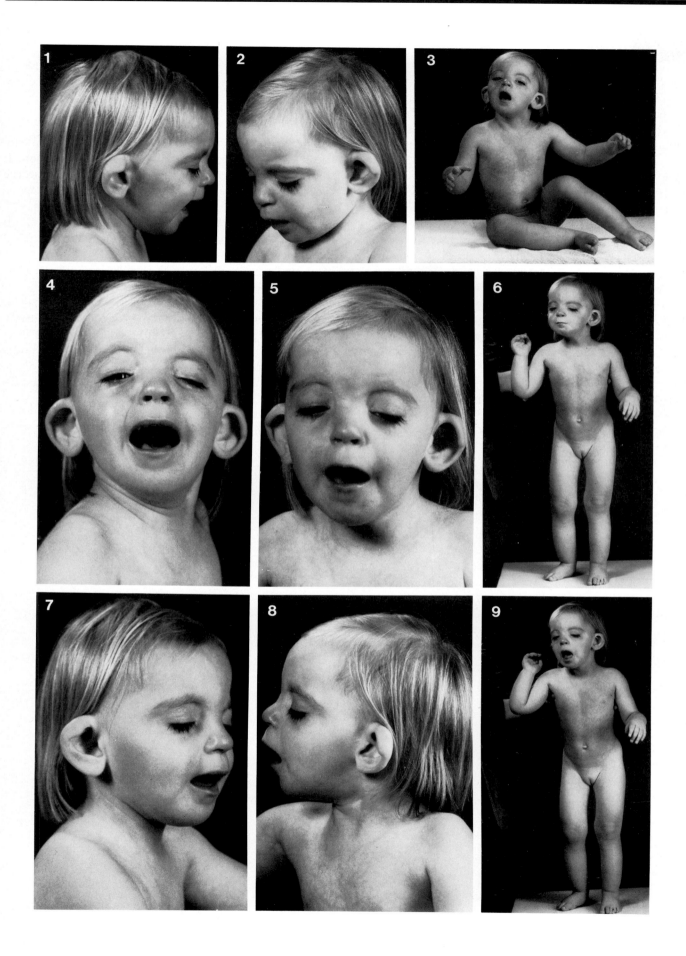

97

Mietens Syndrome
(Mietens–Weber Syndrome)

H.-R.W

A malformation–retardation syndrome with short stature, short forearms held in flexion, unusual facies, corneal clouding and moderate mental retardation.

Main signs:
- Flexion contractures of the elbows with dislocation of the head of the radius and abnormally short forearms (1–4).
- Short stature.
- Unusual facies with bilateral corneal clouding, nystagmus, strabismus and narrow, pointed nose with hypoplastic alae nasi (1 and 2).
- Mental retardation (IQ 70–80).

Supplementary findings: Pes planus and valgus, moderately severe flexion contractures of the knees (2), hip dysplasia, pectus excavatum and clinodactyly may also be present.

Manifestation: Prenatally and postnatally.

Aetiology: Genetically determined syndrome. Mode of inheritance not known, most likely autosomal recessive.

Frequency: Very rare.

Course, prognosis: Intelligence may be difficult to evaluate because of defective vision and limited arm function. If vascular anomalies prove to be part of the syndrome, the prognosis must be guarded.

Treatment: Ophthalmologic and orthopaedic care. All measures to promote the developmentally retarded child.

Illustrations:

1 and 2 Two of four affected siblings. Short stature; mental retardation. Corneal clouding; strabismus. Narrow nose with hypoplastic alae nasi. Abnormally short forearms with flexion contractures of the dislocated elbows. Flexion contractures of the knees; pes planus and valgus. The girl has a history of a ruptured aneurysm of the right anterior cerebral artery.
3 Radiograph of a 5-month-old sibling.
4 Radiograph of the boy shown in 1.

References:
Mietens C, Weber H: A syndrome characterized by corneal opacity, nystagmus, flexion of the elbows, growth failure and mental retardation. *J Pediatr* 1966, **62**:624.
Warring III G O, Rodrigues M M: Ultrastructure and successful keratoplasty of sclerocornea in Mietens' syndrome. *Am J Ophthalmol* 1980, **90**:469.

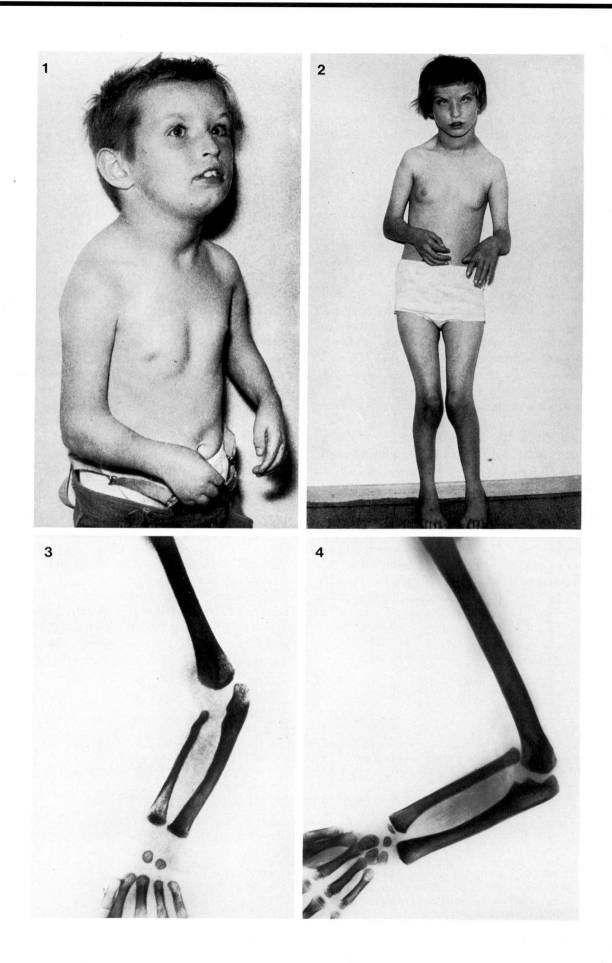

H.-R.W

A genetically determined, very variable malformation–retardation syndrome with characteristic facial dysmorphism, primordial short stature and marked reduction anomalies of the extremities.

Main signs:
- Characteristic facies with bushy eyebrows which meet over the bridge of the nose (synophrys), thick lashes, hypertelorism, antimongoloid slant of the palpebral fissures; anteverted nares with short nose, long or prominent philtrum, narrow lips and down-turned corners of the mouth. Frequently micrognathia; low-set, malformed ears. Low anterior and posterior hairlines. Microbrachycephaly. Low, hoarse, expressionless voice.
- Intra-uterine growth retardation in most patients. Usually considerably impaired psychomotor development. Initial, marked muscular hypertonia, which may interfere with feeding.
- Hypertrichosis on the face, trunk and the extensor surfaces of the extremities.
- Severe growth deficiency in most patients.
- Short hands and feet, proximally displaced thumbs, short fifth finger, simian crease. With marked reduction, retrogression of the rays from the ulnar side with monodactyly and arm stumps in extreme cases; lower extremities generally not as severely affected.

Supplementary findings: Cylindrical trunk, small nipples. Cutis marmorata. Myopia, nystagmus, strabismus. Not infrequently, cleft palate. Cardiac defects, possible diaphragmatic defects, renal anomalies. Undescended testes, hypospadias, hypoplastic genitalia and many more anomalies.

Manifestation: At birth.

Aetiology: The vast majority of cases are sporadic (possible new mutations). However, there have been observations that would seem to support autosomal dominant inheritance (and possible gonadal mosaicism) as well as some cases (less numerous) that do not completely rule out autosomal recessive transmission. Possible heterogeneity. The spectrum of phenotypic variation is very broad. The non-uniform chromosome anomalies occasionally reported are considered concomitant findings. Gene or genes possibly localized on the long arm of chromosome 3

Frequency: Not rare; approximately 250 patients were published by 1971; recent estimate: 1:10 000 to 1:30 000.

Course, prognosis: No progression. Infections pose a threat to severely retarded or markedly hypertonic children, especially in infancy. Probably generally decreased life expectancy. Low empirical risk of recurrence.

Treatment: Symptomatic.

Illustrations:
1–4 Patient 1 at age 10 years and 6 months. Birth weight 2450 g, length 39 cm. Subsequent linear growth just below the third percentile. Frequent infections in infancy. At 12 years, onset of grand mal epilepsy. Mental retardation. Head circumference 49 cm, corresponding to that of a 3-year-old girl.
5 Patient 2 as a neonate with a severe right-sided reduction anomaly (monodactyly).
6 and 7 Patient 3 at age 7 months; weight 5000 g; length 58 cm; head circumference 36.5 cm (birth: weight 1770 g, length 41 cm, head circumference 28.5 cm). Marked muscular hypertonia and severe psychomotor retardation; feeding possible only with a stomach tube; seizures.

References:
Hawley P P, Jackson L G, Kurnit D M: Sixty-four patients with Brachmann-de-Lange syndrome: a survey. *Am J Med Genet* 1985, **20**:453–459.
Opitz J M: Editorial comment: the Brachmann-de-Lange syndrome. *Am J Med Genet* 1985, **22**:89–102.
Mosher G A, Schulte R L, Kaplan P A *et al*: Brief clinical report: pregnancy in a woman with Brachmann-de-Lange syndrome. *Am J Med Genet* 1985, **22**:103–107.
Robinson L K, Wolfsberg E, Jones K L: Brachmann-de-Lange syndrome: evidence for autosomal dominant inheritance. *Am J Med Genet* 1985, **22**:109–115.
Fryns J P, Dereymaeker A M *et al*: The Brachmann-de-Lange syndrome in two siblings of normal parents. *Clin Genet* 1987, **31**:413–415.
Bonorden St W, Reinken L: Ein interdisziplinär koordiniertes Therapiekonzept am Beispiel des Cornelia de Lange-Syndroms. *Klin Pädiatr* 1988, **200**:457–462.
Filippi G: The de Lange syndrome... 15 cases. *Clin Genet* 1989, **35**:343–363.
Pankau R *et al*: Das Brachmann-de-Lange-Syndrom... *Mschr Kinderheilk* 1990, **138**:72–76.
Ireland M *et al*: A de novo translocation... in Cornelia de Lange syndrome. *J Med Genet* 1991, **28**:639–640.
Jackson L G: de Lange syndrome (Editorial). *Am J Med Genet* 1992, **42**:377–378.
Shaffer L G *et al*: Genetic syndromes... de Lange syndrome. *Am J Med Genet* 1993, **47**:383–386.
Chodirker B N, Chudley A E: Male-to-male transmission of mild Brachmann-de-Lange syndrome. *Am J Med Genet* 1994, **52**:331–333.
Holder S E *et al*: Partial trisomy 3q causing mild Cornelia de Lange phenotype. *J Med Genet* 1994, **31**:150–152.
Kousseff B, Newkirk P *et al*: Brachmann-de-Lange syndrome — 1994 update. *Arch Pediatr Adolesc Med* 1994, **148**:751–755.
Opitz J M: Brachmann-de-Lange syndrome — a continuing enigma. *Arch Pediatr Adolesc Med* 1994, **148**:1206–1210.

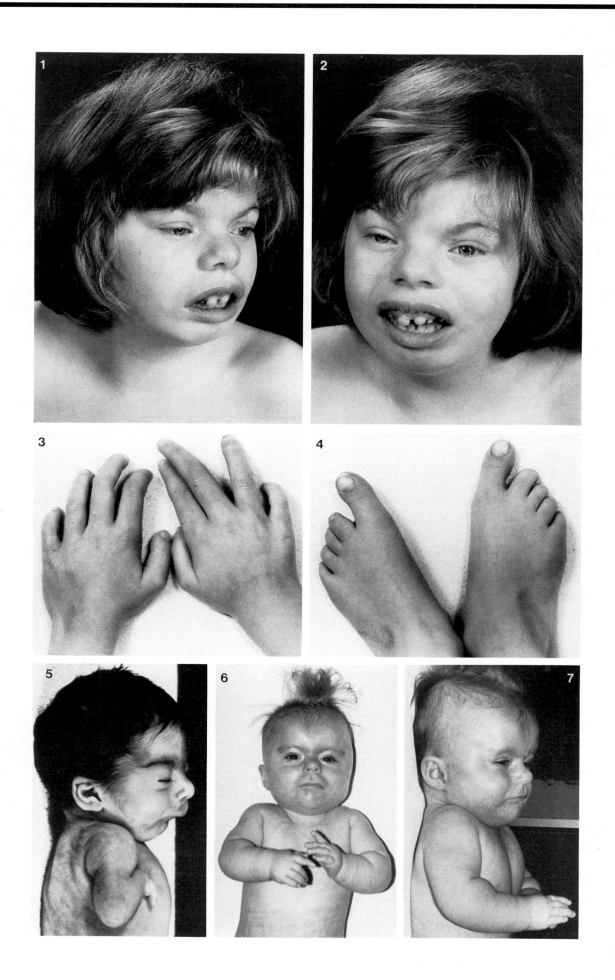

H.-R.W

A form of hypothyroidism of delayed onset and mainly skeletal manifestations, with short stature as the principal sign.

Main signs:
- Variably severe, for the most part proportionate, short stature with thick-set appearance; thorax often broad and bell-shaped; frequent dorsal kyphosis and lumbar lordosis and pronounced muscle contours, especially of the thighs (**1, 3, 4**).
- Often, distinctly waddling gait.
- Radiologically, general delay of ossification and epiphyseal dysgenesis, the latter most pronounced in the hip joints as a multicentric crumbly appearance of the capital femoral epiphysis. Also flattening of the vertebral bodies. All in all, a picture that most resembles that of polyepiphyseal dysplasia (**5–7**). Sella turcica frequently enlarged.
- Mental development may seem normal; skin and hair may be unremarkable; obesity, constipation and so on may be completely absent and the conventional diagnostic laboratory tests (e.g. thyroxine levels) may not yield clearly abnormal results.

Supplementary findings: Delayed dentition. Unequivocal clarification by means of thyroid-stimulating hormone determination (including thyroxine-releasing hormone test). Ectopic thyroid tissue frequently demonstrable.

Comment: This mild form of hypothyroidism with ectopic thyroid glands is not always picked up by newborn thyroid-stimulating hormone screening.

Manifestation: Clinical diagnosis is practically impossible before the third year of life.

Aetiology: Unclear. As a rule, sporadic occurrence. Girls more frequently affected (70:30).

Frequency: Not so rare.

Course, prognosis: Favourable with early diagnosis and prompt initiation of replacement therapy.

Differential diagnosis: This disorder should no longer be confused with the epiphyseal and spondylo-epiphyseal osteodysplasias.

Treatment: Immediate initiation of replacement therapy with L-thyroxine leads to rapid normalization of the pathological laboratory values, rapid advancement of ossification, catching-up of growth and, in some patients, to distinct improvement of intellectual performance.

Illustrations:
1–3, 5–7 A girl aged 11 years and 6 months; height 117.5 cm below the third percentile.
4 A girl aged 4 years and 6 months. Short stature (94 cm), below the third percentile.
8 Radiograph of a 6-year-old female patient.
9 Radiograph of the same girl as in 8, 6 months after initiation of replacement therapy.

References:
Oldigs H D, Schnakenburg Kl v, Wiedemann H-R: Zum Krankheitsbild der oligosymptomatischen Hypothyreose. *Med Welt* 1981, **32**:885.
Dessart Y, Chaussain J L *et al*: Le nanisme hypothyrioidien isolé. Etude de 18 observations. *Arch Fr Pédiatr* 1983, **40**:375–378.
Rochiccioli P, Dutau G *et al*: L'ectopie thyreoidienne, cause d'erreur du dépistage néonatal de l'hypothyroidie. *Arch Fr Pédiatr* 1983, **40**:405–406.
Grant G A, Carson D J *et al*: Congenital hypothyroidism missed on screening. *Arch Dis Child* 1986, **61**:189–197.
Eberle A J: Congenital hypothyroidism presenting as apparent spondyloepiphyseal dysplasia. *Am J Med Genet* 1993, **47**:464–467.
Wiedemann H-R: Oligosymptomatic hypothyroidism presenting as apparent spondyloepiphyseal dysplasia. *Am J Med Genet* 1994, **50**:385.

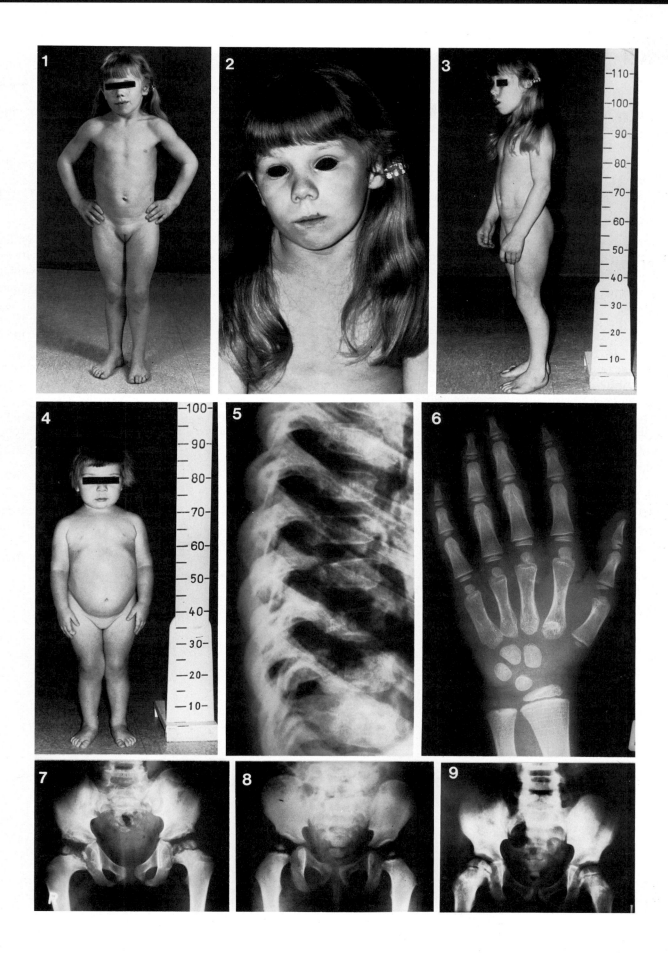

100 Short Stature associated with Vitiligo and, in one case, Chronic Hypoparathyroidism

H.-R.W

A combination of short stature and vitiligo in three siblings, one of whom also has chronic 'idiopathic' hypoparathyroidism.

Main signs:

- Short stature: height of the 16-year-old girl (**2**) on the 15th percentile for her age, height of her 12-year-old brother (**1**) below the third percentile, and of her 10-year-old sister, on the third percentile.
- Vitiligo: typical depigmented patches below the knees in the 16 year old (**5**), also symmetrically on the iliac crests (**2**), below the larynx and on the lower back. The same affecting her brother on the eyelids, chin, inner surfaces of the upper arms, penis, distal lower legs, the backs of the feet and other locations (**1, 4, 6, 7**). The same on the trunk of their younger sister.
- Chronic idiopathic hypoparathyroidism (established biochemically and endocrinologically and controlled therapeutically with dihydrotachysterol) only in the mentally retarded, irritable boy; pseudohypoparathyroidism ruled out; to date, no evidence of autoimmune disease. Both girls of normal intelligence, normocalcaemic and euparathyroid.

Supplementary findings: Additional anomalies in the boy: asymmetric brachycephaly, dysplastic auricles, hypertelorism, epicanthic folds and broad nasal bridge (**3**).

Manifestation: Short stature in the first decade of life. Vitiligo appearing in the 11th, 9th and 10th years of life respectively. First seizure of the boy at 3 months; the first clinical evidence of characteristic tetanic spasms not until some years later.

Aetiology: Uncertain.

Course, prognosis: Normal life expectancy with adequate treatment of hypoparathyroidism.

Comment: The short stature in these patients is familial (father 1.67 m; mother 1.52 m; further people with of short stature in the mother's sibship). Generalized vitiligo as present in these siblings is considered an autosomal dominant defect with variable expression.

Primary idiopathic hypoparathyroidism presenting in early childhood occurs in an X-linked recessive and in an autosomal dominant form, among others.

Combinations of vitiligo with diverse endocrinopathies, including chronic idiopathic hypoparathyroidism, are known.

The association of short stature and generalized vitiligo in the siblings shown here, one of whom has chronic hypoparathyroidism, will for now be considered as a chance combination.

Illustrations:

1, 3, 4, 6, 7 A 12-year-old boy with early-onset chronic idiopathic hypoparathyroidism, generalized vitiligo and (familial) short stature.

2, 5 One of his two euparathyroid sisters with short stature and generalized vitiligo, at age 16 years.

References:

Lerner A B, Nordlund J J: Vitiligo. What is it? Is it important? *JAMA* 1978, **239**:1183.

McBurney, E I: Vitiligo. Clinical picture and pathogenesis. *Arch Intern Med* 1979, **139**:1295.

Betterle C, Mirakian R *et al*: Antibodies to melanocytes in vitiligo. *Lancet* 1984, **I**:159.

Halder R M *et al*: Vitiligo in childhood... *J Am Acad Dermatol* 1987, **16**:948–954.

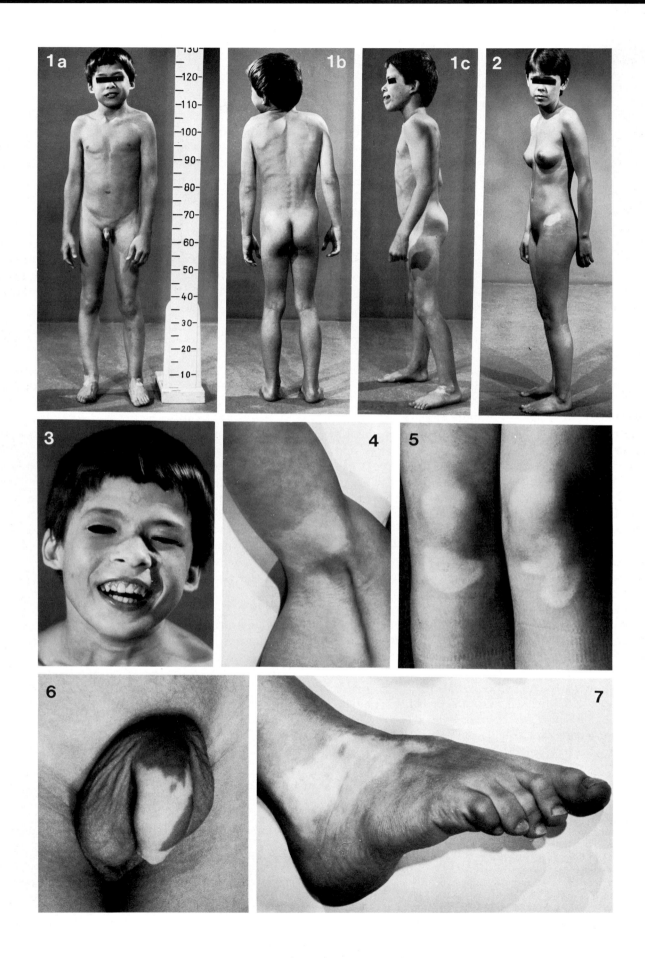

101 Pseudohypoparathyroidism (PHP)

(Albright's Hereditary Osteodystrophy Syndrome)

KI. Kruse/
H.-R.W

A hereditary syndrome comprising short stature, obesity, round face, brachydactyly caused by abnormally short metacarpals, metatarsals and phalanges, mental retardation and, in some patients, seizures.

Main signs:
- Short, stocky physique with short neck, short extremities and round face (1). Adult height between 1.38 and 1.52 m, although occasionally taller than this.
- Obesity - usually moderately severe.
- Short hands and/or feet due to abnormal shortness of one or more metatarsals and metacarpals - especially IV or V, III and I - and/or distal phalanges (especially of the thumb) (3-5).
- Mental retardation of variable severity (not always present).
- Associated endocrinopathies, especially primary hypothyroidism and primary hypogonadism.

Supplementary findings: Manifestations of abnormal mineral metabolism including tetanic spasms or convulsions, delayed eruption of teeth, enamel defects and ectopic calcification (e.g. in subcutaneous tissues, especially of the extremities and joints, 2; lenses of the eyes; the basal ganglia of the brain). Biochemically, typical findings of hypocalcaemia/hyperphosphataemia, high serum level of immunoreactive parathormone and parathormone resistance (diminished response of the kidneys to parathormone as determined by cyclic adenosine monophosphate and phosphate excretion). Normocalcaemic phases also possible.
A PHP type Ib (receptor defect?) and a PHP type II (post receptor defect), in each case, without clinical anomalies, are differentiated from classic PHP with Albright osteodystrophy (type Ia).

Manifestation: Early childhood but also frequently later in childhood. (Obesity, seizures, subcutaneous calcifications, 'osteomata cutis', accelerated bone age, osteoporosis and coarse osseous trabeculations possibly as early as the first months of life.)

Aetiology: Autosomal dominant inheritance of PHP type Ia, in which activity of the adenyl cyclase-stimulating G protein (Gsa) is reduced by approximately 50%. In some patients, diverse point mutations have been detected of the Gsa gene, which is localized on chromosome 20 in the region 20q12-q13.2. Sex ratio of affected girls to boys is 2:1. PHP type Ia is generally only inherited from the mother, the pseudo-PHP only from the father (genomic imprinting). The pseudo-PHP is characterized by the clinical signs of a hereditary Albright osteodystrophy, without demonstrable disturbance of calcium–phosphate metabolism. Note that the Gsa protein is also reduced by 50%.

Frequency: Low, although there are several hundred patients documented in the literature.

Course, prognosis: Normal life expectancy. Not possible to predict whether mental retardation will occur.

Differential diagnosis: Shortening of the fourth and fifth metacarpals may also occur, for instance, in the Ullrich–Turner syndrome (103), which should not be difficult to exclude based on the total clinical picture. Fibrodysplasia ossificans progressiva (252) should also be considered. See also acrodysplasia (102).

Treatment: Symptomatic (for hypocalcaemia, calcitrol; for hypothyroidism, levothyroxine).
Genetic counselling after detailed clinical assessment.

Illustrations:
1 The 'round face' of a typically affected boy.
2 Subcutaneous calcium deposits above the right iliac wing.
3, 4, 6 Typical shortening of (respectively) fingers, metacarpals and toes.
5 A radiograph of the hands of an 11-year-old girl.

References:
Spranger J W, Langer Jr L O, Wiedemann H-R: Bone dysplasias. An atlas of constitutional disorders of skeletal development. Stuttgart and Philadephia: G Fischer and W B Saunders; 1974.
Fitch N: Albright's hereditary osteodystrophy: a review. Am J Med Genet 1982, 11:11–29.
Tsang R C et al: The development of pseudohypoparathyroidism. AJDC 1984, 138:654–658.
Halal F et al: Differential diagnosis in young women with oligomenorrhea and the pseudopseudohypoparathyroidism variant of Albright's hereditary osteodystrophy. Am J Med Genet 1985, 21:551–568.
Kruse K: Hypoparathyreoidismus und Pseudohypoparathyreoidismus. Neue Aspekte... Mschr Kinderheilk 1988, 136:652–666.
Weinstein L S et al: A heterozygous -4p deletion in the Gsa gene (GNAS1) in a patient with Albright hereditary osteodystrophy. Genomics 1992, 13:1319–1321.
Schuster V et al: Normokalzämischer Pseudohypoparathyreoidismus Typ Ia und Pseudopseudohypoparathyreoidismus in einer Familie mit hereditärer Albright-Osteodystrophie. Mschr Kinderheilk 1994, 142:192–198.

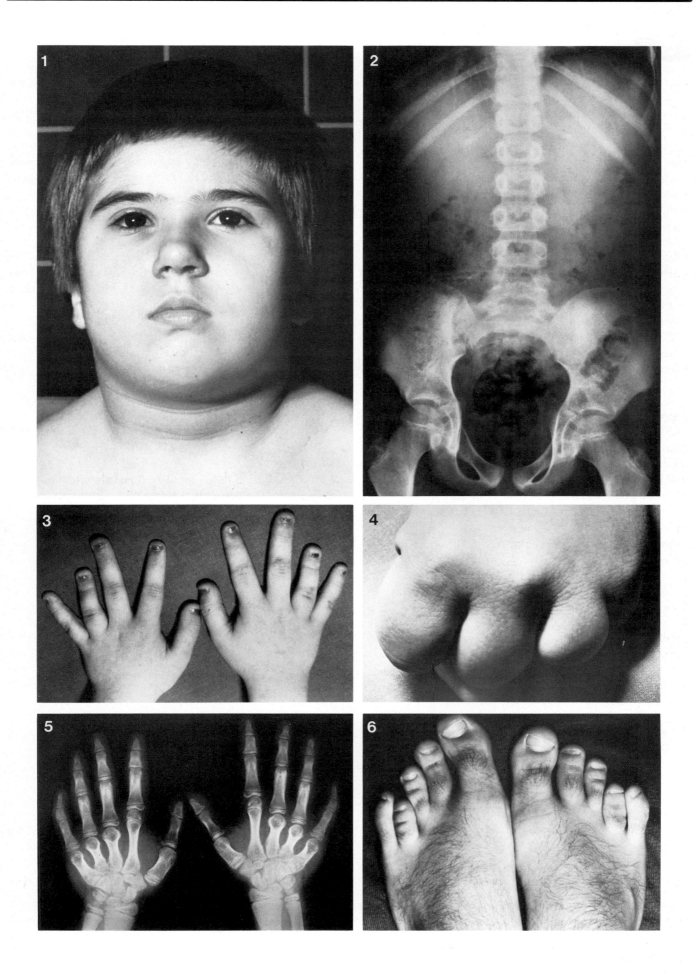

211

102 Acrodysplasia

(Acrodysostosis, Type Maroteaux–Malamut; Maroteaux–Malamut Syndrome; 'PNM Syndrome' from peripheral dysplasia, nasal hypoplasia and mental retardation)

H.-R.W

A syndrome of peripheral dysostosis, growth deficiency, hypoplasia of the nose and mental retardation.

Main signs:

- Considerably shortened hands and feet with short, stump-like fingers and toes; loose, wrinkled soft tissue on the dorsal surfaces and short, broad nails (**1**).
- Often small at birth; postnatal growth deficiency increasingly apparent. Relatively short forearms held in flexion with restricted extension at the elbows (**1**).
- Characteristic facies: hypoplasia of the nose with low nasal bridge; also, nose usually short and flat with a broad tip, which may have a median dimple; anteverted nares; long philtrum (**1**). In some patients, hypoplasia of the upper jaw, hypertelorism, epicanthic folds, prognathism, dysodontiasis, wide mandibular angle.
- Mental retardation (of very variable severity) in about 75% of patients.

Supplementary findings: Radiologically, hyperplasia of the first ray of the foot; severely shortened metacarpals and metatarsals with deformed epiphyses and shortened phalanges with cone-shaped epiphyses; frequent bowing and other malformations of the bones of the forearm (**2**).

Punctate calcification ('stippling') of the epiphyses of the spine, hands, feet and large joints in newborns and infants. Acceleration of bone age.

Hearing defect in approximately two-thirds of the patients.

Manifestation: At birth or later, with increasingly apparent signs.

Aetiology: Most patients have occurred sporadically with increased paternal age. Probable presence of a dominant gene mutation.

Frequency: Low (50 patients described).

Course, prognosis: Complicated by mental retardation, growth deficiency, increasing impairment of the hands, feet and elbows and by the facial disfigurement. Apparently normal life expectancy.

Comment: Pseudohypoparathyroidism (*101*) and acrodysplasia have been considered by some to represent different grades of severity of essentially the same clinical picture.

Treatment: Symptomatic. Plastic or cosmetic surgery may be indicated for patients with marked facial deformity.

Illustrations:

1 and 2 A 1.17 m tall, 15-year-old girl with psychomotor retardation, the first child of nonconsanguineous parents. The patient shows the full clinical picture.

References:

Robinow M, Pfeiffer R A, Gorlin R J *et al*: Acrodysostosis. *Am J Dis Child* 1971, **121**:195.

Ablow R C, Hsia Y E, Brandt I K: Acrodysostosis coinciding with pseudohypoparathyroidism and pseudopseudohypoparathyroidism. *Am J Röntgenol* 1977, **128**:95.

Niikawa N, Matsuda I *et al*: Familial occurrence of a syndrome with mental retardation, nasal hypoplasia, peripheral dysostosis... *Hum Genet* 1978, **42**:227–232.

Butler M G, Rames L J *et al*: Acrodysostosis... with review of literature... *Am J Med Genet* 1988, **30**:971–980.

Hernández R M, Miranda A *et al*: Acrodysostosis in two generations... *Clin Genet* 1991, **39**:376–382.

Viljoen D, Beighton P: Epiphyseal stippling in acrodysostosis. *Am J Med Genet* 1991, **38**:43–45.

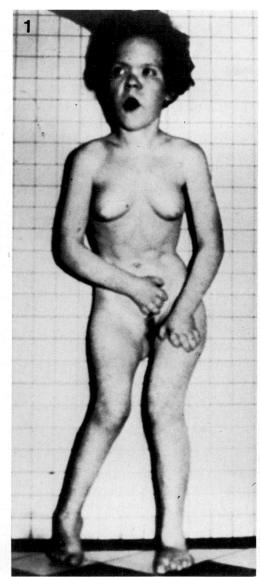

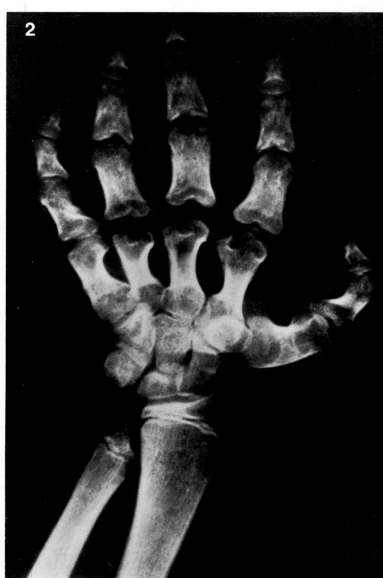

H.-R.W

A malformation syndrome characterized especially by short stature, failure of puberty to occur, webbed neck, lymphoedema of the hands and feet and characteristic facies, all of which can be attributed to complete or partial absence of the X chromosome in phenotypic females.

Main signs:

- Short stature, usually from birth, adult height (untreated) usually approximately 145 cm. Failure of puberty to occur (along with insignificant pubertal growth spurt); absence of spontaneous breast development, poor development of further secondary sexual characteristics, primary amenorrhoea. Neck webbing, redundant skin folds or oedema of the neck; shield chest (**1, 7**). Tendency to obesity.
- Cubitus valgus; at birth, lymphoedema of the dorsal surfaces of the hands and feet which usually regresses by late infancy (**9**); shortening of the fourth and fifth metacarpals; narrow, dysplastic, sometimes spoon-shaped or short nails (**9 and 10**).
- Somewhat expressionless ('sphinx') face. Ptosis of the eyelids, epicanthic folds (**1, 2, 4**); micrognathia (**1**), high and narrow hard palate with malpositioned teeth; low posterior hairline (**6**).

Supplementary findings: Gonadal dysgenesis with rudimentary 'streak' ovaries; renal anomalies (for the most part horseshoe kidney, unilateral renal agenesis); cardiac defect (usually coarctation of the aorta). Intellectual development within normal limits. Increased pigmented naevi and dermatofibromas (**4 and 5**); prominent veins, especially on the arms; retarded bone age and osteoporosis; possible hearing defect (tendency to recurrent otitis). Low oestrogen, high gonadotropin levels. Chromosomal findings are diagnostic.

Manifestation: At birth, however, the child may not come to medical attention until later on.

Aetiology: Either complete (in the majority of patients) or partial absence of an X chromosome. More precisely, complete or partial monosomy for the short arm of the X chromosome in all or a proportion of the body cells.

Frequency: Approximately 1:3000 female births. No increased risk of recurrence for the affected family.

Prognosis: Dependent on the cardiac and renal anomalies. Increased tendency to thyroid disorders and diabetes.

Differential diagnosis: Noonan syndrome (*105*), Klippel–Feil phenotype (*163*).

Treatment: Early treatment to promote growth (apparently best accomplished with a combination of human growth hormone and oxandrolone) by an experienced paediatric endocrinologist. The latter can also determine an adequate schedule for therapy to develop the secondary characteristics and to initiate vaginal bleeding.
Cardiac or renal surgery may be indicated. Plastic surgery (where indicated). Information and psychosocial therapy.

Illustrations:

1–4 Typical 'sphinx-like' facial expression in children of 3 months, 30 months, 9 years and 13 years.

4 and 5 A child with very marked neck webbing, pigmented naevi.

6 The same child as in 3; low posterior hairline.

7 and 8 A 7-year-old girl; shield chest, increased intermamillary distance, somewhat masculine habitus; height approximately corresponding to that of a girl aged 4 years and 6 months.

9 A 9-day-old newborn; marked lymphoedema, short dysplastic nails.

10 A 1-day-old newborn; narrow, hyperconvex nails.

References:

Palmer C G, Reichmann A: Chromosomal and clinical findings in 100 females with Turner syndrome. *Hum Genet* 1976, **35**:35.

Ranke M B, Pflüger H *et al*: Turner syndrome: spontaneous growth in 150 cases... *Eur J Pediatr* 1983, **141**:81–88.

Schwanitz G, Tietze H U *et al*: Gonadendysgenesie – Variationsbreite klinischer, hormoneller, zytogenetischer... *Befunde Klin Pädiatr* 1983, **195**:422–429.

Carr R F, Ochs R H *et al*: Fetal cystic hygroma and Turner's syndrome. *AJDC* 1986, **140**:580–583.

McCauley E, Sybert V P *et al*: Psychosocial adjustment of adult women with Turner syndrome. *Clin Genet* 1986, **29**:284–290.

Rosenfeld R G, Hintz R L *et al*: Three-year results of a randomized prospective trial of methionyl human growth hormone and oxandrolone in Turner syndrome. *J Pediatr* 1988, **113**:393–400.

Heinrichs C *et al*: Craniosynostosis in the Ullrich–Turner syndrome (Letter). *Am J Med Genet* 1991, **40**:252.

Wiedemann H-R, Glatzl J: Follow-up of Ullrich's original patient with 'Ullrich–Turner' syndrome. *Am J Med Genet* 1991, **41**:134–136.

Sylvén L *et al*: Life with Turner's syndrome... *Acta Endocrinol* 1993, **129**:188–194.

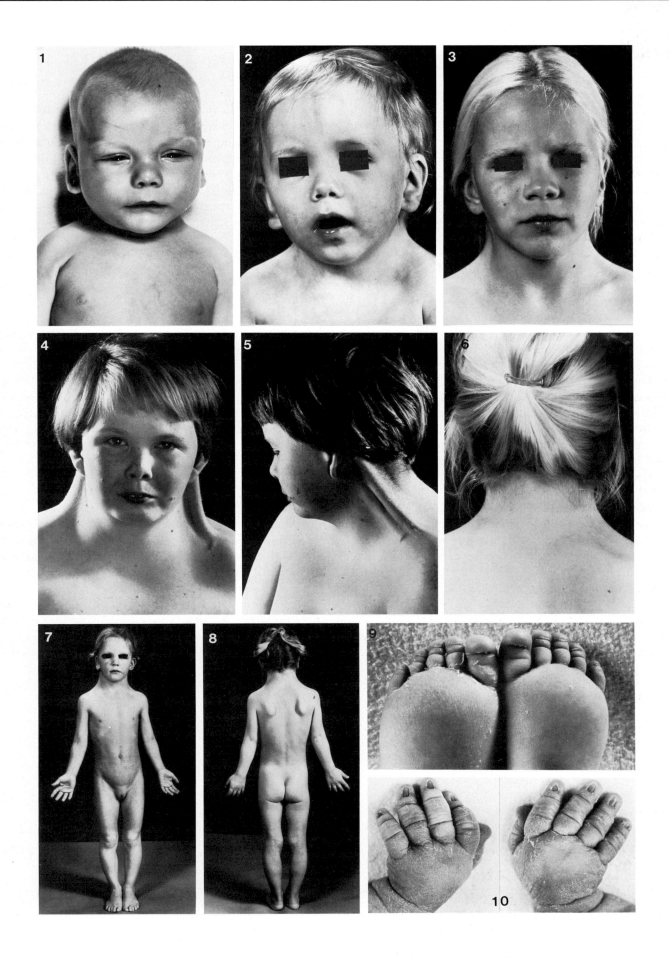

215

H.-R.W/J.K.

A malformation syndrome occurring in males, with growth deficiency, unusual facies, typical genital appearance and other anomalies.

Main signs:
- Short stature, frequently with a long trunk.
- Round face, characterized by a prominent forehead with large widow's peak, hypertelorism, sometimes slight antimongoloid slant of the palpebral fissures and unilateral or bilateral ptosis, hypoplasia of the mid-face, short and broad nose with anteverted nostrils and long broad philtrum, anomalies of the external ear, horizontal groove directly under the lower lip; prognathism (**1, 3**).
- Shawl-like scrotal folds cranially enclosing the base of the penis, cryptorchidism (**2, 4**).
- Short hands (with simian creases) and feet (metatarsus adductus; stubby toes). Short fingers caused by hypoplasia of the distal phalanges, often with mild cutaneous syndactyly and an especially short fifth finger with often only one flexion crease. Unusual hyperextensibility of the proximal interphalangeal joints when the hands are extended at the metacarpophalangeal joints and the distal interphalangeal joints are flexed.

Supplementary findings:
'Receding hairline', antimongoloid slant of the palpebral fissures, broad feet with thickening of the toes. Umbilical anomalies. Pectus excavatum. Inguinal hernias.

Occasional anomalies of the cervical vertebral bodies, craniosynostoses.

Mild mental retardation in approximately 10% of patients.

Manifestation: At birth; retarded growth in height (usually normal birth measurements) during first year of life.

Aetiology: X-linked recessive inheritance assumed to play the main role, because mothers and other female family members of affected boys often show partial manifestations of the syndrome (especially of the face and hands and possibly also slight short stature). However, autosomal dominant (see captions to illustrations) and autosomal recessive inheritance have also been considered. Possible heterogeneity.

Frequency: Apparently not so low; over 130 patients were reported between 1970 (when the first patient was reported) and 1993.

Prognosis: Good. Although initial growth is at or below the third percentile, satisfactory height is usually attained after a normal puberty.

Differential diagnosis: Noonan syndrome (*105*), which does not include the penoscrotal anomaly but includes pulmonary stenosis, pterygium, mental retardation. Robinow syndrome (*113*); BBB/G syndrome (*214*)

Treatment: Symptomatic. Genetic counselling.

Illustration:
1 and 2 Patient 1 at age 9 months (length 66 cm, corresponding to that of a 5-month-old boy). Broad, short hands, undescended testes. Bilateral simian creases. Premature closure of the sagittal suture (also present in his similarly affected sister). The father of both children shows mild signs of the syndrome.
3 and 4 Patient 2 at 3 years and 9 months. Height 95 cm, corresponding to that of a 3-year-old boy. Postherniorrhaphy on the right; seizure disorder.

References:
Hoo J J: The Aarskog (facio-digito-genital) syndrome. *Clin Genet* 1979, 16:269.
Berry C, Cree J, Mann Tr: Aarskog's syndrome. *Arch Dis Child* 1980, 55:706.
Grier R E, Farrington Fr H *et al*: Autosomal dominant inheritance of the Aarskog syndrome. *Am J Med Genet* 1983, 15:39–46.
Meinecke P: Das Aarskog-Syndrom. *Pädiatr Prax* 1983, 28:675–684.
Vooren M J van de, Niermeijer M F *et al*: The Aarskog syndrome... *Clin Genet* 1983, 24:439–445.
Bawle E, Tyrkus M *et al*: Aarskog syndrome... *Am J Med Genet* 1984, 17:595–602.
Nielsen K. Br: Aarskog syndrome... *Clin Genet* 1988, 33:315–317.
Teebi A S, Naguib K K *et al*: New autosomal recessive faciodigitogenital syndrome. *J Med Genet* 1988, 25:400–406.
Teebi A S, Rucquoi J K, Meyn M S: Aarskog syndrome: report of a family with review and discussion of nosology. *Am J Med Genet* 1983, 46:501–509.
Tsukahara M, Fernandez G I: Umbilical findings in Aarskog syndrome. *Clin Genet* 1994, 45:260–265.

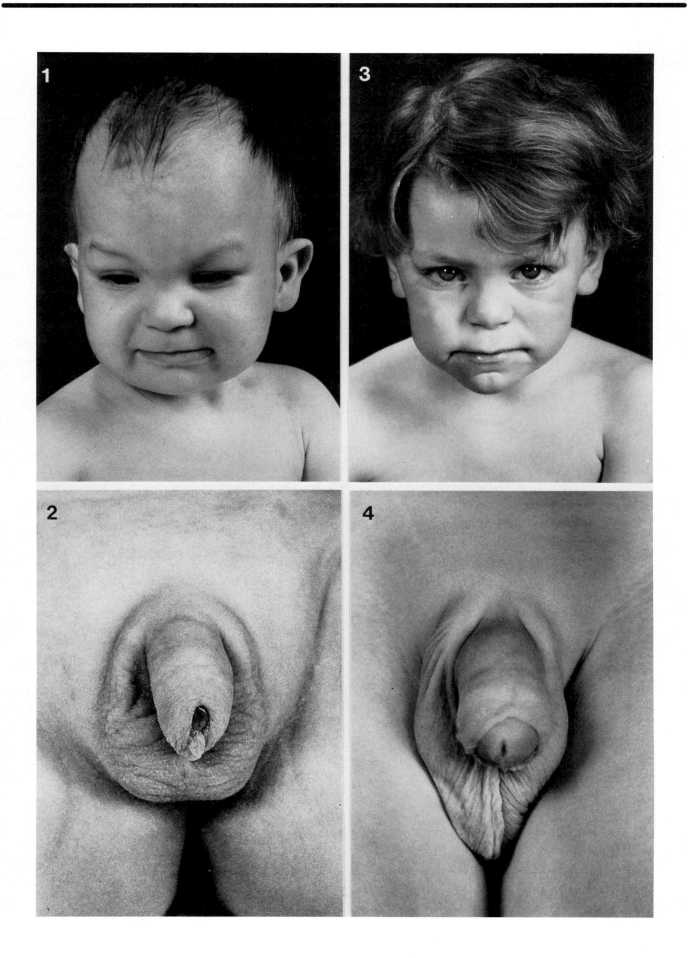

105 Noonan Syndrome

(Pseudo–Ullrich–Turner Syndrome)

H.-R.W

A probably heterogeneous malformation–retardation syndrome occurring in both sexes (without chromosomal aberration) with characteristic facies, growth deficiency, cardiac defect, and multiple other (usually less severe) anomalies.

Main signs:

- Usually mild, proportionate short stature.
- Not infrequently mild to moderate mental retardation; occasionally hearing defects.
- Typical facies (1, 2, 4, 6), mainly characterized by hypertelorism, antimongoloid slant of the palpebral fissures, epicanthus, ptosis, down-turned corners of the mouth and micrognathia.
- Low posterior hairline, webbed neck or redundant skin of the lateral neck (1,7); low-set ears with unusual rims; high palate.
- Shield chest with pectus carinatum and/or excavatum.
- Pulmonary stenosis (valvular, supravalvular, peripheral), rarely atrial septal or other defect.
- Frequently multiple pigment anomalies such as café-au-lait spots.

Supplementary findings: Cryptorchidism; undescended testes; possibly small testes (after puberty). Delayed puberty in some patients; fertility possible in both sexes. Occurrence of renal anomalies.

Cubitus valgus; short radially curved fifth fingers; broad, short finger nails (5); lymphoedema of the backs of the hands and feet in some patients.

Hypertrophic cardiomyopathy and, much less frequently, pulmonary lymphangiectasia may be present; chylothorax in isolated cases. A bleeding diathesis may be present.

Manifestation: At birth, however, the child may not come to medical attention until later in childhood.

Aetiology: Genetically determined syndrome; probable heterogeneity. Extremely variable expression. Occurrence of autosomal dominant inheritance (a gene locus on 12q) and probably other modes of inheritance. Many cases are sporadic. If both parents normal, empirical recurrence risk of approximately 5%.

Frequency: Common (many hundreds of patients); estimated at between 1:2500 and 1:1000 liveborn infants.

Course, prognosis: Essentially dependent on the possible cardiac defect and the mental development.

Treatment: Cardiac surgery, cryptorchidism surgery or removal of webs may be indicated; hormone replacement. Genetic counselling. Psychosocial care.

Differential diagnosis:

- Ullrich–Turner syndrome (103): marked growth retardation, usually normal intellect, failure of puberty to occur, frequent renal anomalies and coarctation of the aorta as the usual cardiac defect. Chromosomal anomaly.
- Multiple lentigines syndrome (LEOPARD syndrome, 178): usually normal intelligence, skin covered by freckles, abnormal ventricular conduction on electrocardiogram, possible hearing defect, autosomal dominant transmission.
- Aarskog syndrome (104).
- Neurofibromatosis–Noonan syndrome (182).

Illustrations:

1 and 2 Patient 1 with typical facies, at age 16 years and 9 months. Height 151 cm (average height of a child at age 12 years and 6 months). Menarche at 14 years. Intelligence just within the normal range.

3–5 Patient 2 at age 6 years. Height 111 cm (third percentile). Birth measurements and heights at ages 11 months and 27 months within the norm. Testes not descended until after the second year of life. Infundibular and valvular pulmonary stenosis. Mild mental retardation.

6–7 Patient 3 at age 3 weeks. Definite psychomotor retardation at 6 months. Mild supravalvular pulmonary stenosis, marked septation of the left ventricle. Malrotation II.

References:

Allanson J E, Hall J G *et al*: Noonan syndrome: the changing phenotype. *Am J Med Genet* 1985, **21**:507–514.

Mendez H M M, Opitz J: Noonan syndrome: a review. *Am J Med Genet* 1985, **21**:493–506.

Ranke M B, Heidemann P *et al*: Noonan syndrome: growth and clinical manifestations in 144 cases. *Eur J Pediatr* 1988, **148**:220–227.

Witt D R, McGillivray B C *et al*: Bleeding diathesis in Noonan syndrome. *Am J Med Genet* 1988, **31**:305–317.

Neri G *et al*: The Noonan-CFC controversy (Editorial). *Am J Med Genet* 1991, **39**:367–370 .

Editorial: Noonan's syndrome. *Lancet* 1992, **340**(1): 22–23.

Sharland M *et al*: Absence of linkage of Noonan syndrome to the neurofibromatosis type I locus. *J Med Genet* 1992, **29**:188–190.

Sharland M *et al*: Genetic counseling in Noonan syndrome. *Am J Med Genet* 1993, **45**:437–440.

Thomas B C *et al*: Long-term treatment with growth hormone... *Acta Paediatr* 1993, **82**:853–855.

Elsawi M *et al*: Genital tract function in men with Noonan syndrome. *J Med Genet* 1994, **31**:468–470.

Burgt van der I, Berends E *et al*: Clinical and molecular studies in... Noonan syndrome. *Am J Med Genet* 1994, **53**:187–191.

Jamieson C R, Burgt van der I *et al*: Mapping a gene for Noonan syndrome to the long arm of chromosome 12. *Nature Genet* 1994, **8**:357–360.

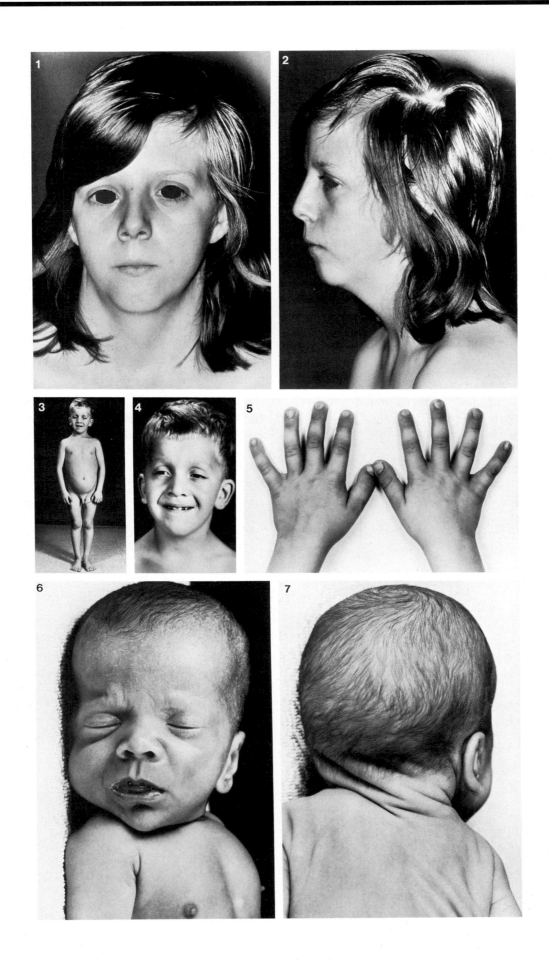

H.-R.W

A syndrome of facial dysmorphism, short stature and considerable mental retardation.

Main signs:
- Facies flat and broad with wide, low-set nasal bridge, hypertelorism, short 'pug' nose and high philtrum. Short, narrow palpebral fissures; epicanthic folds (left more pronounced than right). High narrow palate. Low-set dysplastic ears (1–6). Similarity of the boy's facial features to his father's (7) and his father's father's.
- Primordial short stature, well below the third percentile. Short neck, thickset trunk, stubby hands and feet. Unusual stocky build during infancy and early childhood with extremities at first appearing too short and later too long (3 and 4)
- Severe primary mental retardation.

Supplementary findings: Severe alternating convergent strabismus. Left lower extremity shorter (2.5 cm) and thinner than the right.
  Mild clinodactyly of the little fingers (8).

Manifestation: At birth.

Aetiology: Unclear.

Course, prognosis: Overshadowed by the degree of mental retardation.

Comment: The clinical picture brought to mind several well-known syndromes but could not be classified under any of them. Maternal alcoholism *non aderat*.

Treatment: Symptomatic.

Illustrations:
1, 3 and 5 The affected child at age 3 years and 6 months.
2, 4, 6–8 The same child at 6 years and 10 months.
7 Together with his father. The third child of young, non-consanguineous, healthy but small parents (father 1.64 m; mother 1.52 m). Two older siblings healthy and of normal height. Proband born 10 days before the expected date of delivery after a normal pregnancy, birth measurements 2600 g and 44 cm. At 6 years and 9 months, 104.5 cm. Major internal organs normal (blunted renal pelves on intravenous pyelography). Ocular fundi and electroencephalogram normal. Pneumoencephalogram: cysterna interventricularis et cavum septi pellucidi communicans. Blood chemistry and endocrinological investigations normal. Chromosomal analysis (banding technique) normal.

Note: Similar observation was reported to me from another medical genetics department.

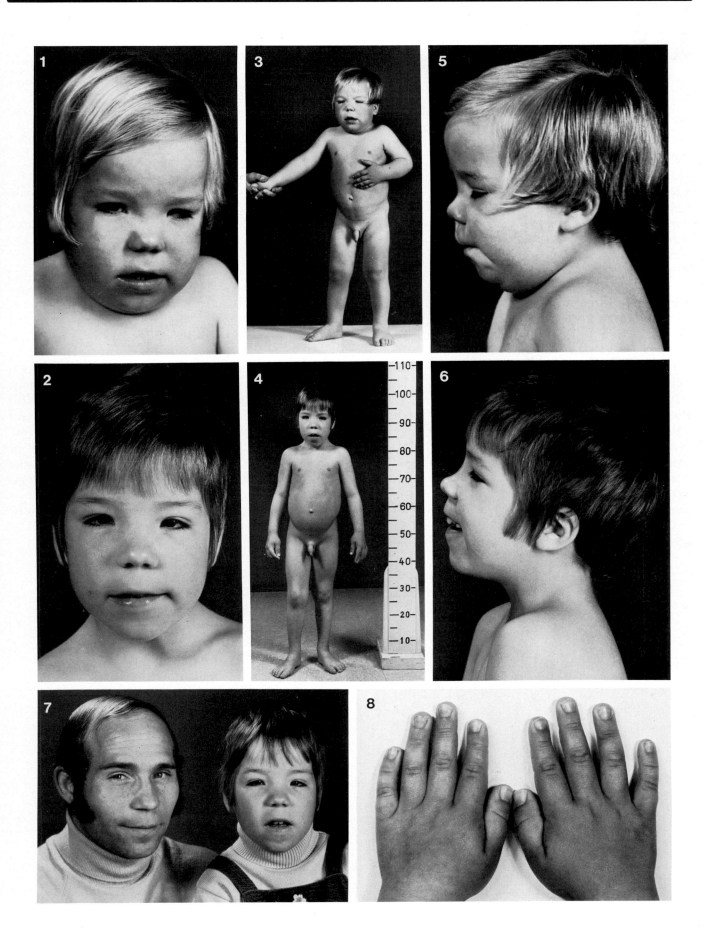

107 Osteopetrosis, Malignant Form

J.K.

Early form with deafness, blindness, hepatosplenomegaly, anaemia and sclerosis of all bones. Synonym: osteosclerosis.

Main signs:
- Deafness.
- Blindness.
- Hepatosplenomegaly caused by haemogenesis.
- Severe anaemia caused by osteosclerosis of the bone marrow: pancytopaenia, extramedullary haematopoiesis, lymphadenopathy.
- Uniformly thick sclerosis of all bones.

Supplementary findings: Cranial sclerosis leads to macrocephaly and hydrocephalus and constricts the cranial nerves, which in turn leads to blindness, retinal atrophy, deafness, paresis of the facial nerve and squinting. Delayed dentition, severe caries. Growth and developmental retardation.

On radiographs additionally: club-like widening of the metaphyses; obliteration of the bone-marrow canals; sclerotic, normally formed epiphyses; mastoid processes and paranasal sinus only minimally aerated.

Metacarpals and metatarsals appear block-shaped with 'bone in bone' appearance.

Manifestation: Generally identifiable at birth.

Aetiology: Autosomal recessive inheritance.

Approximately 100 cases published. One out of 200 000 newborns.

Pathogenesis: Impaired osteoclast function.

Course, prognosis: Survival until 6 years of age is only possible in 30% of patients. Death as a result of anaemia or secondary infections. Better prognosis after allogenic bone-marrow transplantation. Variability within and among families.

Differential diagnosis: Albers–Schönberg syndrome, carbonic anhydrase-II defect with tubular acidosis.

Treatment: Bone-marrow transplantation.

Illustrations:

1a–c A 14-week-old male infant, relative macrocephaly, hepatosplenomegaly, anaemia, generalized sclerosis of all bones.

1d and e The same patient 9 months after bone-marrow transplantation. Remission of the sclerosis: evidence of medullary spaces and normal density of the cortex; the 'bone in bone' structures in the tarsal region are becoming smaller.

2a and b Sibling aged 3 months, generalized sclerosis. Vertebral column with 'bone in bone' structure.

References:

Loria-Cortes R, Quesada-Calvo E, Cordero-Chaverri E: Osteopetrosis in children: a report of 26 cases. *J Pediatr* 1977, **91**:43–47.

Coccia P F, Krivit W, Cervenka J *et al*: Successful bone-marrow transplantation for infantile malignant osteopetrosis. *N Engl J Med* 1980, **302**:701–708.

Sieff C A, Chessells J M, Levinsky R J *et al*: Allogenic bone-marrow transplantation in infantile malignant osteopetrosis. *Lancet* 1983, **I**:437–441.

Fischer A, Friedrich W, Levinsky R, Vossen J, Griscelli C, Kubanek B, Morgan G, Wagemaker G, Landais P: Bone-marrow transplantation for immunodeficiency and osteopetrosis: European Survey, 1968–1985. *Lancet* 1986, **II**:1080–1084.

Bollerslev J: Osteopetrosis: a genetic and epidemiologic study. *Clin Genet* 1987, **31**:86–90.

Gerritsen E J A, Vossen J M *et al*: Autosomal recessive osteopetrosis: variability of findings at diagnosis and during the natural course. *Pediatrics* 1994, **93**:247–253.

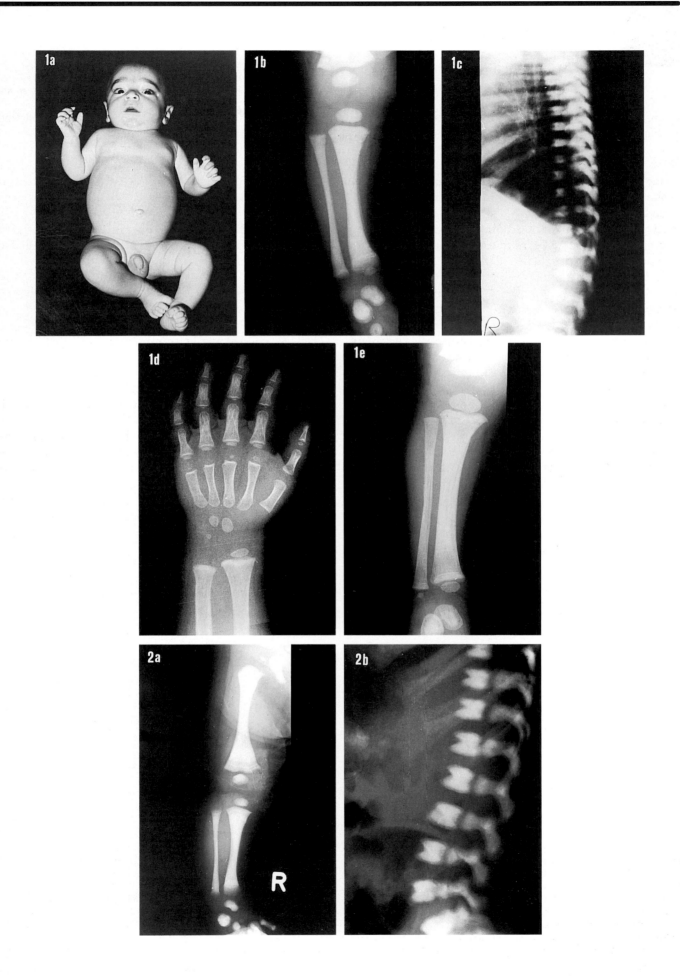

108 Pyknodysostosis
(Maroteaux, Lamy)

H.-R.W

A characteristic hereditary disease of the skeleton with typical facial dysmorphism, short stature and osteosclerosis.

Main signs:
- Short stature from early childhood mainly caused by shortness of the extremities. Adult height between 1.30 and 1.55 m.
- Large, long and narrow cranium with prominent forehead (4 **and** 5), delayed closure of fontanelles and sutures (7), in part until adulthood; relatively small facial part of the cranium with prominent nose, hypoplasia of the lower jaw, micrognathia and marked flattening or even extension of the submaxillary angle (7). Mild exophthalmos in some patients; bluish sclera.
- Short, stubby hands (8) and feet, especially the fingers and toes, with abnormal, very brittle nails (8).
- Frequently increased tendency to fractures (6).

Supplementary findings: Dysodontiasis (anomalies of eruption, malocclusion and others). On radiographs, generalized osteosclerosis. Hypoplasia of the clavicles. Dysplasia or acro-osteolysis of the distal phalanges of the fingers and toes (9), especially of the index fingers.

Manifestation: From infancy.

Aetiology: Monogenic, autosomal recessive disorder.

Frequency: Low. To date, approximately 170 patients described in the literature.

Course, prognosis: Life expectancy normal or only slightly reduced. Tendency to fractures varies from patient to patient. Fractures heal well.

Differential diagnosis: Cleidocranial dysplasia (*19*), mandibulo-acral dysplasia and, readily distinguishable, osteopetrosis (*107*).

Treatment: Early orthodontic supervision as needed.

Illustrations:
The same child at age 30 months (1, 4), 5 years (2, 5), and 10 years (3); growth deficiency respectively of 4, 5, 9.5 and 16 cm compared with the median for age.
7 Skull radiograph at 3 years and 6 months: increased density of the base of the skull; increased density and bossing of the frontal and occipital bones; anterior fontanelle and lambdoid suture wide open; hypoplasia of the mandible with absence of the angle.
9 Radiograph of the hand at 8 years: osteosclerosis; acro-osteolysis of the distal phalanges.
6 Radiograph of the lower leg of an adult with pyknodysostosis showing several spontaneous fractures.

References:
Wiedemann H-R: Pyknodysostose. *Fortschr Röntgenstr* 1965, **103**:590.
Spranger J W, Langer Jr L O, Wiedemann H-R: *Bone dysplasias. An atlas of constitutional disorders of skeletal development.* Stuttgart and Philadephia: G Fischer and W B Saunders; 1974.
Srivastava K K, Bhattacharya A K, Galatius-Jensen F *et al*: Pycnodysostosis (report of four cases). *Aust Radiol* 1978; **22**:70.
M de Almeida L: A genetic study of pycnodysostosis. In: Papadatos C J, Bartsocas C S. (eds.): *Skeletal dysplasias* 1982;195–198.
Beighton P, Cremin B J: Sclerosing bone dysplasias. 1980.
Kumar R, Misra P K *et al*: An unusual case of pycnodysostosis. *Arch Dis Child* 1988, **63**:558–559.
Mills K L G, Johnston A W: Pycnodysostosis. *J Med Genet* 1988, **25**:550–553.
Figueiredo J, Reis A *et al*: Porencephalic cyst in pycnodysostosis. *J Med Genet* 1989, **26**:782–784.
Edelson J G, Suliman O *et al*: Pycnodysostosis, orthopedic aspects with a description of 14 new cases. *Clin Orthopaed* 1992, **280**:263–276.

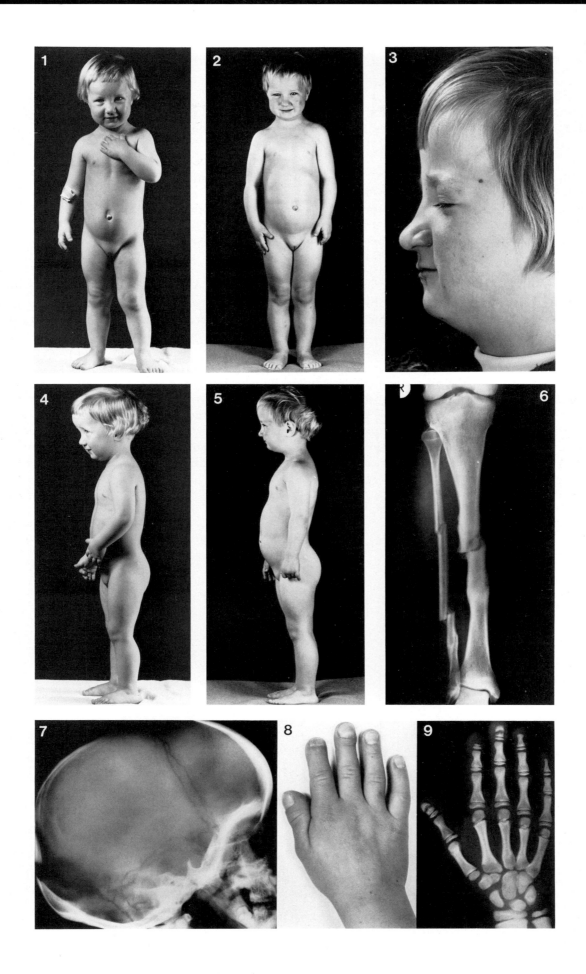

109 Dyschondrosteosis

(Léri–Weill Syndrome)

A syndrome of short forearms with Madelung's deformity and distinct shortening of the lower leg, resulting in disproportionate ('mesomelic') short stature.

Main signs:
- Reducible dorsal subluxation of the distal ulna (Madelung's deformity, **1 and 2**) in both arms with limitation of movement.
- Generally obvious short stature, disproportionate because of striking relative shortness of the slightly bowed forearms and in some patients also of the lower legs.

Supplementary findings: Occasionally short hands and feet; exostoses on the proximal tibia and fibula; hyperlordosis; bow legs or knock knees.

Radiologically: shortening, bowing, broadening and increased separation of the bones of the forearm, dorsal subluxation of the head of the ulna, pyramid-like compression of the carpal ossification centres at the wrist.

Manifestation: From infancy but more frequently somewhat later in childhood with short stature and wrist deformity; development of the full radiological picture of the Madelung's deformity by puberty.

Aetiology: Autosomal dominant disorder, with more severe expression but only 50% penetrance in females. Male:females approximately 4:1.

Heterozygote clinical picture of Langer-type mesomelic dysplasia (*110*).

Frequency: Relatively low.

Course, prognosis: Normal life expectancy. Adult height between 135 and 150 cm.

Treatment: Orthopaedic measures in patients with increased fatigability and wrist pain (e.g. leather supports; surgery in exceptional cases). Genetic counselling.

Illustrations:
1 and 2 A 15-year-old girl with dyschondrosteosis.
1 Reducible dorsal subluxation of the distal end of the ulna and bayonet-like volar displacement of the hand ('Madelung's deformity').
2 Shortening, bowing and broadening of the radii; increased ulnar deviation of the distal radial epiphyses; ulna slender distally; angulation of the carpal bones.

References:

Spranger J, Wiedemann H-R: Dyschondrosteose. In: Opitz, H, Schmid, F. (eds): *Handbuch der Kinderheilkunde* 1967, **6**:204.

Spranger J W, Langer Jr L O, Wiedemann H-R: *Bone dysplasias. An atlas of constitutional disorders of skeletal development.* Stuttgart and Philadephia: G Fischer and W B Saunders; 1974.

Lichtenstein J R, Sundaram M, Burdge R: Sex-influenced expression of Madelung's deformity in a family with dyschondrosteosis. *J Med Genet* 1980, **17**:41.

Koch H L: Die Dyschondrosteose Léri-Weill. *Fortschr Röntgenstr* 1983, **138**:603–606.

Hecht R, Hecht B K: Linkage of skeletal dysplasia gene... (Letter). *Am J Med Genet* 1984, **18**:779–780.

Castillo S, Youlton R, Be C: Dyschondrosteosis is controlled by X and Y linked loci (Abstract). *Cytogenet Cell Genet* 1985, **40**:601–602.

Jackson L G: Dyschondrosteosis: clinical study of a sixth generations family (Abstract). *Proc Greenwood Genet Ctr* 1985, **4**:147–148.

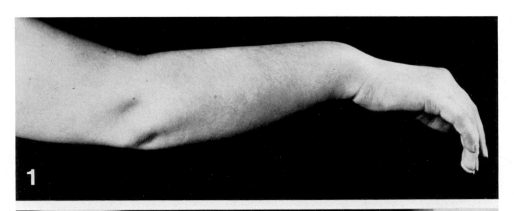

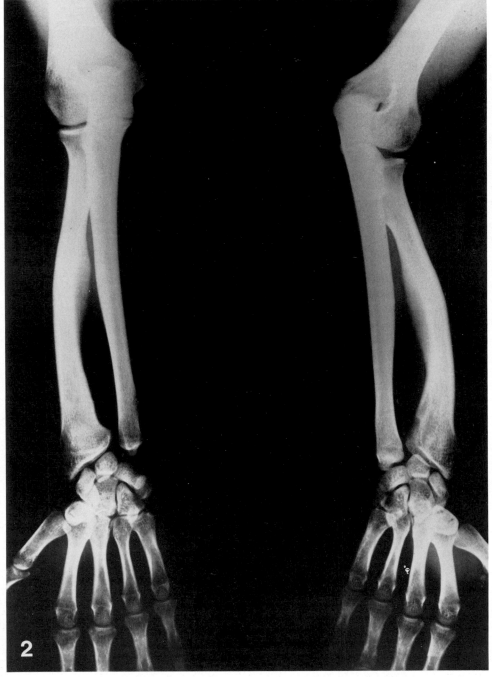

H.-R.W

A hereditary disproportionate dwarfism caused by severe shortening of the forearms and lower legs with characteristic radiological findings.

Main signs:
- 'Mesomelic dwarfism' caused by shortening (and bowing) of the forearms and lower legs with distinct ulnar deviation of the hands, possibly also malpositioning of the feet and limited movement at the elbows, wrists and possibly ankles (1).
- Radiologically, profound symmetrical shortening, bowing and broadening of the bones of the forearms and lower legs (2 and 3) with unusual hypoplasia of the distal ulnae (3) and proximal fibulae (2).

Supplementary findings: Not infrequently, hypoplasia of the mandible. Increased lumbar lordosis.
Normal mental development.

Manifestation: At birth.

Aetiology: Autosomal recessive disorder. Homozygosity of a gene that, in heterozygous individuals, causes dyschondrosteosis (*109*). Typically, both parents therefore suffer from dyschondrosteosis.

Frequency: Low.

Course, prognosis: Normal life expectancy. Adult height about 1.30 m.

Differential diagnosis: Other types of mesomelic dysplasia (*111, 112, 147*) and dyschondrosteosis (*109*); acrodysplasia (*102*).

Treatment: Physiotherapy; orthopaedic treatment may be indicated in some patients. Genetic counselling. Prenatal diagnosis.

Illustration:
1–3 A toddler, the first living child of non-consanguineous parents after three spontaneous abortions and two interrupted pregnancies (indications not clear). Both parents: dyschondrosteosis. Height of the proband at approximately the third percentile.

References:
Spranger J W, Langer Jr L O, Wiedemann H-R: *Bone dysplasias. An atlas of constitutional disorders of skeletal development.* Stuttgart and Philadephia: G Fischer and W B Saunders; 1974.
Esperitu C, Chen H, Wooley P V: Mesomelic dwarfism as the homozygous expression of dyschondrosteosis. *Am J Dis Child* 1975, **129**:375.
Kunze J, Klemm T: Mesomelic dysplasia, type Langer — a homozygous state for dyschondrosteosis. *Eur J Pediatr* 1980, **134**:269.
Goldblatt J, Wallis C *et al*: Heterozygous manifestations of Langer mesomelic dysplasia. *Clin Genet* 1987, **31**:19–24.
Evans M I, Zador I E *et al*: Ultrasonographic prenatal diagnosis... of Langer mesomelic dwarfism. *Am J Med Genet* 1988, **31**:915–920.

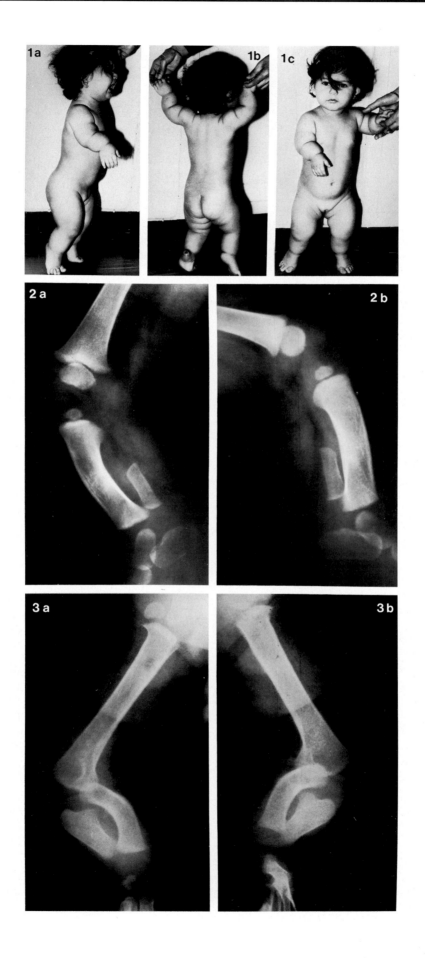

111 Nievergelt Syndrome
(Syndrome of Mesomelic Dysplasia, Nievergelt-Type)

H.-R.W

An autosomal dominant syndrome with severe shortening and deformity of the lower legs, occasionally also of the forearms, with characteristic radiograph findings in the lower extremities.

Main signs:
- Short lower legs (**1 and 2**) with occasional shortening of the forearms; sometimes atypical club feet. Movement may be limited at the elbows as a result of radio-ulnar synostosis; subluxation of the head of the radius.
- Radiologically (**3 and 4**) an almost triangular or rhomboid configuration of the short, broad tibiae (sometimes also of the radii), and to a lesser degree of the fibulae (possibly also of the ulnae). Development of synostoses of the tarsals. Radio-ulnar synostoses in some patients.

Manifestation: At birth.

Aetiology: Autosomal dominant disorder with very variable expression.

Frequency: Extremely low; only eight confirmed patients described since the original report (1944).

Course, prognosis: As a rule, general health is otherwise unimpaired.

Differential diagnosis: Other forms of congenital shortening of the lower legs and forearms can be differentiated radiologically.

Treatment: Surgical correction of club feet, in some patients. Further conservative operative orthopaedic measures and general aids and care for the physically handicapped.
  Genetic counselling.

Illustrations:
1 and 2 A 7-year-old boy; height 1.05 m, with prosthesis for walking 1.23 m; length of lower leg about 11 cm (upper leg 36 cm); genu valgus and curved legs, malpositioning of the feet, deformities of the toes. Arms normal.
3 and 4 Radiographs of the same patient: severe shortening and somewhat rhomboidal broadening of the bones of the lower legs, oblique course of the terminal metaphyseal plates; synostoses of the tarsal bones.

References:
Solonen K A, Sulamaa M: Nievergelt syndrome and its treatment. *Ann Chir Gynaec Fenn* 1958, **47**:142.
Spranger J W, Langer Jr L O, Wiedemann H-R: *Bone dysplasias. An atlas of constitutional disorders of skeletal development.* Stuttgart and Philadephia: G Fischer and W B Saunders; 1974.
Young L W, Wood B P: Nievergelt syndrome. *Birth Defects Orig Art Ser* 1975, **11/5**:81.
Hess O M, Goebel N H, Streuli R: Familiärer mesomeler Kleinwuchs (Nievergelt-Syndrom). *Schweiz med Wschr* 1978, **108**:1202.
Petrella R, Ladman M D *et al*: Mesomelic dysplasia with absence of fibulae and hexadactyly: Nievergelt syndrome or new syndrome? *Am J Med Genet* 1990, 37:10–14.

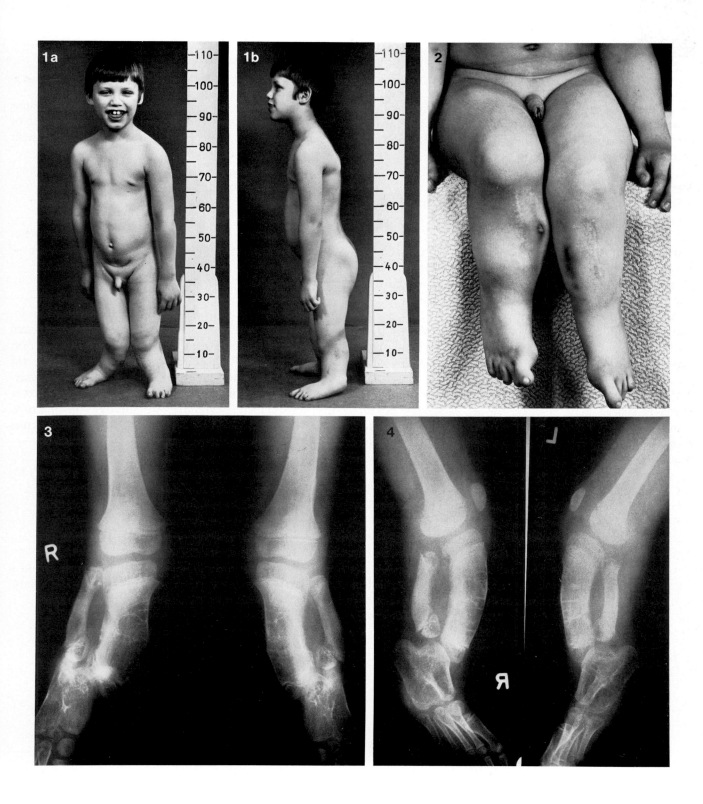

H.-R.W

A syndrome of mesomelic dysplasia with short stature, delayed ossification of the cranial vault, unusual facies, short neck, cardiac defect and symmetrical flexion contractures of the fingers and toes.

Main signs:
- Short, slightly bowed forearms. Lower extremities do not appear short but are likewise bowed (**1, 8, 10**). Short stature, below the third percentile.
- Bilateral, mostly symmetrical, flexion contractures of fingers II–V; bilateral fifth-finger clinodactyly. Pes valgus and planus with mild malpositioning of the toes with flexion contractures (**4 and 5**).
- Large, round cranium with alopecia, except for a cockscomb-like abundant, bristly growth of hair over the region of the sagittal suture (**1–3**). Frontal and sagittal sutures still completely open at age 9 months, wide open anterior fontanelle.
- Unusual facies: broad, slightly prominent forehead; widely spaced eyes; slightly low-set ears; very broad, low nasal bridge; blue sclera; high narrow palate; microretrognathia (**1–3**).
- Short neck; loose nuchal skin, which can be drawn out as a pterygium.
- Cardiologically: complete right bundle-branch block; large atrial septal defect, secundum type.
- Glandular hypospadias; bilateral cryptorchidism.

Supplementary findings: Normal mental and motor development.

Radiologically: subluxation of the elbows, bones of the forearms slightly bowed and short, with the right ulna showing a thornlike excrescence (**9, 11**). Tibiae a little short, slightly curved anteriorly. Fibulae relatively too long, thin, with marked anterior bowing and elevation of the distal ends (**8, 10**). Increased curvature and slight broadening of the clavicles.

Manifestation: At birth; short stature apparent in the toddler.

Aetiology: A genetic basis certain; mode of inheritance not clear.

Frequency: Low.

Course, prognosis: Favourable to date. Direct surgical closure of the atrial septal defect at age 10 years. Present height (130 cm) is between the third and 10th percentile. Pterygium colli. Both testes surgically placed into the scrotum. Ultrasound shows cystic renal anomalies bilaterally (examination revealed both parents to be normal in this respect); no evidence of tubular dysfunction. Diagnosis of orthodontist: absence of a number of dental roots; delayed dentition.

Differential diagnosis: The Robinow syndrome (*113*) shows similarities, however, it can be readily excluded.

Treatment: Symptomatic.

Illustrations:
1–11 The first child of healthy, young, non-consanguineous parents, after two miscarriages. Birth measurements 3000 g and 51 cm.

References:
Löhr H, Wiedemann H-R: Mesomelic dysplasia — associated with other abnormalities. *Eur J Pediatr* 1981, **137**:313.

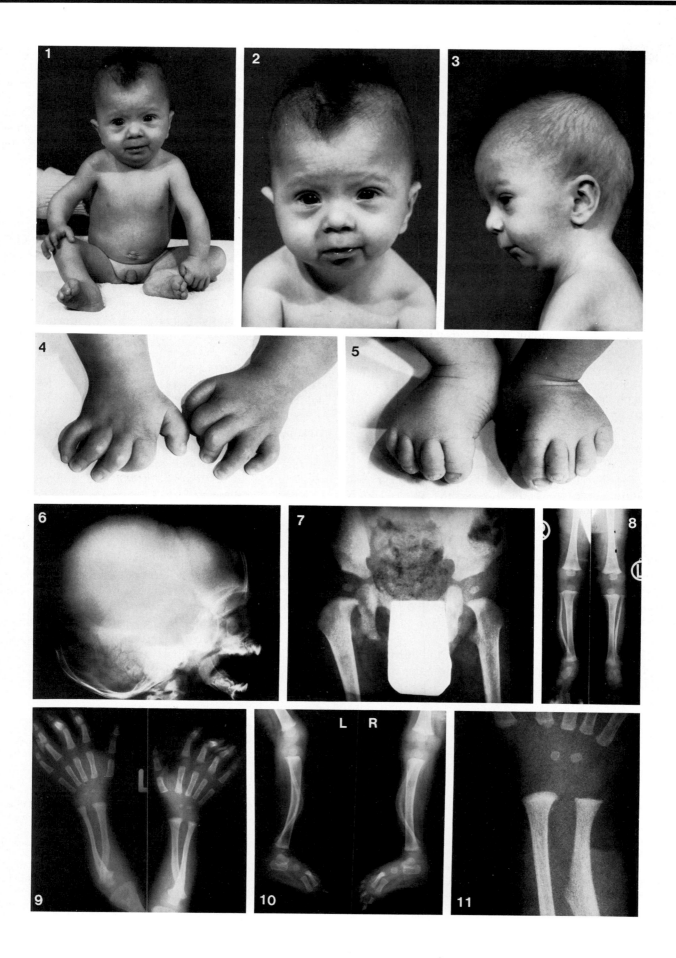

113 Robinow Syndrome

(Foetal Face Syndrome; Mesomelic Dysplasia, Robinow Type; Robinow–Silverman–Smith Syndrome)

H.-R.W

A syndrome of unusual facies, short forearms, genital hypoplasia and short stature.

Main signs:
- 'Foetal face': a disproportionately large cranium with large anterior fontanelle and prominent forehead, the face being relatively small and flat with hypertelorism, wide palpebral fissures and correspondingly large-appearing eyes, antimongoloid slant of the palpebral fissures; mid-face hypoplasia, pug nose, long philtrum, relatively large triangular mouth with down-turned corners, micrognathia (**1**).
- Mesomelic dysplasia of the upper extremities, the forearms being short. Brachydactyly with fifth-finger clinodactyly. Lower legs comparatively less affected or normal.
- Micropenis, with testes and scrotum usually unremarkable (**1**); hypoplasia of the clitoris and labia minora. Possible partial primary hypogonadism that may be caused by androgen receptor defect.
- Short stature.

Supplementary findings: Mental development normal in over 80% of patients.

Radiologically, bowing of the radius with subluxation of the capitulum; obvious shortening of the ulna. Clefts of the distal phalanges of the fingers in some patients; dysplasia of the nails.

Frequent anomalies of the vertebral column and ribs (hemi- or block vertebrae, fusion), in some patients resulting in scoliosis. Frequent dental anomalies and gingival hyperplasia.

Cryptorchidism not infrequent. Inguinal hernias. Cystic kidneys reported.

Manifestation: At birth. Growth retardation: birth lengths within normal limits but falling to below the third percentile during the first years of life.

Aetiology: Genetically determined but variable syndrome. Autosomal dominant inheritance established. An autosomal recessive form, clinically indistinguishable, also occurs. Heterogeneity.

Frequency: Low; around 50 patients described.

Course, prognosis: With respect to general health, good for most patients. Less favourable for development of the penis. Adult height may be about normal. Penis development poor. Fertility of female patients normal, reduced in males.

Differential diagnosis: Other forms of mesomelic dysplasia should not be difficult to rule out.

A disturbingly striking overlap with the features of Aarskog syndrome (*104*), which however shows a peculiar type of scrotal dysplasia, as opposed to genital hypoplasia (in both sexes).

Treatment: Symptomatic. Orthopaedic measures for some patients. Possible early trial testosterone therapy to modify the micropenis, which may otherwise be treated by constructive plastic surgery. Psychological guidance. Genetic counselling.

Illustrations:

1 A mentally normal 8-year-old boy, the third child of healthy, non-consanguineous parents after two healthy children. Birth measurements 3200 g, 49 cm, head circumference 39 cm. Present height below the third percentile; cranial circumference in relation to his height, 98th percentile; frontal bossing. Micropenis of maximum 3 cm length (after plastic surgery). Brachydactyly, clinodactyly; radiologically, slight clefts of the distal phalanges of the thumbs.

References:
Giedion A, Battaglia G F, Bellini F *et al*: The radiological diagnosis of the fetal face (= Robinow) syndrome (mesomelic dwarfism and small genitalia). *Helv Paediat Acta* 1975, **30**:409.
Vogt J, Reinwein H, Fink M *et al*: Das Robinow-Syndrom. *Pädiatr Prax* 1979, **21**:103.
Lee P A, Migeon Cl J, Brown T R *et al*: Robinow's syndrome. Partial primary hypogonadism in pubertal boys, with persistence of micropenis. *Am J Dis Child* 1982, **136**:327.
Shprintzen R J, Goldberg R B *et al*: Male-to-male transmission of Robinow's syndrome. *AJDC* 1982, **136**:594–597.
Bain M D, Winter R M *et al*: Robinow synmdrome without mesomelic 'brachymelia': a report of five cases. *J Med Genet* 1986, **23**:350–354.
Glaser D, Herbst J, Roggenkamp K *et al*: Robinow syndrome with parental consanguinity. *Eur J Pediatr* 1989, **148**:652–653.
Schönau E, Pfeiffer R A *et al*: Robinow or 'fetal face' syndrome in a male infant with... androgen receptor deficiency. *Eur J Pediatr* 1990, **149**:615–617.
Teebi A S: Autosomal recessive Robinow syndrome. *Am J Med Genet* 1990, **35**:64–68.
Wiens L *et al*: Robinow syndrome... with cystic kidney disease. *Clin Genet* 1990, **37**:481–484.
Schorderet D F *et al*: Robinow syndrome... *Eur J Pediatr* 1992, **151**:586–589.

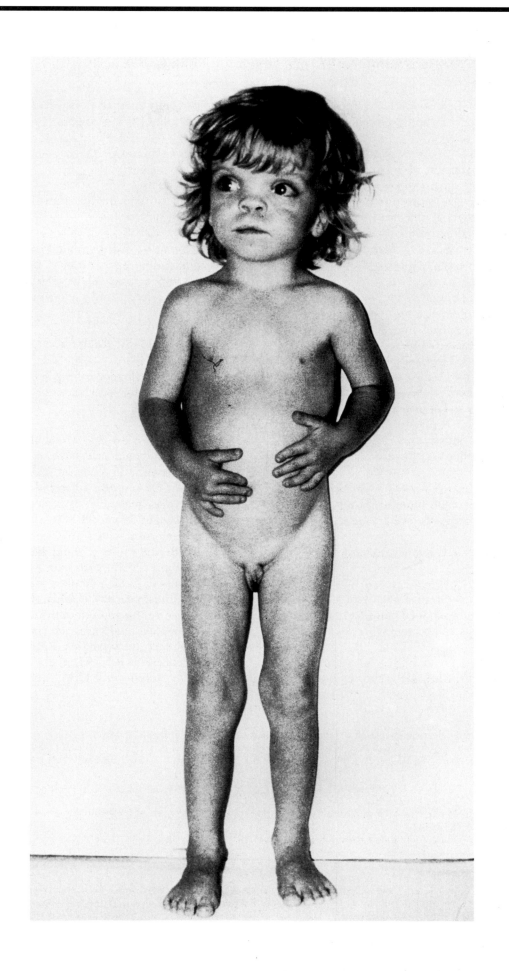

114 Peters'-Plus Syndrome
(Krause–Kivlin Syndrome, Pillay Syndrome)

J.K.

A growth deficiency syndrome with rhizomelia, Peters' anomaly, round face, thin upper lip and psychomotor retardation.

Main signs:
- Occasionally polyhydramnios; birth between 35th and 40th week of pregnancy; prenatal dystrophy; weight 2300 g, length 43 cm, approximately the third percentile. Circumference of the head variable (third to 97th percentile). Feeding problems (84%).
- Micromelic, disproportionate, rhizomelic growth deficiency, retarded bone age, clinodactyly of the fifth fingers. Brachycarpia.
- Facial dysmorphism: round, wide face, thin upper lip, short hypoplastic columella, prominent forehead, thin, narrow palpebral fissures, anteverted nostrils, downslanting labial commissure, micrognathia.
- Corneal clouding caused by the Peters' anomaly: secondary glaucoma, defects of the Descemet membrane, the posterior stroma and endothelium of the cornea. Adhesion between both cornea and lens and cornea and iris. Flattening of the anterior chamber, anterior polar cataract. Hypertelorism.
- Narrow external auditory canal. Microtia.
- Urogenital anomalies: duplication of the ureter, hypospadias, cleft prepuce, cryptorchidism, hypoplastic clitoris and labia. Recurrent pyelonephritis.
- Cardiac anomalies: single umbilical artery, ventricular septal defect, atrial septal defect.
- Sacral cysts, sinus.
- Psychomotor retardation in early infancy. Microcephaly (20%).

Supplementary findings: Strabismus, nystagmus, cleft lip, cleft palate. Triangular-shaped face. Hydrocephalus. Agenesis of the corpus callosum. Hyperextensible limbs. Pre-auricular tags.

Manifestation: At birth. Rhizomelic shortening detectable *in utero* by ultrasound.

Aetiology: Autosomal recessive disorder. Siblings of both sexes reported. Low consanguinity rate.

Pathogenesis: Unknown.

Frequency: Forty-seven patients. Nine families with 52 siblings, nine of which being patients. In 31 couples, 19 miscarriages, nine stillbirths.

Course, prognosis: In early childhood, developmental and speech retardation. Later, normal intelligence not unusual. The oldest patient is age 17 years with normal intelligence. Recurrent otitis media and pyelonephritis. Eventual height: 128–155 cm.

Differential diagnosis: Robinow syndrome (*113*)

Treatment: Ophthalmological measures. Corneal transplantation. Antibiotics for recurrent otitis and pyelonephritis.

Illustrations:
1–6 Male patient. 1–3 Age 27 months. 4–6 Age 7 years: Hydramnios, omphalocoele, birth weight and height -3 SD, head circumference 35.5 cm, left-side cleft lip and palate, clouding of the cornea bilaterally (Peters' anomaly). Inguinal hernias bilaterally. Artial septal defect (secundum type). 1–3 Height 74 cm (-4 SD), arm span 65 cm, round face, hypertelorism, telecanthus, strabismus, nystagmus, broad nasal bridge, long philtrum. Micrognathia. 4–6 Height 96.5 cm (-5 SD), arm span 87 cm, head circumference 54 cm (+1.4 SD), hooked nasal tip, short upper extremities, brachydactyly, clinodactyly bilaterally, brachytarsia. 7 Age 5 years and 6 months, unilateral cleft lip and palate, unilateral clouding of the cornea, prominent forehead, round face, micrognathia. Recurrent cystitis.
7 from Hennekam R C M et al. The Peters'-Plus syndrome. *Clin Dysmorphol* 1993, 2:283–300.

References:
Pillay V K: Ophthalmo-mandibulo-melic dysplasia: an hereditary syndrome. *J Bone Joint Surg* 1964, 46A:858–862.
Krause U, Koivisto M, Rantakallio P: A case of Peters syndrome with spontaneous corneal perforation. *J Paediatr Ophthalmol* 1969, 6:145–149.
van Schooneveld M J, Delleman J W, Beemer F A, Bleeker-Wagemakers E M: Peter's plus: a new syndrome. *Ophthalmol Paediatr Genet* 1984, 4:141–145.
Kivlin J D, Fineman R M, Crandall A S, Olson R J: Peter's anomaly as a consequence of genetic and non-genetic syndromes. *Arch Ophthalmol* 1986, 104:61–64.
Saal H M, Greenstein R M, Weinbaum P J, Poole A E: Autosomal recessive Robinow-like syndrome with anterior chamber cleavage anomalies. *Am J Med Genet* 1988, 30:709–718.
Thompson E M, Winter R M: A child with sclerocornea, short limbs, short stature, and distinct facial appearance. *Am J Med Genet* 1988, 30:719–724.
de Almeida J C C, Reis D F *et al*: Short stature, brachydactyly, and Peters' anomaly (Peters' plus syndrome): confirmation of autosomal recessive inheritance. *J Med Genet* 1991, 28:277–279.
Frydman M, Weinstock A L, Cohen A H, Savir H, Varsano I: Autosomal recessive Peters anomaly, typical facial appearance, failure to thrive, hydrocephalus, and other anomalies: further delineation of the Krause–Kivlin syndrome. *Am J Med Genet* 1991, 40:34–40.
Hennekam R C M, van Schooneveld M J, Meinecke P: The Peters'-plus syndrome: description of 16 patients and review of the literature. *Clin Dysmorphol* 1993, 2:283–300.
Thompson E M, Winter R M, Baraitser M: Kivlin syndrome and Peters'-plus syndrome: are they the same disorder? *Clin Dysmorphol* 1993, 2:301–316.
Camera G, Centa A, Pozzolo S, Camera A: Peters'-plus syndrome with agenesis of the corpus callosum: report of a case and confirmation of autosomal recessive inheritance. *Clin Dysmorphol* 1993, 2:317–321.

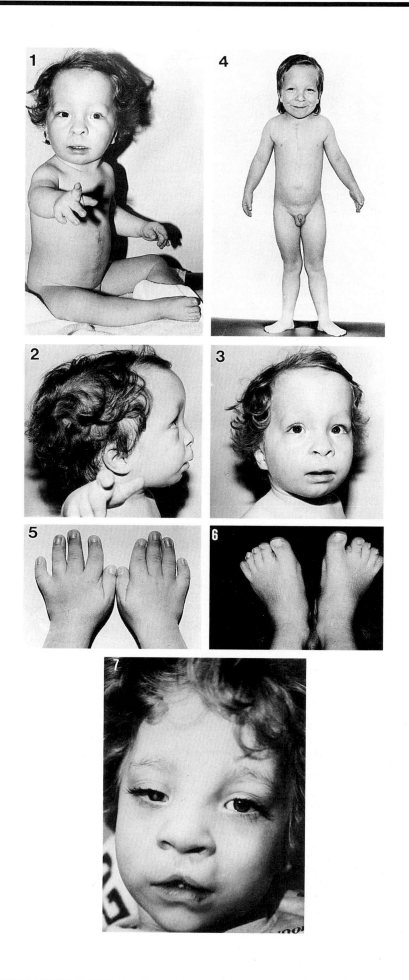

J.K./H.-R.W

An extremely severe congenital skeletal dysplasia with macrocephaly, extreme micromelia and a variable degree of hydrops.

Main signs:
- Macrocephaly, 'absent neck'. Short trunk with distended abdomen. Extremely short extremities, usually with varus positioning of the lower extremities.
- Hydropic appearance (**1a**).

Supplementary findings: Normal number of fingers and toes. Radiologically, more or less absent ossification of the vertebral bodies (but vertebral arches calcified) and sacrum and of the pubic bones and ischia (**1b**). Minimal ossification of the cranial bones, with occipital defect. Short ribs without fractures but with terminal splaying. Moderate elongation of the clavicles, hypoplastic scapulae. Short humeri with stellate calcification, minimal calcification of the radii and ulnae. Triangular configuration of the femora, tibiae and fibulae, likewise stellate. Hands and feet not calcified.

Usually premature birth. Death in immediate postnatal period.

Manifestation: At birth.

Aetiology: Autosomal recessive mode of inheritance. Possible collagen II defect.

Frequency: Low; a total of 20 patients have been described to date.

Course, prognosis: If not stillborn, death shortly after delivery.

Differential diagnosis: Achondrogenesis IA, II (*116*) and hypochondrogenesis.

Treatment: Genetic counselling. With subsequent pregnancies, prenatal diagnosis with ultrasound.

Illustrations:

1a and b A child born 6 weeks prematurely (pregnancy complicated by hydramnios); length 28 cm.

References:

Wiedemann H-R, Remagen W, Hienz H A, Gorlin R J, Maroteaux P: Achondrogenesis within the scope of connately manifested generalized skeletal dysplasias. *Z Kinderheilk* 1974, **116**:223.

Spranger J W, Langer Jr L O, Wiedemann H-R: *Bone dysplasias. An atlas of constitutional disorders of skeletal development.* Stuttgart and Philadephia: G Fischer and W B Saunders; 1974.

Kozlowski K, Masel J, Morris L *et al*: Neonal death dwarfism. *Aust Radiol* 1977, **21**:164.

Schulte M J, Lenz W, Vogel M: Letale Achondrogenesis: Eine Übersicht über 56 Fälle. *Klin Pädiat* 1978, **191**:327.

Andersen P R Jr: Achondrogenesis type II in twins. *Br J Radiol* 1981, **54**:61.

Chen H, Lin T, Yang S S: Achondrogenesis: a review... *Am J Med Genet* 1981, **10**:379.

Smith W L, Breitweiser Th D, Dinno N: In utero diagnosis of achondrogenesis, type I. *Clin Genet* 1981, **19**:51.

Whitley Ch B, Gorlin R J: Achondrogenesis... genetic heterogeneity. *Radiology* 1983, **148**:693–698.

Maroteaux P, Stanescu V *et al*: Hypochondrogenesis. *Eur J Pediatr* 1983, **141**:14–22.

Borochowitz Z, Ornoy A *et al*: Achondrogenesis II — Hypochondrogenesis: variability versus heterogeneity. *Am J Med Genet* 1986, **24**:273–288.

Kozlowski K, Tsuruta T *et al*: A new type of achondrogenesis. *Pediatr Radiol* 1986, **16**:430–432.

Horton W A, Machado M A *et al*: Achondrogenesis type II... *Pediatr Res* 1987, **22**:324–329.

Borochowitz Z, Lachman R *et al*: Achondrogenesis type I:... identification of two distinct subgroups. *J Pediatr* 1988, **112**:23–31.

Dilmen U, Kaya I S *et al*: Achondrogenesis type II. *Pediatr Radiol* 1988, **19**:53.

Spranger J, Maroteaux P: The lethal osteochondrodysplasias. In: *Advances in human genetics* 1990, **19**:1–130.

Freisinger P, Stanesen V *et al*: Achondrogenesis type I B (Fraccaro): study of collagen in the tissue and in chondrocytes cultured in agarose. *Am J Med Genet* 1994, **49**:439–446.

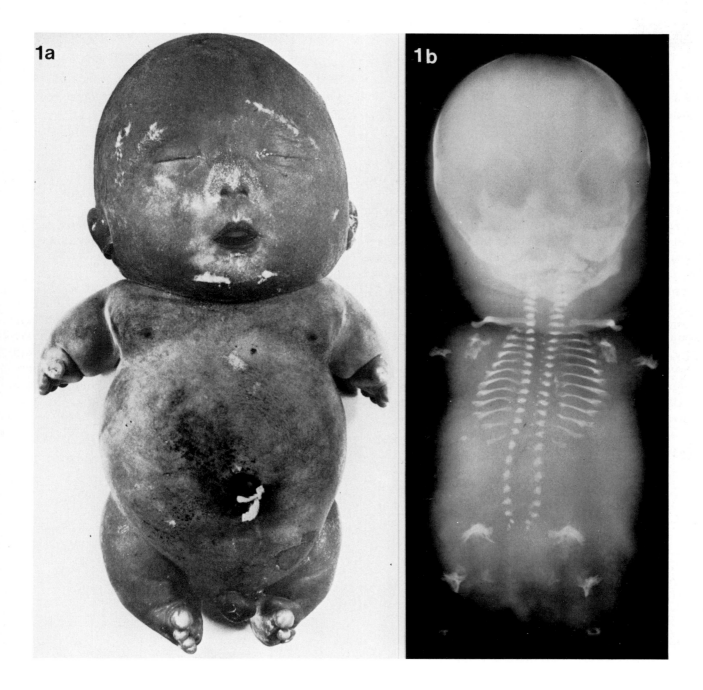

116 Achondrogenesis Type II
(Langer–Saldino)

J.K.

A lethal osteochondrodysplasia with short trunk and grossly shortened extremities.

Main signs:
- Severe neonatal growth deficiency with premature birth, hydrops and severe shortening of the trunk, neck and extremities.
- On radiographs, short ribs with terminal splaying. Ossification defects of the pubis and ischium. Short, broad femora and metaphyseal irregularities. The vertebral arches are ossified but ossification of the vertebral bodies is severely impaired. In severe forms, there is no ossification of the entire vertebral column and sacrum.

Supplementary findings: Variable radiological findings.

Manifestation: Prenatal and at birth.

Aetiology: Heterogeneity. Generally new mutations.

Observations in siblings point to autosomal recessive inheritance or germline mosaicism.

Pathogenesis: Collagen-II defect.

Course, prognosis: Fatal within the uterus or shortly after birth. The mild forms survive for several weeks.

Differential diagnosis: Achondrogenesis type I A, achondrogenesis type I B (Fraccaro, *115*), hypochondrogenesis.

Illustrations:
1–7 41st week of pregnancy, male, lived for 55 min. Macrosomia: length 39 cm, weight 3890 g, head circumference 44 cm. Congenital hydrops. Minimal ossification of the vertebral column with complete absence of the vertebral bodies and arches. Shortened long bones with metaphyseal widening and bowing of the femora. Horizontal ribs, no ossification of the pubis and ischium, small ilium, with terminal splaying of the ribs.

References:
Chen H, Liu C T, Yang S S: Achondrogenesis: a review with special consideration of achondrogenesis type II (Langer-Saldino). *Am J Med Genet* 1981 **10**:379–394.
Whitley C B, Gorlin R J: Achondrogenesis: new nosology with evidence of genetic heterogeneity. *Radiology 1983*, **148**:693–698.
Borochowitz Z, Ornoy A, Lachman R, Rimoin D L: Achondrogenesis II-hypochondrogenesis: variability versus heterogeneity. *Am J Med Genet* 1986, **24**:273–288.
Feshchenko S P, Rebrin I A, Sokolnik V P, Sher B M, Sokolov B P, Kalinin V N, Lazjuk G I: The absence of type II collagen and changes in proteoglycan structure of hyaline cartilage in a case of Langer-Saldino achochondrogenesis. *Hum Genet* 1989, **82**:49–54.

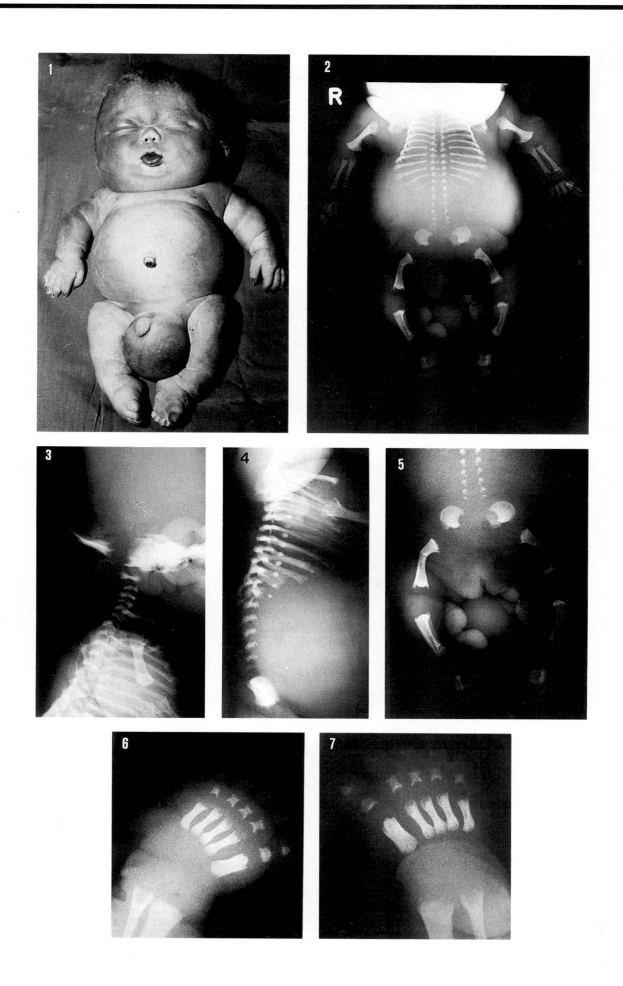

117 Boomerang Dysplasia

J.K.

A lethal osteochondrodysplasia with gross shortening and bowing of all extremities.

Main signs:
- Disproportionate neonatal growth deficiency, less than 40 cm, relative macrocephaly, short trunk, narrow thorax.
- Shortening of all extremities, anterior bowing of the lower extremities. Equinovarus position of the feet.
- Craniofacial dysmorphism: epicanthus medialis bilaterally, broad nasal bridge, severe hypoplasia of the alae nasi and of the nasal septum (small oval nostrils), prominent philtrum, small mandible.

Supplementary findings: On radiographs, boomerang-like, triangular or oval form of the long bones. Absent radii and fibulae. Ossification anomalies of the cervical and thoracic vertebral column. Hypoplastic ilium, absent os pubis.

Manifestation: Prenatal and at birth.

Aetiology: Possibly autosomal recessive inheritance.

Pathogenesis: Unknown.

Course, prognosis: Association with hydramnios, premature birth, death *in utero* or during the neonatal period.

Differential diagnosis: Atelosteogenesis.

Illustrations:
1 Premature female, 26th week of pregnancy, head circumference 25 cm, weight 805 g, length 27 cm, lived for 86 min. Disproportionate tetramicromelia and syndactyly. Relative macrocephaly, broad forehead, micrognathia.
2 Humerus, ulna, radius and fibula present only in cartilaginous form. Distally reduced ossification of the vertebral column.

References:

Kozlowski K, Tsuruta T, Kameda Y, Kan A, Leslie G: New forms of neonatal death dwarfism: report of 3 cases. *Pediatr Radiol* 1981, **10**:155–160.
Tenconi R, Kozlowski K, Largaiolli G: Boomerang dysplasia: a new form of neonatal death dwarfism. *Fortschr Geb Röntgenstr* 1983, **138**:378–380.
Kozlowski K, Sillence D, Cortis-Jones R, Osborn R: Boomerang dysplasia. *Br J Radiol* 1985, **58**:369–371.
Winship I, Cremin B, Beighton P: Boomerang dysplasia. *Am J Med Genet* 1990, **36**:440–443.
Hunter A G W, Carpenter B F: Atelosteogenesis I and Boomerang dysplasia: a question of nosology. *Clin Genet* 1991, **39**:471–480.
Greally M T, Jewett T, Smith W L Jr, Penick G D, Williamson R A: Lethal bone dysplasia in a fetus with manifestations of atelosteogenesis I and Boomerang dysplasia. *Am J Med Genet* 1993, **47**:1086–1091.

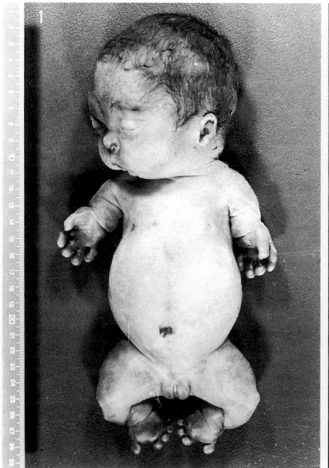

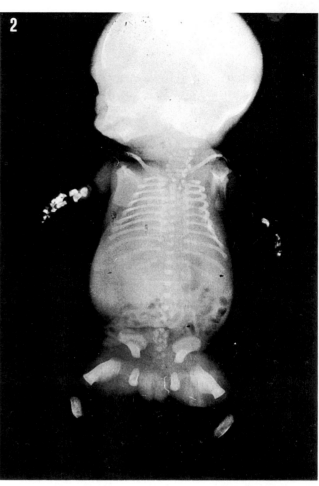

118 Thanatophoric Dysplasia Type 1
(Maroteaux, Lamy, Robert)

J.K./H.-R.W

A severe congenital skeletal dysplasia with disproportionately large cranium, narrow thorax and marked micromelia.

Main signs:
- Macrocephaly (with wide fontanelles and sutures), with low nasal bridge and exopthalmos.
- Relatively normal trunk length with narrow thorax.
- Micromelia with numerous ring-shaped skin folds (**1a**).
- Length at birth 36–46 cm, head circumference 32–40 cm.

Supplementary findings:
Radiologically: short ribs with narrow thorax; marked platyspondyly with abnormal configuration of the vertebral bodies; narrow, short and flat pelvis; long bones shortened, poorly shaped and, in part, considerably bowed (the shape of the femur has been compared with that of a telephone receiver) (**1b**). Immediate development of the respiratory distress syndrome.

Cerebral malformations: abnormal gyration in the temporal lobe region, dysgenesis of the parahippocampus, agenesis of the Ammon's horn, periventricular heterotopia and polymicrogyria temporally, megalencephaly.

Manifestation: At birth (frequently hydramnios).

Aetiology: Sporadic occurrence; possible autosomal dominant new mutation. Impaired endochondral ossification.

Frequency: Low (1:40 000–1:45 000 births; up to 1990, more than 100 observations were reported in the literature.

Course, prognosis: As a rule, death shortly after birth. Rarely, survival for up to 200 days and, with respiratory aids, up to 5 years. However, such patients have severe psychomotor disturbance, extreme short stature and failure to thrive.

Early ultrasound diagnosis should be carried out in subsequent pregnancies.

Differential diagnosis: The appearance of the children is very suggestive of the Parrot syndrome (achondroplasia, *130*) in older individuals. However, the physical signs and radiological findings in newborns with the usual heterozygotic (and even with the rare homozygotic) achondroplasia are considerably milder.

Type II and several 'variants' of thanatophoric dysplasia, in addition to other severe congenital skeletal dysplasias, must be ruled out.

Illustrations:
1a and b A child (8-month gestation) who died on the second day of life and a radiograph of the same.

References:
Spranger J W, Langer Jr L O, Wiedemann H-R: *Bone dysplasias. An atlas of constitutional disorders of skeletal development.* Stuttgart and Philadephia: G Fischer and W B Saunders; 1974.
Connor J M, Connor R A C *et al*: Lethal neonatal chondrodysplasias... *Am J Med Genet* 1985, 22:243–253.
Martinez-Frias M L, Ramos-Arroyo M A *et al*: Thanatophoric dysplasia: an autosomal dominant condition? *Am J Med Genet* 1988, 31:815–820.
Young I D, Patel I, Lamont A C: Thanatophoric dysplasia in identical twins. *J Med Genet* 1989, 26:276.
Spranger J, Maroteaux P: The lethal osteochondrodysplasias. In: *Advances in human genetics 19.* H. Harris, K. Hirschhorn (eds.). New York – London: Plenum 1990.
MacDonald I M, Hunter A G W, MacLeod P M, MacMurray S B: Growth and development in thanatophoric dysplasia. *Am J Med Genet* 1989, 33:508–512.
Coulter C L, Leech R W, Brumback R A, Schaefer G B: Cerebral abnormalities in thanotophoric dysplasia. *Child Nerv Syst* 1991, 7:21–26.

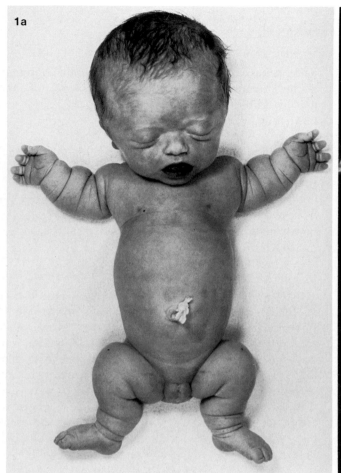

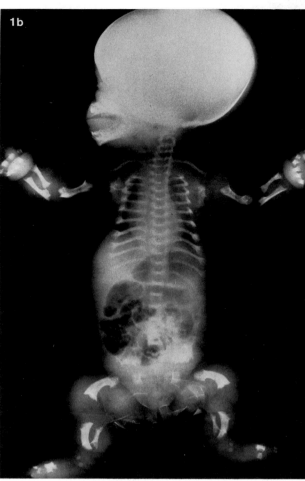

J.K./H.-R.W

A form of thanatophoric dysplasia with cloverleaf skull, characterized by straight or minimally bowed femora and less markedly flattened vertebral bodies.

Main signs:
- Macrocephaly with cloverleaf-like deformity (large cranium with upward and outward protrusions; depressed nasal bridge, exophthalmos, and downward displacement of the ears, almost to the horizontal) (**1–5**).
- Trunk of near-normal length, with narrow, often bell-shaped thorax and protruding abdomen (**2, 6**).
- Micromelia with numerous skin folds; extremities held away from the trunk, femora abducted and externally rotated; very small fingers and toes (**2, 6**).

Supplementary findings:
- Below average size in many patients.
- Radiologically, short ribs with narrow thorax, unremarkable clavicles. Flattening of the vertebral bodies. However, height of L2 (second lumbar) is 50% or more of the height of the adjacent L2–3 intervertebral disc.
- Characteristic pelvic shape of thanatophoric dysplasia. Shortening and partial bowing of the long bones, although the femora may be straight for the most part. The fibulae are shorter than the tibiae. Very short, broad phalanges of the fingers and toes (**6**).
- Immediate development of the respiratory distress syndrome.

Manifestation: At birth (frequently hydramnios).

Aetiology: With the exception of one set of siblings, all patients have to date been sporadic; parental consanguinity never demonstrated with certainty. Mode of inheritance is still unclear. For the time being, the risk of recurrence may be considered very low.

Frequency: Low; 25 patients have been reported in the literature.

Course, prognosis: As a rule, death shortly after birth from respiratory insufficiency.
Early ultrasound diagnosis indicated in subsequent pregnancies.

Diagnosis, differential diagnosis: The cloverleaf skull is aetiologically and pathogenically heterogeneous. It occurs in the following syndromes: Apert's syndrome (*9*), Carpenter's syndrome (*11*), Pfeiffer's syndrome (*8*), Crouzon syndrome (*6*), osteoglophonic dysplasia, amniotic constriction grooves (*219*), camptomelic dysplasia (*129*), in association with other unknown syndromes, chromosomal disorders and in isolation.
Plate 118 shows an example of type I thanatophoric dysplasia (with markedly bowed femora and severe platyspondyly). Here, a very mild cloverleaf skull configuration is present only as an exception.

Illustrations:
1–6 A characteristically affected male newborn, born at term. Birth measurements: 47 cm, 3540 g, 39 cm (head circumference). Death at 5 days of age from respiratory insufficiency.

References:
Partington M W, Gonzalez-Crussi F, Khakee S G *et al*: Cloverleaf skull and thanatophoric dwarfism. Report of four cases, two in the same sibship. *Arch Dis Child* 1971, 46:656–664.
Gemelli M, Galatioto S, Longo M *et al*: Nanismo tanatoforo con cranio a trifoglio. *Min Ped* 1982, **34**:977–982.
Horton W A, Harris D J, Collins D L: Discordance for the Kleeblattschädel anomaly in monozygotic twins with thanatophoric dysplasia. *Am J Med Genet* 1983, 15:97–101.
Isaacson Gl, Blakemore K J, Chervenak Fr A: Thanatophoric dysplasia with cloverleaf skull. *Am J Dis Child* 1983, 137:896–898.
Elejalde B R, de Elejalde M M: Thanatophoric dysplasia: fetal manifestations and prenatal diagnosis. *Am J Med Genet* 1985, 22:669–683.
Langer L O Jr, Yang S S, Hall J G *et al*: Thantophoric dysplasia and cloverleaf skull. *Am J Med Genet Suppl* 1987, 3:167–179.
Norman A M, Rimmer S, Landy S, Donnai D: Thanatophoric dysplasia of the straight-bone type (type 2). *Clin Dysmorphol* 1992, 1:115–120.
Corsello G, Maresi E, Rossi C, Giuffré L, Cittadini E: Thanatophoric dysplasia in monozygotic twins discordant for cloverleaf skull: prenatal diagnosis, clinical and pathological findings. *Am J Med Genet* 1992 42:122–126.

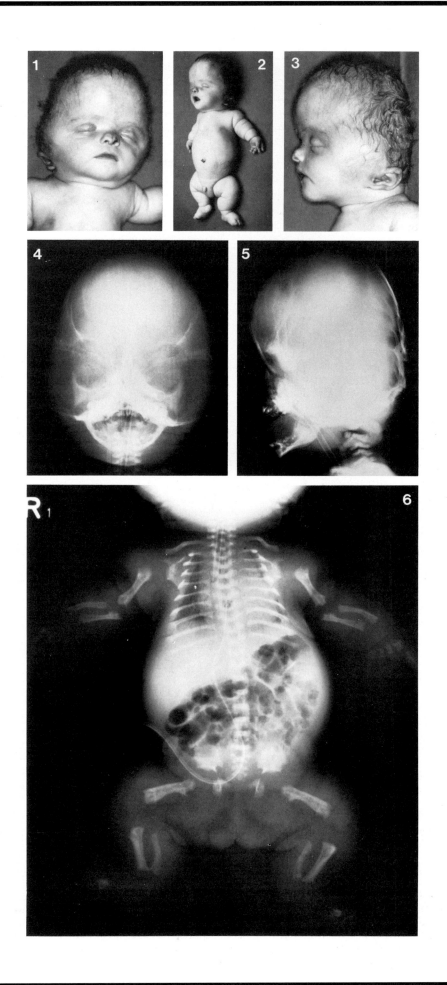

J.K.

A lethal osteochondrodysplasia with micromelia and markedly delayed skeletal maturation ('opsismo').

Main signs:
- Rhizomelic shortening of the extremities, especially distinctive brachycarpia and brachytarsia.
- Craniofacial dysmorphism: Protruding forehead, anterior fontanelle wide open, short nose with depressed flat bridge, long upper lip. Dysplastic ears with lateral deviation of the upper auricle.
- Distinctive, generalized muscular hypotonia.

Supplementary findings: Especially characteristic on radiographs is the marked delay in skeletal maturation: marked reduction in the height of the vertebral bodies, markedly shortened shafts of the long bones with widened, irregular metaphyses. Square-shaped iliac wings.

Manifestation: Prenatal and at birth.

Aetiology: Autosomal recessive inheritance. We observed three affected foetuses of different sexes in one consanguineous marriage.

Pathogenesis: Overproduction of type-I collagen instead of type-II collagen.

Course, prognosis: Death in the first 3 years of life.

Differential diagnosis: Radiological differentiation from other lethal osteochondrodysplasias.

Treatment: Symptomatically with recurrent infections of the respiratory tract.

Illustrations:
1–6 One out of three children died postnatally: 34th week of pregnancy, length 33 cm, weight 2285 g, head circumference 33.5 cm. Micromelia, depressed, flat nasal bridge. Brachycarpia and brachytarsia.
7–11 Delayed skeletal maturation, platyspondylia, diaphyseal shortening of the long bones and widened, irregular metaphyses. Square configuration of the pelvis.

References:

Maroteaux, P, Stanescu, V, Stanescu, R, Le Marec, B, Moraine, C, Lejarraga, H: Opsismodysplasia: a new type of chondrodysplasia with predominant involvement of the bones of the hand and the vertebrae. *Am J Med Genet* 1984, **19**:171–182.
Beemer F A, Kozlowski K S: Additional case of opsismodysplasia supporting autosomal recessive inheritance. *Am J Med Genet* 1994, **49**:344–347.
Maroteaux P, Stanescu V, Stanescu R: Four recently described osteochondrodysplasias; opsismodysplasia. In: Papadatos C J, Bartsocas C. (eds.): *Skeletal dysplasias.* New York: 1982; 347–348.

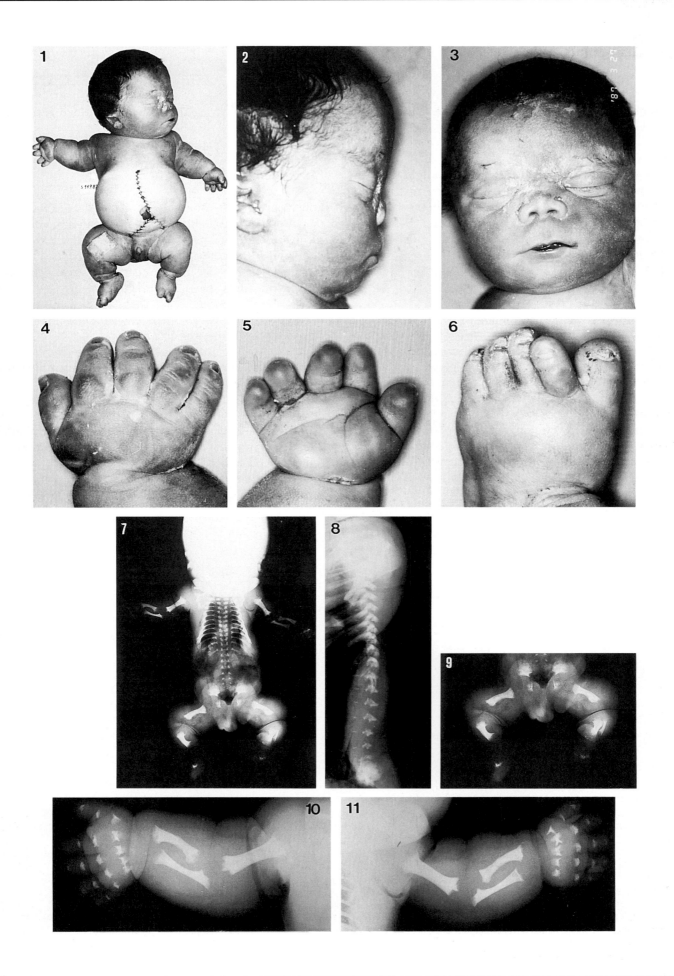

249

Asphyxiating Thoracic Dysplasia
(Jeune Syndrome)

J.K.

A short-rib syndrome with or without polydactyly and high lethality.

Main signs:
- Long, narrow thorax with pectus carinatum.
- Respiratory insufficiency in the newborn, sometimes becoming more marked in the first month of life with infections of the upper respiratory tract, tachypnoea, cyanosis, minimal expansion of the bony thorax (abdominal respiratory type).
- Relatively short extremities compared with the long thorax. Rarely, polydactyly.

Supplementary findings: Radiologically, short, horizontal ribs with widening of the anterior parts. Distally, markedly shortened and thickened long bones with irregular metaphyses. Cone-shaped epiphyses of the middle phalanges (only developing in surviving infants). Small wings of the ilium, tricorn configuration of the lower edge. Beginning at school age, renal insufficiency with proteinuria and arterial hypertonia, nephronophthisis, polycystic kidneys. In adulthood, cystic and fibrous transformation of the liver (rarely, congenital fibrosis of the liver) and pancreas; in isolated cases, retinitis pigmentosa.

Manifestation: In the neonatal period. Prenatal diagnosis is possible with ultrasound in severly affected patients.

Aetiology: Autosomal recessive inheritance.

Pathogenesis: Unknown.

Course, prognosis: Some children die in the neonatal period. Most children do not survive early infancy. Following survival of the first few months of life, the prognosis is determined by kidney insufficiency. In survivors, respiratory insufficiency decreases and the thoracic configuration remains unchanged. Normal intelligence.

Differential diagnosis: Chondro-ectodermal dysplasia (Ellis-van Creveld syndrome, *135*).

Treatment: At the appropriate time, active immunization against influenza, measles, pertussis.

Illustrations:
1 Male infant at age 7 weeks with mild thoracic dysplasia.
2 and 3 Severe thoracic anomaly with short ribs. Lived for only 21 h after birth.
4 Distally shortened long bones, widened, irregular metaphyses, small wings of the ilium, tricorn configuration of the lower edge.

References:
Friedman J M, Kaplan H G, Hall J G: The Jeune syndrome (asphyxiating thoracic dystrophy) in an adult. *Am J Med Genet* 1975, **59**:857–862.
Cortina H, Beltran J, Olague R, Ceres L, Alonso A, Lanuza A: The wide spectrum of the asphyxiating thoracic dysplasia. *Pediatr Radiol* 1979, 8:93–99.
Donaldson M D C, Warner A A, Trompeter R S, Hayccock G B, Chantler C: Familial juvenile nephronophthisis, Jeune's syndrome, and associated disorders. *Arch Dis Child* 1985, **60**:426–434.
Elejalde B R, Mercedes de Elejalde M, Pansch D: Prenatal diagnosis of Jeune syndrome. *Am J Med Genet* 1985, 21:433–438.
Turkel S B, Diehl E J, Richmond J A: Necropsy findings in neonatal asphyxiating thoracic dystrophy. *J Med Genet* 1985, 22:112–118.
Schinzel A, Savoldelli G, Briner J, Schubiger G: Prenatal sonographic diagnosis of Jeune syndrome. *Radiology* 1986, 154:777–778.
Giorgi P L, Gabrielli O, Bonifazi V, Catassi C, Coppa G V: Mild form of Jeune syndrome in two sisters. *Am J Hum Genet* 1990, **35**:280–282.
Rinaldi S, Dionisi-Vici C, Goffredo B, Dallapiccola B, Rizzoni G: Jeune syndrome associated with cystinuria: report of two sisters. *Am J Med Genet* 1990, 7:301–303.
Harms K, Klinge O, Speer Ch P: Variabilität des Jeune-Syndroms. *Monatsschr Kinderheilkd* 1993, **141**:868–873.

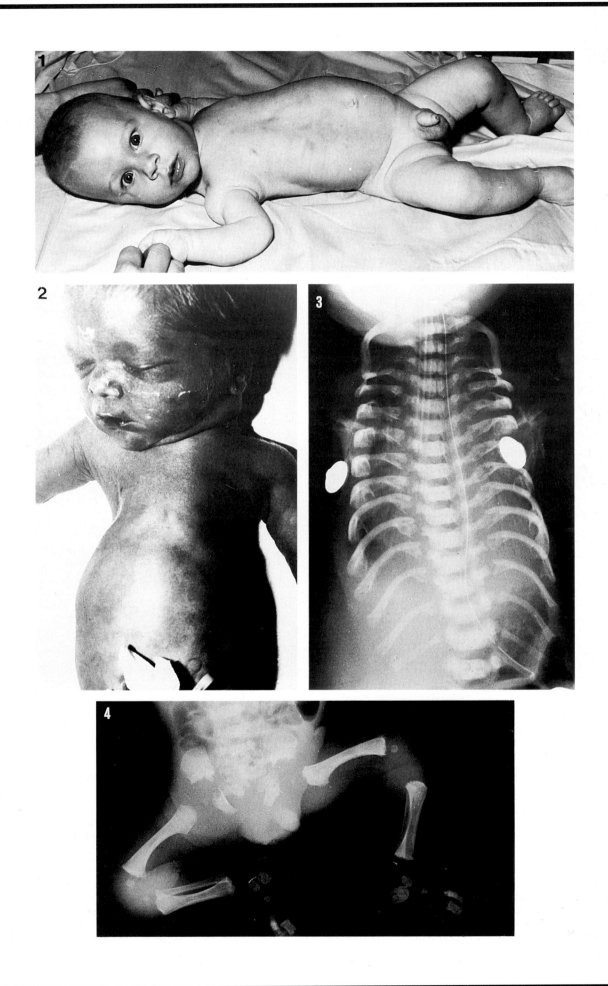

122 Saldino–Noonan Type of Short Rib-Polydactyly Syndrome
(Saldino–Noonan Syndrome)

J.K./H.-R.W

A syndrome leading to perinatal death with constriction of the thorax, very short ribs, brachymelia, polydactyly, anogenital anomalies and characteristic radiological changes.

Main signs:
- Severe narrowing of the thorax (with hypoplasia of the lungs) and distended abdomen (1). Respiratory insufficiency.
- Brachymelia and usually postaxial polydactyly (1).
- Anal atresia and genital hypoplasia or malformation.
- Usually congenital hydrops.
- Radiologically: short, horizontal ribs, anomalies of the scapulae and the pelvis, marked metaphyseal irregularities of the long bones, which are considerably shortened and other abnormalities. (1b).

Supplementary findings: Round, flat face; absence of nails. At autopsy, anomalies of the heart, kidney, pancreas and other organs are frequent.

Manifestation: At birth.

Aetiology: Autosomal recessive disorder.

Frequency: Low; by 1987 over 60 observations had been reported; primarily female newborns.

Course, prognosis: Poor. If not stillborn, the infant dies shortly after birth from respiratory insufficiency.

Differential diagnosis: There are other rare short rib–polydactyly syndromes. In addition, the Ellis-van Creveld syndrome (135) and trisomy 13 (47) should be considered, along with asphyxiating thoracic dysplasia (121).

Treatment: Symptomatic. Genetic counselling; prenatal diagnosis with ultrasound in subsequent pregnancies.

Illustrations:
1a and b A typically affected premature newborn (35.5 cm; 1300 g), the first child of young parents after one terminated pregnancy and a spontaneous abortion. Death immediately *post partum*. Postaxial polydactyly of the hands and feet. (Unusual additional finding: multiple frenula between the upper lip and the alveolar process, as in Ellis-van Creveld syndrome, 135).

References:

Spranger J W, Langer Jr L O, Wiedemann H-R: *Bone dysplasias. An atlas of constitutional disorders of skeletal development.* Stuttgart and Philadephia: G Fischer and W B Saunders; 1974.

Krepler R, Weißenbacher G, Leodolter S et al: Nicht lebensfähiger, mikromeler Zwergwuchs... *Mschr Kinderheilk* 1976, **124**:167.

Richardson M M, Beaudet A L, Wagner M L et al: Prenatal diagnosis of recurrence of Saldino–Noonan dwarfism. *J Pediatr* 1977, **91**:467.

Rupprecht E, Gurski A: Kurzrippen-Polydaktylie-Syndrom Typ Saldino–Noonan bei zwei Geschwistern. *Helv Paediat Acta* 1982, 37:161.

Johnson V P, Petersen L P et al: Midtrimester prenatal diagnosis of... Saldino–Noonan syndrome. *Birth Defects, Orig Art Ser* 1982, **18**:(3A):133–141.

Grote W, Weisner D et al: Prenatal diagnosis of... Saldino–Noonan at 17 weeks' gestation. *Eur J Pediatr* 1983, 140:63–66.

Toftager-Larsen K, Benzie R J: Fetoscopy in prenatal diagnosis of... Saldino–Noonan... *Clin Genet* 1984, **26**:56–60.

Bernstein R, Isdale J et al: Short rib-polydactyly syndrome: a single or heterogenous entity? *J Med Genet* 1985, **22**:46–53.

Sillence D, Kozlowski K et al: Perinatally lethal short rib-polydactyly syndromes... *Pediatr Radiol* 1987, 17:474–480.

Garcia H, Drescher H, Kuchelmeister K, Lenz W, Roessner A: Short rib-polydactyly syndromes. *Klin Pädiat* 1988, **200**:140–144.

Erzen M, Stanescu R, Stanescu V, Maroteaux P: Comparative histology of the growth cartilage in short-rib polydactyly syndromes type I and III and in chondroectodermal dysplasia. *Ann Génét* 1988, 31:144–150.

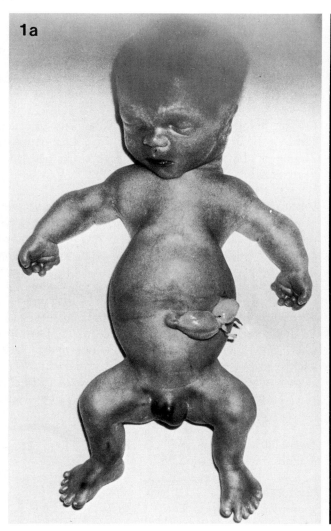

1a

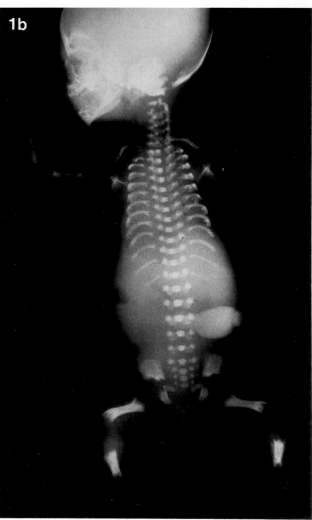

1b

123 Chondrodysplasia Punctata, Autosomal Recessive Type
(Chondrodysplasia Punctata, Rhizomelic Type)

J.K./H.-R.W

A hereditary disorder with primordial growth deficiency, distinctive facies, not infrequently ichthyosiform skin changes and regularly severe psychomotor retardation.

Main signs:
- Disproportionate short stature with predominantly symmetrical shortening of the arms and upper legs and multiple joint contractures (**1**).
- Flat face; very full cheeks; broad, depressed nasal bridge. Altogether somewhat mongoloid appearance (**1**). Very short, broad neck.
- In 25%, ichthyosiform skin changes, alopecia.
- Marked psychomotor retardation, tetraplegia, usually mild microcephaly.

Supplementary findings: Bilateral cataracts almost always present, occasional optic atrophy.

Radiologically, usually severe symmetrical shortening, metaphyseal flaring and punctate calcification of the ends of the humerus or femur (**2**). Dysplasia of the pelvis. Little or no punctate calcification ('stippling') in the vertebral column; dorsal and ventral ossification centres of the vertebral bodies (on lateral view) not joined. (Disappearance of the calcium spots usually during the first year of life; fusion of the vertebral ossification centres.)

Manifestation: At birth.

Aetiology: Autosomal recessive disorder; peroxisomal enzyme defect: disturbance of plasmalogen synthesis, phytanic acid oxidation, severe catalase deficiency. Markedly increased peroxisomes.

Frequency: Very low (about 60 observations in the literature). 1:100 000 live births.

Course, prognosis: Poor. The great majority of affected children die in infancy, usually of infections. More than 20 patients have survived the first year. The oldest is 16 years of age.

Differential diagnosis: Other types of chondrodysplasia punctata (124, 126), a milder autosomal recessive form (Sheffield type) and an autosomal recessive form with pseudohermaphroditism. X-linked recessive inheritance must also be considered, along with other conditions that show or may show stippled epiphyses on radiograph in the newborn period, such as trisomy 18 (*48*) and Down (*49*) syndromes, CHILD (*127*), Smith–Lemli–Opitz (*281*) or Zellweger (*291*) syndromes, foetal alcohol syndrome (*275*) and coumarin ('Warfarin') embryopathy (*125*), anticonvulsive syndrome (*255*), GM1 gangliosidosis (*71*), I-cell disease (*72*), MPS II (*65*), acrodysostosis (*102*), Keutel syndrome (*128*), hypothyroidism, vitamin-K-epoxide-reductase deficiency.

Treatment: Symptomatic. Genetic counselling. Prenatal diagnosis with ultrasound.

Illustrations:
1 and 2 A newborn. Early death from pneumonia and hypoplastic lungs. Right clubfoot.

References:
Spranger J W, Langer Jr L O, Wiedemann H-R: *Bone dysplasias. An atlas of constitutional disorders of skeletal development.* Stuttgart and Philadephia: G Fischer and W B Saunders; 1974.
Gilbert E F, Opitz J M, Spranger J W *et al*: Chondrodysplasia punctata – rhizomelic form. *Eur J Pediatr* 1976, **123**:89.
Heymans H S A, Oorthuys J W E *et al*: Rhizomelic chondrodysplasia punctata: another peroxismal disorder. *N Engl J Med* 1985, **313**:187–188.
Heymans H S A, Oorthuys J W E *et al*: Peroxismal abnormalities in rhizomelic chondrodysplasis punctata. *J Inher Metab Dis* 1986, **9**:329–331.
Poulos A, Sheffield L *et al*: Rhizomelic chondrodysplasia punctata… *J Pediatr* 1988, **113**:685–690.
Bick D, Curry C J R *et al*: Male infant with ichthyosis, Kallmann syndrome, chondrodysplasia punctata, and an Xp chromosome deletion. *Am J Med Genet* 1989, **33**:100–107.
Nivelon A, Nivelon J L, Mabille J P, Maroteaux P *et al*: New autosomal recessive chondrodysplasia – pseudohermaphrodism syndrome. *Clin Dysmorphol* 1992, **1**:221–227.
Stoll C, Dott B, Roth M, Alembik Y: Birth prevalence rates of skeletal dysplasias. *Clin Genet* 1989, **35**:88–92.
Wardinsky T D, Pagon R A *et al*: Rhizomelic chondrodysplasia punctata and survival beyond one year: a review of the literature and five case reports. *Clin Genet* 1990, **38**:84–93.
Norman A M, Jivani S, Kingston H M: Chondrodysplasia punctata: further evidence of heterogeneity. *Clin Dysmorphol* 1992, **1**:161–164.
Heikoop J C, Wanders R J A *et al*: Genetic and biochemical heterogeneity in patients with rhizomelic form of chondrodysplasia punctata — a complementation study. *Hum Genet* 1992, **89**:439–444.
Hughes J L, Poulus A *et al*: Ultrastructure and immunocytochemistry of hepatic peroxisomes in rhizomelic chondrodysplasia punctata. *Eur J Pediatr* 1992, **151**:829–836.
Toriello H V, Higgins J V, Miller T: Provisionally unique autosomal recessive chrondrodysplasia punctata syndrome. *Am J Med Genet* 1993, **47**:797–799.

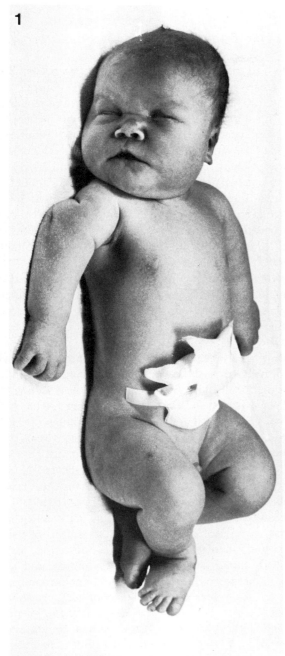

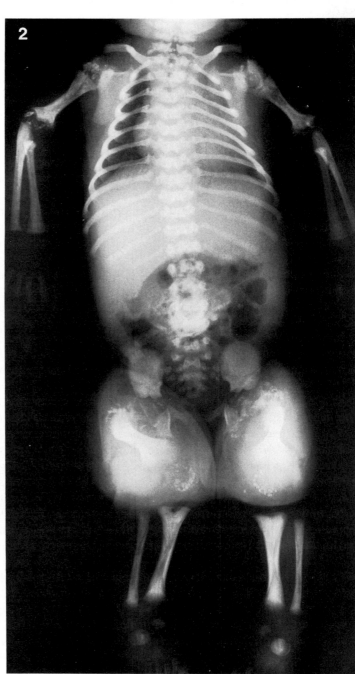

124 Chondrodysplasia Punctata, X-Linked Recessive Type with Terminal Xp22.3 Deletion

(Chondrodysplasia Punctata with Brachytelephalangism)

J.K.

A sex-linked recessive hereditary contiguous-gene syndrome with growth deficiency, chondrodysplasia punctata ichthyosis, Kallmann syndrome, ocular albinism and mental retardation.

Main signs:

- Facial dysmorphism: mid-face hypoplasia, prominent forehead, naevus flammeus, saddle nose, small short nose with anteverted nostrils, 'pouting' mouth.
- Short, plump, wide paw-like hands; short, plump fingers; shortening of the distal phalanges. Ulnar deviation of the metacarpal joint (hypoplasia of the distal ulna). Simian crease. Broad feet.
- Ichthyosis, manifest from the sixth month of life (steroid sulphatase deficiency), sparse unruly hair, thin dystrophic nails.
- Microgenitalia: short phallus, hypoplastic scrotum (Kallmann syndrome).
- Ocular albinism.
- Mental retardation: IQ 50–70, minimal speech development. The retardation is evidently dependent on the size of the chromosomal deletion.
  Microcephaly (third percentile). Hyperactivity.
- Proportionate short stature with radiologically identifiable, extensive, punctate calcifications, distributed bilaterally and symmetrically throughout the skeletal system (paravertebral, laryngeal, tracheal, sacral, and coccygeal) and the epiphyseal region of all long bones, including the tarsal phalanges. Short metacarpals and phalanges, hoodlike calcifications on the proximal epiphyses of the metacarpals. Markedly shortened distal phalanges. Vertebral segregational disorder.

Supplementary findings: Hydramnios. Postnatal respiratory insufficiency caused by laryngomalacia (cartilage hypoplasia), which leads to tracheal collapse. Hypertelorism, strabismus, nystagmus, high myopia, choroidal atrophy. Cardiomyopathy. Mild joint contractures, absent 12th ribs, spina bifida. Thyroid ectopia with hypothyroidism. Anosmia. Impaired hearing (combined conductive-hearing and sensorineural disorder).

Manifestation: Prenatal and postnatal.

Aetiology: X-linked recessive inheritance. Contiguous gene syndrome: the smallest cytogenic deletions (here: Xp22.3 →) can lead to the association of different mendelian disorders. Female carriers have an increased spontaneous abortion rate (20%), are twice as likely to produce female offspring, are 12 cm shorter (154 cm) than non-carriers (166 cm), show broad wrists and short arms. Significantly increased paternal age.

Frequency: Up to 1993, 34 male patients and 24 symptomatic female carriers were reported from 11 families.

Prognosis: Increased postnatal mortality caused by tracheal collapse, pneumonia, bronchiolitis, sudden infant death syndrome. General failure to thrive in the first year of life. Mild growth deficiency (third percentile). Slight to moderately severe retardation.

Treatment: After birth, intubation followed by artificial ventilation. Antibiotics. Symptomatic treatment according to clinical requirements. Prenatal diagnosis in the second trimester by ultrasound.

Illustrations:

1–3 Male aged 3 years and 8 months, characteristic facies, growth deficiency, shortened extremities, plump appearance, small phallus, hypoplastic scrotum. Dry, scaling skin. **4** Age 4 years and 2 months, height 78 cm (20 cm below third percentile), weight 10 kg, head circumference 49 cm (0.5 cm below third percentile). **5 and 6** Age 3 years and 8 months, brachycarpia, shortened distal phalanges, short nails, ichthyosis. **7** Age 2 months, brachytarsia, short metatarsals. **8 and 9** Age 2 months, shortened metacarpals and phalanges with hoodlike calcifications. **10 and 11** Age 4 years and 2 months, short metacarpals, some cone-shaped epiphyses, dysplastic distal phalanges. Dysplasia of the distal ulna with angulation between ulna and radius. Skeletal age 12–18 months. **12** In the lower lumbar and sacral region, numerous rather coarse, irregular calcareous patches. On the ischia there are hoodlike, confluent, patchy calcifications. On the, as yet uncalcified, capital femoral epiphyses, confluent calcareous patches, with a comma-shaped configuration. **13 and 14** On the day of birth; fissuration of the middle thoracic vertebral bodies. Extensive fine-grained calcifications, which surround the vertebral bodies, the transverse processes and the spines of the vertebrae. Punctate calcifications also of the lower thoracic and lumbar spine but more intensive in the lateral parts of the vertebrae and in the intervertebral discs.

References:

Petit C, Melki J *et al*: An interstitial deletion in Xp22.3 in a family with X-linked recessive chondrodysplasia punctata and short stature. *Hum Genet* 1990, **85**:247–250.

Ballabio A, Zollo M *et al*: Deletion of the distal short arm of the X chromosome (Xp) in a patient with short stature, chondrodysplasia punctata, and X-linked ichthyosis due to steroid sulfatase deficiency. *Am J Med Genet* 1991, **41**:184–187.

Wulfsberg E A, Curtis J, Jayne C H: Chondrodysplasia punctata: a boy with X-linked recessive chondrodysplasia punctata due to an inherited X-Y translocation with a current classification of these disorders. *Am J Med Genet* 1992, **43**:823–828.

Bennett C P, Berry A C *et al*: Chondrodysplasia punctata: another possible X-linked recessive case. *Am J Med Genet* 1992, **44**:795–799.

Pryde P G, Bawle E *et al*: Prenatal diagnosis of nonrhizomelic chondrodysplasia punctata (Conradi–Hünermann syndrome). *Am J Med Genet* 1993, **47**:426–431.

Meindl A, Hosenfeld D *et al*: Analysis of a terminal Xp22.3 deletion in a patient with six monogenic disorders: implications for the mapping of X-linked ocular albinism. *J Med Genet* 1993, **30**:838–842.

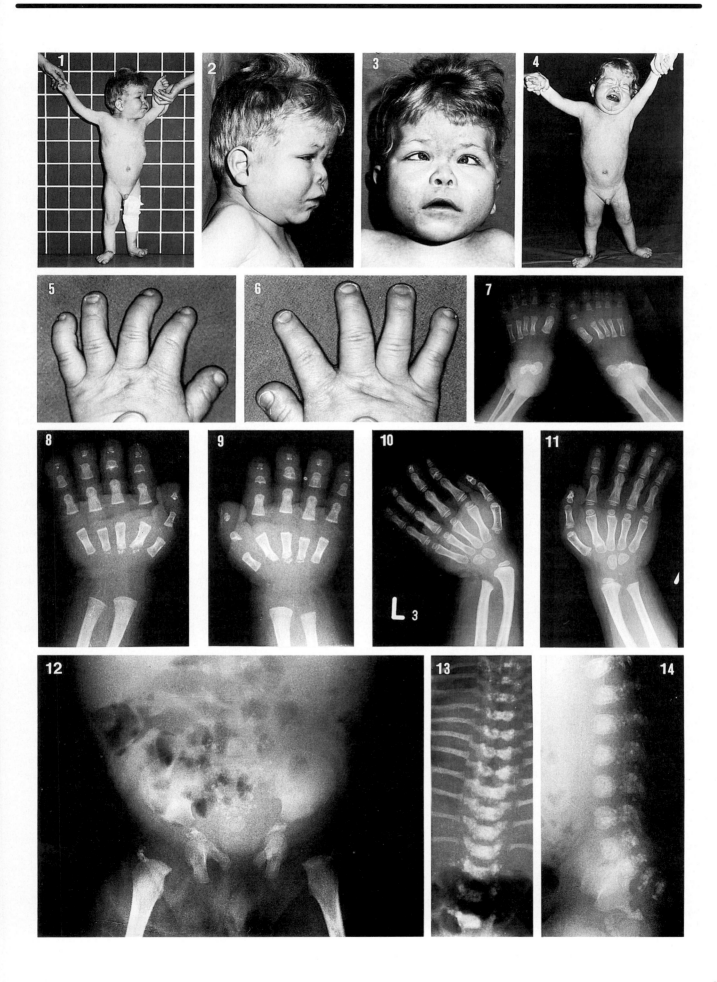

125 Coumarin Embryopathy
(Warfarin Embryopathy)

H.-R.W

An embryopathy that can present a variably severe phenocopy of a chondrodysplasia punctata (stippled epiphyses).

Main signs:
- Hypoplasia of the midface; low, broad nasal bridge, initially with anteverted nares and with generally obvious notches between the tip of the nose and the alae nasi (**1–3**).
- Prenatal growth retardation and postnatal short stature with symmetric or slightly asymmetric shortening of the extremities, especially the proximal portions (**4**).
- In infancy, radiological punctate or stippled calcifications, especially of the carpal and tarsal bones, along the vertebral column and in the proximal femur. Eventual disappearance of these calcifications (**7**).

Supplementary findings: Frequently, initial respiratory difficulties (possibly caused by choanal stenosis). Frequent subsequent development of hyperlordosis or kyphosis, scoliosis (**4 and 5**). Limited movement of the large joints. Brachydactyly, syndactyly (**6**). Hypoplasia of the nails. Mental impairment in some patients.

Manifestation: At birth.

Aetiology: Coumarin exposure of the mother in the first trimester of pregnancy, especially between the sixth and the ninth weeks. (Subsequent or prolonged exposure can cause marked central nervous system damage, especially to the eyes and vision.)

Frequency: Low; perhaps 50 patients are known.

Course, prognosis: Increased mortality in the perinatal period and in the first year of life, dependent on severity. The nose improves in appearance with the passage of time (**1–3**).

Differential diagnosis: Chondrodysplasia punctata and occasionally some of the numerous other disorders that may show epiphyseal stippling on radiograph during the newborn period and infancy.

Treatment: Symptomatic, including orthopaedic care.

Illustrations:
1–7 The same patient at age 2 months (**1, 7**, left side), 13 months (**7**, right side), 8 years (**2, 4**) and 31 years (**3, 5, 6**).
At 2 months, length and weight below the third percentile, short upper arms and thighs, bent legs and stippling of the vertebral column, most of the epiphyses of the bones of the arms and legs and the tarsals and carpals. Height at 8 years and 6 months: 105 cm (below the third percentile); right extremities somewhat shorter than the left; scoliosis, flattening of the vertebral bodies from T6 down; limited extension at both knees and elbows. At 31 years, disproportionate short stature of 154 cm; scoliosis, lordosis; brachydactyly, syndactyly. Normal intelligence.
In 1954, the clinical picture was considered that of chondrodysplasia calcificans; subsequently that of an autosomal dominant type. When, in 1985, the patient's wife was expecting their first child and was very concerned about the 50% risk, the patient's mother's medical records from 1953 were checked. These showed that she had received coumarin therapy during the sixth to ninth and 11th to 13th weeks of gestation. Subsequent birth of a healthy child.

References:
Hall J G, Pauli R M, Wilson K M: Maternal and fetal sequelae of anticoagulation during pregnancy. *Am J Med* 1980, **68**:122–140.
Whitfield W F: Chondrodysplasia punctata after warfarin in early pregnancy. *Arch Dis Child* 1980, **55**:139–142.
Kleinebrecht J: Zur Teratogenität von Cumarin-Derivaten. *Dtsch Med Wschr* 1982, **107**:1929–1931.
Chong M K B *et al*: Follow-up study of children whose mothers were treated with warfarin during pregnancy. *Br J Obstet Gynaecol* 1984, **91**:1070–1073.
Kaplan L C: First trimester warfarin exposure and Dandy–Walker malformation... *Proc Greenwood Genet Ctr* 1986, **5**:167.
Tamburrini O, Bartolomeo-De Iuri A, Di Guglielmo G L: Chondrodysplasia punctata after warfarin. *Pediatr Radiol* 1987, **17**:323–324.
Hosenfeld D, Wiedemann H-R: Chondrodysplasia punctata in an adult recognized as vitamin K antagonist embryophathy. *Clin Genet* 1989, **35**:376–381.

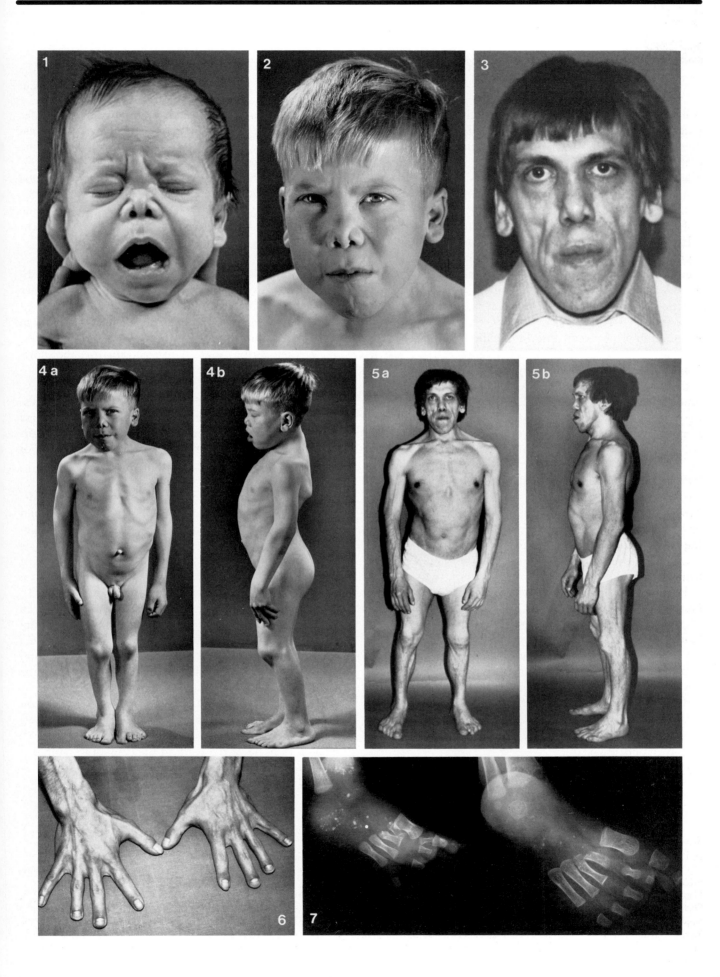

J.K./H.-R.W

A dysplasia syndrome affecting only females with a mosaic pattern of skin changes and anomalies of the skeleton and eyes, generally with asymmetric distribution.

Main signs:
- Asymmetric skeletal anomalies with congenital shortening of the long bones (most frequently the femur, then the humerus) (**2**); dysplasia and contracture of joints (hip, knee, ankle and others) and in some patients, dysplasia of the vertebral column, with secondary scoliosis. Unusual facies with low, broad nasal bridge, slight mongoloid slant of the palpebral fissures, possible marked asymmetry of the facial skeleton. Hexadactyly in some patients (**3**).
- Congenital ichthyosiform erythroderma (**4, 7**) with patchy and striated areas of hyperkeratosis. Later, patchy and striated atrophy of the skin, especially affecting the hair follicles (particularly of the forearm); patchy areas of alopecia (**6, 8**) and areas of brittle, tortuous, coarse, lackluster hair (**6**); eyebrows and eyelashes sparse, growing in different directions (**6**). Older children frequently affected with ichthyosis (**5**).
- Congenital or early cataracts in approximately two-thirds of patients, may be unilateral or bilateral; if bilateral, usually one eye more severely affected than the other (**1**); also microphthalmia and microcornea.

Supplementary findings: Systemic streaky pigmentation anomalies in some patients; nails may be flat, with tendency to split horizontally (**3**).

Frequent short stature, in part, secondary to scoliosis. Normal intellect.

Radiologically, 'stippling' (punctate calcifications) in various areas of the skeleton, especially the epiphyses of the long bones, also paravertebral and tracheal. Early disappearance of the stippling; diagnosis also possible in its absence.

Mental development usually normal, sometimes slightly retarded.

Manifestation: At birth.

Aetiology: Presumably an X-linked dominant disorder with lethal effect of the gene on male embryos. The presence of mild cutaneous signs in the mothers of some probands (**9**) suggests there is also an incomplete manifestation of this hereditary form. Most cases are sporadic and should represent new mutations. Gene locus: Xq28.

Frequency: Low. By 1990, over 50 patients could be identified, exclusively in females.

Course, prognosis: Good on the whole (patients handicapped by growth deficiency, scoliosis and sometimes ocular defects).

Spontaneous regression of the congenital ichthyosiform erythroderma during infancy with development of systemic atrophoderma. Severely affected foetuses die shortly after birth.

Differential diagnosis: See *123* and, for the X-linked recessive forms, *124*. A systemic anomaly of pigmentation may suggest the Bloch–Sulzberger syndrome (*187*) (transmitted by the same mode of inheritance), which should not be difficult to exclude by careful observation.

Treatment: Symptomatic (ophthalmologic, orthopaedic and so on). Careful examination of the mother for mild signs of the disorder. Genetic counselling. Prenatal diagnosis.

Illustrations:
1–6 An affected girl as a newborn (**4**), at 6 months (**1, 3**), at 6 years (**2**) and as an adolescent. Asymmetric thorax and asymmetrical shortening of the extremities; postaxial hexadactyly of the left hand. As a newborn, multiple foci of calcium in the epiphyses of the left leg and in the costal cartilages. Foci of alopecia and typical changes of the scalp hair.
7 and 8 An affected girl as a newborn (also 'stippling' on radiograph, skeletal asymmetry and unilateral cataract) and as an adolescent.
9 Foci of alopecia of the scalp of the proband's mother.

References:
Manzke H, Christophers E, Wiedemann H-R: Dominant sex-linked inherited chondrodysplasia punctata: a distinct type of chondrodysplasia punctata. *Clin Genet* 1980, **17**:107.
Happle R: X-gekoppelt dominante Chondrodysplasia punctata. *Mschr Kinderheilk* 1980, **128**:203.
Happle R, Phillips R J S *et al*: Homologous genes for X-linked chondrodysplasia punctata in man and mouse. *Hum Genet* 1983, **63**:24–27.
Mueller R F, Crowle P M *et al*: X-linked dominant chondrodysplasia punctata... *Am J Med Genet* 1985, **20**:137–144.
Kozlowski K, Bates E H *et al*: Dominant X-linked chondrodysplasia punctata. *AJDC* 1988, **142**:1233–1234.
Herman G E, Walton S J: Close linkage of the murine locus bare patches to the X-linked visual pigment gene: implications for mapping human X-linked dominant chondrodysplasia punctata. *Genomics* 1990, **7**:307–312.

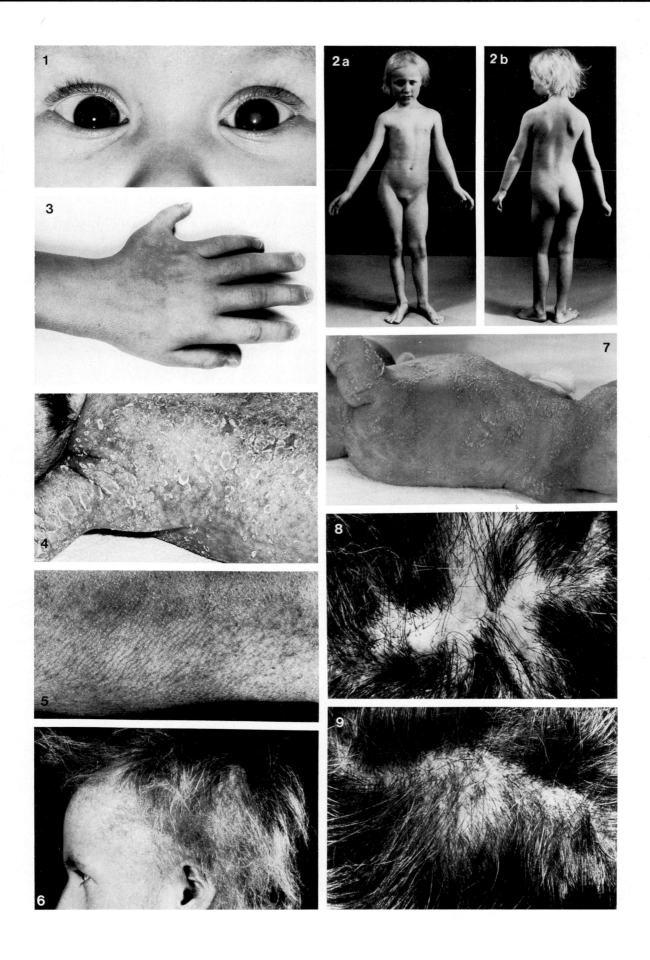

127 CHILD Syndrome
(Syndrome of Congenital Hemidysplasia with Ichthyosiform Naevus and Limb Defects)

H.-R.W

A syndrome of unilateral 'ichthyosiform' erythroderma ('CHILD naevus') and ipsilateral defects of variable severity of the limbs and skeleton.

Main signs:
- Ichthyosiform erythroderma, which, more or less completely, affects one-half of the body and is sharply outlined along the midline of the trunk (**1, 7**). Variable progression, the extent may parallel the severity of the skeletal and visceral defects. The face is usually spared. The nails may develop severe hyperkeratoses (**3 and 4**).
- Ipsilateral skeletal hypoplasia (**2**). Practically any part of the skeleton may be affected, in most patients the long bones are involved, varying from mere hypoplasia of phalanges to absence of a whole extremity. A hand or foot may be severely deformed.

Supplementary findings: The right side has been affected in the vast majority of patients observed to date (smaller anomalies may also occur contralaterally).

Secondary scoliosis in some patients (**2a**).

Ipsilateral anomalies of the internal organs (heart, lungs, kidneys or others) or of the nervous system may occur.

On radiograph: in a few patients examined in the early postnatal period, epiphyseal calcium spots were demonstrated ipsilaterally in the limbs, the pelvis or elsewhere.

Manifestation: At birth. The CHILD naevus may develop later, during the first months of life.

Aetiology: Based on an X-linked dominant gene with lethal effect in males (functional X-linked mosaic in an unusual lateralization pattern).

Frequency: Low; 29 observations to date; 28 females and 1 male.

Course, prognosis: The dermatosis may remain constant in severity or may transiently vary in severity; it may affect new areas of skin, but may also show continuing spontaneous regression.

Otherwise the prognosis depends on the presence and severity of internal and skeletal defects.

Differential diagnosis: With chondrodysplasia punctata of the X-linked dominant type (*126*), the dermatosis occurs on both sides of the body in a different pattern and (in older children) with signs of dermal atrophy.

The Schimmelpenning–Feuerstein–Mims 'syndrome' (*173*) shows a different type of dermatosis.

Treatment: No effective treatment for the dermatosis is known. Remedial measures, such as orthopaedic, prosthetic or plastic surgery. Treatment of internal organ anomalies in some patients. Handicap aids. Genetic counselling.

Illustrations:
1–6 An affected girl at ages 4 months (**1 and 2**), 1 year (**3–5**) and 3 years (**6**). Hypoplasia of the extremities on the right (**2**) with flexion contracture of the elbow. Right-sided hypoplasia of the mandible, scapula, ribs, pelvis and right vertebral bodies (note also vertebral clefts) with secondary scoliosis (**2**). Dermatosis manifest at 2 months, sharply outlined along the mid-line of the trunk (**1**), the only areas spared being part of the face and head and the palmar and plantar surfaces. Right renal aplasia. Dermatosis for the most part resistant to therapy but eventual spontaneous regression (**5 and 6**). Development of severe hyperkeratosis of and around the nails (**3 and 4**).
7 and 8 A 4-year-old girl with similar skeletal involvement and corresponding localized, medially outlined dermatosis in the right lumbar region (**7**) and an affected area on the left hand (**8**).

References:
Happle R, Koch H, Lenz W: The CHILD Syndrome. *Eur J Pediatr* 1980, **134**:27.
Happle R: X-chromosomal vererbte Dermatosen. *Hautarzt* 1982, **33**:73–81.
Christiansen J V, Petersen H O *et al*: The CHILD-syndrome... *Acta Derm Venereol* 1984, **64**:165–168.
Happle R: The lines of Blaschko... *Curr Probl Dermatol* 1987, **17**:5–18.
Hebert A A *et al*: The CHILD syndrome... *Arch Derm* 1987, **123**:503–509.
Happle R: Ptychotropism as a cutaneous feature of the CHILD syndrome. *J Am Acad Dermatol* 1990, **23**:763–766.

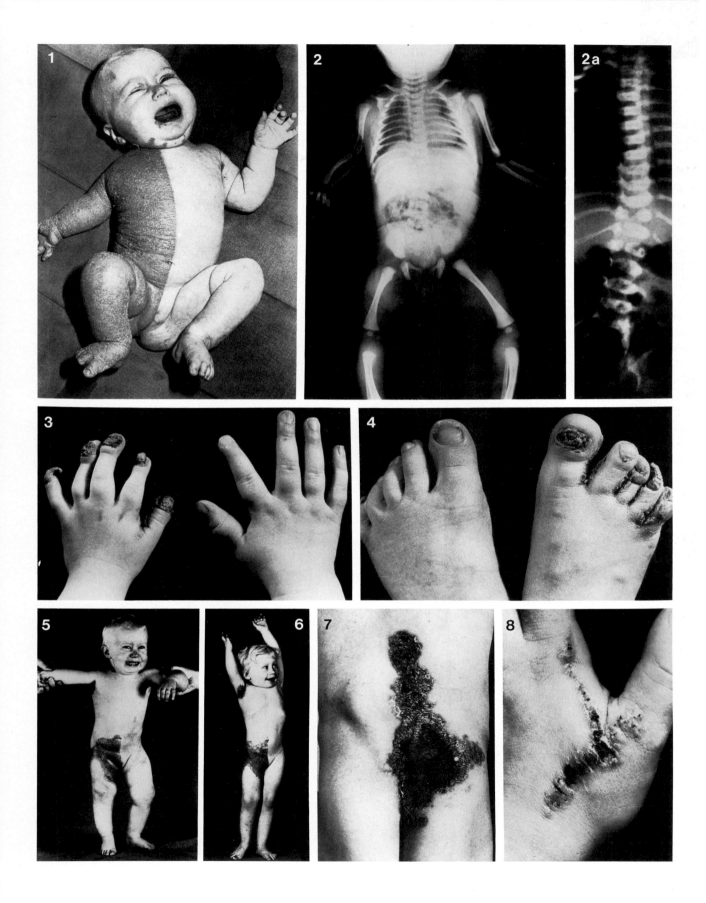

H.-R.W

A characteristic syndrome of brachytelephalangism, abnormal cartilage calcification, impaired hearing and distinctive appearance.

Main signs:
- Abnormally short distal phalanges of the fingers (**4**).
- Abnormal calcification of cartilage in the tracheo-bronchial tree, in the epiphyses of the long bones (stippled epiphyses) and in the nose and ears (**3**).
- Hearing defect of a mixed or conductive nature.
- Facies characterized by hypoplasia of the mid-face with abnormally shaped nose (**1** and **2**).

Supplementary findings: Increased susceptibility to infections of the respiratory tract, bronchiectasis or bronchial asthma (10 out of 11 affected children). Anomalies of the cardiovascular system (peripheral pulmonary stenosis, septal defect) in eight out of 11 patients. Mental retardation (seven out of 11); short stature (six out of 11).

Manifestation: At birth and later.

Aetiology: Autosomal recessive disorder.

Frequency: Low; to date only 11 patients in the literature.

Course, prognosis: Mainly dependent on the involvement of the thoracic organs.

Diagnosis, differential diagnosis: The syndrome must be considered in children with 'stippled epiphyses'.

Treatment: Cardiac surgery in some patients; otherwise symptomatic.

Illustrations:
1–4 Typical findings in a 13-year-old girl.

References:

Keutel J, Jörgensen G, Gabriel P: A new autosomal recessive syndrome: peripheral pulmonary stenoses, brachytelephalangism; neural hearing loss and abnormal cartilage calcification/ossification. In Bergsma D. (ed.) The *Clinical delineation of birth defects: the cardiovascular system.* Baltimore: Williams and Wilkins Co for the National Foundation — March of Dimes. BD: OAS 1982, **VIII**(5):60–68.

Fryns J P, van Fleteren A, Mattelaer P *et al*: Calcification of cartilages, brachytelephalangy and peripheral pulmonary stenosis. Confirmation of the Keutel syndrome. *Eur J Pediatr* 1984, **142**:201–203.

Cormode E. J, Dawson M, Lowry R B: Keutel syndrome: clinical report and literature review. *Am J Med Genet* 1986, **24**:289–294.

Khosroshahi H E, Uluoglu Ö *et al*: Keutel syndrome: a report of four cases. *Eur J Pediatr* 1989, **149**:188–191.

Ziereisen F, De Munter C *et al*: The Keutel syndrome. Report of a case and review of the literature. *Pediatr Radiol* 1993, **23**:314–315.

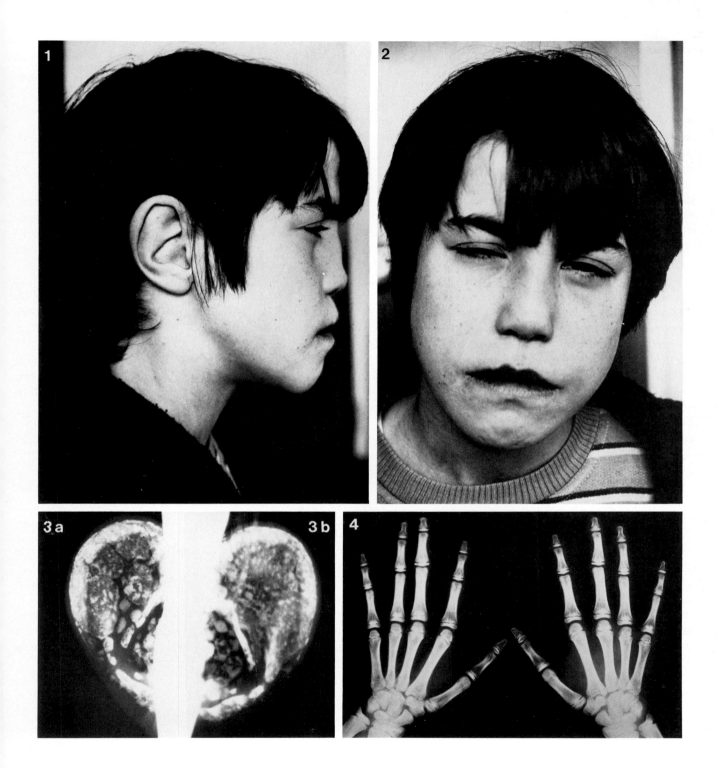

Camptomelic Dysplasia
(Camptomelic Syndrome)

J.K./H.-R.W

A clinical picture of congenital symmetrical bowing and shortening of the lower extremities (with club feet), unusual facies and usually early death of the child from respiratory insufficiency, to be differentiated from other disorders with congenital bowing of the long bones.

Main signs:
- Micromelic growth deficiency with disproportionate body at birth because of shortened extremities, especially the lower extremities, which show symmetrical anterior bowing (1) with pretibial dimples and club feet. Arms may be shortened in some patients, and are only occasionally bowed.
- Unusual facies: low nasal bridge, hypertelorism, narrow palpebral fissures, long philtrum, Robin sequence (micrognathia, glossoptosis, cleft palate, 39), usually relatively small mouth, anomalies of the external ears.
- Frequent macrodolichocephaly, head circumference 36 cm at birth (in 90%); wide open fontanelles (1).
- Narrow thorax; in most patients, respiratory problems with hypoplasia of the lungs.
- Radiologically short, broad, bowed tibiae; bowed femora of normal width. Absence of the distal femoral and proximal tibial epiphyses. Severe hypoplasia of the scapulae, fibulae, clavicles, 11 rib pairs and other bones.

Supplementary findings: Birth usually at term with moderate low birth weight; hydramnios relatively frequent.
Muscular hypotonia. Possible dislocation of the hips, elbows, halluces, fingers (with mild brachydactyly of the hands). Additionally: ureterostenosis, hypoplasia of the larynx, absence of camptomelia also observed.
Phenotypic females often show a male karyotype.
At autopsy, frequent hydronephrosis, cardiac anomalies and anomalies of the olfactory nerve and trachea.

Manifestation: At birth.

Aetiology: Usually sporadic occurrence; distinct preponderance of females affected (1:2.3); among these, frequently individuals with a male karyotype and absence of the HY-antigen. After karyotyping, the sex ratio is reversed (male:female = 2:1). Autosomal recessive inheritance. Seven sets of affected siblings reported. Pathogenically, the malformations of the lower extremities are attributed to vascular malformations (absence of the anterior tibial artery and dorsalis pedis artery).

Frequency: Low; over 100 patients had been reported by 1983. Incidence between 0.05:10 000 and 2:10 000 liveborn children.

Course, prognosis: Unfavourable; patients have respiratory and feeding problems and usually die within a few weeks of birth; in exceptional cases, survival into adulthood.

Differential diagnosis: Other skeletal dysplasias with congenital bowing of the long bones.

Treatment: Symptomatic. Genetic counselling and prenatal diagnosis with ultrasound in future pregnancies.

Illustrations:
1a–c Patient 1: An 8-day-old male infant with pretibial pitting on the left.
2a and b Patient 2: An 8-day-old female infant with pretibial pitting bilaterally.
3a and b Patient 3: 37th week of pregnancy, female; lived for only 2 h and 30 min. Hypoplasia of the upper rib pairs and scapula, hypoplastic acetabula, bowing of the femora and tibiae.

References:
Hall Br D, Spranger J: Campomelic dysplasia. Am J Dis Child 1980, 134:285.
Bricarelli Fr D, Fraccaro M, Lindsten J et al: Sex-reversed XY females with campomelic dysplasia are HY negative. Hum Genet 1981, 57:15.
Noyal P, Vermeulin G et al: La dysplasie campomélique. Arch Fr Pédiatr 1982, 39:621–624.
Balcar I, Bieber Fr R: Sonographic... findings in campomelic dysplasia. AJR 1983, 14:481–482.
Houston C St, Opitz J M et al: The campomelic syndrome: review, report of 17 cases... Am J Med Genet 1983, 15:3–28.
Cooke Cl T, Mulcahy M T et al: Campomelic dysplasia with sex reversal... Pathology 1985, 17:526–529.
Kapur S, Vloten A. van: Isolated congenital bowed long bones. Clin Genet 1986, 29:165–167.
Nogami H, Oohira A et al: Congenital bowing of long bones... Teratology 1986, 33:1–7.
Pazzaglia U E, Beluffi G: Radiology and histopathology of the bent limbs in campomelic dysplasia... Pediatr Radiol 1987, 17:50–55.
Gillerot Y, Vanheck C A, Foulon M. et al: Campomelic syndrome: manifestations in a 20 week fetus and case history of a 5 year old child. Am J Med Genet 1989, 34:579–592.
Friedrich U, Schaefer E, Meinecke P: Campomelic dysplasia without overt campomelia. Clin Dysmorphol 1992, 1:172–178.
Young I D, Zuccollo J M et al: Campomelic dysplasia associated with a de novo 2q:17q reciprocal translocation. J Med Genet 1992, 29:251–252.
Lynch S A, Gaunt M L, Minford A M B: Campomelic dysplasia: evidence of autosomal dominant inheritance. J Med Genet 1993, 30:683–686.
Rodriguez J I: Vascular anomalies in campomelic syndrome. Am J Med Genet 1993, 46:185–192.
Normann E K, Pedersen J C, Stiris G, van der Hagen C B: Campomelic dysplasia — an underdiagnosed condition? Eur J Pediatr 1993, 152:331–333.

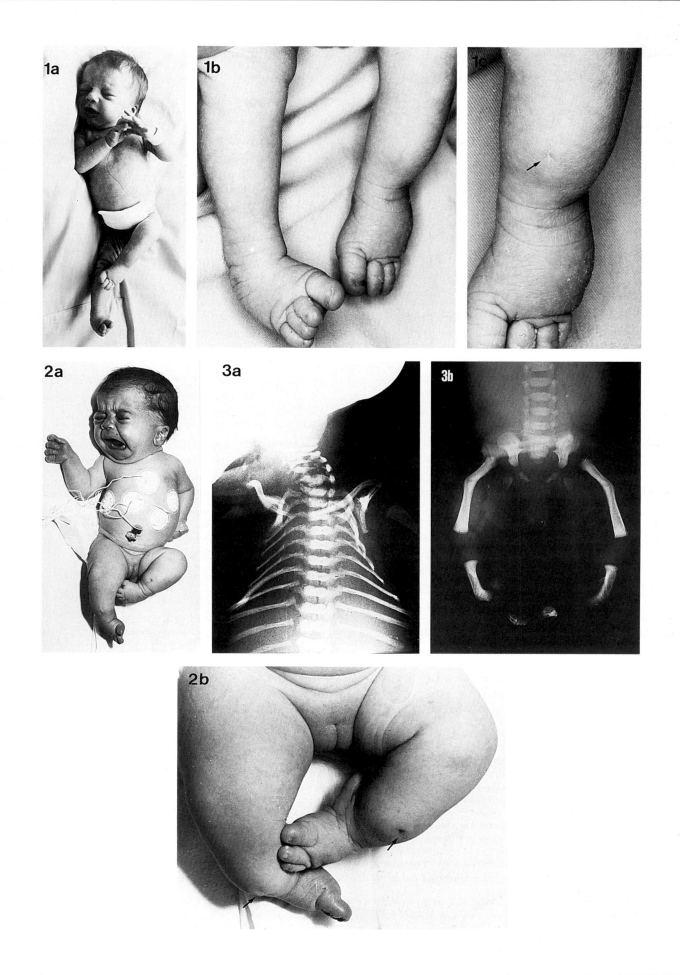

130 Achondroplasia
(Chondrodystrophia Foetalis, Parrot Syndrome)

H.-R.W/J.K.

A 'classic' generalized skeletal dysplasia with disproportionate short stature, large head, typical facial dysmorphism, and characteristic X-ray findings.

Main signs:
- Primordial disproportionate short stature; the proximal parts of the extremities (upper arm, thigh) more severely shortened than the trunk (3-7). Average adult height for women 124 cm; for men 131 cm. Ulnar deviation of the hands, splayed fingers ('trident hand', 8). Limited extension at the elbows; genu varus, rarely valgus (3, 5, 6).
- Head too large for the body and occasionally also for age, especially the cerebral cranium, which shows striking growth in the first years of life (men, around 60 cm and women, around 57 cm). Coarse facial features, depressed nasal bridge, prognathism, and hypoplasia of the midface (1, 3-7).
- Flat thorax, frequently bell-shaped. Thoracolumbar kyphosis, lumbosacral lordosis (4, 5, 7).
- Delayed motor development due to initial muscular hypotonia, normal mental development. Occasional hearing impairment (conductive or sensorineural).

Supplementary findings: Large cranium with frontoparietal bossing and relatively short base. Small foramen magnum, progressive narrowing of the lumbar spinal canal caudally (which, combined with progressive lumbosacral lordosis, may lead to corresponding signs of compression).

Broad flat pelvis, narrow pelvic inlet (generally dystocia), flat acetabula (9). Long bones shortened, but with normal width (2), fibulae relatively too long.

Aetiology: Autosomal dominant disorder. Gene locus: short arm of chromosome 4 (4p16.3). 80-90% of cases are new mutations (usually with above-average paternal age). Risk of recurrence after an affected child is generally around 5%; with siblings affected (germline mosaicism), risk of recurrence 20-35%; in the rare cases of familial occurrence, a labile premutation with reduced 'phenotrance' is still assumed.

Affected homozygotes are rare; in these cases early death usual with extremely severe skeletal dysplasia.

Frequency: About 1:20 000 to 1:25 000.

Prognosis: Increased mortality in all age groups. Under 4 years from brain stem compression; subsequently, up to about 25 years, from central nervous system causes or respiratory disorders (due to thoracic deformities, airway obstruction, or neurological defects [see above]); later from cardiac problems.

Differential diagnosis: Thanatophoric dysplasia (118/119), hypochondroplasia (144), pseudochondroplasia (148), and others.

Treatment: Symptomatic. Ultrasound of the skull at regular intervals after birth and during infancy is recommended. Attention to hearing. Best measures possible to prevent obesity and kyphosis. Possible osteotomies and specific surgery for signs of neurological compression. Orthopedic care; aids for the physically handicapped. Genetic counseling. Prenatal diagnosis with ultrasound or early application of DNA-based techniques.

Illustrations:
1 A 7-month-old infant.
2 X-ray of the left hand of a toddler.
3-5 An 8-year-old boy.
6-9 A 15-year-old boy.

References:

Spranger J W, Langer Jr L O, Wiedemann H-R: *Bone dysplasias. An atlas of constitutional disorders of skeletal development.* Stuttgart and Philadephia: G Fischer and W B Saunders; 1974.

Horton W A, Rotter J I *et al*: Standard growth curves for achondroplasia. *J Pediatr* 1978, 93:435–438.

Hall J G, Golbus M S, Graham C B. *et al*: Failure of early prenatal diagnosis in classic achondroplasia. *Am J Med Genet* 1979, 3:371.

Bland J D, Emery J L: Unexpected death of children with achondroplasia... *Dev Med Child Neurol* 1982, 24:489–492.

Hall J G, Horton W *et al*: Head growth in achondroplasia... *Am J Med Genet* 1982, 13:105.

Stokes D C, Phillips J A *et al*: Respiratory complications of achondroplasia. *J Pediatr* 1983, 102:534–541.

Opitz J M: 'Unstable premutation' in achondroplasia: penetrance vs phenotrance. *Am J Med Genet* 1984, 19:251–254.

Reiser C A, Pauli R M *et al*: Achondroplasia: unexpected familial recurrence. *Am J Med Genet* 1984, 19:245–250.

Thompson J N, Schaefer G B *et al*: Achondroplasia and parental age. *N Engl J Med* 1986, 314:521–522.

Dodinval P, Marec B. Le: Genetic counseling in unexpected familial recurrence of achondroplasia. *Am J Med Genet* 1987, 28:949–954.

Hecht J T, Francomano C A *et al*: Mortality in achondroplasia: *Am J Hum Genet* 1987, 41:454–464.

Editorial: Leg lengthening in achondroplasia. *Lancet* 1988, I:1032.

Nelson F. W *et al*: Neurological basis of respiratory complication in achondroplasia. *Ann Neurol* 1988, 24:89–93.

Correll J: Surgical correction of short stature... *Acta Paed Scand (Suppl)* 1991, 377:143–148.

Horton W A *et al*: Growth hormone therapy in achondroplasia. *Am J Med Genet* 1992, 42:667–670.

Brinkmann G *et al*: Cognitive skills in achondroplasia. *Am J Med Genet* 1993, 47:800–804.

Velinov M *et al*: The gene for achondroplasia maps to... chromosome 4p. *Nature Genet* 1994, 6:314–317.

Merrer Le M, Rousseau F *et al*: A gene for achondroplasia-hypochondroplasia maps to chromosome 4p. *Nature Genet* 1994 6:318–321.

Bellus G A, Escallon C S *et al*: First-trimester prenatal diagnosis in a couple at risk for homozygous achondroplasia. *Lancet* 1994, 344(II):1511–1512.

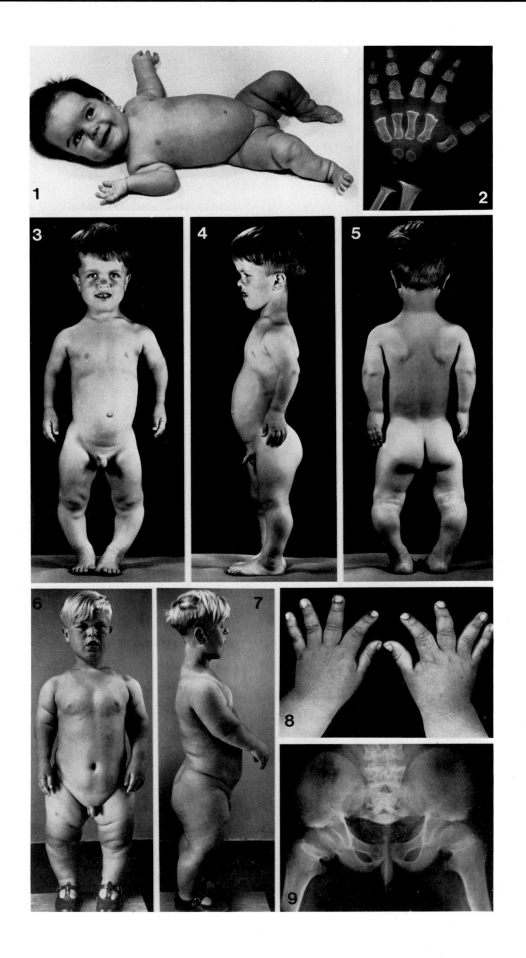

131 Diastrophic Dysplasia

H.-R.W

A characteristic hereditary disorder of severe short stature, club feet, joint contractures, malpositioning of the thumbs and halluces, anomalies of the auricles and cleft palate.

Main signs:

- Short-limbed dwarfism, birth measurements between 38 and 44 cm, with treatment-resistant club feet, joint contractures (especially of the shoulders, elbows, hips and interphalangeal joints) and abduction of the proximally displaced, hyperextensible thumbs ('hitchhiker thumb') and halluces (**1–3, 6**).
- Anomalies of the external ear (development of serosanguineous cystic masses in early infancy; later, thickening, calcification of cartilage and deformity) (**5**). Cleft palate in approximately 25% of patients.
- In most patients, progressive thoracolumbar kyphoscoliosis and cervical kyphosis (**2b, 4**).

Supplementary findings: Tendency to subluxation and dislocation of the joints, promoted by laxity of the muscles and ligaments.

Stridor in approximately 25% of patients.

Possible deafness as a result of fusion or absence of auditory ossicles. Absence of the flexion creases of the fingers caused by intra-uterine joint contractures (**7**).

Radiologically, severe epimetaphyseal changes of the, shortened, long bones and widening of the metaphyses; delayed ossification with deformity especially of the proximal femoral epiphyses; usually distinct fork-like deformity of the distal femoral and distal radial epiphyses and of the metatarsals; hook-shaped changes of the lateral ends of the clavicles, ovoid deformity of first metacarpal in the young child and other anomalies (**8 and 9**).

Manifestation: At birth. (Changes of the external ear usually develop in the first 3 months of life; kyphoscoliosis usually develops after infancy.)

Aetiology: Autosomal recessive disorder with very variable expression: gene locus probably on chromosome 5 (5q31-q34?).

Frequency: More than 300 patients have been reported, especially from Finland.

Course, prognosis: Increased early mortality because of respiratory disorders and in some patients cardiac defects. Later on, increased risk as a consequence of the severe kyphoscoliotic changes. Adult height may be under 1 m, but occasionally may reach 1.40 m. Normal mental development.

Differential diagnosis: Pseudodiastrophic dysplasia (*132*), arthrogryposis (*226*).

Treatment: Symptomatic. Intensive orthopaedic care mandatory. All appropriate aids for the physically handicapped. Genetic counselling. Prenatal diagnosis by ultrasound in subsequent pregnancies.

Illustrations:

1, 3, 6 A boy aged 4 years and 6 months.

2, 4, 8 An 18-month-old girl.

5 A female infant.

Note micromelia, club feet, swelling of the external ear (**5**), hypermobility or abduction (with subluxation in extreme patients) of the thumbs and halluces, early thoracolumbar kyphosis (**2b**) and considerable cervical kyphosis (**4**), blunting and deformity of the hand bones (**8**).

7, 9 Features of other typical patients.

References:

Walter H: Der diatrophische Zwergwuchs. *Adv Hum Genet* 1970, **2**:31.
Spranger J W, Langer Jr L O, Wiedemann H-R: *Bone dysplasias. An atlas of constitutional disorders of skeletal development.* Stuttgart and Philadephia: G Fischer and W B Saunders; 1974.
Horton W A, Rimoin D L, Lachman R S *et al*: The phenotypic variability of diastrophic dysplasia. *J Pediatr* 1978, **93**:609.
Bethem D, Winter R B, Lutter L: Disorders of the spine in diastrophic dwarfism. *J Bone Jt Surg* 1980, **62**(A):529.
Lachman R, Sillence D, Rimoin D *et al*: Diastrophic dysplasia... *Radiology 1981,* **140**:79.
Horton W A, Hall J G, Scott C I *et al*: Growth curves for height for diastrophic dysplasia... *Am J Dis Child* 1982, **136**:316.
Gustavson K H, Holmgren G, Jagell St *et al*: Lethal and non-lethal diastrophic dysplasia. *Clin Genet* 1985, **28**:321–334.
Butler M G, Gale D D, Meaney F J: Metacarpophalangeal pattern profile analysis in diastrophic dysplasia. *Am J Med Genet* 1987, **28**:685–689.
Gollop T R, Eigier A: Prenatal ultrasound diagnosis of diastrophic dysplasia at 16 weeks. *Am J Med Genet* 1987, **27**:321–324.
Krecak J, Starshak R J: Cervical kyphosis in diastrophic dwarfism: CT and MR findings. *Pediatr Radiol* 1987, **17**:321–322.
Gembruch U, Niesen M *et al*: Diastrophic dysplasia: a specific prenatal diagnosis by ultrasound. *Prenat Diagn* 1988, **8**:539–545.
Godbersen G S, Hosenfeld D, Pankau R: Die diastrophische Dysplasie. *HNO* 1990, **38**:256–258.
Hastbacka J, Kaitila I *et al*: Diastrophic dysplasia gene maps to the distal long arm of chromosome 5. *Proc Nat Acad Sci* 1990, **87**:8056–805.
Hastbacka J, Sintonen P *et al*: A linkage map spanning the locus for diastrophic dysplasia (DTD). *Genomics* 1991 **11**:968–973.
Stanescu V *et al*: Non-collagenous protein screening in the human chondrodysplasias... *Am J Med Genet* 1994, **51**:22–28.

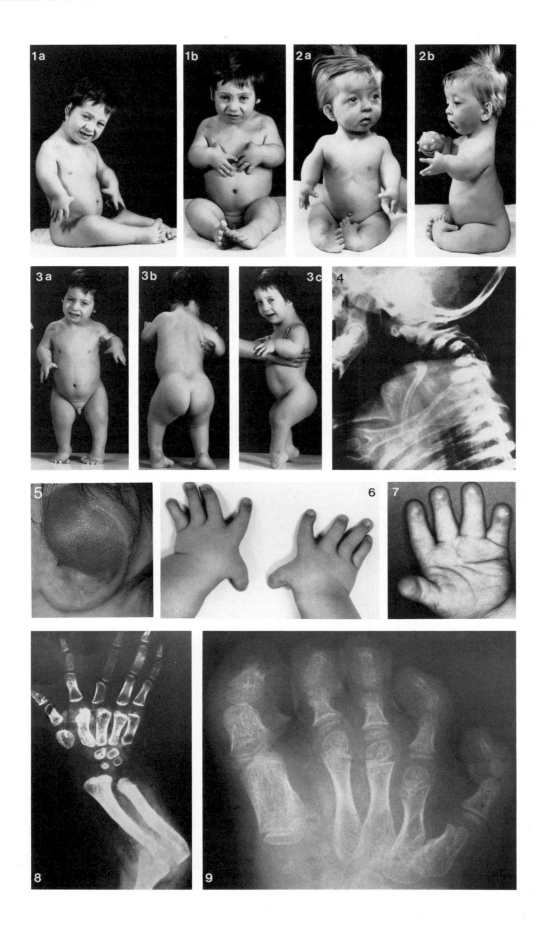

H.-R.W

A syndrome of micromelic short stature, with macrocranium and unusual facies, short neck, club feet, joint contractures and dislocation, large pinnae and cleft palate.

Main signs:
- Congenital micromelic small stature. Large skull. Short neck. Bell-shaped thorax (wider above). Marked lumbar lordosis, almost angular dorsolumbar kyphosis or early scoliosis (**1, 2, 4**).
- Peculiar facies with flat nose, hypertelorism, hypoplasia of the midface and abnormally full cheeks. Cleft palate. Large deformed ears (**1, 2**).
- Club feet. Limited movement at the metacarpal and metatarsal joints, the vertebral column and to a lesser degree the knees and shoulders. Dislocation of both hips, both elbows and, characteristically, several finger joints (**3**).

Supplementary findings: Radiologically, all bones of the extremities shortened and bluntly shaped (**3**). Hypoplasia of the scapulae with dysplasia of the joint fossae; somewhat squarish, deformed ilia. Hypoplasia of the cervical vertebrae; marked platyspondyly of the lower vertebrae with narrowing of the interpedicular and widening of the intervertebral spaces. Short ribs. Multiple interphalangeal and metacarpophalangeal dislocations, but (in contrast to diastrophic dysplasia) normal appearance of the first metacarpals.

Manifestation: At birth.

Aetiology: Autosomal recessive disorder. Molecular defect unknown.

Frequency: Low (only 10 patients known).

Course, prognosis: Increased early mortality. In patients surviving longer, problems arise as a consequence of severe kyphoscoliotic changes.

Differential diagnosis: Diastrophic dysplasia (*131*), arthrogryposis (*226*).

Comment: Although designated pseudodiastrophic dwarfism because of signs overlapping with those of diastrophic dysplasia the similarities are limited to appearance; this syndrome is an independent entity, clinically, radiologically and osteochondro-histologically and histochemically.

Treatment: Symptomatic. Appropriate physiotherapeutic, orthopaedic and, if indicated, neurosurgical care. Genetic counselling. Prenatal diagnosis by ultrasound in future pregnancies.

Illustrations:
1–4 The first child of healthy young non-consanguineous parents. Birth measurements: 3120g, 44cm, and head circumference 38cm. Progression of the kyphoscoliosis. The peculiar facies persisted unchanged. Chromosomal analysis negative. Frequent episodes of fever of unknown origin (normal immunoglobulins). Sudden death at age 8 months.
A female sibling born subsequently showing the same clinical picture died at age 4 days with idiopathic hyperthermia.

References:
Burgio G R, Belloni C, Beluffi G: Nanisme pseudodiastrophique. Etude de deux soeurs nouveaunées. *Arch Franç Péd* 1974, **31**:681.
Gorlin R J, Pindborg J J, Cohen M M Jr: *Syndromes of the head and neck.* 2nd Ed. New York: McGraw-Hill 1976.
Kozlowski K, Masel J, Morris L, Kunze D: Neonatal death dwarfism (a further report). *Fortschr Röntgenstr* 1978, **129**:626.
Stanescu V, Stanescu R, Maroteaux P: Etude morphologique et biochimique du cartilage de croissance dans les osteochondrodysplasies. *Arch Franç Péd Suppl* 1977, **1**:34.
Horton W A, Rimoin D L *et al*: The phenotypic variability of diastrophic dysplasia. *J Pediatr 1978*, **93**:609–613.
Canki N, Sernec-Logar B *et al*: Le nanisme pseudodiastrophique... *J Génét Hum* 1979, **27**:247–252.
Gustavson K L, Holmgren G *et al*: Lethal and non-lethal diastrophic dysplasia... *Clin Genet* 1985, **28**:321–334.
Eteson D J, Beluffi G, Burgio G R *et al*: Pseudodiastrophic dysplasia: a distinct newborn skeletal dysplasia. *J Pediatr* 1986, **109**, 635–641.
Canki-Klain N, Stanescu V *et al*: Pseudodiastrophic dysplasia. Evolution with age and management. *Ann Génet* 1990, **33**:129–136.
Bertrand J G, Tyazi A *et al*: La dysplasie pseudodiastrophique. *Ann Pédiatr* 1991, **38**:19–22.

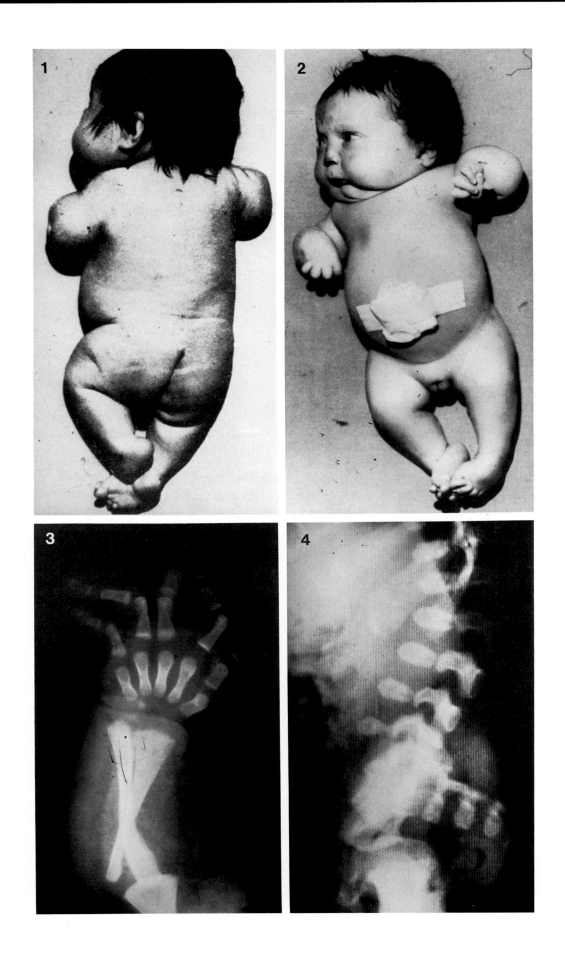

H.-R.W

An inherited disorder leading to severe short stature with 'turnabout of proportions' during the course of childhood (initially, relatively short extremities; subsequently, more obvious shortening of the trunk) combined with limitation of movement of the large joints and frequently with a tail-like formation of the sacral area.

Main signs:
- In the newborn and young child, a relatively long trunk with narrow thorax and short extremities (**1, 3**).
- In the older child (and adults), 'truncal short stature' as a result of platyspondyly (**8**) and usually also severe progressive kyphoscoliosis, extremities now appearing abnormally long (**5, 7**)
- Often a tail-like appendage medially over the sacral area (**3c, 5b, 7b**).
- Restricted movement at the generally prominent large joints (**1, 5, 7**)

Supplementary findings: Secondary deformities of the thorax. Hyperextensible finger joints.
   Radiologically, anisospondyly and platyspondyly (**8**), striking anomalies in the size and form of the pelvic bones and proximal femora (**4**), severe epimetaphyseal disorders of the shortened long bones with broadening of the metaphyses and marked irregularities of the epiphyseal ossification centres (**2, 6**).

Manifestation: At birth and later by the change of proportions.

Aetiology: Monogenic disorder; possible heterogeneity. Occurrence of autosomal dominant and perhaps also autosomal recessive transmission. Possibly three differentiable types:
- Relatively favourable form with autosomal dominant transmission;
- Non-lethal form with autosomal recessive transmission;
- Lethal form with death shortly before or after delivery and unknown transmission.
Molecular defect unknown.

Frequency: Relatively low.

Course, prognosis: Increased early mortality as a consequence of the congenitally narrowed thorax. Later, patients at risk from the effects of severe kyphoscoliosis. In severe cases, adult height may between 1.10 and 1.20 m. Normal mental development.

Differential diagnosis: Particularly Kniest-type osteodysplasia (*138*) and mucopolysaccharidosis IV (*67*).

Treatment: Symptomatic. Intensive orthopaedic supervision and for some patients therapy. All appropriate handicap aids. Genetic counselling.

Illustrations:
1 The same child at ages 15 months, 3 years, (**1c**) and 4 years (**1b**).
3, 5 A girl at 10 months and again at 7 years ('turnabout of proportions').
6–8 A 7-year-old child, with radiographs of hand (**6**) and spine (**8**).
2, 4 Radiographs of a newborn.

Note: The early onset of manifest kyphosis in **3a** and the severe progression in **5**. 'Tail formations' in **3c, 5b, 7**.

References:
Maroteaux P, Spranger J, Wiedemann H-R: Der metatropische Zwergwuchs. *Arch Kinderheilk* 1966, **173**:211.
Spranger J W, Langer Jr L O, Wiedemann H-R: *Bone dysplasias. An atlas of constitutional disorders of skeletal development.* Stuttgart and Philadephia: G Fischer and W B Saunders; 1974.
Miething R, Stöver B, Noeske H: Metatroper Zwergwuchs. *Mschr Kinderheilk* 1980, **128**:153.
Beck M, Roubicek M *et al*: Heterogeneity of metatropic dysplasia. *Eur J Pediatr* 1983, **140**:231–237.
Boden S D, Kaplan F S *et al*: Metatropic dwarfism. *J Bone Jt Surg* 1987, **69**(**A**):174–184.
Shohat M, Lachman R, Rimoin D L: Odontoid hypoplasia with vertebral cervical subluxation and ventriculomegaly in metatropic dysplasia. *J Pediatr* 1989, **114**:239–243.

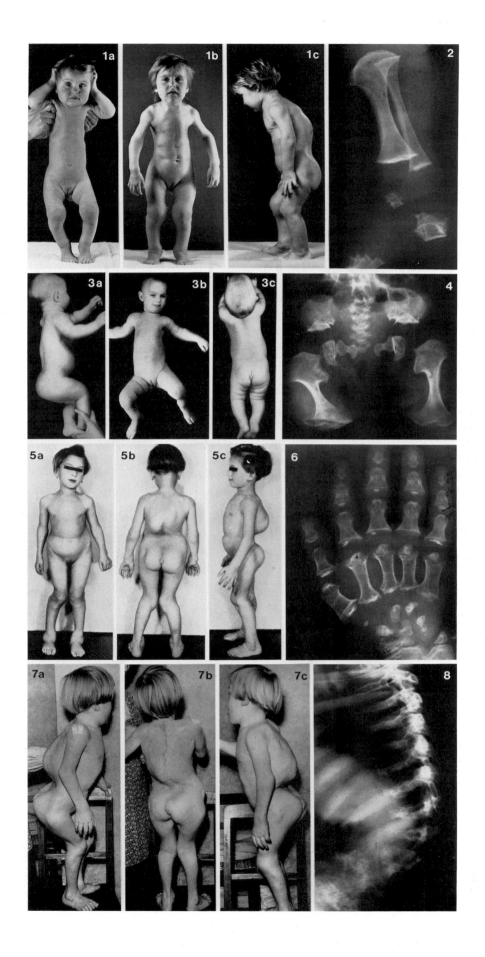

J.K.

A rare familial, neonatally lethal, rhizomelic chondrodysplasia with broad, dumb-bell-shaped long bones and pear-shaped vertebral bodies.

Main signs:
- Mild brachycephaly, wide open fontanelles and suture.
- Facial dysmorphism: round face, hypertelorism, large prominent eyes, flat nasal bridge, anteverted nostrils, microstomia.
- Short neck, flat thorax. Rhizomelic shortening of the arms and legs. Absence of the flexion and extension creases of the fingers.
- Death from respiratory insufficiency in the neonatal period.
- Radiographical findings: wide fontanelles and cranial sutures. Long, thin clavicles. Short ribs with wide anterior ends. Cervical to lumbar vertebral bodies flat (platyspondyly). In the upper and mid-vertebral column, ossification of only the anterior parts of the vertebral bodies. In the lower thoracic spine and the lumbar region, the increased anterior ossification of the vertebral bodies lends them a pear-shaped appearance on lateral view. In the anteroposterior view, sagittal mid-line clefts of the vertebral bodies with broad defects of midline ossification. Hypoplastic pelvis with ovoid ilium, flat acetabulum with medially placed notch. The pubic and ischial bones are short and broad. The long bones are also short and broad with dumb bell-like distension of the metaphyses. Short fibulae.

Manifestation: Prenatally and postnatally.

Aetiology: Autosomal recessive inheritance probable. Take note of possible consanguinity.

Frequency: Five patients were known by 1988 (one male, four female). Male twins were reported in one case.

Prognosis: Unfavourable: death in the newborn period from respiratory insufficiency in spite of intensive medical measures.

Differential diagnosis: Metatropic dysplasia (*133*), Kniest-type osteodysplasia (*138*), atelosteogenesis and SED congenita (*136*), thanatophoric dysplasia (*118, 119*), achondrogenesis (*115, 116*), boomerang dysplasia (*117*), 'Schneckenbecken' dysplasia (dysplasia with a snail-like radiographic appearance of the pelvis).

Illustrations:
1–7 Typical features of an affected neonate.

References:
Whitley C B, Langer Jr, L O, Ophoven J *et al*: Fibrochondrogenesis: lethal, autosomal recessive chondrodysplasia with distinctive cartilage histopathology. *Am J Med Genet* 1984, **19**:265–275.
Eteson E J, Adomian G E, Ornoy A *et al*: Fibrochondrogenesis: radiologic and histologic studies. *Am J Med Genet* 1984, **19**:277–290.
Bankier A, Fortune D, Duke J, Sillence D O: Fibrochondrogenesis in male twins at 24 weeks gestation. *Am J Med Genet* 1991, **38**:95–98.

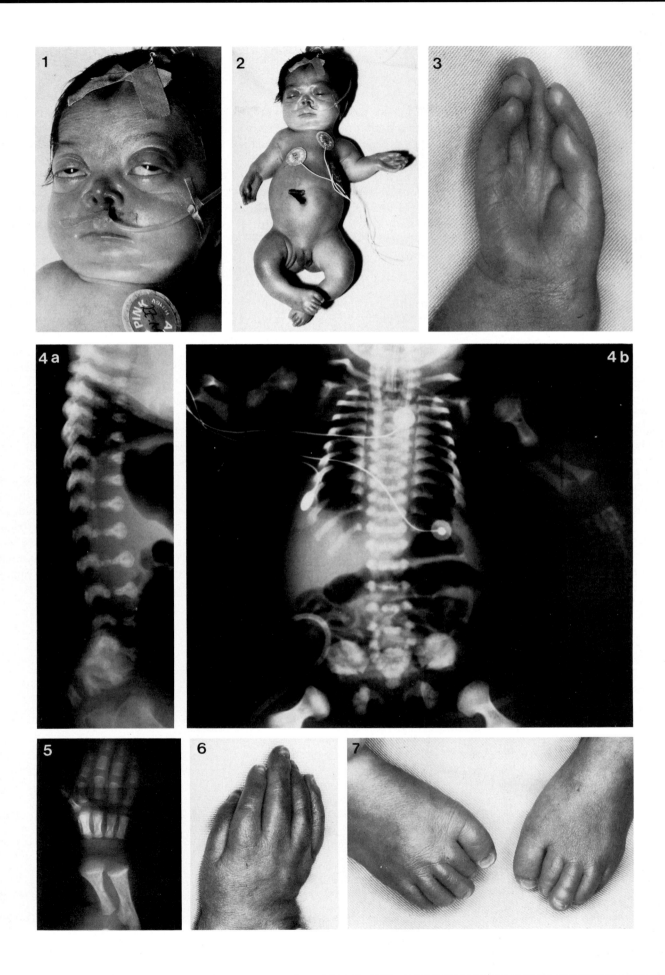

H.-R.W

A syndrome of congenital micromelic short stature with postaxial polydactyly, hypoplasia of the nails and abnormal frenula between the upper lip and the alveolar process.

Main signs:
- Disproportionate, micromelic short stature with more marked shortness of the extremities distally (**1 and 2**).
- Postaxial hexadactyly of the hands, occasionally also of the feet (**1, 2, 4, 5**). Also heptadactyly and syndactyly.
- Hypoplasia and dysplasia of the nails (**4 and 5**).
- Short upper lip, joined to the alveolar ridge by numerous, generally accessory frenula (**3**).
- Dysodontiasis (possible congenital teeth; partial anodontia; small, early or late-erupting teeth; malpositioning of teeth).
- In at least one-half of the patients, congenital cardiac anomaly (usually large atrial septal defects).
- Frequently genital anomalies.

Supplementary findings: In some patients, narrow thorax (**1**); later, genu valgus.

Radiologically, dysplasia of the pelvis and of several larger epiphyses; markedly increasing hypoplasia of the distal phalanges; possible bony fusion of metacarpals or phalanges or of the capitate and hamate; many other anomalies.

Manifestation: At birth.

Aetiology: Autosomal recessive disorder with variable expression of the pleiotropic gene.

Frequency: Low (apart from the Lancaster County Amish in the USA, for whom there are at least five patients out of 1 000 births); altogether about 250 patients known to date.

Course, prognosis: In infancy, markedly increased mortality as a consequence of pulmonary complications (because of short ribs) or cardiac defect. Adult height variable (between 1.05 and 1.60 m).

Differential diagnosis: The fully expressed syndrome should not cause diagnostic difficulties. A few specific short-rib polydactyly syndromes (121, 122) would need to be excluded in the newborn.

Treatment: Symptomatic. Orthopaedic treatment of polydactyly and genu valgus. Early dental care. Surgical correction of cardiac defect may be indicated. Genetic counselling. Prenatal diagnosis.

Illustrations:

1 A typically affected infant with hexadactyly; death at 24 days from respiratory insufficiency.

2–5 A 9-month-old boy, the first child of healthy, young, nonconsanguineous parents. The characteristically disproportionate development is more marked on the left side (**2, 4, 5**); ulnar deviation of the left hand; clinodactyly of the fifth and sixth fingers bilaterally. Considerable hypoplasia of the left wing of the ilium with dysplasia and subluxation of the hip. Bilateral talipes calcaneus and pes valgus. Delayed dentition. Small penis.

References:

McKusick V A, Egeland J A, Eldridge R *et al*: Dwarfism in the Amish. I. The Ellis–van Creveld syndrome. *Bull Johns Hopkins Hosp.* 1964, **115**:306–336.

Spranger J W, Langer Jr L O, Wiedemann H-R: *Bone dysplasias. An atlas of constitutional disorders of skeletal development.* Stuttgart and Philadephia: G Fischer and W B Saunders; 1974.

Milgram J W, Bailey J A: Orthopaedic aspects of the Ellis–van Creveld syndrome. *Bull Hosp Joint Dis* 1975, **36**:11.

Oliveira E, Silva D, Janovito D *et al*: Ellis–van Creveld syndrome: report of 15 cases... *J Med Genet* 1980, **17**:349.

Rosemberg S, Carneiro P C, Zerbini M C N *et al*: Chondroectodermal dysplasia (Ellis–van Creveld) with anomalies of CNS and urinary tract. *Am J Med Genet* 1983, **15**:291–295.

Serotkin A, Stamberg J *et al*: Duplication 17q mosaicism: an infant with features of Ellis–van Creveld syndrome. *J Med Genet* 1988, **25**:258–269.

Zangwill K M, Boal D K B *et al*: Dandy-Walker malformation in Ellis–van Creveld syndrome. *J Med Genet* 1988, **31**:121–129.

Fryns J P: Postaxial polydactyly as heterozygote manifestation in Ellis–van Creveld syndrome? *Am J Med Genet* 1991, **39**:500.

Qureshi F *et al*: Skeletal histopathology in... Ellis–van Creveld syndrome. *Am J Med Genet* 1993, **45**: 471–476.

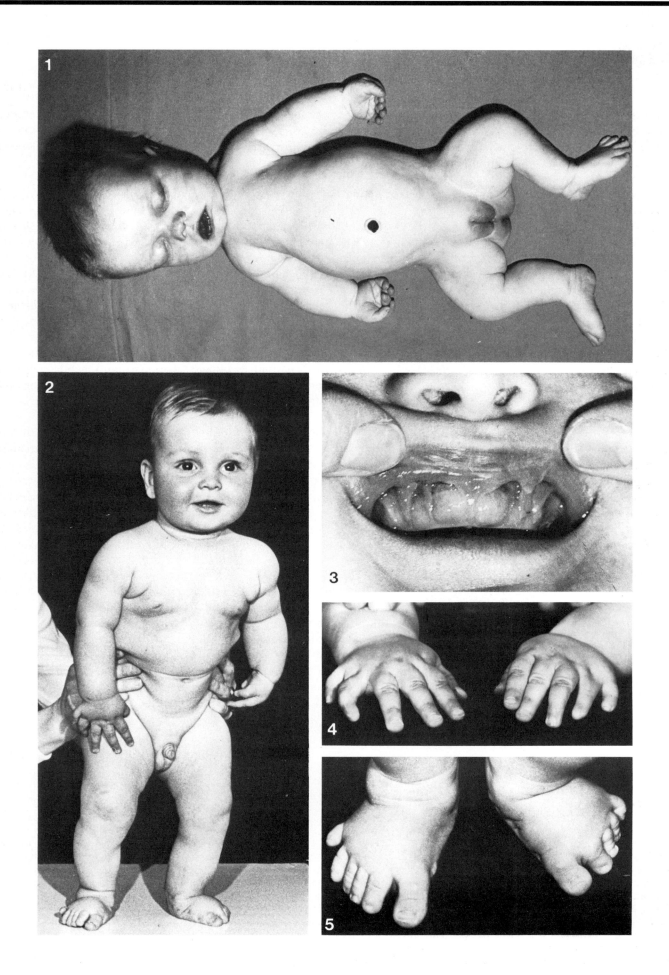

136 Spondylo-epiphyseal Dysplasia Congenita
(SED Congenita)

H.-R.W

An autosomally-dominant hereditary syndrome of disproportionate short stature with severe shortening of the vertebral column; barrel-shaped chest; deep lumbar lordosis and severe dysplasia of the epiphyses, especially those near the trunk; practically normal cranium, hands and feet; frequently in combination with myopia or retinal detachment.

Main signs:

- Disproportionate short stature with shortening especially of the vertebral column. Short neck, compressed-appearing trunk with barrel-shaped chest and pectus carinatum, lumbar hyperlordosis, possible kyphoscoliosis of the thoracic spine (**1a–d**).
- Relatively long extremities. Frequent waddling gait with severe hip dysplasia and marked coxa vara. Frequent genu valgus (less frequently varus). Normal-sized hands and feet (**1**).
- Impaired vision because of myopia or retinal detachment in approximately 50% of the patients.

Supplementary findings: Flat face (occasional hypertelorism) (**1a, 1d**). Occasional cleft palate.

Fully mobile, sometimes hyperextensible joints (with the possible exception of hips, shoulders, and elbows). Lax ligaments. Muscular hypotonia in infancy. Occasionally club feet.

Delayed motor, normal mental development.

Sensorineural hearing impairment not unusual.

Radiologically, delayed ossification (**3**), especially in the pelvic bones and hip joints (with severe coxa vara), flattening and diverse irregularities of the vertebral bodies with hypoplasia of the odontoid process, epimetaphyseal dysplasia of the long bones, relatively normal bones of the hands and feet.

Manifestation: At birth.

Aetiology: Autosomal dominant inheritance with markedly variable expression. Frequently new mutations. Assumed gene locus: 12q13.11-q13.2. Collagen structural defect, type II.

Frequency: Not particularly rare.

Course, prognosis: As retinal detachment may occur relatively early, regular examination by an ophthalmologist is indicated. Danger of compression of the cervical medulla, from hypoplasia of the odontoid and laxity of the ligaments, which requires preventive orthopaedic care.
Adult height between 90 and 130 cm. Increasing arthritis of the large joints and corresponding handicaps in adulthood.

Differential diagnosis: The Morquio syndrome (later manifestation and other differences; 67) and Stickler syndrome (302), among others, need to be ruled out.

Treatment: Symptomatic. Early treatment of club feet when present; closure of cleft palate as required; careful neurological supervision and preventive orthopaedic measures in view of the danger of spinal cord compression; coagulation treatment may be indicated for retinal detachment. All available aids and supports for the physical handicaps. Genetic counselling. Prenatal diagnosis (by DNA analysis of chorionic villi, otherwise by ultrasound).

Illustrations:

1a–d The same child at 6 months (height 14 cm below the average for age) and 7 years and 3 months (height deficit approximately 40 cm). Early kyphoscoliosis. Hypoplasia of the odontoid, with previously normal movement at the atlanto-occipital joint. Cleft palate.

2 Hand radiograph of a 4-year-old female patient (father similarly affected).

3 A hand radiograph of the child in **1** at age 5 years.

References:

Spranger J W, Langer Jr L O, Wiedemann H-R: *Bone dysplasias. An atlas of constitutional disorders of skeletal development.* Stuttgart and Philadephia: G Fischer and W B Saunders; 1974.

Luthardt T, Reinwein H, Schönenberg H, Spranger J, Wiedemann H-R: Dysplasia spondyloepiphysaria congenita. *Klin Pädiat* 1975, **187**:538.

Kozlowski K, Masel J, Nolte K: Dysplasia spondyloepiphysealis congenita Spranger-Wiedemann. *Aust Radiol* 1977, **21**:260.

Horton W A, Hall J G, Scott C I *et al*: Growth curves for height for diastrophic dysplasia, spondyloepiphyseal dysplasia congenita... *Am J Dis Child* 1982, **136**:316.

Reardon W, Hall C M *et al*: New autosomal dominant form of spondylo-epiphyseal dysplasia presenting with atlanto-axial instability. *Am J Med.Genet* 1994, **52**:432–437.

Spranger J, Winterpacht A, Zabel B: The type II collagenopathies: a spectrum of chondrodysplasias. *Eur J Pediatr* 1994, **153**:56–65.

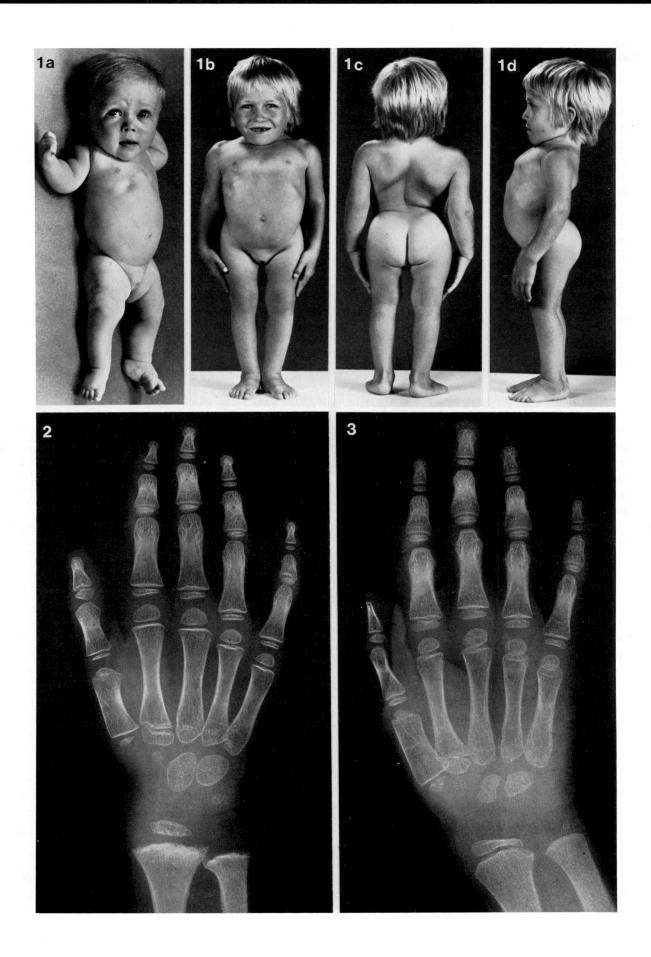

J.K./H.-R.W

A familial syndrome manifest between the fourth and 12th years of life with short stature, short vertebral column, prominent sternum, increased lumbar lordosis and waddling gait with femoral epiphyseal dysplasia.

Main signs:

- Disproportionate short stature with shortened vertebral column; platyspondyly, increasing lumbar lordosis, sternal protrusion, broad thorax.
- Extremities clinically normal, hands and feet of normal size, narrow hips. Premature osteo-arthritic complaints in the hip, knee, shoulder and ankle joints. Waddling gait.

Supplementary findings: Calcification of the vertebral column may result in limitation of movements. Some patients show hyperextensible joints; a few have shown corneal dystrophy (of the autosomal recessive, so-called Toledo type). Rarely poikiloderma and colour blindness. Unimpaired mental development.

Manifestation: Between the fourth and 12th years of life. Usually clinically recognized between the sixth and eighth years of life. Occasional early suspicion of 'hip disorder'.

Aetiology: Heterogeneity: usually X-linked recessive transmission (Xq22.2-q22.1) but autosomal dominant and autosomal recessive inheritance have also been described. Chondroitin sulphate synthesis defect?

Frequency: Up to now, a rarely diagnosed disorder.

Course, prognosis: Adult height of the patients between 125 and 160 cm. Osteoarthritis of the hips and knees and calcification in the region of the vertebral column worsen the prognosis for freedom of movement in later years. Nevertheless, approximately normal life expectancy.

Differential diagnosis: Several authors have classified SED tarda into four groups, A–D:

- brachyrachia (A)
- brachyolmia (B)
- classic X-linked recessive SED tarda (C)
- autosomal dominant and autosomal recessive SED tarda (D).

It is important to consider Morquio syndrome (97) in the differential diagnosis.

Treatment: Orthopaedic care, physiotherapy.

Illustrations:

1 A patient 7 years and 9 months old with short stature and hyperlordosis.

2 Slightly reduced height of the vertebral bodies, flattening of the anterior marginal crests; suggestion of tongue-like anterior extensions of L1–4.

3 Flattening of the epiphyses of metacarpals II–IV; clinodactyly of the little fingers.

4 Pelvis and hip joints of the boy at age 4 years.

References:

Spranger J, Langer L O, Wiedemann H-R: *Bone dysplasias.* Stuttgart: Gustav Fischer Verlag, 1974.

Byers P H, Holbrook K A, Hall J G *et al*: A new variety of spondyloepiphyseal dysplasia characterized by punctate corneal dystrophy and abnormal dermal collagen fibrils. *Hum Genet* 1978, 40:157–169.

de Pina Neto J M, Bonfim M D, Ferrari I: Classic X-linked spondyloepiphyseal dysplasia tarda in a woman with normal karyotype. In: *Skeletal dysplasias.* C J Papadatos, C S Bartsocas (eds.). New York: Alan Liss 1982; 127–132.

Al-Awadi S A, Farag T I, Naguib K *et al*: Spondyloepiphyseal dysplasia tarda with progressive arthropathy. *J Med Genet* 1984, 21:193–196.

Harrod M E J, Friedman J M, Currarino, G *et al*: Genetic heterogeneity in spondyloepiphyseal dysplasia congenita. *Am J Med Genet* 1984, 18:311–320.

Iceton J A, Horne G: Spondylo-Epiphyseal dysplasia tarda. The X-linked variety in three brothers. *J Bone Jt Surg* 1986, 68B:616–619.

Kohn G, Elrayyes E R, Makadmah I *et al*: Spondyloepiphyseal dysplasia tarda: a new autosomal recessive variant with mental retardation. *J Med Genet* 1987, 24:366–377.

Szpiro-Tapia S, Sefiani A *et al*: Spondyloepiphyseal dysplasia tarda: linkage... from the distal short arm of the X chromosome. *Hum Genet* 1988, 81:61–63.

Sewell A C, Wern C, Pontz B F: Brachyolmia: a skeletal dysplasia with an altered mucopolysaccharide excretion. *Clin Genet* 1991, 40:312–317.

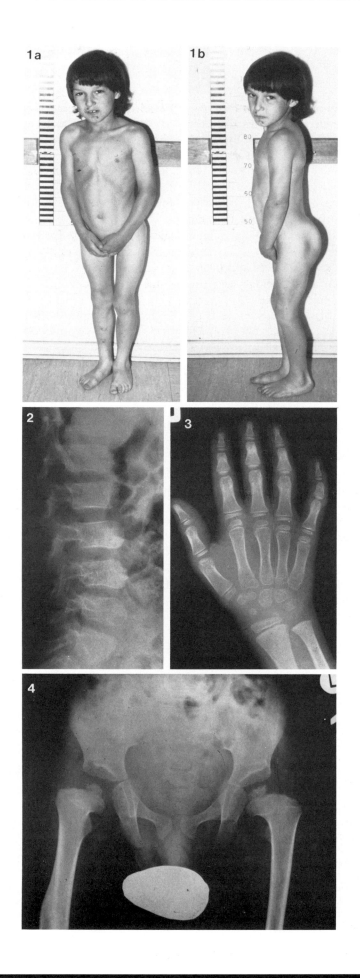

138 Kniest-Type Osteodysplasia
(Kniest Syndrome, Kniest Disease)

H.-R.W

An inherited disorder of disproportionate short stature with kyphoscoliosis, flat facies, often with hearing and visual impairment and characteristic radiograph findings.

Main signs:
- Disproportionate short stature with short trunk, wide thorax, marked lumbar lordosis and thoracic kyphoscoliosis and short extremities, which appear swollen at the joints and too long relative to the trunk (**1**). Final height between about 105 and 155 cm.
- Flat facies, possibly with widely spaced eyes and proptosis caused by flat orbits, flat nasal bridge and (in approximately 50% of patients) cleft palate.
- Frequently limited movement at the joints (especially marked at the hips); long fingers.
- Frequent hearing impairment (conductive or sensorineural defect), frequent high-grade myopia with retinal degeneration and danger of glaucoma, cataract and retinal detachment with loss of sight.

Supplementary findings: Often umbilical and inguinal hernias. Radiologically, striking anomalies in shape and size of the pelvic and femoral bones. Platyspondyly with ventrally tapering vertebral bodies, short clavicles, marked changes of the long bones, broadening of the metaphyses and marked irregularities of the epiphyses and metaphyses in the form of honeycombed, porous translucencies and delayed ossification (especially of the femoral heads).

Manifestation: At birth (short, deformed extremities, disorders of joint mobility) and later, delayed motor development.

Aetiology: Autosomal dominant disorder with extremely variable expression. In many cases, new mutations; low risk of recurrence for the parents. Gene locus on 12q13.11-q13.2 suspected. Type 2 collagen structural defect. Heterogeneity cannot be excluded with certainty.

Frequency: Low.

Course, prognosis: Except for rare, very severe forms, life expectancy is probably about average but with moderate to severe physical handicaps: articular, respiratory, and in some patients ocular and auditory.

Differential diagnosis: Mainly metatropic dysplasia (*133*) and spondylo-epiphyseal dysplasia congenita (*136*). Morquio syndrome (*67*) and diastrophic and pseudodiastrophic dysplasias (*131, 132*) should be fairly easy to rule out. Stickler dysplasia (*302*) could be regarded as the mildest form of Kniest-type osteodysplasia.

Treatment: Starting at an early age, regular follow-up with ophthalmological and audiometric examinations. Closure of cleft palate and speech therapy if required. Orthopaedic care of joint contractures and kyphoscoliosis. All appropriate aids for the physically handicapped.
  Genetic counselling. Severe cases can be prenatally diagnosed by ultrasound.

Illustrations:
1–3, 5, 6 A typically affected infant.
4 A 7 year old with Kniest syndrome and his healthy twin brother.

References:
Spranger J W, Langer Jr L O, Wiedemann H-R: *Bone dysplasias. An atlas of constitutional disorders of skeletal development.* Stuttgart and Philadephia: G Fischer and W B Saunders; 1974.
Lachman R S, Rimoin D L, Hollister D W *et al*: The Kniest syndrome. *Am J Roentgenol* 1975, **123**:805.
Kniest W, Leiber B: Kniest–Syndrom. *Mschr Kinderheilk* 1977, **125**:970.
Silengo M C, Davi G F *et al*: Kniest disease... *Pediatr Radiol* 1983, **13**:106–109.
Wynne-Davies R, Hall C M *et al*: *Atlas of skeletal dysplasias.* Edinburgh: Churchill-Livingstone 1985.
Maumenee I H, Traboulsi E I: The ocular findings in Kniest dysplasia. *Am J Ophthalmol* 1985, **100**:155–160.
Farag T I *et al*: A family with spondyloepimetaphyseal dwarfism... *J Med Genet* 1987, **24**:597–601.
Poole A R *et al*: Kniest dysplasia... *Am J Clin Invest* 1988, **8**:579–589.
Oestreich A E, Prenger E C: MR demonstrates cartilaginous megaepiphyses of the hips in Kniest dysplasia... *Pediatr Radiol* 1992, **22**:302–303.
Majewski R, Spranger J: Dyssegmentale Dysplasie... *Med Genetik* 1994, **6**:15–19.
Spranger J, Winterpracht A, Zabel B: The type II collagenopathies: a spectrum of chondrodysplasias. *Eur J Pediatr* 1994, **153**:56–65.
Stanescu V *et al*: Non-collagenous protein screening in the human chondrodysplasias... *Am J Med Genet* 1994, **51**:22–28.
Wilkins D J, Bogaert R *et al*: A single amino acid substitution... in the type II collagen triple helix produces Kniest dysplasia. *Hum Mol Genetm* 1994, 3:1999–2005.

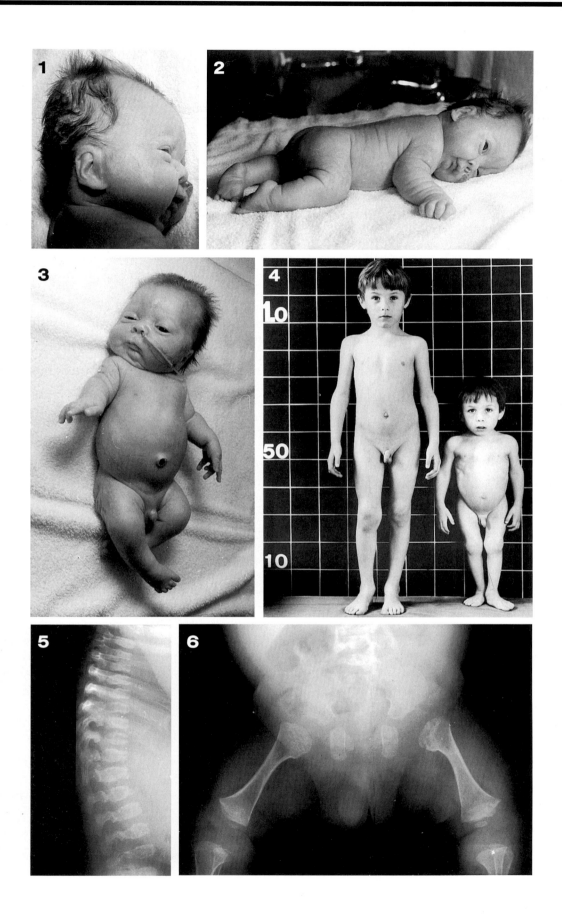

J.K./H.-R.W

A familial disorder with deficient calcification of the bones, absent calcification of the calvaria (craniotabes), late closure of the anterior fontanelle, craniosynostosis, premature loss of deciduous teeth, bowed long bones, fractures, hypercalcaemia, and nephrocalcinosis.

Main signs:
Very variable expression (lethal congenital [or foetal], infantile, late infantile–juvenile and adult forms).
- Absent calcification of the calvaria (craniotabes), late fontanelle closure, craniosynostosis, oxycephaly.
- Fractures and bowing of the long bones, genu valgum.
- Rickets-like radiological changes: absent calcification of the skeletal system of varied severity, rachitic rosary, broad metaphyses, 'notching' or 'fraying' of the ends of the long bones.

Biochemically: decreased or absent alkaline phosphatase; frequent hypercalcaemia; hypercalciuria; increased phospho-ethanolamine and pyrophosphate excretion in the urine.

Supplementary findings: Muscular hypotonia, failure to thrive, respiratory disorders, seizures, anaemia, nephrocalcinosis, exophthalmos, increased intracranial pressure, vomiting, bone pains, increased tendency to infections, growth retardation. Caries, premature loss of teeth, premature craniosynostosis.

Manifestation: Foetal form: intra-uterine. Prenatal diagnosis from absent calcification of the cranium (differentiate from anencephaly), decreased alkaline phosphatase in amniotic fluid and cells.
   Infantile form: at birth and thereafter.
   Late infantile–juvenile form: after the third year of life.
   Adult form: After puberty. History of 'rickets'.

Aetiology: As a rule, autosomal recessive inheritance. Diagnosis of heterozygotes difficult (decreased alkaline phosphatase, increased phospho-ethanolamine excretion in the urine). Late and milder forms tend to have autosomal dominant inheritance. Gene localized to chromosome 1p36.1-p34. With the lethal congenital form, genetic defect for the nonspecific tissue phosphatases from the liver and bones. Impaired connective tissue and endochondral ossification.

Frequency: By 1972 more than 120 patients had been diagnosed. Adult form is frequently not recognized.

Course, prognosis: Foetal form: intra-uterine death, stillbirth.
   Infantile form: lethal in 50% of patients. Fractures, bowing, failure to thrive, rachitic signs, seizures, premature craniosynostosis, hypercalcaemia, nephrocalcinosis.
   Juvenile form: good chance of survival, orthopaedic and dental problems. Early loss of teeth, rachitic signs, short stature.
   Adult form: spontaneous fractures. Osteoporosis, ectopic calcifications.
   No clear boundaries between the individual forms.

Treatment: To date, no effective means of treatment. Vitamin D therapy is contraindicated (hypercalcaemia). Orthopaedic measures. Prenatal diagnosis.

Differential diagnosis: Achondrogenesis (*115, 116*) and thanatophoric dysplasia (*118, 119*) with the neonatal forms. Osteogenesis imperfecta (*204, 205*).

Illustrations:
1a and b Foetal form, intra-uterine death. Absent calcification of the skull; barely mineralized, thin ribs. Vertebral bodies and pelvic bones barely distinguishable. Partial calcification of the long bones, flaring of the metaphyses.
2a A 5-month-old infant, early craniostenosis, thoracic in-drawing. **2b** Defective calcification of the skeleton, osteomalacia.

References:
Terheggen H G, Wischermann A: Die kongenitale Hypophosphatasie. *Monatsschr Kinderheilkd* 1984, **132**:512–522.
Fallon M D *et al*: Hypophosphatasia: clinicopathologic comparison of the infantile, childhood, and adult forms. *Medicine* 1984, **63**:12–24.
Ornoy A, Adomian G E, Rimoin D L: Histologic and ultrastructural studies on the mineralization process in hypophosphatasia. *Am J Med Genet* 1985, **22**:743–758.
Warren R C *et al*: First trimester diagnosis of hypophosphatasia with a monoclonal antibody to the liver/bone/kidney isoenzyme of alkaline phosphatase. *Lancet* 1985, **II**:856–858.
Whyte M P, Magill H L, Fallon M D *et al*: Infantile hypophosphatasia: normalization of circulating bone alkaline phosphatase activity followed by skeletal remineralization. *J Pediatr* 1986, **108**:82–88.
Moore C A, Ward J C *et al*: Infantile hypophosphatasia: autosomal recessive transmission to two related sibships. *Am J Med Genet* 1990, **36**:15–22.
Shohat M, Rimoin D L *et al*: Perinatal lethal hypophosphatasia; clinical, radiologic and morphologic findings. *Pediatr Radiol* 1991, **21**:421–427.
Macfarlane J D, Kroon H M, van der Harten J J: Phenotypically dissimilar hypophosphatasia in two sibships. *Am J Med Genet* 1992, **42**:117–121.
Kishi F, Matssura S *et al*: Prenatal diagnosis of infantile hypophosphatasia. *Prenat Diagn* 1991, **11**:305–309.
Brock D J. H, Barron L: First-trimester prenatal diagnosis of hypophosphatasia: experience with 16 cases. *Prenat Diagn* 1991, **11**:387–391.

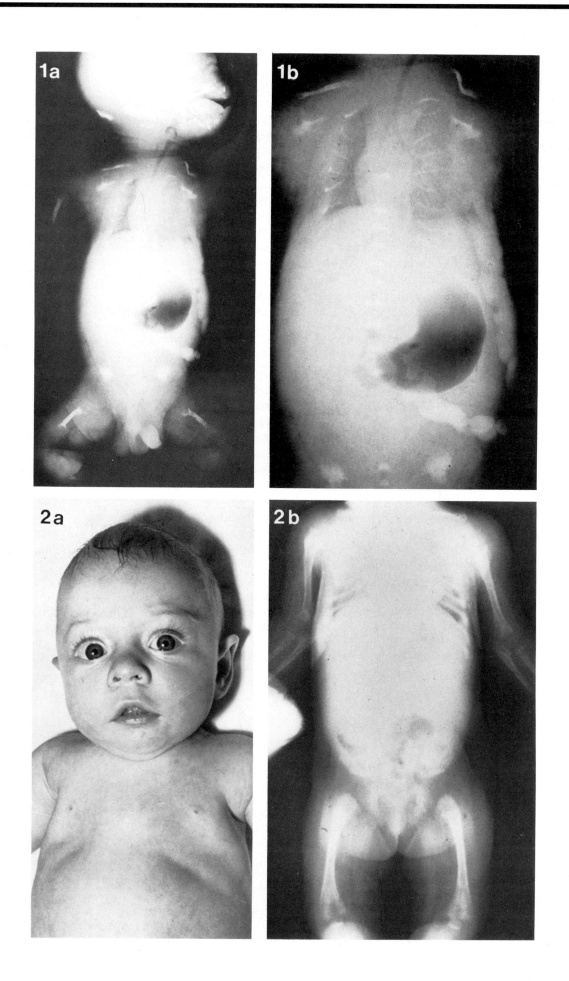

140 Familial Hypophosphataemic Rickets

(So-called Vitamin D-Resistant Rickets; Phosphate Diabetes)

H.-R.W/

K. Kruse

A hereditary metabolic disorder with short stature and rachitic bone changes.

Main signs:
- Moderately short stature with abnormalities of the lower extremities; pronounced bow legs, less frequently knock knees (**1, 2, 4**). Waddling gait, coxa vara. In childhood, also´ other rachitic bone changes (rachitic rosary, enlargement of the wrists and ankles and so on).
- Dental changes such as defects of enamel and dentin, delayed eruption, dental abscesses, early loss.
- In adulthood, possibility of bone pain, abnormal curvature of the spine, osteomalacia, calcifications around the tendons, ligaments and joint capsules and sensorineural hearing impairment.
- Occasionally, craniosynostosis.

Supplementary findings: Radiologically, changes as in vitamin D-deficiency rickets (**3**), However, the pelvic and spinal regions are spared.

Hypophosphataemia, hyperphosphaturia (these, together with slightly short stature, are the only signs of the mild form of the disorder); increased serum alkaline phosphatase, normal serum calcium and parathormone.

Manifestation: Biochemically, during the first 6 months of life. Clinically, usually between 6 and 18 months or later.

Aetiology: X-linked dominant disorder, which is triggered by a genetic defect localized on the distal part of the short arm of the X chromosome; correspondingly milder manifestations of the disease in affected girls. Combined disorder of phosphate reabsorption and of regulation of 1,25-(OH)2D secretion in the proximal renal tubules.

Frequency: Approximately 1:25 000.

Course, prognosis: Improvement of the signs of florid rickets with the physiological slowing and the cessation of growth. Adult height between 1.30 and 1.60 m. Frequent back and joint pain and complaints of stiffness in adulthood.

Differential diagnosis: Vitamin-deficiency rickets (here, elevated parathormone and low 25-hydroxy-vitamin D in serum; no positive family history) and other forms of rickets (*141*), metaphyseal chondrodysplasia syndrome, Schmid type (*145*) and cartilage-hair hypoplasia (*147*).

Treatment: Clinically and biochemically, good results from daily administration of vitamin D analogs (1a-OHD3, 1,25-(OH)2D3) with careful monitoring of blood chemistries. Many authors have seen a positive effect on growth.

Correction of the leg deformities by orthopaedic surgery preferably after cessation of growth.

Illustrations:

1 and 2 Two children (different parents) at ages 5 and 3 years. Both have a height deficit of 9 cm.

3 The radiological bone changes of a 1-year-old patient.

4 A father and daughter with phosphate diabetes; the short stature of the child led to diagnostic clarification; the father has a history of corrective surgical procedures.

References:

Stanbury J B, Wyngaarden J B, Fredrickson D S *et al: The metabolic basis of inherited disease.* New York: McGraw-Hill 1983; 1743.

Carlsen N L T, Krasilnikoff P A, Eiken M: Premature cranial synostosis in X-linked hypophosphatemic rickets... *Acta Paediatr Scand* 1984, **73**:149–154.

Mimouni F, Mughal Z *et al:* Picture of the month: X-linked dominant hypophosphatemic rickets. *AJDC* 1988, **142**:191–192.

Scriver C R, Tenenhouse H S: X-linked hypophosphataemia: a homologous phenotype in humans and mice with unusual organ-specific gene dosage. *J Inherited Metab Dis* 1992, **15**:610–624.

Steendijk R, Hauspie R C: The pattern of growth and growth retardation of patients with hypophosphataemic vitamin D-resistant rickets: a longitudinal study. *Eur J Pediatr* 1992, **151**:422–427.

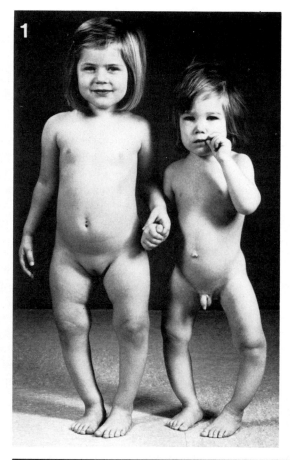

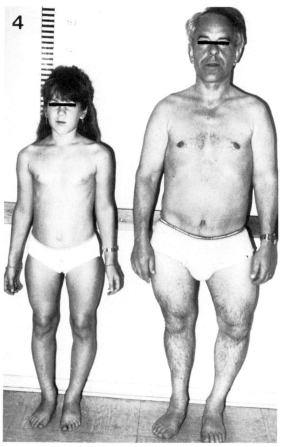

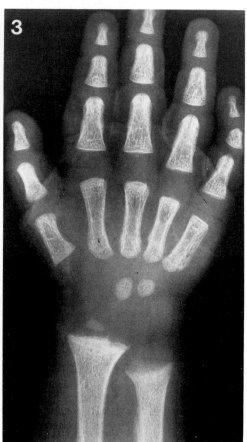

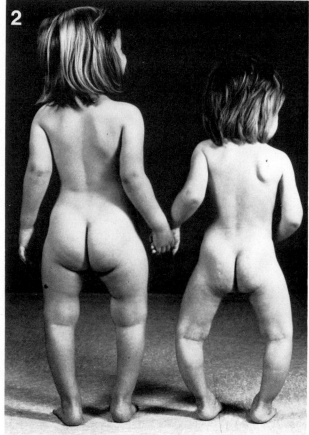

141 Vitamin D–Dependent Rickets Type ll

J.K.

A rare rachitic disorder with resistance to 1,25-dihydroxy vitamin D and alopecia

Main signs:
- The alopecia generally develops between the third and sixth month of life; rarely already manifest at birth. It correlates with the severity of the disorder and is always present in those patients who cannot become normocalcaemic, despite high exogenic administration of calciferol.
- Onset of rickets in the first year of life with muscular hypotonia, generalized asthaenia, delayed motor development, defects of the tooth enamel, pathologic fractures. As the condition progresses, bowing of the bones, seizures, tetany, short stature, thickening of the wrists, positive Chvostek's and Trousseau's signs.

Supplementary findings: Radiologically, no differentiation from other forms of rickets. Laboratory tests reveal hypocalcaemia, hypophosphataemia, increased excretion of cyclical adenosine monophosphate in the urine. In serum, the parathormone levels (secondary hyperparathyroidism), alkaline phosphatase and 1,25-dihydroxyvitamin D are elevated. 25-hydroxyvitamin D is normal. Additionally: amino-aciduria.

Manifestation: Alopecia generally develops between the third and sixth months of life, clinical signs of rickets after the sixth month of life.

Aetiology: Sporadic occurrence in 50% of all affected individuals. The multiplicity of sibling disorders from consanguineous marriages indicates autosomal recessive inheritance. Genetic localization: 12q12-q14.

Pathogenesis: End-organ resistance to 1,25-dihydroxy vitamin D.

Course, prognosis: In patients who respond to the treatment, the prognosis for growth, development and reproduction is good. The prognosis is still unclear in the case of total resistance to treatment.

Differential diagnosis: Differentiation from other genetically determined rachitic disorders, for example phosphate diabetes (*140*)

Treatment: In many patients, up to 20µg/day of 1,25(OH)$_2$D together with oral administration of calcium corrects the hypocalcaemia, secondary hyperparathyroidism and rickets. However, some patients do not respond at all.

Illustrations:

1–4 Male infant, 8 months old, with total alopecia, including eyelashes and eyebrows. Severe treatment-resistant hypocalcaemia.

5 Radiological diagnosis of rickets on admission to hospital at 7 months.

6 Rickets unchanged 2 months later (despite attempted oral treatment with vitamin D and calcium).

References:

Eil C, Liberman U A, Rosen F J, Marx S J: A cellular defect in hereditary vitamin-D-dependent rickets type II: defective nuclear uptake of 1,25-dihydroxyvitamin D in cultured skin fibroblasts. *N Engl J Med* 1981, **304**:1588–1591.

Manadhar D S, Sarkawi S, Hunt M C J: Rickets with alopecia-remission following a course of 1-alpha-hydroxy vitamin D (3) therapy. *Eur J Pediatr* 1984, **148**:761–763.

Balsan S, Garabedian M, Larchet M, Gorski A M, Cournot G, Tau C, Bourdeau A, Silve C, Ricour C: Long-term nocturnal calcium infusions can cure rickets and promote normal mineralization in hereditary resistance to 1,25-dihydroxyvitamin D. *J Clin Invest* 1986, 77:1661–1667.

Hughes M R, Mallay P J, Kieback D G, Kesterson R A, Pike J W, Feldman D, O'Malley B W: Point mutations in the human vitamin D receptor gene associated with hypocalcaemic rickets. *Science* 1988, **242**:1702–1705.

Malloy P J, Hochberg Z, Tiosan, D, Pike J W, Hughes M R, Feldman F: The molecular basis of hereditary 1,25-dihydroxyvitamin D3 resistant rickets in seven related families. *J Clin Invest* 1990, **86**:2071–2079.

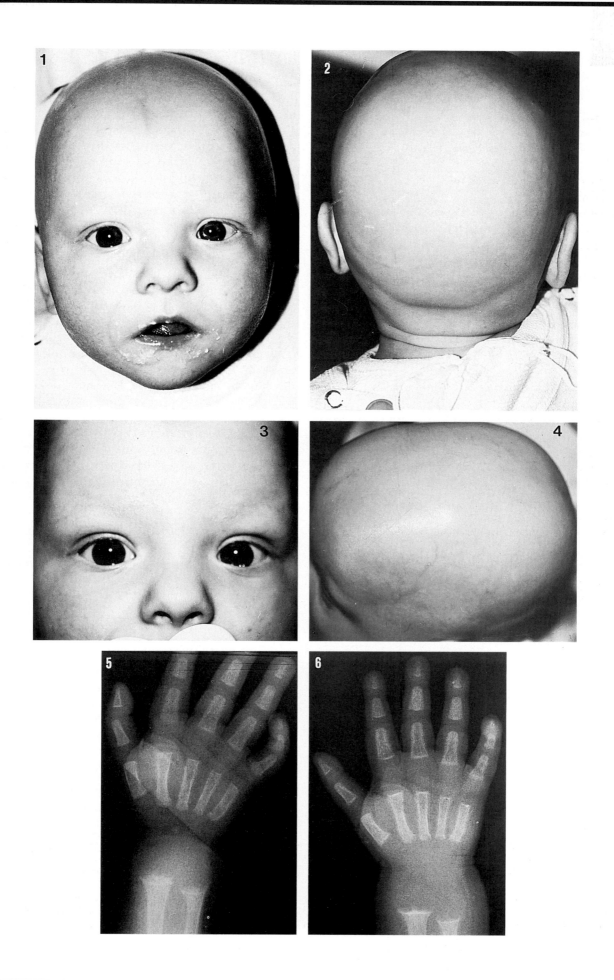

An Unusual Syndrome of Short Stature with Striking Distal Inhibition of Ossification

H.-R.W

A syndrome of short stature, severe infantile scoliosis and other skeletal anomalies, with severely delayed ossification of the bones of the hands and feet.

Main signs:
- Marked short stature.
- Marked infantile scoliosis with corresponding abnormal proportions and other secondary changes (11–13).
- On radiograph, markedly delayed ossification in bones of the hands and feet ('empty wrist') (6 and 7).

Supplementary findings: Normal mental development for age.
   Radiologically, numerous wormian bones of the skull (3 and 4). Possible evidence of malformations of the vertebral column or other regions.

Manifestation: At birth or in early childhood.

Aetiology: Not established (possible receptor defect in the bone matrix). Genetic basis probable.

Course, prognosis: Unclear, certainly very dependent on the skeletal problems and whether the scoliosis is amenable to therapy.

Treatment: Adequate orthopaedic care.

Illustrations:
1–13 A boy 4 years and 6 months old, the sixth child of healthy, consanguineous Turkish parents. A similarly affected sister: mental development normal for age; short stature; severe right convex scoliosis of the thoracic spine, allegedly since 3 years of age, with wedge-shaped vertebrae and synostoses; torsion defect of the lower leg. Other living siblings healthy.

   In the proband, the deformities of the spine and thorax (bulging rib cage on the right) were said to be present at birth. Normal mental, delayed motor development. Currently, short stature, well below the third percentile, with short neck, abnormal orientation of the ribs, extremities relatively too long and severe right convex scoliosis of the thoracic spine (sloping of shoulders and pelvis). Round cranium and numerous wormian bones in the sagittal and especially the lambdoid sutures. Mild coxa vara; torsion defect of the upper and lower leg; lateral dislocation of the patellae; pes adductus with various positional anomalies of the toes. Radiologically, practically 'empty' wrists and markedly delayed ossification of the metacarpals and phalanges but approximately normal epiphyses for age at the pelvis and knees. Also, marked delay in development of the bones of the feet. Exhaustive laboratory examinations (including endocrinological tests) were normal.

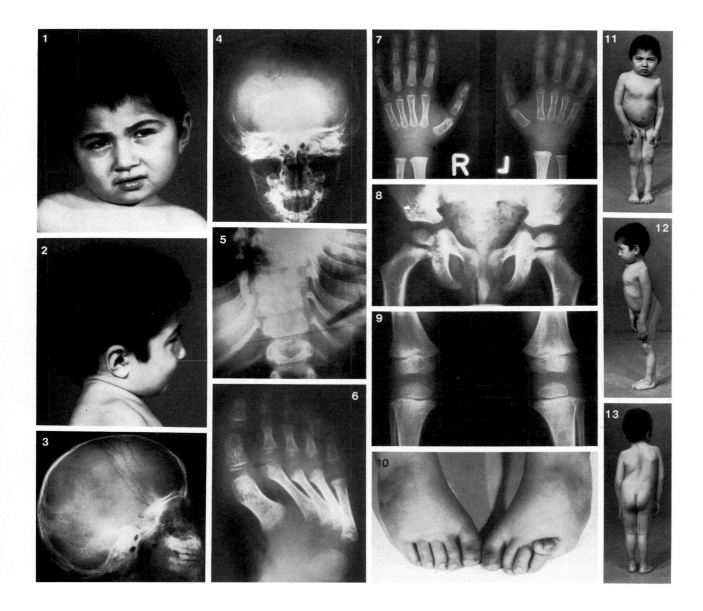

H.-R.W

An unusual syndrome with multiple congenital joint dysplasias, short stature and telangiectatic erythema of the face.

Main signs:
- Congenital, not completely symmetrical anomalies of the joints and skeleton: dysplasia of the hips, limited extension of the knees and small club feet, bilateral malformation of the distal humeri with dislocation of the humero-ulnar and radio-ulnar joints, relatively short forearms, limited mobility of the wrists, camptodactyly and sometimes clinodactyly of fingers II–V (4, 6–8). No skin dimples.
- Primary (and secondary) short stature, below the third percentile (at 12 years and 2 months 1.30 m; twin brother: 1.60 m).
- Starting at age 2 years and persisting for more than 6 years, butterfly-like distribution of a paranasally localized telangiectatic erythema of the face, minimally also on the forearms, which may have been aggravated by sunlight (1 and 2; in 3 and 5 at age 12 years, only mild residual spots on the left cheek).

Supplementary findings: Dolichocephaly, long narrow face with prominent nose and slightly receding chin (3, 5).
Kyphoscoliosis, lumbar hyperlordosis (4).
At 12 years, still no signs of onset of puberty.
Radiographs of the hands and feet: hypoplasia of the distal ends of the ulnae with absence of the styloid processes; considerable bilateral brachymesophalangy of fingers II–V, severe brachymesophalangy of toes II–V.

Manifestation: At birth and later.

Aetiology: Undetermined.

Comment: Bloom syndrome (199) is apparently not present. Larsen syndrome (230) could be ruled out. Classification as arthrogryposis multiplex congenita (226) did not seem to be justified here.

Treatment: Intensive orthopaedic–surgical and physiotherapeutic efforts required. Promotion of intellectual development, adequate vocational training and psychological support. Genetic counselling.

Illustrations:
1–8 A mentally normal girl, a twin child (brother normal) of healthy, non-consanguineous parents after two older siblings. Father was 47 years old and mother 40 years old at the proband's birth. Unremarkable family history. Birth measurements 3000 g, 49 cm; no problems of any kind in first year of life.
1 The patient as a young preschool child.
2 As a young schoolgirl.
3–8 At age 12 years and 3 months. Flexion and adduction contractures of the hips with deviation of the thighs to the left; contracted talipes equinovarus. Chromosomal analysis normal.

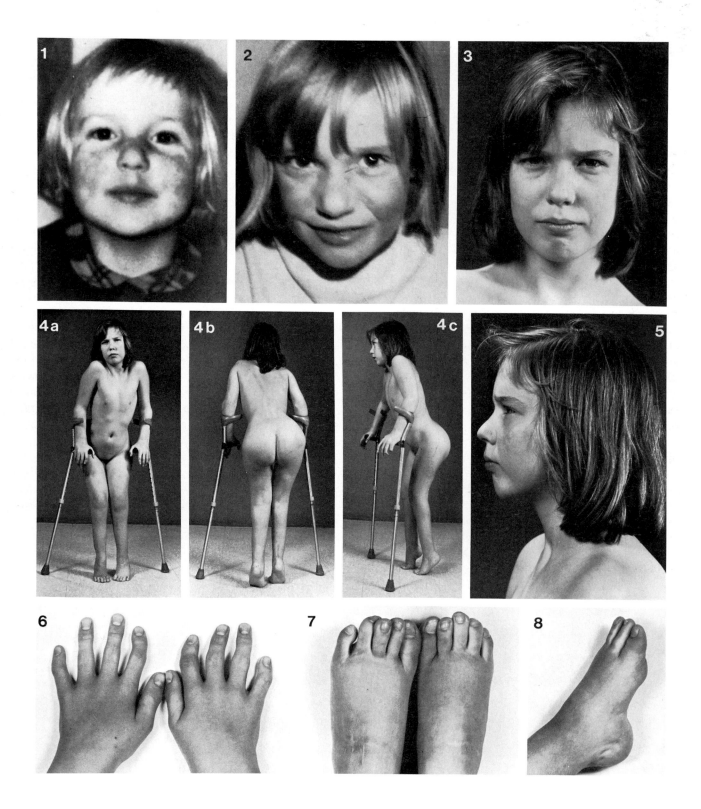

H.-R.W

An achondroplasia-like hereditary condition with micromelic short stature of milder expression.

Main signs:
- Short stature with disproportionately short extremities, which are usually clinically obvious, and broad, short hands (without 'trident' appearance) and feet (1–6). Adult height between 1.25 and 1.55 m.
- Cranium normal or (more frequently) oversized, often with prominent forehead. Bridge of the nose is not low and the facial formation is otherwise essentially normal (1–5).
- Limited movement of the elbows (with regard to full extension and supination). Frequently, increased lumbar lordosis (4b) and genu varus with bow-legs (2, 3, 4a).

Supplementary findings: Radiologically (6 and 7), signs of a somewhat 'attenuated achondroplasia'. Square pelvis with narrow inlet (often leading to dystocia), short and broad femoral necks, disproportionately long fibulae, brachydactyly and so on.

Occasional, usually mild, mental retardation (in approximately 10% of patients).

Manifestation: At birth (length usually approximately 48 cm) and thereafter. Sporadic cases are first noted by family members during the early preschool years.

Aetiology: Hereditary disorder, autosomal dominant, of very variable expression, may even appear very similar to achondroplasia. Also sporadic cases representing new mutations, frequently associated with increased paternal age. Gene locus: short arm of chromosome 4 (4p16.3). Presumed to be an allelic variant of classic achondroplasia.

Frequency: Not particularly rare.

Course, prognosis: Normal life expectancy. Adult height of males between 1.35 and 1.55 m, in females between 1.25 and 1.50 m.

Differential diagnosis: Achondroplasia (*130*; here, typical facial dysmorphism, markedly shortened upper arms, trident hands and so on), metaphyseal chondrodysplasia Schmid type (*145*; here, different radiograph findings) and other forms of short stature.

Treatment: Symptomatic. Possibly growth hormone therapy.
Genetic counselling. Prenatal diagnosis virtually impossible by ultrasound; given a positive family history, can be accomplished by linked DNA markers.

Illustrations:
1–5 Children and adults with hypochondroplasia: a 1-year-old boy; an 11-year-old boy; a mother and daughter; two girls aged 12 and 16 years, respectively.
6 Radiograph of the left hand of a further child at 6 and 13 years.
7 Radiographs of the lower extremities of the girl in 3.

References:
Spranger J W, Langer Jr L O, Wiedemann H-R: *Bone dysplasias. An atlas of constitutional disorders of skeletal development.* Stuttgart and Philadephia: G Fischer and W B Saunders; 1974.
Oberklaid F, Danks M, Jensen F *et al*: Achondroplasia and hypochondroplasia. *J Med Genet* 1979, **16**:140.
Hall Br D, Spranger, J: Hypochondroplasia: clinical and radiological aspects in 39 cases. *Radiology* 1979, **133**:95.
Stoll C, Manini P *et al*: Prenatal diagnosis of hypochondroplasia. *Prenat Diagn* 1985, 5:423–426.
Maroteaux P, Falzon P: Hypochondroplasie. Revue de 80 cas. *Arch Fr Pédiatr* 1988, 45:105–109.
Appan S, Laurent S, Chapman M *et al*: Growth and growth hormone therapy in hypochondroplasia. *Acta Paed Scand* 1990, 79:796–803.
Le Merrer M, Rousseau F *et al*: A gene for achondroplasia-hypochondroplasia maps to chromosome 4p. *Nature Genet* 1994, 6:318–321.

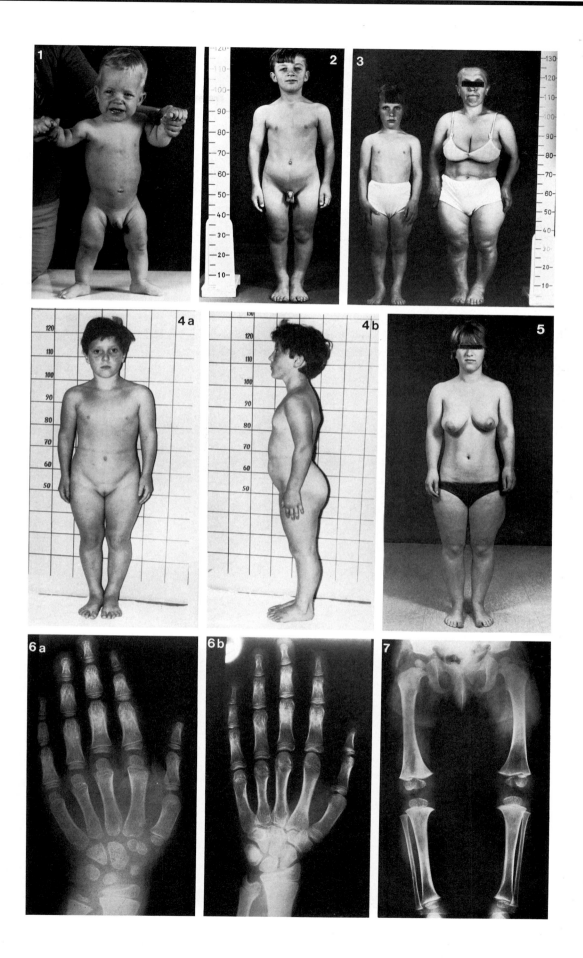

145 Schmid–Type Metaphyseal Chondrodysplasia
(Schmid-Type Dysostosis Metaphysaria)

H.-R.W

An autosomal dominant disorder of short stature, relatively short legs with bowed appearance and a waddling gait, the metaphyses of the long bones appearing similar to pseudorickets on radiographs.

Main signs:
- Short stature with short legs and unremarkable cranium, face, and trunk. Fairly marked bow legs (**1a and b**). Waddling gait. Large joints usually freely mobile. No muscular hypotonia.
- Radiologically, shortening of the long bones with variable rickets-like changes of the metaphyses (but without mineral depletion) especially in the lower extremities, and mostly in the femora (distally greater than proximally). Coxa vara; enlarged epiphyses of the femoral heads in early childhood; short femoral necks (**1c**). Vertebral column not involved.

Supplementary findings: Normal blood and urine analyses.

Manifestations: Second year of life.

Aetiology: Autosomal dominant disorder. Gene locus 6q21-q22.3. Type X collagen structural defect.

Frequency: Low (approximately 55 comparable patients in the literature up to 1988).

Course, prognosis: Favourable. Even though the varus deformity of the lower extremities usually persists, joint function is generally normal. Adult height between 1.30 and 1.60 m.

Differential diagnosis: Syndrome of hereditary vitamin D-resistant rickets and other forms of rickets (*141*), which show appropriate biochemical abnormalities. Cartilage-hair hypoplasia (*147*), Wiedemann–Spranger-type metaphyseal chondrodysplasia (*146*).

Treatment: After closure of the epiphyses, osteotomy to correct the bow legs.
   Vitamin D therapy is contraindicated. Genetic counselling.

Illustrations:
1a–c An affected child at ages 1 year (**a, c**) and 10 years. Micromelic short stature; bowed legs; swelling of some of the joints. Radiograph shows broad, dense metaphyses and irregular borders; separate epiphyseal ossification centres of normal configuration.

References:
Spranger J W, Langer Jr L O, Wiedemann H-R: *Bone dysplasias. An atlas of constitutional disorders of skeletal development.* Stuttgart and Philadephia: G Fischer and W B Saunders; 1974.
Lachman R S, Rimoin D L, Spranger J: Metaphyseal chondrodysplasia, Schmid type... with a review of the literature. *Pediatr Radiol* 1988, 18:93–102.
Dharmavaram R M *et al*: Identification of a mutation in type X4 collagen in a family with Schmid metaphyseal chondrodysplasia. *Hum Mol Genet* 1994, 3:507–510.

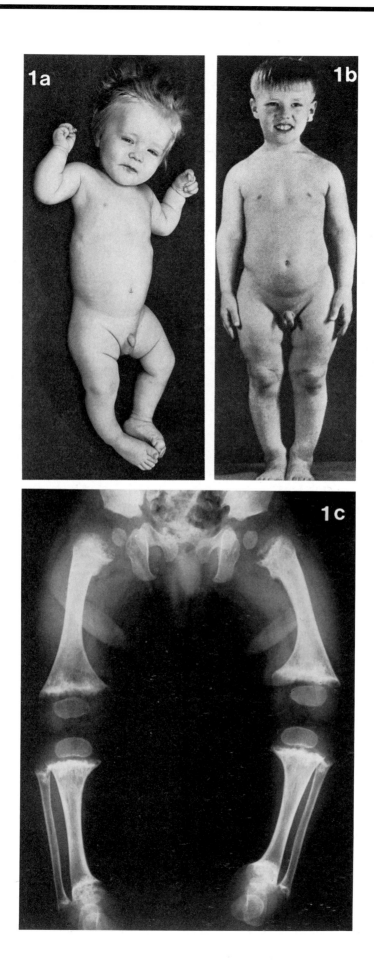

(Metaphyseal Anadysplasia)

H.-R.W

A congenital skeletal dysplasia with micromelic short stature presenting during the first decade of life (the metaphyses of the long bones appearing similar to pseudorickets on radiograph), a somewhat unusual appearance and a good prognosis.

Main signs:

- Congenital disproportionate short stature caused by shortening, especially of the proximal extremities and to bowed legs (1). Short neck (1). Limited movement at the hips; initial swelling of the knees, wrists and ankles.
- Antimongoloid slant of the palpebral fissures (1 and 2).
- Radiologically, marked pseudorachitic structural anomalies of the long bones (3, 7) and on lateral view, deformities of the vertebral bodies in part suggesting a reclining hourglass (5).
- Gradual improvement of proportions, resulting in an unremarkable neck, straightening of the legs, extensive compensation of the initial radiological changes (2, 4, 6, 8) and catch-up of growth.

Supplementary findings: Hypermobility of the shoulder and wrist joints. Unremarkable slender hands and feet. Increased lumbar lordosis.

Somewhat delayed motor development, initially with pronounced waddling gait.

No characteristic metabolic abnormalities.

Manifestation: At birth.

Aetiology: Little doubt of a genetic basis; mode of inheritance not yet completely clear (X-chromosomal?); heterogeneity probable.

Frequency: Low.

Course, prognosis: Favourable. Adult height about normal. Normal life expectancy.

Differential diagnosis: Other metaphyseal chondrodysplasias (Schmid type, *145*), which, however, are easily differentiated because they are usually manifest later in life.

Treatment: Symptomatic.

Illustrations:

1–8 The first child of healthy, tall, well-proportioned, non-consanguineous parents, born 6 weeks prematurely with length 41 cm, birth weight 2000 g (3, 7 at 5 months; 1 at 10 months; 5 at 13 months; 4, 8 at 13 years; 2, 6 at 18 years). Gradual compensation of his growth deficiency during his early school years; adult height 1.66 m.

The proband now has healthy monozygotic twin daughters, aged 14 years, whose appearance closely resembles his own.

References:

Wiedemann H-R, Spranger J: Chondrodysplasia metaphysaria (Dysostosis metaphysaria) — ein neuer Typ? Z *Kinderheilk* 1970, **108**:171.

Maroteaux P, Verloes A, Stanescu V and R: Metaphyseal anadysplasia… Am J Med Genet 1991, **39**:4–10.

Wiedemann H-R: Metaphyseal anadysplasia… Dysmorphol. *Clin Genet* 1992, 6:123–127.

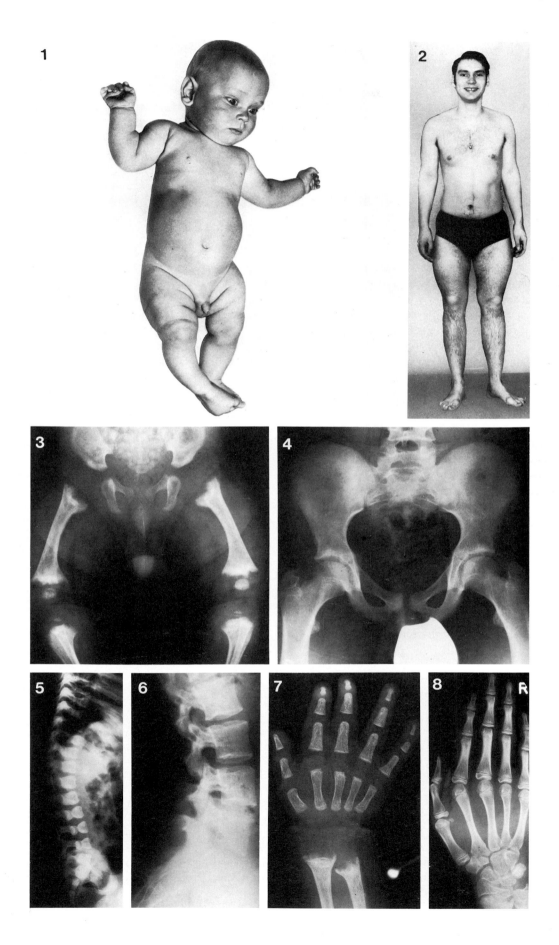

147 Cartilage-Hair Hypoplasia

(Cartilage-Hair Hypoplasia = CHH; Metaphyseal Chondrodysplasia, McKusick Type)

H.-R.W

A hereditary disorder, characteristic when fully expressed, comprising short stature caused by short extremities, combined with fine, sparse hair and short, stubby hands and feet.

Main signs:

- Short stature of the micromelic type with normal cranial and facial configuration (**1a and b**).
- Short, stubby hands and feet (**1a**) with hyperextensible wrist, ankle and finger joints.
- Sparse, fine, light, relatively brittle scalp hair; eyebrows, eyelashes, beard and body hair may show similar characteristics. This sign is not obligatory.

Supplementary findings: Frequently, moderately severe deformity of the thorax and lumbar lordosis. Narrow pelvis. Slightly bowed legs (crura vara). Limited extension at the elbows. Short, sometimes brittle, fingernails and toenails.

Radiologically, shortening and metaphyseal dysplasia of the long bones (**1c**), the metaphyseal irregularities being generally more distinct in the knee region than in the proximal femora. Disproportionately long fibulae, especially distally. At an early age, the distal femoral epiphyses may be large and rounded.

Possible signs of malabsorption in early childhood (tending to improve spontaneously); also Hirschsprung's disease. Severe combined immune defect; T cell defects have been described. Additionally, anaemia.

Decreased intelligence in some patients.

Manifestation: Usually at birth.

Aetiology: Autosomal recessive disorder; very variable expression both within and among families. Possible gene locus 9q13-9q11.

Frequency: Low (apart from special isolates with inbreeding in the USA and Finland).

Course, prognosis: Limited vitality and a decreased average lifespan have been recorded. Adult height between 1.10 and 1.45 m. With pregnancy, caesarian section needed because of narrow pelvis.

Differential diagnosis: Schmid-type metaphyseal chondrodysplasia (*145*) does not show correspondingly short, stubby hands and feet (or nail changes) but shows more pronounced bowing of the legs, radiological abnormalities and a different mode of inheritance.

All forms of rickets can be clinically differentiated from the fully expressed syndrome; in addition, they are easily ruled out biochemically.

Other rare clinical pictures associated with immune deficiency and metaphyseal skeletal anomalies should be considered.

Treatment: Avoidance of smallpox vaccination and, where possible, of exposure to varicella and shingles. Genetic counselling.

Illustrations:

1a–d A now 23-year-old patient with the full picture of cartilage-hair hypoplasia. Short stature since birth; height now 130 cm. Short, broad hands with short nails. Scalp hair short, brittle, thin, sparse and blond. Secondary hair growth sparse. Hyperextensible wrists; limited extension of the elbows.

1c Knee joints with moderate metaphyseal irregularities at 8 years of age.

1d The same joint at 23 years. Both show hypoplasia of the lateral portion of the femoral epiphysis.

References:

Wiedemann H-R, Spranger J, Kosenow W: Knorpel-Haar-Hypoplasie. *Arch Kinderheilk* 1967, **176**:74.
Spranger J W, Langer Jr L O, Wiedemann H-R: *Bone dysplasias. An atlas of constitutional disorders of skeletal development.* Stuttgart and Philadephia: G Fischer and W B Saunders; 1974.
Trojak J E, Polmar S H *et al*: Immunologic studies of cartilage hair hypoplasia... *Johns Hopkins Med J* 1981, **148**:157–164.
van den Burgt I *et al*: Cartilage hair hypoplasia... review. *Am J Med Genet* 1991, **41**:371–380.
Le Merrer M, Maroteaux F: Cartilage hair hypoplasia in infancy... *Eur J Pediatr* 1991, **150**:847–851.
Mäkitie O *et al*: Skeletal growth in cartilage-hair hypoplasia. *Pediatr Radiol* 1992, **22**:434–439.
Mäkitie O, Kaitila I: Cartilage-hair hypoplasia... in 108 Finnish patients. *Eur J Pediatr* 1993, **152**:211–217.

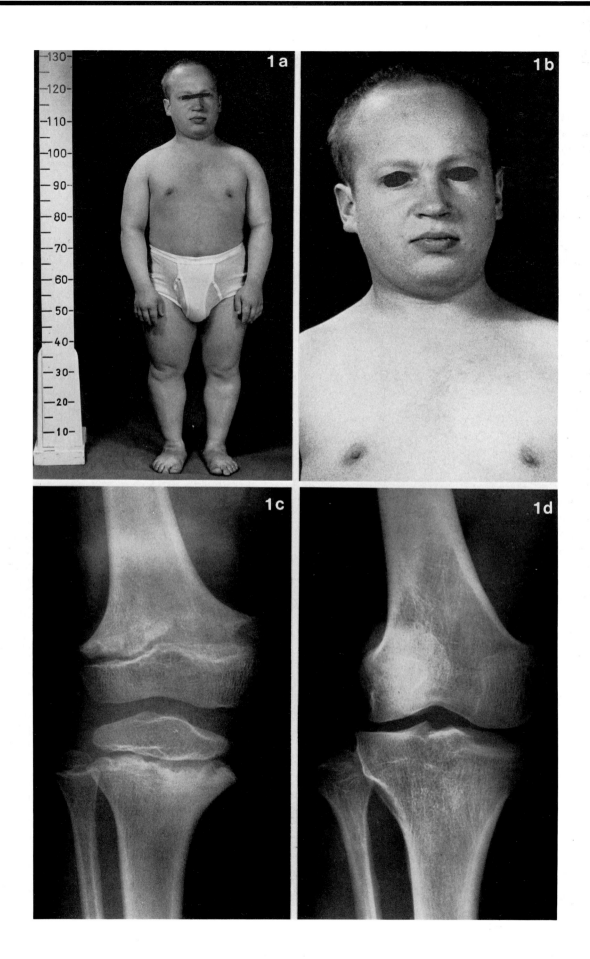

148 Pseudo-achondroplasia
(Spondylo-epiphyseal Dysplasia(s), Pseudo-achondroplastic Type)

H.-R.W/J.K.

In appearance, achondroplasia-like short stature but manifest postnatally, with normal craniofacial skeleton and a marked disorder of epiphyseal ossification on radiograph.

Main signs:
Marked micromelic short stature with disproportionately long trunk. Craniofacial skeleton normal. Lumbar hyperlordosis. Genu valgus or bowing of the legs. Hypermobility of most joints except the elbows (possibly also the hips and the knees) (1–3).

Supplementary findings: Weakness of joint capsules and ligaments. Not infrequently, development of scoliosis.
Normal mental development.
Radiological changes of the vertebral bodies: severe developmental defects of the head of the femur and other epimetaphyseal areas (4 and 5).

Manifestation: During the second year of life or later with the onset of a waddling gait and growth retardation (with corresponding radiological changes).

Aetiology: Monogenic hereditary disorder with severe and mild forms; heterogeneity. Apparently, there are autosomal dominant and perhaps also autosomal recessive types, each with a mild and severe form. These cannot be differentiated at present, neither clinically, radiologically, nor biochemically, except that the growth deficiency would be more marked in the autosomal recessive form. Possible gene localized to the long arm of chromosome 19 (19q12).

Frequency: Not particularly low.

Course, prognosis: Normal life expectancy. Adult height between 0.90 and 1.40 m. Early development of arthritis, especially of the hip and knee joints.

Differential diagnosis: Achondroplasia (*130*), manifested congenitally, abnormal cranial configuration and so on; congenital spondylo-epiphyseal dysplasia (*136*), manifestation at birth; hypochondroplasia (*144*).

Treatment: Symptomatic and orthopaedic. Surgical correction of bow legs towards the end of the growth period. Arthroplasties may be needed eventually.
Psychological support with the best possible education and vocational training.
Genetic counselling.

Illustrations:
1 A 14-year-old boy.
2 and 3 Two girls of about the same age. Height of each well below the third percentile (height difference compared with the average for age: 40 cm for the girl in 3; and 70 cm for the boy in 1).
The boy in 1 was normally proportioned as an infant and could walk without support at 9 months. Manifestation at 2 years.
4 and 5 Radiographs of the child in 3.

References:
Kapits S E, Lindstrom J A, McKusick V A: Pseudoachondroplastic dysplasia: pathodynamics and management. *Birth Defects Orig Art Ser* 1974, **10/12**:341.
Spranger J W, Langer Jr L O, Wiedemann H-R: *Bone dysplasias. An atlas of constitutional disorders of skeletal development.* Stuttgart and Philadephia: G Fischer and W B Saunders; 1974.
Hall J: Pseudoachondroplasia. *Birth Defects Orig Art Ser* 1975, **11/6**:187.
Heselson N G, Cremin B J, Beighton P: Pseudoachondroplasia, a report of 13 cases. *Br J Radiol* 1977, **50**:473.
Maroteaux P, Stanescu R, Stanescu V *et al*: The mild form of pseudoachondroplasia. *Eur J Pediatr* 1980, **133**:227.
Horton W A, Hall J G, Scott C I *et al*: Growth curves for height for diastrophic dysplasia, spondyloepiphyseal dysplasia congenita, and pseudoachondroplasia. *Am J Dis Child* 1982, **136**:316.
Stanescu V, Maroteaux P *et al*: The biochemical defect of pseudoachondroplasia. *Eur J Pediatr* 1982, **138**:221–225.
Young I D, Moore J R: Severe pseudoachondroplasia with parental consanguinity. *J Med Genet* 1985, **22**:150–153.
Wynne-Davies R, Hall C M *et al*: Pseudoachondroplasia:... comparison of autosomal dominant and recessive types... review of 32 patients... *J Med Genet* 1986, **23**:425–434.
Hall J G, Dorst J P *et al*: Gonadal mosaicism in pseudoachondroplasia. *Am J Med Genet* 1987, **28**:143–151.
Nores J M, Maroteaux P: Evolution sur 40 ans d'un cas de pseudo-achondroplasie. *Presse Méd* 1988, **17**(43):2283–2286.
Byers P H: Molecular heterogeneity in chondrodysplasias (Editorial). *Am J Med Genet* 1989, **45**:1–4.
Hecht J T *et al*: Exclusion of human proteoglycan link protein... and type II collagen... genes in pseudoachondroplasia. *Am J Med Genet* 1992, **44**:420–424.
Langer L O *et al*: Patient with double heterozygosity for achondroplasia and pseudoachondroplasia... *Am J Med Genet* 1993, **47**:772–781.
Stanescu V *et al*: Non-collagenous protein screening in the human chondrodysplasias... *Am J Med Genet* 1994, **51**:22–28.
Woods C G *et al*: Two sibs are double heterozygotes for achondroplasia and pseudoachondroplastic dwarfism. *J Med Genet* 1994, **31**:565–569.

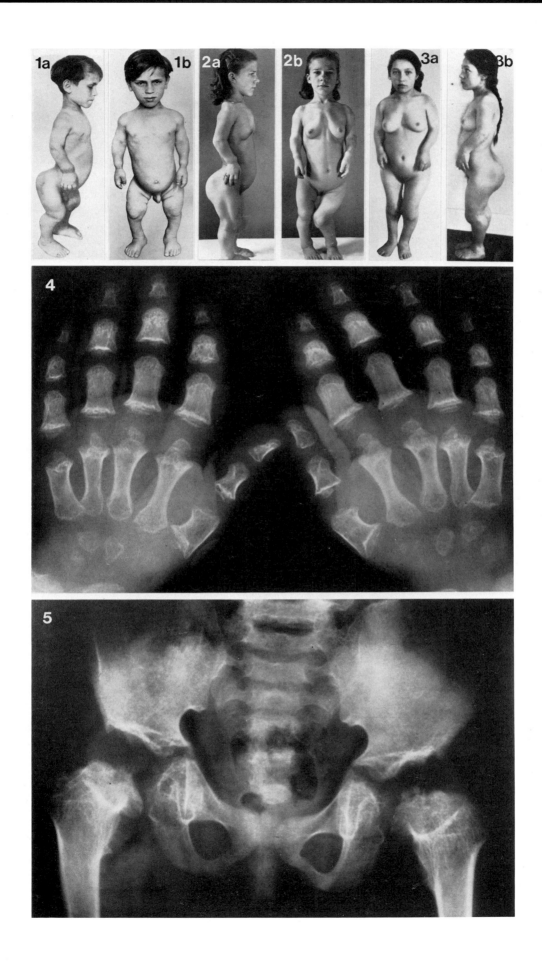

305

149 Progeria

(Gilford Syndrome, Hutchinson–Gilford Syndrome)

H.-R.W

A highly characteristic syndrome comprising postnatal growth deficiency and premature 'ageing'.

Main signs:
- Birth weight approximately 2500 g. Growth deficiency manifesting after the first year of life.
- Concomitant, progressive 'ageing': loss of hair (**3–5**), of subcutaneous fat, including that of the earlobes (**7 and 8**) and of the normal thickness and elasticity of the skin; flexion contractures of the large joints (**1, 6**) and the finger joints; dystrophy of the nails (**9**); prominent scalp veins (**4, 5, 7, 8**). Development of a sharp, beak-like nose jutting out from the small face with receding chin, slightly protruding eyes and a relatively large cranium, defining a 'bird face' (**1, 7**), protruding abdomen.

Supplementary findings: In some patients, skin changes of diffuse scleroderma.

Radiologically, hypoplastic skeleton with persistence of the anterior fontanelle, atrophy of the lateral portions of the clavicles and of the terminal phalanges (acromicria, **10**); coxa valga.

Delayed and irregular dentition.

Absence or delay of sexual development (**1, 6**). High, squeaky voice.

Intelligence in the normal range.

Insulin resistance (possible post receptor defect), increased metabolic rate, serum lipid and collagen anomalies. No growth hormone deficiency.

Aetiology: The usually sporadic occurrence, not infrequently associated with increased paternal age, can only suggest autosomal dominant new mutations. Several pairs of affected siblings (with or without parental consanguinity) may point to an autosomal recessive gene or, rather, to germline mosaicism. The localization of a progeria gene on chromosome 1 has been assumed.

Frequency: Very low; approximately one out of 250 000 live births estimated. Over 100 patients have been described to date (three of them in Germany).

Course, prognosis: Attained height little more than 1.15 m, attained weight barely 15 kg. Usually premature development of atherosclerosis. Death usually in the second decade of life as a result of atherosclerotic complications (coronary occlusion).

Diagnosis, differential diagnosis: Fully expressed clinical picture unmistakable. Rule out the Cockayne (*89*), Hallermann–Streiff–François (*301*), congenital cutis laxa (*152*), de Barsy (*153*) and Wiedemann–Rautenstrauch (*150*) syndromes and mandibulo-acral dysplasia.

Treatment: Only symptomatic treatment is possible (psychological support, possibly a wig and so on)

Illustrations:

1 Progeria in a 17-year-old from H. Gilford (1897/1904).
2–10 A German patient at 10 months (**2**); 18 months (**3**), demonstrating growth deficiency, loss of hair; 3 years and 6 months (**4**); 7 years and 6 months (**5**) and 14 years and 6 months (**6–10**).
6 Height of a 7 year old; no signs of puberty; thin, tense, yellow–brownish, irregularly hyperpigmented skin; sclerosed radial artery; calcification of one of the heart valves; cardiac death at 15 years and 9 months.

References:

Wiedemann H-R: Syndrome mit besonderem 'Altersaspekt': Progerie (Hutchinson–Gilford–Syndrom). *Handbuch der Kinderheilkunde* 1971, 1(1):828.
De Busk F L: The Hutchinson–Gilford progeria syndrome. *J Pediatr 1972*, 80:697.
Brown W T, Darlington G J, Arnold A *et al*: Detection of HLA antigens on progeria syndrome fibroblasts. *Clin Genet* 1980, 17:213.
Dyck J D *et al*: Management of coronary artery disease in Hutchinson–Gilford syndrome. *J Pediatr* 1987, 111:407–410.
Wiedemann H-R: Progeria. In: *Neurocutaneous diseases.* Gomez, M. R. (ed.). Boston: Butterworth 1987; 247–253.
Khalifa M M: Hutchinson–Gilford progeria syndrome... autosomal recessive inheritance. *Clin Genet* 1989, 35:125–132.
Badame A J: Progeria. *Arch Dermatol* 1990, 125:540–544.
Brown W T *et al*: Hutchinson–Gilford syndrome... (Abstract). *Am J Hum Genet* 1990, 47(Suppl.A):50.
Yu Q X, Zeng L H: Progeria... *J Oral Pathol Med* 1991, 20:860–888.
Wagle W A *et al*: Cerebral infarction in progeria. *Pediatr Neurol* 1992, 8:476–477.

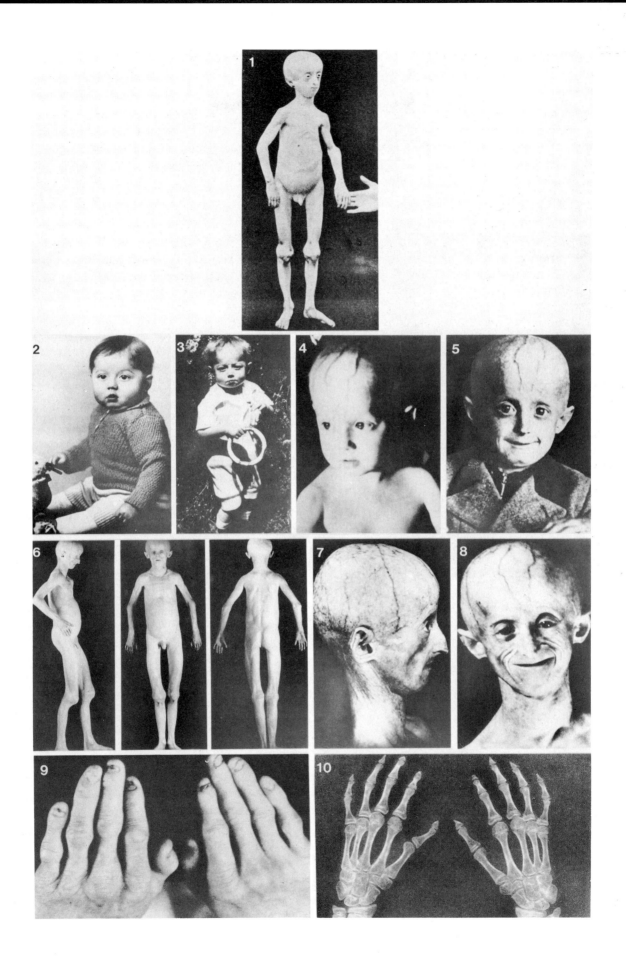

150 Congenital Pseudohydrocephalic Progeroid Syndrome
(Neonatal Progeroid Syndrome, Wiedemann–Rautenstrauch Syndrome)

H.-R.W

A congenitally manifest syndrome comprising prenatal and postnatal growth deficiency, pseudohydrocephalus, small senile-appearing face, 'congenital teeth' and extensive deficiency of adipose tissue.

Main signs:
- Small, somewhat triangular, senile-appearing face and hydrocephaloid cranium with wide-open sutures, persistent anterior fontanelle, prominent venous markings, and sparse scalp hair (1–9). Relatively low-set ears, deep-set eyes, sparse eyebrows and eyelashes (possible entropion). Small upper jaw, protruding chin; 'congenital' incisors.
- Relatively large hands and feet or fingers and toes.
- Striking generalized deficiency of subcutaneous adipose tissue, apart from the possible development of paradoxical caudal accumulations of adipose tissue on the buttocks and flanks or in the anogenital area (10–13).

Supplementary findings: Prenatal dystrophy with birth weights of 2100–2500 g and lengths of 45 to 49 cm, birth at term. Failure to thrive. Deficient growth and development. Loss of both congenital and newly erupted dysplastic teeth.

Progressive development of a beak-like nose in infancy (4–6).

Delayed motor development; appearance of neurological signs such as ataxia, dysmetria and nystagmus has been observed in a number of patients. Mental development generally severely impaired but possibly within normal limits.

Radiologically, possible congenital ossification disorders with tendency to normalize.

Manifestation: At birth.

Aetiology: Hereditary defect with presumably autosomal recessive transmission (two pairs of affected siblings; one child of a consanguineous marriage).

Frequency: Extremely low; to date, barely a dozen published reports; a number of further patients, thought to have this syndrome, have been reported to us.

Course, prognosis: Mainly dependent on the presence and severity of a mental or neurological impairment. There are still no truly long-term observations.

Differential diagnosis: Clinical differentiation of Hallermann–Streiff–François syndrome (301) and congenital generalized lipodystrophy (155) is not difficult. Hutchinson–Gilford syndrome, the true progeria (149), is not as a rule manifest congenitally. The Silver–Russell (82) and de Barsy (153) syndromes should also be considered.

Treatment: Symptomatic.

Illustrations:
1–3 Three different children, all at just a few weeks of age.
4–6 The development of a somewhat beak-like nose (4 and 5: the same child at ages 6 weeks and 8 months, respectively).
7–9 Three children at age 8 months.
10–13 Absent subcutaneous adipose tissue, except for paradoxical accumulations of fat caudally, the latter especially apparent in 13.
(1, 7, 8, 11 from Rautenstrauch et al.)
14 and 15 A 3-week-old female infant: progeroid appearance, pseudohydrocephalus.
16 Thin, atrophic skin through which the vessels are visible.
17 Congenital camptodactyly.

References:
Rautenstrauch T, Snigula F et al: Progeria: a cell culture study and clinical report of familial incidence. Eur J Pediatr 1977, 124:101.
Wiedemann H-R: An unidentified neo-natal progeroid syndrome: follow-up report. Eur J Pediatr 1979, 130:65.
Devos E A, Leroy J G et al: The Wiedemann–Rautenstrauch or neonatal progeroid syndrome. Eur J Pediatr 1981, 136:245.
Snigula F, Rautenstrauch T: A new neonatal progeroid syndrome. Eur J Pediatr 1981, 136:325.
Leung A K C: Natal teeth. AJDC 1986, 140:249–251.
Ohashi H, Eguchi T et al: Neonatal progeroid syndrome... Jpn J Hum Genet 1987, 32:253–256.
Rudin C, Thommen L et al: The neonatal pseudohydrocephalic progeroid syndrome (Wiedemann-Rautenstrauch). Eur J Pediatr 1988, 147:433–438.
Hagadorn J T, Wilson W G et al: Neonatal progeroid syndrome: more than one disease? Am J Med Genet 1990, 35:91–94.
Toriello H V: Wiedemann–Rautenstrauch syndrome. J Med Genet 1990, 27:256–257.
Castiñeyra G, Panal M et al: Two sibs with Wiedemann–Rautenstrauch syndrome: possibilities of prenatal diagnosis by ultrasound. J Med Genet 1992, 29:434–436.
Obregon M G, Bergami G L et al: Radiographic findings in Wiedemann–Rautenstrauch syndrome. Pediatr Radiol 1992, 22:474–475.

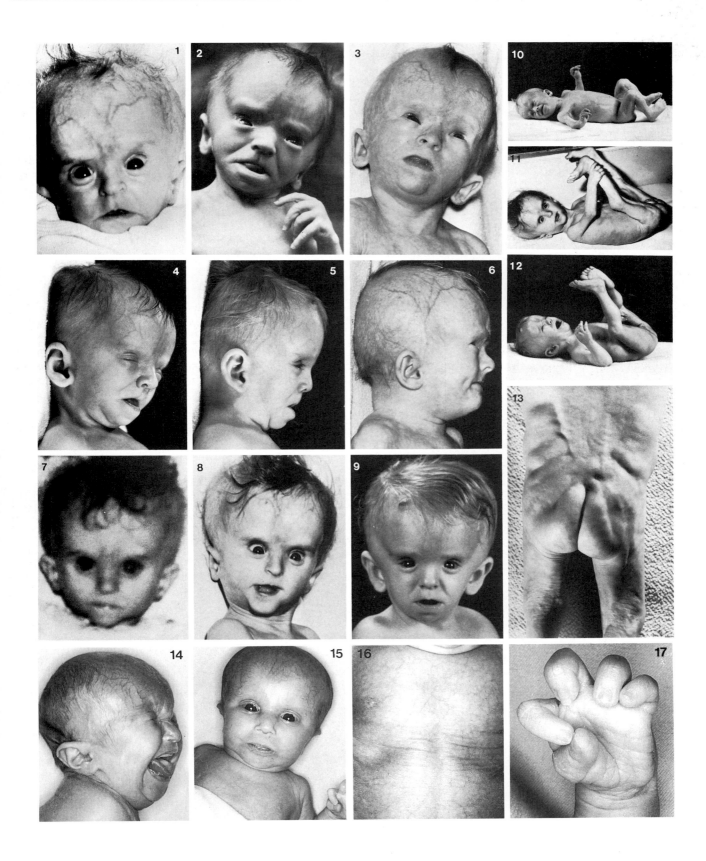

151 Petty–Laxova–Wiedemann Progeroid Syndrome

H.-R.W

A genetically determined, early-onset progeroid syndrome comprising prenatal and postnatal growth deficiency, deficiency of adipose tissue and cutis laxa, umbilical hernia, poor hair growth, wide-open anterior fontanelle, hypoplastic distal phalanges with hypoplasia of the nails.

Main signs:
- Growth deficiency with prenatal onset.
- Progeroid facies with wide-open, persistent anterior fontanelle, wide cranial sutures, protruding cranial veins, sparse hair on the head.
- Generalized reduction of subcutaneous adipose tissue; cutis laxa.
- Severe umbilical hernia.
- Short distal phalanges with hypoplastic or aplastic nails.

Supplementary findings: Relatively small face with broad forehead; small, low-set ears. Short stature.

Manifestation: At birth and thereafter.

Aetiology: Genetic determination virtually beyond doubt; nothing further known.

Frequency: Low. Only three patients known to date, all of them females.

Course, prognosis: Normal to exceptional mental and motor development without neurological abnormalities. The oldest proband died of an undetermined cause approaching her 50th year.

Differential diagnosis: In newborns, one would have to consider Wiedemann–Rautenstrauch syndrome (150).

Treatment: Symptomatic.

Illustrations:
1a and b The characteristically affected patient observed in Germany between 1943 and 1990.
2a and b An extremely similar patient observed in the USA.
1a, 2a, 2b from: E. M. Petty, R. Laxova, H.-R. Wiedemann, Previously unrecognized congenital progeroid disorder. *Am J Med Genet* 1990, 35:383–387.

References:
Petty E M, Laxova R, Wiedemann H-R: Previously unrecognized congenital progeroid disorder. *Am J Med Genet* 1990, 35:383–387.
Wiedemann H-R: Newly recognized congenital progeroid disorder (Letter). *Am J Med Genet* 1992, 42:857.

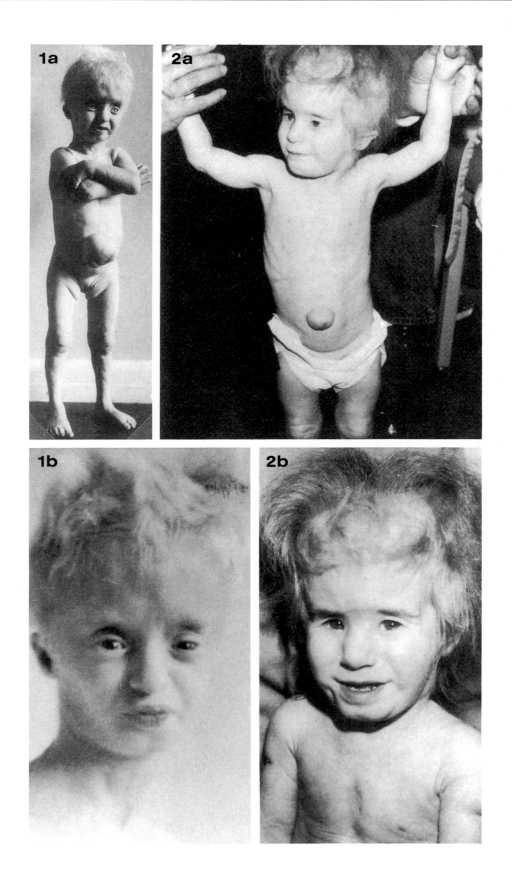

152 Congenital Cutis Laxa Syndrome
(Dermatochalasis Connata)

H.-R.W

A hereditary syndrome comprising congenital cutis laxa with corresponding 'aged' appearance, which may be associated with numerous other defects.

Main signs:
Generalized cutis laxa: too much skin, soft, slack, pendulous and wrinkled (**1–3**), giving (especially in the face) the impression of premature ageing, even senility (**3a**) and possibly a grotesque appearance.

Supplementary findings: Depending on the biological type, the following may be present: congenital microsomia; postnatal growth retardation and general developmental delay; deficiency of subcutaneous adipose tissue and muscle weakness; hypertelorism (**3a**); micrognathia (**1c**) and other skeletal dysmorphism or deformities; delayed closure of the fontanelles; dislocation of the hips; generalized hyperextensibility of the joints and tendency to dislocation. Internal changes may include laxity of the vocal cords, emphysema of the lungs, vascular wall aneurysms and vascular stenoses, multiple gastro-intestinal diverticula, hernias and prolapses. Thus, laxity of the skin may be only one, external sign of a systemic mesenchymal disorder.

Manifestation: At birth and thereafter.

Aetiology: The syndrome (a still poorly delineated 'umbrella' term) comprises a number of monogenic hereditary disorders; thus, heterogeneity. There are probably several autosomal recessive types of different expression and severity, a milder autosomal dominant type and probably also X-linked types.

Formal pathogenesis: Histologically, deficiencies of elastic fibres have been demonstrated repeatedly, partly as a fairly generalized elastolysis (with degeneration and decomposition of elastic fibers and collagen disorders). In many patients, defects of various enzymes or enzyme inhibitors have been demonstrated or abnormalities of copper metabolism, with the basic defect still unknown.

Frequency: Low. Nevertheless, there are well over 100 reports in the literature.

Course, prognosis: Dependent on the type. Potentially early lethal course especially with the recessive types (e.g. as a result of cor pulmonale).

Differential diagnosis: De Barsy syndrome (*153*), which is also regarded as a subtype of cutis laxa. Certain patients from the broad field of the Ehlers–Danlos syndrome (*203*) and others.

Treatment: The use of cosmetic plastic surgery in patients with mild forms of the disorder should be carefully considered.
  Genetic counselling.

Illustrations:
1–3 A congenitally undersized 6-year-old boy (his firstborn brother died *post partum* with the identical clinical picture). Growth deficiency of approximately 15%; markedly delayed closure of the fontanelles; bilateral dislocated hips; generalized weakness of the ligaments, capsules and muscles with further dislocations. Hypoplasia of the iris, tortuous fundal vessels. Sudden death at age 7 years.

References:
Wiedemann H-R: Über einige progeroide Krankheitsbilder und deren diagnostische Einordnung. *Z Kinderheilk* 1969, **107**:91.
Beighton P: Cutix laxa. A heterogenous disorder. *Birth Defects Orig Art Ser* 1974, **10**:126.
Wilsch L, Schmid G, Haneke E: Spätmanifeste Dermatochalasis. *Dtsch med Wschr* 1977, **102**:1451.
Agha A, Sakati N O *et al*: Two forms of cutis laxa presenting in the newborn period. *Acta Paed Scand* 1978, **67**:775.
Sakati N O, Nyhan W L: Congenital cutis laxa and osteoporosis. *AJDC* 1983, **137**:452–454.
Sakati N O, Nyhan W L *et al*: Syndrome of cutis laxa, ligamentous laxity, and delayed development. *Pediatrics* 1984, **72**:903–904.
Fitzsimmons J S, Fitzsimmons E M *et al*: Variable clinical presentation of cutis laxa. *Clin Genet* 1985, **28**:284–295.
Allanson J, Austin W *et al*: Congenital cutis laxa with retardation of growth and motor development... *Clin Genet* 1986, **29**:133–136.
Gardner L I, Sanders-Fay K *et al*: Congenital cutis laxa syndrome... *Arch Dermatol* 1986, **122**:1241–1243.
Rogers J, Danks D: Congenital cutis laxa. *Clin Genet* 1986, **30**:345.
Patton M A, Tolmie J *et al*: Congenital cutis laxa... *J Med Genet* 1987, **24**:556–561.
Taieb A, Aumailley M *et al*: Collagen studies in congenital cutis laxa. *Arch Dermatol Res* 1987, **279**:308–314.
Maldergem L van, Vamos E *et al*: Severe congenital cutis laxa with pulmonary emphysema... *Am J Med Genet* 1988, **31**:455–464.
Goldblatt J, Wallis C *et al*: Cutis laxa... Dysmorphol. *Clin Genet* 1988, **1**:142–144.
Chabrolle J P, Caillez D *et al*: Cutis laxa... *Arch Fr Péd* 1989, **46**:129–132.
Ogur G *et al*: Syndrome of congenital cutis laxa... *Am J Med Genet* 1990, **37**, 6–9.
Damkier *et al*: Cutis laxa: autosomal-dominant inheritance... *Clin Genet* 1991, **39**:321–329.
Biver A, Rijcke De S *et al*: Congenital cutis laxa with ligamentous laxity and delayed development... *Clin Genet* 1994, **42**:318–322.
Davies S, Hughes H E: Costello syndrome: natural history and differential diagnosis of cutis laxa. *J Med Genet* 1994, **31**:486–489.
Imaizumi K *et al*: Male with type II autosomal recessive cutis laxa. *Clin Genet* 1994, **45**:40–43.

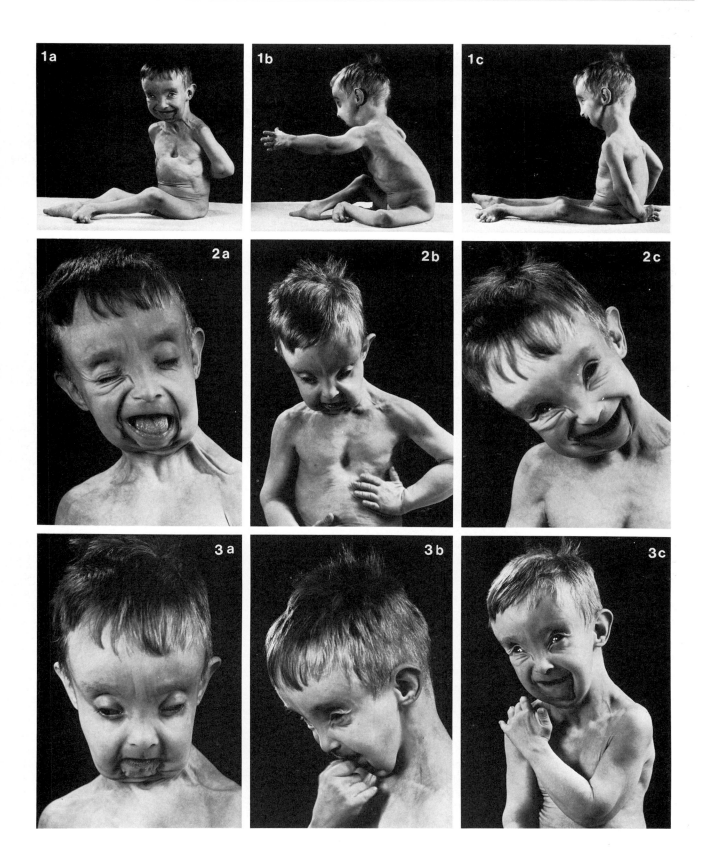

153 De Barsy Syndrome

An autosomal recessive progeroid syndrome with progressive mental impairment, cutis laxa, atrophy of the skin, decrease of subcutaneous adipose tissue, hyperextensibility of the small joints, eye changes and short stature.

Main signs:
- Postnatal onset of growth deficiency.
- Progeroid facies with pronounced nasolabial folds, decrease of subcutaneous adipose tissue,
- Large, dysplastic, prominent ears.
- Corneal clouding, cataract.
- Cutis laxa, skin atrophy with pigment anomalies.
- Mental impairment.

Supplementary findings: Thin lips, hyperextensibility of the small joints, muscular hypotonia with increased tendon reflexes, accentuation of the mid-forehead, microcephaly, short stature, hypertrichosis, synophrys.

Manifestation: Corneal clouding present at birth; cutis laxa apparent by 6 months of age (at the latest).

Aetiology: Autosomal recessive disorder. Reduced elastin synthesis.

Frequency: Low. To date only seven isolated patients and three families reported (with four, three and two affected siblings, respectively).

Course, prognosis: Progressive mental impairment leading to helplessness and confinement to bed.

Differential diagnosis: Can be readily differentiated from Berardinelli–Seip progressive lipodystrophy (*155*), Hutchinson–Gilford progeria (*149*), Wiedemann-–Rautenstrauch neonatal progeroid syndrome (*150*), Cockayne syndrome (*89*), Hallermann–Streiff syndrome (*301*) and cutis laxa syndrome (*152*).

Treatment: Symptomatic.

Illustrations:
1–4 Siblings.
1a and b A 6-month-old male infant; bilateral corneal clouding, hyperelastic, wrinkled atrophic skin.
2 His sister aged 7 years and 6 months, who has had corneal surgery; hypertrichosis; hyperextensibility of the small joints; thin, hyperpigmented atrophic skin.
3 Their 10-year-old sister, the same appearance; mental impairment.
4a and b Their 20-year-old brother; very marked signs of skin ageing; distinct mental impairment.

References:
Kunze J, Majewski F, Montgomery P *et al*: De Barsy syndrome — an autosomal recessive progeroid syndrome. *Eur J Pediatr* 1985, **144**:348–354.
Pontz B F *et al*: Biochemical, morphological and immunological findings in a patient with cutis laxa-associated inborn disorder (De Barsy syndrome). *Eur J Pediatr* 1986, **145**:428–434.
Karnes P S, Shamban A T, Olsen D R, Fazio M J, Falk R E: De Barsy syndrome: report of a case, literature review, and elastin gene expression studies of the skin. *Am J Med Genet* 1992, **42**:29–34.
Freund S, Palitzsch D: De-Barsy–Syndrom. *Monatsschr Kinderheilkd* 1994, **142**:588–591 .

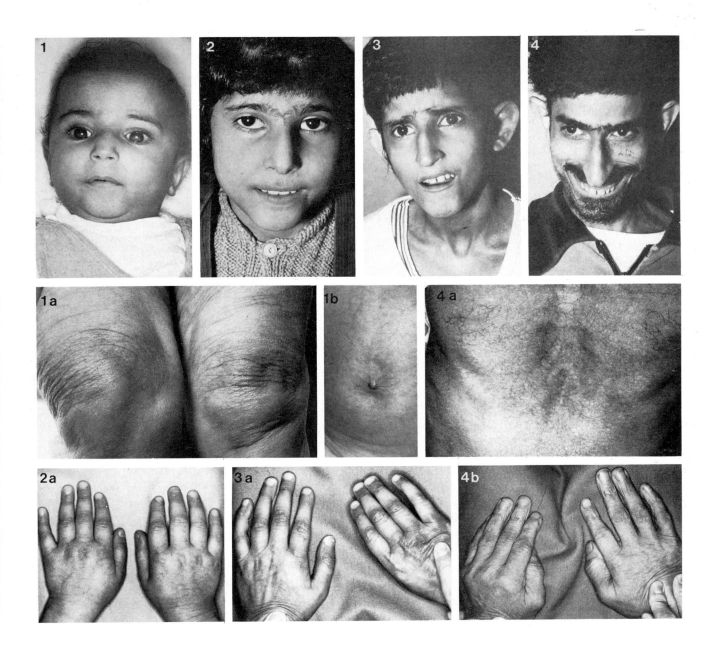

H.-R.W

A syndrome of elderly appearance, extremely lean build, sparse hair growth, joint abnormalities, cardiovascular anomalies and delayed maturation.

Main signs:
- Narrow face, appearing generally 'too old', with hypotelorism, short palpebral fissures; somewhat deep-set eyes; prominent, narrow, slightly aquiline nose; prominent ears; high palate and microretrognathia, particularly in infancy (1–3, 5, 6). Dimpled chin (2, 5).
- Premature closure of the fontanelles with the cranium remaining generally small (52.5 cm at 14 years). Mental development normal for age.
- Extremely sparse development of scalp hair, eyebrows and eyelashes during infancy (1–3). Subsequently also, relatively thin and delicate hair growth; at 14 years still almost no body hair and a deficiency of other signs of maturity (4–6).
- Markedly poor development of musculature and subcutaneous adipose tissue (this 14-year-old boy of normal height (1.60 m) weighs only 35 kg).
- Knee and elbow joints not fully extensible since birth; other large joints hyperextensible. Unusually long fingers and toes, especially in infancy (7 and 8), with 'acrogeria' (7–9); at 14 years, slight flexion contractures of the distally tapered distal phalanges of the fingers. Asymmetrically elevated shoulders with prominent scapulae; increased thoracic kyphosis. Dimples over most of the large joints.
- Cardiac anomaly (ventricular septal defect, subvalvular pulmonary stenosis, both surgically corrected at 14 years, pulmonary vascular anomalies); no decrease of exercise tolerance.

Supplementary findings: Ophthalmological examination normal.

Radiologically, no skeletal malformations; slightly delayed ossification. Blood chemistries normal. Karyotype 46 XY.

Unilateral cryptorchidism.

Manifestation: At birth.

Aetiology: Unknown.

Course, prognosis: Apparently favourable.

Differential diagnosis: Many similarities with the observation of Ruvalcaba *et al*, however, the progeroid manifestations occurred considerably later in their patients.

Note: A child closely resembling my proband was reported to me by F. Majewski in 1993.

Treatment: Symptomatic.

Illustrations:
1–9 The second child of young, healthy, apparently non-consanguineous parents (first child unremarkable). Pregnancy normal; birth at term with normal measurements.
1–3, 7, 8 The proband at age 6 months;
4–6, 9 At age 14 years.
2 The remainder of an ossified cephalohaematoma on the left.

References:
Ruvalcaba R H A, Churesigaew S, Myhre S A *et al*: Children who age rapidly — Progeroid syndromes. *Clin Pediatr* 1977, 16:248.

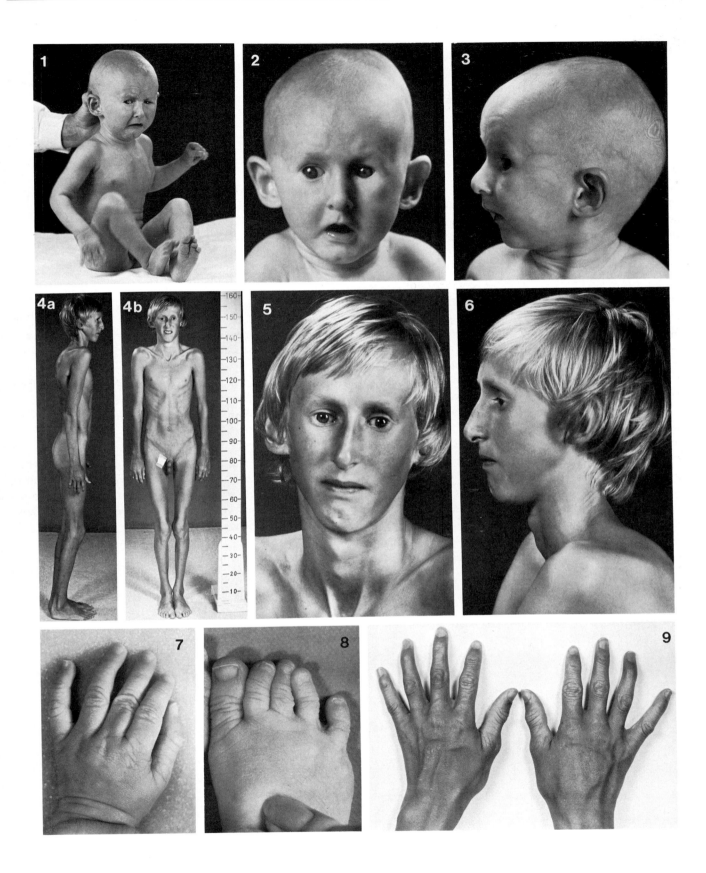

155 Congenital Generalized Lipodystrophy
(Berardinelli–Seip Syndrome)

H.-R.W

A hereditary disorder with generalized deficiency of adipose tissue beginning at an early age, muscular hypertrophy, tall stature, acromegaly, encephalopathy and other anomalies.

Main signs:
- Generalized lipoatrophy (**1 and 2**).
- Muscular hypertrophy, possibly giving the child an athletic appearance.
- Hyperpigmentation, acanthosis nigricans; overabundant curly scalp hair (**2**) or generalized hypertrichosis; dilated cutaneous veins (**1b, 2b**).
- Long or macrosomic at birth or several years of postnatal tall stature. Acromegaloid facial dysmorphism, relatively large ears, abnormally large hands and feet (**1b, 2b**); possible hypertrophy of the penis or clitoris, and polycystic ovaries.
- 'Encephalopathy' of a nonprogressive nature, with approximately 50% of the patients showing mental retardation (mild to severe) associated with demonstrable partial dilation of the cerebral ventricles or cisterns.

Supplementary findings: Hepatomegaly (fatty liver) in most patients; cardiomegaly, nephromegaly also frequent.

Postnatal tall stature is accompanied by corresponding acceleration of ossification and dentition.

Increased metabolic rate. Disorder of fat and carbohydrate metabolism; extreme insulin resistance, hyperlipaemia.

Development of nonketotic diabetes mellitus with lipoatrophy (starting at about the beginning of the second decade of life).

Manifestation: At birth and thereafter.

Aetiology: Autosomal recessive disorder. Possible insulin receptor defect.

Frequency: Low (fewer than 100 observations in the literature).

Course, prognosis: Premature closure of the epiphyses; normal adult height. Onset of puberty at about the expected age. Prognosis complicated by hypertrophic cardiomyopathy and possibility of diabetic vascular complications.

Differential diagnosis: Acquired generalized lipodystrophy; partial lipodystrophies.

Treatment: Symptomatic, including psychological support and, when indicated, cosmetic measures.
Genetic counselling.

Illustrations:
1 and 2 Typically affected siblings (15 months and 6 years old). Tall stature; bone age of the 6 year old equivalent to a 12 year old; hepatomegaly in both children; enlargement of the third ventricle and the basal cistern respectively on pneumo-encephalogram.

References:
Seip M: Generalized lipodystrophy. *Ergeb Inn Med Kinderheilk N F* 1971, 31:59.
Wiedemann H-R: Dienzephale Syndrome des Kindesalters. *Pädiat Prax* 1972, 11:95.
Oseid S, Beck-Nielsen H *et al*: Decreased binding of insulin to its receptor in... congenital generalized lipodystrophy. *N Engl J Med* 1977, 296:245–248.
Huseman C A, Johanson A J *et al*: Congenital lipodystrophy... with polycystic ovarian disease. *J Pediatr* 1979, 95:72–74.
Bjørnstad P G, Semb B K H *et al*: Echocardiographic assessment of cardiac function and morphology in patients with generalized lipodystrophy. *Eur J Pediatr* 1985, 144:355–359.
Lestradet C, Massol J *et al*: Lipodystrophie généralisée congénitale. *Arch Fr Pédiatr* 1985, 42:705–707.
Mørk N J, Rajka G *et al*: Treatment of acanthosis nigricans with etretinate... in... generalized lipodystrophy. *Acta Derm Venereol* 1986, 66:173–174.
Rheuban K S, Blizzard R M *et al*: Hypertrophic cardiomyopathy in total lipodystrophy. *J Pediatr* 1986, 109:301–302.

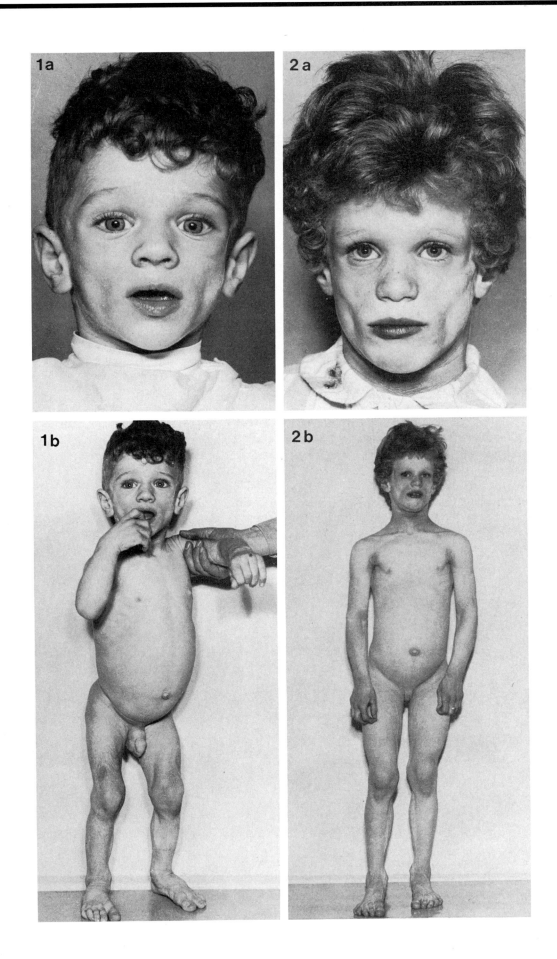

H.-R.W

A lipodystrophy beginning in the lower extremities and subsequently affecting the upper extremities and the face, associated with juvenile diabetes mellitus.

Main signs:
- Lipoatrophy of insidious onset in the second or third year of life (proband I is the child in **1**) and in the fourth year of life (proband II is the child in **4**), affecting the right foot and lower leg, beginning distally in proband I and both feet, lower legs and lower thighs, beginning distally in proband II. In the meantime, proband II shows advanced lipoatrophy of the upper thighs and new areas on both hands, the distal half of both forearms and in the buccal areas bilaterally (right side more than the left; already disfigured). Possible corresponding onset in the buccal area in proband I.
- Easily controlled insulin-dependent diabetes mellitus in both children (manifest in proband I at 3 years and 6 months and in proband II at 13 months with precoma).

Supplementary findings: In areas of lipoatrophy, thin skin with very prominent veins (**1–6**). Normal musculature.

In part, the lipoatrophy has been directly preceded by 'transient itchy flushing of the skin' as well as painless nodular indurations of the tissues.

Differentiating laboratory findings in the children. In proband II, conforming with the greater acuteness of the process, considerably increased gamma globulins and immunoglobulin G; C_3 complement elevated.

Manifestation: Early childhood.

Aetiology: Not clear. Genetic basis assumed, the patients being monozygotic twins. The precise nature of the process is still not known.

Frequency: Highly unusual course for a lipodystrophy; the association with juvenile diabetes mellitus is also unusual.

Course, prognosis: Further progression of the lipoatrophy can be expected.

Differential diagnosis: Other forms of lipodystrophy.

Treatment: Only symptomatic treatment possible (including immunosuppression).

Illustrations:
1–6 Four-year-old monozygotic twin brothers of normal mental development, in whom subjective wellbeing is unaffected; no further internal or neurological findings. No acceleration of growth in height, ossification or dentition. They are the second and third children of young, healthy, non-consanguineous parents; a 16-year-old brother of the father has had insulin-dependent diabetes mellitus since 12 years of age.

References:
Peters M S, Winkelmann R K: Localized lipoatrophy (atrophic connective tissue disease panniculitis). *Arch Dermatol* 1980, **116**:1363.
Billings J K, Milgraum S S *et al*: Lipoatrophic panniculitis: a possible autoimmune inflammatory disease of fat. *Arch Dermatol* 1987, **123**:1662–1666.

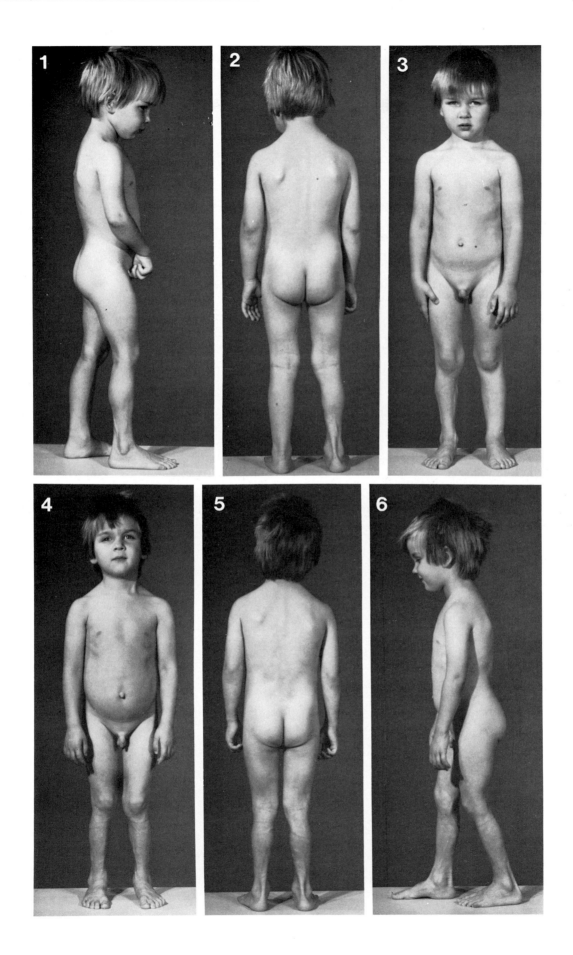

H.-R.W

A syndrome comprising severe wasting of adipose tissue, pseudo-anaemic pallor and vomiting with good food intake, a feeling of wellbeing to euphoria; behaviour ranges from lively to hyperactive.

Main signs:
- Progressive emaciation (**1**) in spite of good food intake (even hyperphagia).
- Undiminished alertness, ranging from sprightliness to euphoria.
- Liveliness to hyperactivity.
- Vomiting (occasional or frequent). Striking pallor without anaemia.
- Nystagmus (in at least 50% of patients).

Supplementary findings: Excitability, tremor, sweating. Diabetes insipidus in some patients.

Possible accelerated growth with acromegalic features (hands, feet, genitalia) (**1a**).

Characteristically, definite neurological signs tend to be absent for a long time.

Manifestation: From early infancy to about the end of the second year of life (rarely later).

Aetiology: A slowly growing glioma in the anterior hypothalamus (usually an astrocytoma).

Frequency: Relatively low. Approximately 200 patients described in the literature.

Course, prognosis: To a great extent depends on how soon recognized and on the treatment. Average survival of untreated patients after first manifestation, approximately 12 months.

Diagnosis: When suspected, ultrasound, computerized tomography scan, or further neuroradiological examinations in addition to cerebrospinal fluid protein determination and cell count.

Treatment: Where indicated, surgery or cobalt radiotherapy (which may prolong life considerably).

Illustrations:
1a–c A 2-year-old boy with 'diencephalic lipodystrophy' of several months' duration (underweight by 3.4 kg in relation to height; wasting, 'tobacco-pouch buttocks'). Cranium normal for age (but appearing relatively large). Large ears, thick protruding lips, large penis and large feet. Pseudo-anaemic pallor. Lively, friendly behaviour (**1a**). Neurological examination superficially unremarkable. Suspected tumour on brain scan and angiography. Operatively confirmed hypothalamic spongioblastoma.

References:
Wiedemann H-R: Dienzephale Syndrome des Kindesalters. *Pädiat Prax* 1972, **11**:95.
Burr I M, Slonim A E, Danish R K, Gadoth N, Butler I J: Diencephalic syndrome revisited. *J Pediatr* 1976, **88**:439.
Andler W, Stolecke H, Sirang H: Endocrine dysfunction in the diencephalic syndrome of emaciation in infancy. *Helv Paediat Acta* 1978, **33**:393.
Drop S L S, Guyda H J, Colle E: Inappropriate growth hormone release in the diencephalic syndrome of childhood: case report and a 4 year endocrinological follow-up. *Clin Endocrinol* 1980, **13**:181.
Waga S, Shimizu T *et al*: Diencephalic syndrome of emaciation (Russell's syndrome). *Surg Neurol* 1982, **17**:141–146.
Blanc J F, Chatelan P *et al*: Diagnostic échographique d'une tumeur diencéphalique cachectisante. *Arch Fr Pédiatr* 1983, **40**:575–577.
Albright A L, Price R A *et al*: Diencephalic gliomas in children. *Cancer* 1985, **55**:2789–2793.
Namba S, Nishimoto A *et al*: Diencephalic syndrome of emaciation (Russell's syndrome). Long term survival. *Surg Neurol* 1985, **23**:581–588.
Baracchini A, Chiaravalloti G *et al*: Sindrome diencefalica. *Minerva Pediatr* 1993, **45**:407–410.

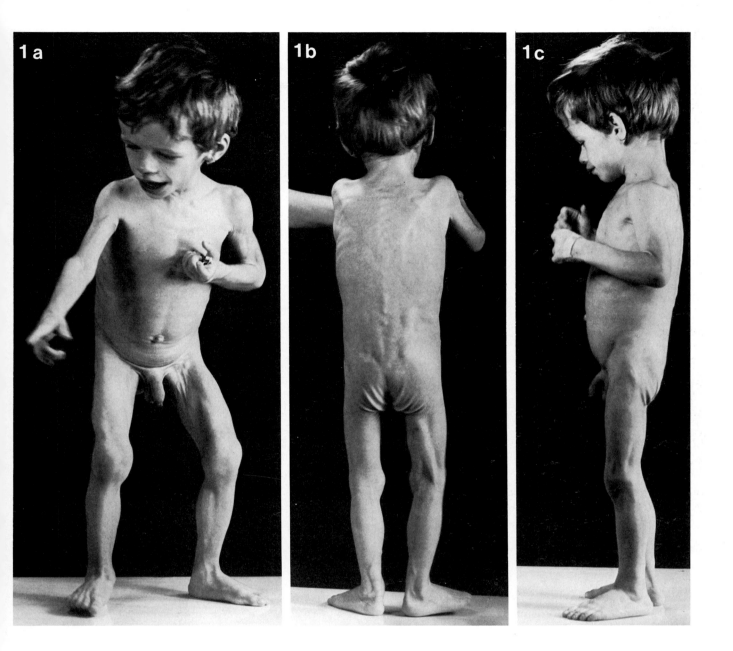

J.K./H.-R.W

A syndrome comprising mental retardation, short stature, obesity and hypogonadism, following initial marked muscular hypotonia in infancy.

Main signs:
Short stature (3–6), increasing obesity with hyperphagia, psychomotor retardation (usually severe); hypogenitalism: scrotal hypoplasia and frequent cryptorchidism (3, 5, 6, 7) or absence of the labia minora and underdevelopment of the labia majora; hypogonadism in both sexes.

Supplementary findings: A relatively narrow, prominent forehead, frequent strabismus, almond-shaped eyes in some patients and a triangular, open mouth may yield typical facies in young children. Hypoplasia of enamel in some patients; early severe caries (8 and 9).
Small hands and feet (acromicria) (10 and 11). Frequent hypopigmentation. Frequent development of kyphoscoliosis.
Development of prediabetic metabolism; later, nonketotic diabetes (usually after the second decade).

Manifestation: Congenital muscular hypotonia (possibly after weak foetal movements *in utero* and breech presentation, frequently low birth weight) often with extreme hypokinesia (1 and 2) and respiratory and feeding problems. Gradual improvement of muscle tone during the second half of the first year of life. Obesity, hyperphagia and growth retardation manifest after infancy.

Aetiology: In 95% of patients, loss of paternal alleles from the region 15q11-13: because of deletion in 65% and maternal disomy in 30% (both chromosomes 15 come from the mother). Like Angelman syndrome, subject to genomic imprinting (maternal allele loss in this case); genes for both syndromes are close together but not identical. Risk of recurrence under 1%, providing no parental chromosomal changes (e.g. translocation).

Frequency: Not low, at least 1:10 000 births.

Course, prognosis: Obesity is often very difficult to control and may increase to a grotesque extent. Decreased life expectancy. Often, delayed or incomplete puberty; no voice change in males. Frequent psychosocial problems in adolescence and adulthood. Infertility.

Diagnosis, differential diagnosis: In 95% of patients, diagnosis can be confirmed by molecular–genetic techniques (microsatellite markers). Initially, other forms of early manifest muscular hypotonia ('floppy infant') must be ruled out. Later, diagnosis facilitated by the two-phase course, that is the history of congenital muscular atony and initial failure to thrive. Thus, Bardet–Biedl syndrome (*159*) (which additionally has polydactyly, retinitis pigmentosa), Fröhlich adiposogenital dystrophy (with no mental retardation but progressive central nervous system signs) and Cohen syndrome (*160*) can be readily eliminated.

Treatment: Limitation of the hyperphagia as far as possible, especially in view of the disposition to diabetes. Special nursery schools, special schooling and so on may be indicated.

Illustrations: 1 and 2 A 4-month-old infant with severe muscular hypotonia, asthenia, hypokinesia and hyporeflexia; weak crying, sucking, and swallowing; expressionless face with triangular, open ('fish') mouth; micrognathia; psychomotor retardation. **3, 7** The same child at age 5 years. **3–6** Four children aged 5, 5, 6 and 7 years, all mentally retarded, with short stature, respectively 6, 5, 9, 11, and 24 cm less than the average for age. Cryptorchidism in all three boys. Hyperglycemia of the boy in **6** after age 4 years and manifest diabetes after age 6. **8** Same child as in **6**. **10 and 11** A hand and a foot of a Prader–Willi patient (right) compared with those of a healthy child of the same age (left).

References:

Prader A, Labhart A, Willi H: Ein Syndrom von Adipositas, Kleinwuchs, Kryptorchismus und Oligophrenie nach myatonieartigem Zustand im Neugeborenenalter. *Schweiz med Wschr* 1956, 86:1260.

Schinzel A: Approaches to the prenatal diagnosis of the Prader–Willi syndrome. *Hum Genet* 1986, 74:327.

Greenswag L R: Adults with Prader–Willi syndrome: a survey of 232 cases. *Dev Med Child Neurol* 1987, 29:145–152.

Lee P D K, Wilson D M, Rountree L *et al*: Linear growth response to exogenous growth hormone in Prader–Willi syndrome. *Am J Med Genet* 1987, 28:865–871.

Wenger S L, Hanchett J M, Steele M W *et al*: Clinical comparison of 59 Prader–Willi patients with and without the 15(Q12) deletion. *Am J Med Genet* 1987, 28:881–887.

Caldwell M L, Taylor R L: *Prader–Willi syndrome.* Berlin, Heidelberg, New York: Springer 1988; 120.

Greenswag L R, Alexander R C: *Management of Prader–Willi syndrome.* Berlin, Heidelberg, New York: Springer 1988; 250.

Whitman B Y, Accardo P: Emotional symptoms in Prader–Willi syndrome adolescents. *Am J Med Genet* 1987, 28:897–905.

Zellweger H: Can women with the Prader–Labhart–Willi syndrome (PLWS) reproduce? Does the deletion (15)(qll-13) occur in individuals not affected with PLWS? *Am J Med Genet* 1988, 29:669–672.

Knoll J H M, Nicholls R D *et al*: Angelman and Prader–Willi syndromes share a common chromosome 15 deletion but differ in parental origin of the deletion. *Am J Med Genet* 1989, 32:285–290.

Dittrich B, Robinson W P, Knoblauch H *et al*: Molecular diagnosis of the Prader–Willi and Angelman syndromes by detection of parent-of-origin specific DNA methylation in 15q11-13. *Hum Genet* 1992, 90:313–315.

Nicholls R D: Genomic imprinting and candidate genes in the Prader–Willi and Angelman syndromes. *Curr Opin Genet Dev* 1993a, 3:445–456.

Nicholls R D: Genomic imprinting and uniparental disomy in Angelman and Prader–Willi syndromes: a review. *Am J Med Genet* 1993b, 46:16–25.

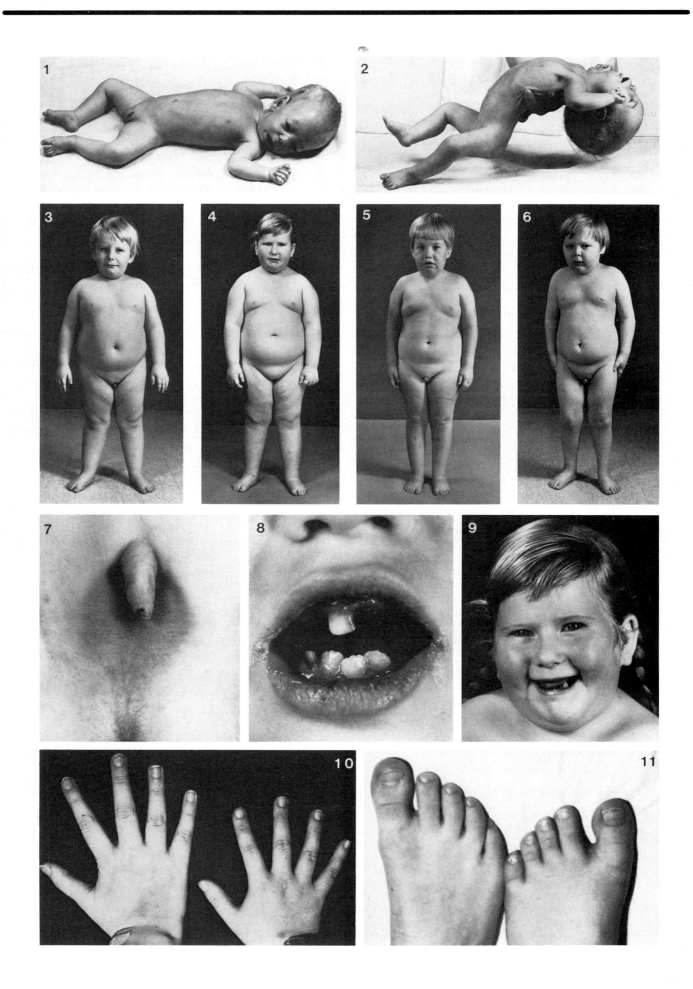

H.-R.W

A hereditary disorder with polydactyly, hypogenitalism, obesity, impaired vision and mental retardation.

Main signs:
- Obesity, mainly of the trunk, usually of early onset, frequently increasing (**1, 6**).
- Hypogenitalism (with normal and decreased gonadotropin levels), small genitalia (**4**), undescended testes, bifid scrotum, hypospadias. Little or no development of the secondary sex characteristics. Amenorrhoea.
- Distinct mental impairment. Occasionally defective hearing.
- Ulnar or fibular polydactyly, varying from rudimentary appendages to functioning sixth fingers or toes (**2 and 3**), usually of the feet. In most patients, also middle syn- or brachydactyly.

Supplementary findings: Short stature, usually moderate.
Retinitis pigmentosa (but also sine pigmento) as a very consistent characteristic; nystagmus; other ophthalmological findings possible.
Frequent small, cystic–dysplastic, poorly functioning kidneys with progressive decrease of function (with uremia in extreme cases); also malformations of the heart and urinary tract, fibrosis of the liver, diabetes mellitus.

Manifestation: Hexadactyly and possibly increased body weight at birth, retinopathy and distinct truncal obesity in early childhood, hypogenitalism from birth onwards.

Aetiology: Autosomal recessive disorder of variable expression. Heterogeneity. Gene loci on chromosome 3 or on the long arm of chromosome 11?
Even with heterozygotes, special attention should be paid to obesity, renal disorders, hypertension and diabetes mellitus.

Frequency: Less than 1:160 000.

Course, prognosis: Determined by the degree of mental retardation and by the progression of the retinopathy and neuropathy.

Diagnosis, differential diagnosis: Symptomatic overlap with a number of other syndromes. The Prader–Willi syndrome (*158*), which is much more frequent, does not show polydactyly and retinopathy.

Treatment: Symptomatic; regular ophthalmological follow-up, urinary cultures, measurement of blood pressure. Kidney transplantation where indicated.
Genetic counselling.

Illustrations:
1–6 The same patient at ages 7 and 33 years. Overweight since infancy. Mild mental retardation. Rudimentary sixth rays of the hands and feet. Retinitis pigmentosa. Hypogenitalism.

References:
Pagon R A, Haas J E *et al*: Hepatic involvement in the Bardet–Biedl syndrome. *Am J Med Genet* 1982, **13**:373–381.
Schachat A P, Maumenee I H: Bardet–Biedl syndrome and related disorders. *Arch Ophthalmol* 1982 **100**:285–288.
Linné T, Wikstad I, Zetterström R: Renal involvement in the Laurence–Moon–Biedl syndrome. *Acta Paediatr Scand* 1986, **75**:240–244.
Harnett, J D, Green J S *et al*: The spectrum of renal disease in Laurence–Moon–Biedl syndrome. *N Engl J Med* 1988, **319**:615–618.
Ritchie G, Jequier S, Lussier-Lazaroff: Prenatal renal ultrasound of Laurence–Moon–Biedl syndrome. *Pediatr Radiol* 1988, **19**:65–66.
Editorial: Laurence–Moon and Bardet–Biedl syndromes. *Lancet* 1978, **II**:1178.
Green J S *et al*: The cardinal manifestations of Bardet–Biedl syndrome... *N Engl J Med* 1989, **321**:1002–1009.
Croft J B *et al*: Obesity, hypertension, and renal disease in relatives of Bardet–Biedl syndrome sibs. *Am J Med Genet* 1990, **36**:37–42.
Gershoni-Baruch R *et al*: Cystic kidney dysplasia... Bardet–Biedl syndrome. *Am J Med Genet* 1992, **44**:269–273.
Elbedour Kh, Zucker N *et al*: Cardiac abnormalities in the Bardet–Biedl syndrome. *Am J Med Genet* 1994, **52**:164–169.
Leppert M *et al*: Bardet–Biedl syndrome... chromosome 11q... *Nature Genet* 1994, **7**:108–112.
Sheffield V C, Carmi R *et al*: Identification of a Bardet–Biedl syndrome locus on chromosome 3... *Hum Mol Genet* 1994, **3**:1331–1337.

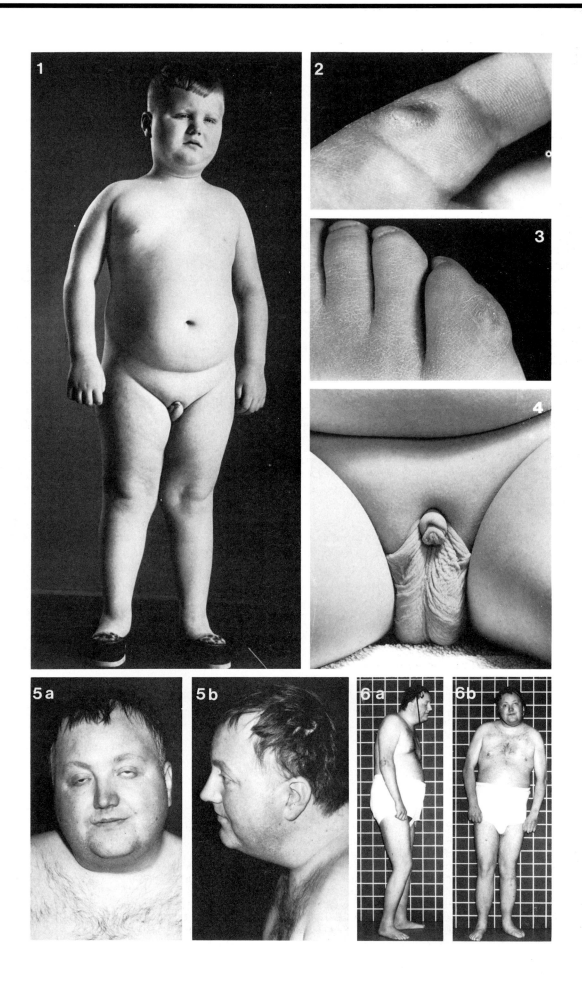

H.-R.W

A syndrome of characteristic facies, mental retardation with microcephaly, muscular hypotonia, short stature, obesity and anomalies of the hands and feet.

Main signs:
- Facies: possible slight antimongoloid slant of the palpebral fissures with broad, prominent nasal bridge; fairly prominent ears; prominence of the premaxilla, middle incisors and upper lip with high narrow palate, short philtrum, and open mouth; micrognathia (1–3).
- Mild microcephaly in approximately 50% of patients. Mental retardation (IQ between 30 and 70) practically without exception. Not infrequently, seizures. Friendly manner.
- Hypotonic and flaccid musculature and joints.
- Short stature in about 70%.
- Mild to moderate truncal obesity in approxiamtely 70% of patients (1).

Supplementary findings: Hands and feet strikingly narrow with long, thin fingers and toes; possible syndactyly, simian crease. Cubitus valgus, genu valgum.

Possible strabismus, myopia, chorioretinal dystrophy, and other ocular anomalies; abnormal electroretinogram.

Possible development of scoliosis, mitral valve prolapse, hiatus hernia.

Possible granulocytopaenia (may be intermittent) and perhaps also defective coagulation.

Manifestation: At birth and later. Onset of obesity usually in mid-childhood.

Aetiology: Hereditary disorder with variable expression; possible autosomal recessive connective tissue disease. Gene on the long arm of chromosome 8.

Frequency: Relatively low; at least 100 patients known up to 1994.

Differential diagnosis: Primarily, Prader–Willi syndrome (*158*) and Bardet–Biedl syndrome (*159*).

Treatment: Symptomatic.

Illustrations:
1–3 The first and second children of healthy, young, nonconsanguineous parents. The 11-year-old girl and her 10-year-old brother are slightly microcephalic, mentally retarded, of short stature and obese and show the characteristic facies. The boy is hypotonic; the girl has had a focal seizure disorder since early childhood.

References:
Cohen M M Jr, Hall B D, Smith D W *et al*: A new syndrome with hypotonia, obesity, mental deficiency, and facial, oral, ocular, and limb anomalies. *J Pediatr* 1973, **83**:280 .
Ferré P, Fournet J P, Courpotin C: Le syndrome de Cohen… *Arch Fr Pédiat* 1982, **39**:159.
Goecke T, Majewski F, Kauther K D *et al*: Mental retardation… (Cohen syndrome). *Eur J Pediatr* 1982, **138**:338–340.
Friedman E, Sack J: The Cohen syndrome. Report of five cases and a review of the literature. *J Craniofac Genet Biol* 1982, **2**:193–200.
Norio R, Raitta C *et al*: Further delineation of the Cohen syndrome… *Clin Genet* 1984, **25**:1–14.
North C, Patton M A *et al*: The clinical features of the Cohen syndrome… *J Med Genet* 1985, **22**:131–134.
Young I D, Moore J R: Intrafamiliar variation in Cohen syndrome. *J Med Genet* 1987, **24**:488–492.
Méhes K, Kosztolányi G *et al*: Cohen syndrome: a connective tissue disorder? *Am J Med Genet* 1988, **31**:131–133.
Higgins J J, Kaneski C R *et al*: Pyridoxine-responsive hyper-β-alaninemia associated with Cohen's syndrome. *Neurology* 1994, **44**:1728–1732.
Schlichtemeier T L, Tomlinson G E *et al*: Multiple coagulation defects and the Cohen syndrome. *Clin Genet* 1994, **45**:212–216.
Tahvanainen E, Norio R *et al*: Cohen syndrome gene assigned to the long arm of chromosome 8… *Nature Genet* 1994, **7**:201–204.

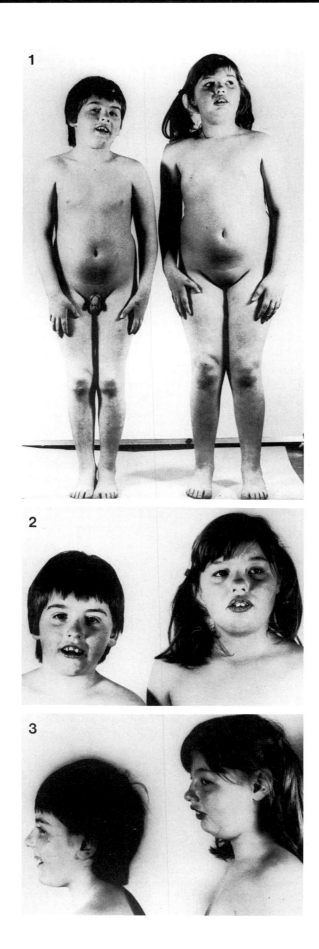

J.K.

A characteristic complex of malformations with ocular defects, costovertebral malformations, infantile nodding spasms, agenesis of the corpus callosum and progressive psychomotor retardation, occurring only in females.

Main signs:

- Limited virtually exclusively to females (to date only two boys reported with Aicardi syndrome; of these, one Australian with 47XXY karyotype).
- Microphthalmia. Numerous pathognomonic lacunar chorioretinopathic foci; usually peripapillary and bilateral, less often peripheral. The foci are pigment-free; the lacunae, pale to ivory-coloured.
- Costovertebral malformations, fusion of vertebral bodies, hemivertebrae, clefts, absent ribs, fused ribs.
- Infantile spasms within the first 2–4 months of life; rarely as early as the first days of life. Clinically, variable pattern of seizures, possibly with focal signs.
- Partial or total agenesis of the corpus callosum.
- Progressive psychomotor retardation, asymmetric hypotonic tetraplegia or diplegia. Microcephaly in 75% of patients.

Supplementary findings: Cortical heterotopia, polygyria and microgyria, deformity of the ventricles, as in the Dandy–Walker syndrome, in some patients.

Normal electroretinogram.

Absent pupillary reaction; strabismus, nystagmus, cataract, synechiae of the iris, ptosis.

Characteristic electroencephalogram pattern: so-called burst-suppression pattern (groups of high theta and delta waves with enclosed hypersynchronic potentials, interrupted by stretches of flat activity of only a few seconds).

Manifestation: At birth. Seizures beginning in the second to fourth months of life.

Aetiology: Probably an X-linked dominant disorder with lethality in males. The Australian with XXY bears out this assumption. All patients have been single observations in their families. New mutations. Six pairs of dizygotic twins, with only one child affected in each; female siblings observed once.

Frequency: Over 200 patients have been described to date.

Course, prognosis: Progressive psychomotor retardation, decreased vision. The oldest known patient is 14 years old. Patients generally die by 5 years of age from respiratory infections.

Differential diagnosis: The oculovertebral syndrome of Weyers–Thier, which has dysplasia of the roof of the orbit, no lacunar chorioretinopathy, no sex limitation, no seizure disorder, no anomalies of the corpus callosum.

Treatment: Symptomatic treatment of the salaam spasms. Measures to promote development: physiotherapy, occupational therapy, visual training.

Illustrations:

1 A typically affected female newborn; short neck, microphthalmia on the right.
2 Her chest radiograph, showing hemivertebrae, tilted and oblique vertebrae, fused vertebrae, unequal number of ribs on the two sides, scoliosis.

Malformations also of the cervical vertebrae.

References:

Bertoni J M, v Loh S, Allen R J: The Aicardi syndrome: report of 4 cases and review of the literature. *Ann Neurol* 1979, 5:475–482.
Köhler B, Bayer H, Osswald H: Das Aicardi-Syndrom. *Pädiat Prax* 1983/84, 29:45–58.
Yamamoto N *et al*: Aicardi syndrome: report of 6 cases and a review of Japanese literature. *Brain Dev* 1985, 7:443–449.
Besenski N, Bosnjak V *et al*: Cortical heterotopia in Aicardi's syndrome... *Pediatr Radiol* 1988, 18:391–393.
Donnenfeld A E, Packer R J *et al*: Clinical cytogenetic, and pedigree findings in 18 cases of Aicardi syndrome. *Am J Med Genet* 1989, 32:461–467.
Molina J A, Mateos F *et al*: Aicardi syndrome in two sisters. *J Pediatr* 1989, 115:282–283.
Neidich J A, Nussbaum R L *et al*: Heterogeneity of clinical severity and molecular lesions in Aicardi syndrome. *J Pediatr* 1990, 11:911–917.
Nielsen K B, Anvret M *et al*: Aicardi syndrome: early neuroradiological manifestations and results of DNA studies in one patient. *Am J Med Genet* 1991, 38:65–68.
Ohtsuka Y, Oka E *et al*: Aicardi syndrome: a longitudinal clinical and electroencephalographic study. *Epilepsia* 1993, 34:627–634.
Tsao C, Sommer A, Hamoudi A B: Aicardi syndrome, metastatic angiosarcoma of the leg, and scalp lipoma. *Am J Med Genet* 1993, 45:594–596.

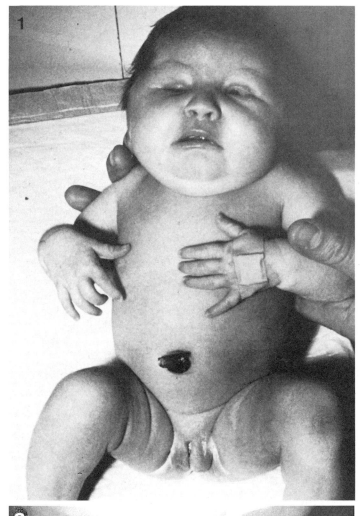

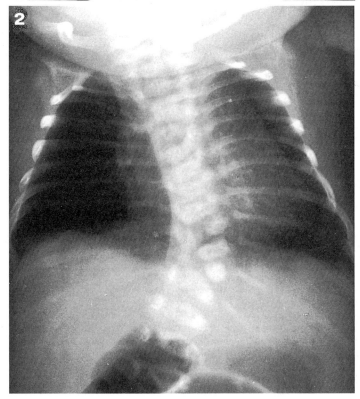

162 Spondylocostal Dysostosis

(Spondylocostal Dysplasia, Spondylothoracic Dysplasia/Dysostosis, Costovertebral Dysplasia, Jarcho–Levin Syndrome, Polydysspondyly, Occipito-Facio-Cervico-Thoraco-Abdomino-Digital Syndrome)

An aetiologically heterogeneous clinical picture with vertebral and rib anomalies due to a disorder of segmentation in the axial skeleton.

Main signs:

- Shortened trunk; opisthotonus position of the head; short neck; broad, asymmetrical, barrel-shaped thorax; protuberant abdomen; diastasis recti; slender, elongated extremities; hypotonic musculature.
- Multiple hemi-, wedge-shaped and block vertebrae; spina bifida.
- Rib anomalies: particularly of number and shape, as well as synostoses.

Supplementary findings: Additional malformations occur very occasionally: renal anomalies (aplasia, hydronephrosis, mega-ureter, double ureter, horseshoe kidney), cardiac defect (tetralogy of Fallot, pulmonary stenosis). Scoliosis, lordosis, camptodactyly, polydactyly, syndactyly, club feet.

Manifestation: At birth.

Aetiology: Heterogeneous. Very often autosomal recessive but also autosomal dominant inheritance described; part of a genetic malformation syndrome (costovertebral segmentation defect with mesomelia = COVESDEM). The following disorders also show vertebral segmentation defects: Klippel–Feil anomaly (163), the VATER symptom complex (311), VACTERL-plus H syndrome (312), Goldenhar syndrome (30), cardiofacial symptom complex (33); sporadic cases. Possible receptor defect in sclerotome development. Recently subdivided into spondylothoracic dysostosis (vertebral anomalies, fan-shaped widening of the ribs, defects of the neural tube, high mortality, autosomal recessive inheritance) and spondylocostal forms (malformations of the vertebral bodies, dramatic malformations of the ribs, short stature). No 'crab-like' chest. In most cases autosomal recessive, occasionally autosomal dominant.

Frequency: Over 200 published reports of patients.

Course, prognosis: Normal mental development; stable vertebral column but also perinatal or early infantile death from cardiopulmonary complications. The oldest patient is age 11 years.

Differential diagnosis: Differentiation from the Klippel–Feil 'syndrome' (163) with its anomalies and synostoses in the cervical spine region. The VATER association (311) shows additional malformations.

Treatment: Orthopaedic care. Prenatal diagnosis?

Illustrations:

1a A characteristically affected male newborn. **1b** Severe skeletal changes in the thoracic region of this child.
2 Radiograph of the trunk region of another newborn with this syndrome.

References:

Gassner M, Grabs S G: Kostovertebrale Dysplasie. Ein Rezeptordefekt der Sklerotomentwicklung? *Schweiz med Wschr* 1982, **112**:791–797.
Pfeiffer R A, Hansen H G, Böwing B *et al*: Die Spondylocostale Dysostose. Bericht über 5 Beobachtungen einschließlich Geschwister und einen atypischen Fall. *Monatsschr Kinderheilk* 1983, **131**:28–34.
Aymé S, Preus M: Spondylocostal/spondylothoracis dysostosis: the clinical basis for prognosticating and genetic counseling. *Am J Med Genet* 1986, **24**:599–606.
Ohashi H, Sugio Y *at al*: Spondylocostal dysostosis: report of three patients. *Jpn J Hum Genet* 1987, **32**:299–307.
Tolmie J L, Whittle M J, McNay M B *et al*: Second trimester prenatal diagnosis of the Jarcho–Levin syndrome. *Prenat Diagn* 1987, 7:129–134.
Lorenz P, Rupprecht E: Spondylocostal dysostosis: dominant type. *Am J Med Genet* 1990, **35**:219–221.
Karnes P S, Day D, Berry S A, Piermont M E M: Jarcho–Levin syndrome: four new cases and classification of subtypes. *Am J Med Genet* 1991, **40**:264–270.
Romeo M G, Distefano G *et al*: Familial Jarcho–Levin syndrome. *Clin Genet* 1991, **39**: 253–259.
Giacoia G P, Say B: Spondylocostal dysplasia and neural tube defects. *J Med Genet* 1991, **28**:51–53.
Satar M, Kozanoglu M N, Atilla E: Identical twins with an autosomal recessive form of spondylocostal dysostosis. *Clin Genet* 1992, **41**:290–292.
La Grutta A, Corsello G, Benigno V, Bianco A *et al*: Spondylo-costal dysostosis in two siblings. *Klin Pädiat* 1992, **204**:48–55.
Schulman M, Gonzales M T, Bye M R: Airway abnormalities in Jarcho–Levin syndrome: a report of two cases. *J Med Genet* 1993 **30**:875–876.
McCall C P, Hudgins L, Cloutier M, Greenstein R M, Cassidy, S. B: Jarcho–Levin syndrome: unusual survival in a classical case. *Am J Med Genet* 1994, **49**:328–332.
Van Thienen M-N, van der Auwera B J: Monozygotic twins discordant for spondylocostal dysostosis. *Am J Med Genet* 1994, **52**:483–486.
Martinez-Frias M-L, Bermejo E *et al*. Severe spondylocostal dysostosis associated with other congenital anomalies: a clinical/epidemiologic analysis and description of ten cases from the Spanish registry. *Am J Med Genet* 1994, **51**:203–212.

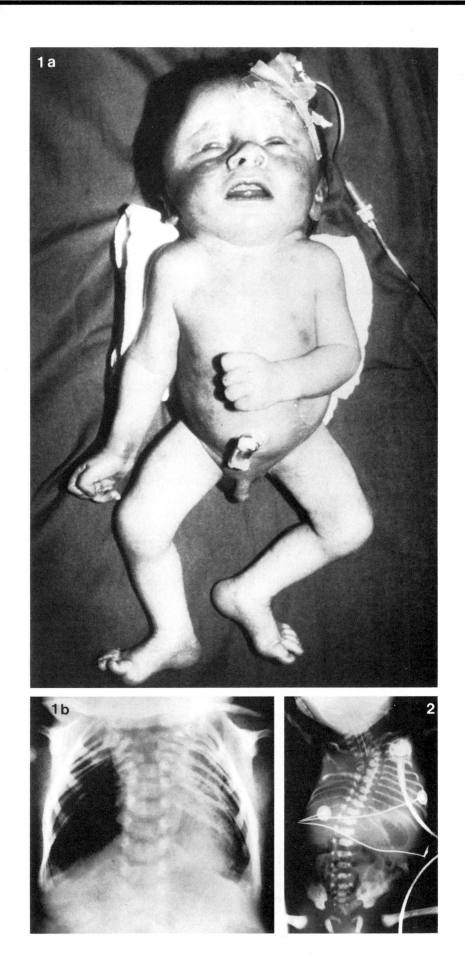

163 Klippel–Feil 'Syndrome'

H.-R.W/J.K.

A malformation complex particularly of the cervical spine with short neck and possible impairments of mobility, posture and neurological function.

Main signs:

- Short neck (**1a and b**) to 'absent neck', with low nuchal hairline. Usually, limited (painless) movement of the head, especially sidewards (**1a**). Thorax may be barrel-shaped, with high rounded hump. Possible elevation of the shoulders.
- Radiologically: block vertebrae for a variable extent of the cervical spine (possible wedge-shaped or hemivertebrae or anomalies of the neural arches), sometimes with malformations of the lower spine or ribs (**2 and 3**) and scoliosis.

A classification into different types according to the nature, severity and localization of the malformations has been undertaken:

Type I: extensive fusion of the cervical and upper thoracic vertebral bodies.

Type II: fusion of only one or two cervical vertebral bodies but beyond this, hemivertebrae, atlanto-occipital fusion.

Type III: cervical and lower thoracic and lumbar fusions.

Supplementary findings: Kyphoscoliosis in 60%, spina bifida occulta in 45%, malformations of the urogenital system in 55% (renal agenesis, ectopic kidneys, hydronephrosis and so on), genital anomalies (absent vagina, uterus). Hypospadias. Anomalies of the ribs in 30%. Ophthalmic defects (microphthalmia, ptosis, coloboma, nystagmus and so on). Torticollis. Cleft palate. Cardiac defect in 8%. Neurological complications. Pains, spasticity, hyperreflexia, paraesthesia. Associated malformations: clefting of the vertebral column, syringomyelia, hydrocephalus, sternal anomalies, situs inversus viscerum. Megacolon, intestinal atresia. Short stature, mental retardation.

Manifestation: At birth and later, depending on the severity of the malformations.

Aetiology: Not uniform. Mostly isolated cases (may represent a disruption sequence caused by embryonic vascular disturbance of the subclavian artery). Autosomal dominant and recessive transmission also observed.

Frequency: Over 350 reports published.

Prognosis: Dependent on the severity of the anatomical disorder.

Differential diagnosis: Ullrich–Turner syndrome (*103*), Noonan syndrome (*105*), foetal alcohol syndrome (*275*), Crouzon syndrome (*6*), Goldenhar syndrome (*30*), Wildervanck syndrome (*164*), VATER symptom complex (*311*), cardiofacial symptom complex (*33*).

Treatment: For the most part symptomatic orthopaedic treatment. Early auditory evaluation and adequate therapy if indicated.

Illustrations:

1a and b A 6-month-old male infant with short neck, limited sideways movement of the head, somewhat barrel-shaped chest, otherwise normal psychomotor development.

2 Antero-posterior cervical spine radiograph of the same boy, showing hemivertebrae and partial block vertebrae at the junction of the cervical and thoracic spines; bilateral hypoplasia of the upper ribs.

3 Lateral radiograph of the cervical spine of a 12-year-old girl with Klippel–Feil syndrome. Extensive block vertebrae with partial inclusion of the neural arches and spinal processes.

References:

Gunderson C H, Greenspan R H, Glaser G H, Lubs H A: The Klippel–Feil syndrome: genetic and clinical reevaluation of cervical fusion. *Medicine* 1967, **46**:491.

Palant D I, Carter B L: Klippel–Feil-syndrome and deafness. *Am J Dis Child* 1972, **123**:218.

Helmi C, Pruzansky S: Craniofacial and extracranial malformations in the Klippel–Feil syndrome. *Cleft Palate J* 1980, **17**:65.

Fragoso R, Cid-Garcia A *et al*: Frontonasal dysplasia in the Klippel–Feil syndrome... *Clin Genet* 1982, **22**:270–273.

Silva E O de: Autosomal recessive Klippel–Feil syndrome. *J Med Genet* 1982, **19**:130–134.

Nagib M G, Maxwell R E *et al*: Klippel–Feil syndrome in children: clinical features and management. *Child Nerv Syst* 1985, **1**:255–263.

Brill C B, Peyster R G *et al*: Isolation of the right subclavian artery with subclavian steal in a child with Klippel–Feil anomaly... *Am J Med Genet* 1987, **26**:933–940.

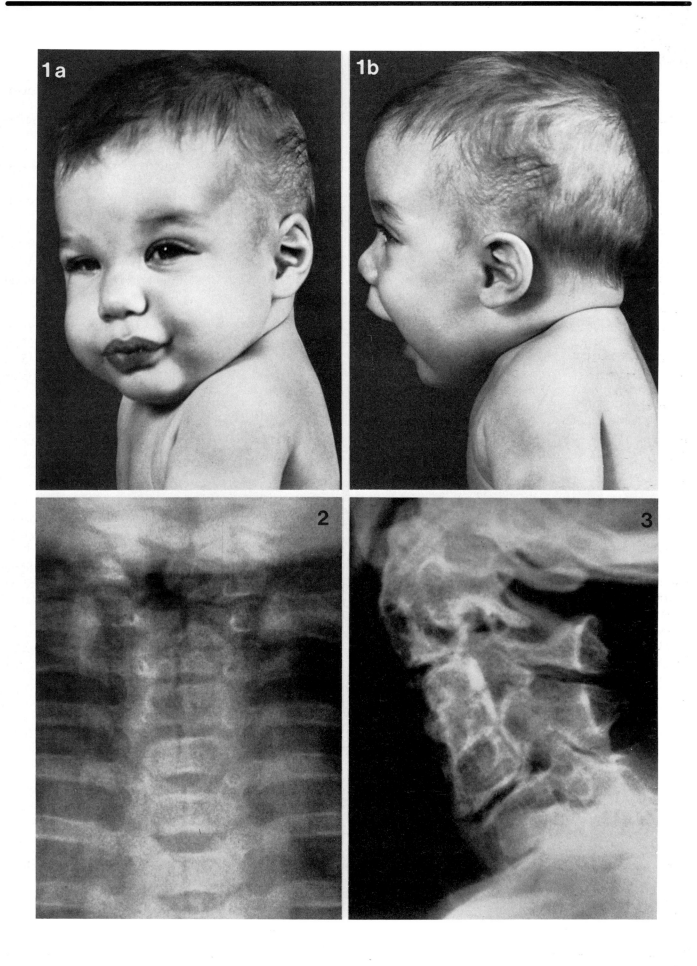

164 Wildervanck Syndrome
(Cervico-Oculo-Acoustic Syndrome)

H.-R.W/J.K.

A complex of anomalies including short neck (similar to that in Klippel–Feil syndrome), facial anomalies and hearing impairment, occurring almost exclusively in females.

Main signs:
- Those of the Klippel–Feil syndrome (*163*).
- Usually, facial asymmetry, possibly with torticollis, uni- or less frequently bilateral paralysis of the abducent nerve and bulbar retraction (Duane syndrome), hypoplasia of the upper jaw, micrognathia, narrow or possibly cleft palate.
- Unilateral or bilateral, moderate to severe, conductive hearing impairment, sensorineural hearing impairment or a combination of the two. Occurrence of outer and inner ear malformations: pre-auricular tags, malformed ears, atresia of the external auditory canal, malformed or absent ossicles, hypoplasia of the labyrinth.

Supplementary findings: Mental development normal as a rule. Unilateral epibulbar dermoids may occur (and heterochromia iridis, cleft palate, pterygium colli and renal aplasia have been noted in individual patients). Spina bifida occulta, Sprengel's deformity, hemivertebrae, anomalies of the ribs, kyphoscoliosis.

Manifestation: At birth; hearing impairment possibly later.

Aetiology: Genetic situation not clear. As the vast majority of patients are female, sex-linked dominant inheritance has been considered, although multifactorial inheritance is also a possibility. Sex ratio: seven male to 75 female patients.

Frequency: Not particularly rare (approximately 1:3000 deaf children); several hundred reports in the literature.

Course, prognosis: Favourable for life expectancy, after a potentially difficult neonatal course.

Diagnosis, differential diagnosis: Differentiation from the Goldenhar 'syndrome' (*30*) can be very difficult, if not impossible, as in the patient presented here. Similar difficulties encountered in ruling out the Klippel–Feil 'syndrome' (*163*). Exclusion of mandibulofacial dysostosis (*28*) not difficult.

Treatment: Initial care as with the Pierre Robin sequence may be indicated. Early evaluation of hearing and, when indicated, prompt application of special hearing and speech aids. Orthopaedic surgery, cosmetic surgery or orthodontic corrective measures may be required.

Illustrations:
1–6 A 6-year-old girl with a faciovertebral anomaly complex. Bony malformation at the atlanto-occipital junction, block formation of second to fourth cervical vertebrae and synostoses of the spinous processes to C6. Low nuchal hairline. Marked limitation of movement of the neck. Mild facial asymmetry, relatively narrow and somewhat oblique left palpebral fissure (no epibulbar dermoid). Hypoplasia of the upper jaw (which has a double row of teeth), narrow palate, immobile soft palate, well-corrected horizontal clefts of the cheeks. Unremarkable external ears. Conductive hearing impairment.

References:
Sherk H H, Nicholson J T: Cervico-oculo-acusticus syndrome. *J Bone Jt Surg* 1972, 54(**A**):1776.
Konigsmark B W, Gorlin R J: *Genetic and metabolic deafness.* Philadelphia: Saunders 1976.
Wildervanck L S: The cervico-oculo-acusticus syndrome. In: *Handbook of clinical neurology.* Vinken, P. J, Bruyn, G. W, Myrianthopulos, N. C. (eds.). 1978, **21**:123–130. Amsterdam: North-Holland Publ.
Strisciuglio P, Raia V *et al*: Wildervanck's syndrome with bilateral subluxation of lens and facial paralysis. *J Med Genet* 1983, **20**:72–73.
Corsello G, Carcione A, Castr L, Giuffrè L: Cervicooculo-acusticus (Wildervanck's) syndrome: a clinical variant of Klippel–Feil sequence? *Klin Pädiatr* 1990, 1990, **202**:176–179.

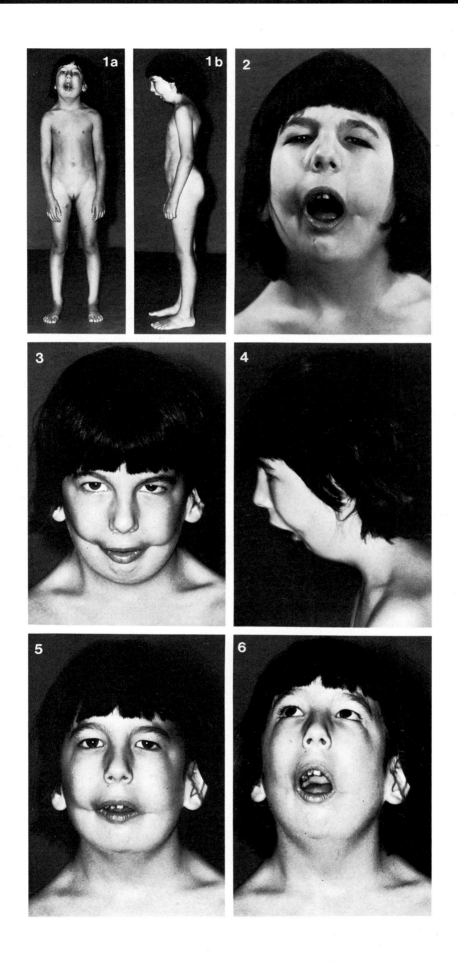

165 Aplastic Abdominal Musculature 'Syndrome'
(Prune Belly 'Syndrome' or Sequence)

H.-R.W.

A condition seen in males at birth with a slack, wrinkled abdominal wall, undescended testes and urinary-tract anomalies. (Analogous dysplasia of the abdominal muscles occurs only rarely in females.)

Main signs:
- A thin, slack and (especially in early life) wrinkled and shrivelled ('prune-like') abdominal wall with persistent furrow-like umbilicus (1, 3), protruding over 'wobbly' abdominal organs. (Basis: hypoplasia and aplasia of the abdominal wall musculature, not necessarily symmetrical.)
- Bilateral cryptorchidism.
- Fairly extensive, marked anomalies of the urinary tract: megacystis, mega-ureter, cystic dysplasia of the kidneys, hydronephrosis (4).

Supplementary findings: Frequently, malrotation or other additional abnormalities (e.g. of hips, feet, heart or elsewhere).

Manifestation: Intra-uterine or at birth.

Aetiology: Not clear. Probably heterogeneous pathological complex (polytropic field defect). One theory is that it results from intra-uterine urethral obstruction, to which male foetuses are far more susceptible. A few familial observations. The risk of recurrence in further offspring is a few per cent at the most.

Frequency: Approximately 1:40 000 live births. Well over 800 patients described in the literature.

Course, prognosis: Dependent on the severity of the anomalies. A large proportion of those affected die within the first years of life.

Differential diagnosis: Cantrell sequence (pentalogy of Cantrell).

Treatment: Exact assessment of the urodynamics. Prompt primary decompression may be required, for example, by cystostomy. Measures to prevent urinary tract infection. Follow-up care by a paediatric urologist.

Genetic counselling. Prenatal diagnosis with chromosomal analysis ('prune belly' also occurs with trisomies) and with ultrasound in subsequent pregnancies (looking for megacystis and foetal ascites). The question of possible antenatal decompression requires very careful consideration.

Illustrations:

1 A very severely affected male newborn; lethal form.

2 A 3-day-old male infant with hypoplasia of the abdominal wall, hydronephrosis and hydro-ureter; death at 6 weeks.

3 and 4 A further male infant. The second child of healthy parents (the first pregnancy resulted in a stillbirth at 7 months, cause not known). Birth of the proband after a normal pregnancy; extensive aplasia of the abdominal wall musculature, megacystis, mega-ureter and undescended testes. Resection of a urethral polyp at 4 months. Apart from initial urinary tract infections, normal development of the child, who has since reached school age; his renal collecting system and total renal tubular function are now normal and his testes, following surgery, are in a normal position.

4 Urogram in the neonatal period showing extreme mega-ureter.

References:

Pagon R A, Smith D W, Shephard Th H: Urethral obstruction malformation complex: a cause of abdominal muscle deficiency and the 'prune belly'. *J Pediatr* 1979, **94**:900 and *ibid* **96**:776–777 (letters to the editor).
Aaronson I A, Cremin B J: Prune belly syndrome in young females. *Urol Radiol* 1979/80, **1**:151.
Kösters S, Horwitz H, Ritter R: Typische röntgenologische Veränderungen an Nieren und Harntrakt beim Bauchmuskelaplasie-Syndrom. *Pädiat prax* 1979/80, **22**:125.
Straub E, Spranger J: Etiology and pathogenesis of the Prune Belly Syndrome. *Kidney Int* 1981, **20**:695–699.
Lubinsky M, Rapoport P: Transient fetal hydrops and 'prune belly' in one identical female twin. *N Engl J Med* 1983, I:256–257.
Oliveira G, Boechat M I, Ferreira M A: Megacystis-microcolon-intestinal hypoperistalsis syndrome in a newborn girl whose brother had prune belly syndrome: common pathogenesis? *Pediatr Radiol* 1983, **13**:294–296.
Belohradsky B H, Henkel C: Das Prune-Belly-Syndrom. *Ergeb Inn Med Kinderheilk* 1984, **52**:157–205.
Burton B K, Dillard R G: Prune belly syndrome: observations supporting the hypothesis of abdominal overdistension. *Am J Med Genet* 1984, **17**:669–672.
Moerman P, Fryns J-P, Goddeeris P *et al*: Pathogenesis of the prune-belly syndrome: a functional urethral obstruction caused by prostatic hypoplasia. *Pediatrics* 1984, **73**:470–475.
Nakayama D K, Harrison M R, Chinn D H *et al*: The pathogenesis of prune belly. *AJDC* 1984, **138**:834–836.
Kawamoto K, Ikeda T, Matsuo T. *et al*: Prune belly syndrome: report of twelve cases and possible pathogenesis. *Cong Anom* 1985, **25**:1–15.
Greskovich F J III, Nyberg L M Jr: The prune belly syndrome: a review... *J Urol* 1988, **140**:707–713.
Buntix I M, Bourgeois N *et al*: Acardiac amorphous twin with prune belly syndrome in the co-twin. *Am J Med Genet* 1991, **39**:453–457.
Reinberg Y, Shapiro E *et al*: Prune belly syndrome in females... *J Pediatr* 1991, **118**:395–398.

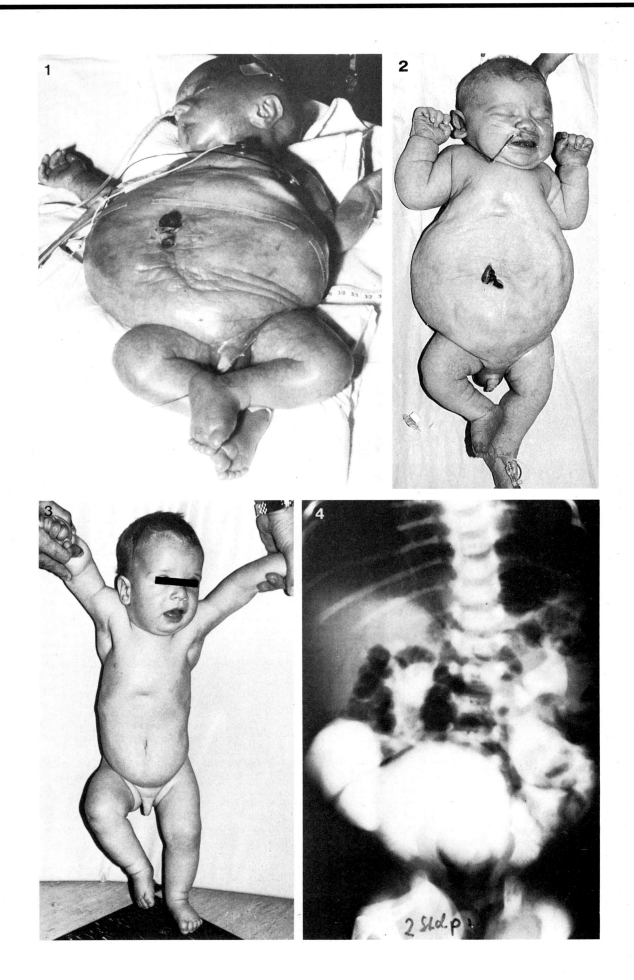

166 Autosomal Recessive Polycystic ('infantile') Kidney Disease

K. Zerres
H.-R.W

A clinical picture of early abdominal distension, palpable 'giant tumours', often rapidly progressive course in the neonatal period and fibrosis of the liver of variable severity with portal hypertension and arterial hypertension.

Main signs:
- Protuberant and bulging abdomen with markedly enlarged kidneys (**1 and 2**).
- Liver fibrosis of varying degrees of severity, with hepatomegaly and signs of portal hypertension to the extent of bleeding from oesophageal varices.
- In the very severe form, 'Potter syndrome' as the result of oligohydramnios or ahydramnios or respiratory insufficiency resulting from upward displacement of the diaphragm and hypoplasia of the lungs.
- Fairly rapid development and progression of renal insufficiency, arterial hypertension.

Supplementary findings: Ultrasound evidence of kidney enlargement with high echogenicity; intravenous pyelogram shows radially arranged, narrow collecting tubules filled with contrast medium (**2**). Larger single cysts not typical, at least not in the neonatal period; eventual loss of a uniform picture. Presence or development of corresponding urinary, serum and circulatory abnormalities.

Manifestation: Possible prenatal manifestation as 'Potter syndrome'; otherwise in neonatal period. Rarely presents in childhood or adolescence; not until adulthood only in exceptional cases.

Aetiology: Autosomal recessive disorder. Various clinical forms probably caused by multiple alleles.

Frequency: Not clear; between 1:40 000 and 1:60 000.

Course, prognosis: Life expectancy distinctly reduced depending on the age at presentation: the earlier the presentation, the poorer the prognosis.

Comment, differential diagnosis: Differentiation from early presentation of the autosomal dominant ('adult') form is occasionally possible solely by a positive family history (ultrasound examination of both parents) or by demonstration of hepatic fibrosis.

Treatment: Symptomatic. In later stages, dialysis or transplantation may be required.

Genetic counselling. Prenatal diagnosis may be attempted by ultrasound in future pregnancies, although this is often unsuccessful in the first half of pregnancy.

Illustrations:

1 and 2 The first child of young, healthy, non-consanguineous parents. Birth at about term after a normal pregnancy, 3170 g; breech presentation, markedly protuberant abdomen and symmetrical, firm kidney 'tumours' extending from the costal arch into the true pelvis. Intravenous pyelogram on the seventh or eighth day of life: after 2 h, widely separated, markedly dilated renal collecting systems vaguely recognizable and 19 h after injection, clearly visible renal parenchymal shadows 10 cm and 6 cm in diameter, with axes converging caudally (**2**). Cystography: unremarkable efferent urinary tract.

During a 10-week hospital stay, initial oedema, elevation of urinary nitrogen, haematuria, erythrocyturia, leukocyturia and mild proteinuria. With symptomatic treatment, clearing of these signs and subsequent good progress.

1 The proband at 3 years and 4 months. At 5 years and 7 months, 112.5 cm and 20.5 kg (average for age); palpably enlarged kidneys, liver 3 cm below the costal margin; urine negative; blood pressure with medication normal, occasionally up to 135/80 mmHg. The boy has in the mean time started attending school and has three healthy younger brothers.

References:

Blyth H, Ockenden B G: Polycystic disease of kidneys and liver presenting in childhood. *J Med Genet* 1971, 8:257.
Zerres K: Genetics of cystic kidney disease. Criteria for classification and genetic counseling. *Pediatr Nephrol* 1987, 1:397–404.
Neumann H P H, Zerres Kl *et al*: Late manifestation of autosomal-recessive polycystic kidney disease in two sisters. *Am J Nephrol* 1988, 8:194–197.
Kaplan B S, Fay I *et al*: Autosomal recessive polycystic kidney disease. *Pediatr Nephrol* 1989, 3:43–49.
Zerres K: Autosomal recessive polycystic kidney disease. *Clin Invest* 1992, 70:794–801.

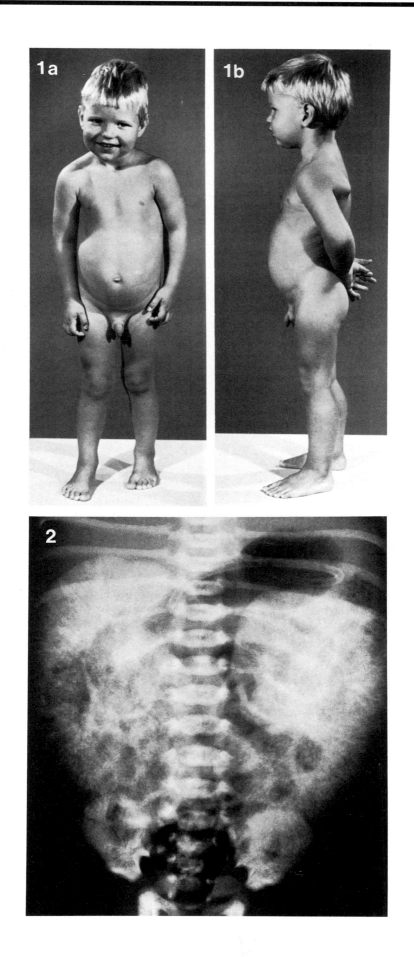

167 Gaucher's Disease Type 1
('Classic', chronic visceral form of Gaucher's disease)

H.-R.W

A chronic lysosomal 'storage' disease which spares the nervous system, with hepatosplenomegaly, dyshematopoiesis and characteristic 'orthopaedic complications'.

Main signs:
- Hepatosplenomegaly, which may be considerable (**1b**).
- Dyshematopoiesis ('splenogenic marrow depression', thrombocytopaenia, leukopaenia, anaemia); pallor, possibly haemorrhages.
- Periodic bone and joint pain, especially in the long bones; pseudo-osteomyelitic or pseudo-arthritic pathologic fractures, sometimes with aseptic necrosis; epiphysiolysis. Usually found in: femur (on radiograph showing an 'Erlenmeyer flask deformity' distally); necrosis of the femoral head is particularly characteristic (**1c, 2**); also destruction of vertebral bodies and other areas.
- In children, frequent short stature, delayed puberty (**1a**).

Supplementary findings: Mental development and nervous system normal.

Yellow–brownish colouration of the skin in some patients, especially of the face, back of the neck, hands and extensor surfaces of the lower legs and, in adults, yellowish spots ('pingueculae') of the sclera.

Elevation of the (tartrate-resistant) serum acid phosphatase; demonstration of Gaucher cells in bone marrow aspirates or other tissue preparations or demonstration of a cerebroside-beta-glucosidase defect in leukocytes, which is simpler and diagnostic.

Manifestation: Possible at any age (from early childhood).

Aetiology: Autosomal recessive disorder especially affecting Jewish individuals (Ashkenazim): homozygote affected 1:2500, heterozygotes 4%. Heterogeneity.

Course, prognosis: Patients may live to an old age.
The sequelae to fractures of the neck of the femur with necrosis of the femoral head are, when damage is irreversible, often considered as the greatest problem in adults.

Treatment: Careful orthopaedic supervision. Exemption from school sports. Promotion of intellectual development and adequate vocational guidance. For acute attacks of pain, immobilization suffices. For previous severe hip damage, possible operative reduction and more extensive revision at a later date. Splenectomy for marked signs of abdominal displacement and marked dyshematopoiesis.

Psychological support. Genetic counselling. Heterozygote test and prenatal diagnosis by enzyme assay. Gene therapy may be possible in the future as a result of progress in molecular genetics.

Illustrations:

1 and 2 A 14-year-old girl (one parent Ashkenazi). 'Coxitis' on the left at age 5 years, further attacks of hip pain at 11 and, bilaterally, at 13 years. Protuberant abdomen caused by both hyperlordosis (**1b**) and upper abdominal organomegaly. Postsplenectomy (typical Gaucher histology); hepatomegaly to the level of the umbilicus. Growth deficiency (here below the third percentile) with overlong extremities; delayed puberty (no menarche to date); bone age retarded by 3 years. 'Limping' for months: dislocated left hip with necrosis of the left femoral head and severe destruction of the neck of the femur (for which a reduction was carried out); storage deposits also in the right femur below the lesser trochanter (**2**); no further skeletal foci found (nor evidence of lung involvement). Enzyme defect demonstrated by leukocyte test.

References:
Any detailed textbook on paediatrics and internal medicine. Additionally: Tjhen K Y, Zillhardt H W: M Gaucher Typ 1. *Pädiat Prax* 1977, **18**:247.
Goldblatt J, Sacks S, Beighton P: The orthopedic aspects of Gaucher disease. *Clin Orthopaed* 1978, **137**:208.
Choy F Y M: Gaucher disease... *Am J Med Genet* 1985, **21**:519–528.
Grabowski G A, Goldblatt J *et al*: Genetic heterogeneity in Gaucher disease... *Am J Med Genet* 1985, **21**:529–549.
Beaudet A L: Gaucher's disease. *N Engl J Med* 1987, **316**:619–620.
Hobbs J R, Jones K H *et al*: Beneficial effect of pretransplant splenectomy on displacement bone marrow transplantation for Gaucher's syndrome. *Lancet* 1987, I:1111–1115.
Matoth Y, Chazan S *et al*: Frequency of carriers of chronic (type I) Gaucher disease... *Am J Med Genet* 1987, **27**:561–565.
Choy F Y M: Intrafamilial clinical variability of type I Gaucher disease... *J Med Genet* 1988, **25**:322–325.
Goldblatt J: Type I Gaucher disease. *J Med Genet* 1988, **25**:415–418.
Zlotogora J, Sagi M *et al*: Gaucher disease type 1 and pregnancy. *Am J Med Genet* 1989, **31**:475–477.

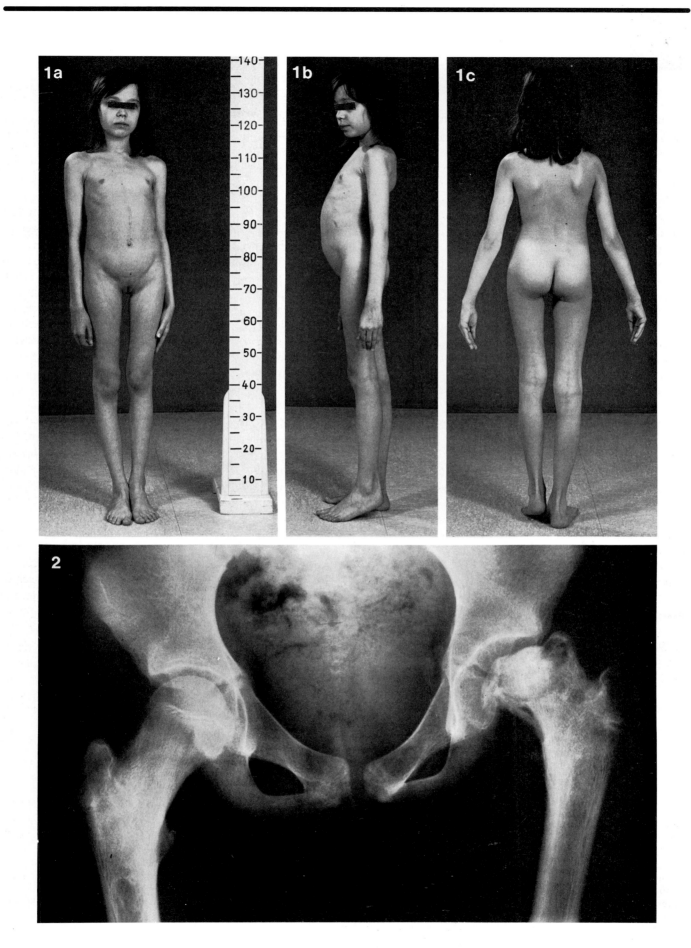

A sequence of hypoplasia or aplasia of the caudal spine of variable severity, with developmental defect of the corresponding spinal segments, and hypoplasia or dysplasia of the pelvis and lower extremities.

Main signs:
- Shortening, narrowing or atypical configuration of the lower part of the trunk, especially apparent dorsally, the buttocks often appearing flat with dimples and a shortened gluteal fold (**1b**). Distinctly disproportionate short stature possible caused by short trunk and relatively long extremities, especially the arms (**1a and b**).
- Weakness and atrophy, with possible malformation or hypoplasia of the legs. Hips frequently dislocated (**2 and 3**). Flexion contractures of the hips and knees. Club feet. Frequent paralysis of the pelvic floor muscles and sphincters with urinary and faecal incontinence; frequent areflexia of the legs (motor and sensory defects need not correspond). Thus, total neurological impairment may vary from a slight disorder of bladder control to total paralysis below the defect.

Supplementary findings: Radiologically, lumbo-sacro-coccygeal vertebral defects of variable severity. Possible malformation and narrowing of the pelvis with narrowly spaced hypoplastic ilia, which are directly apposed dorsally (**2 and 3**). Dislocated hips, femoral hypoplasia possible. Arthrogryposis, club feet.

Possible malformation of the gastro-intestinal tract, the abdominal organs or the heart; polycystic kidneys, hydronephrosis, renal dysplasia, hypospadias. Additionally, growth retardation, hydrocephalus, Pierre Robin sequence, club hand, radial aplasia, polydactyly, myelomeningocoele, exstrophy of the bladder, rectovaginal fistula.

Manifestation: At birth.

Aetiology: Not uniform. Mostly isolated cases. At least 28% of patients have mothers with poorly controlled diabetes; in these, the syndrome falls within the spectrum of a 'diabetic embryopathy' (*299*).

Frequency: 1–5:100 000 liveborn children. Out of 445 patients, 34% had an isolated sacrococcygeal dysgenesis association, 12% had sirenomelia (*44*), 27% VATER association (*311*), and 27% have yet to be classified. For the purposes of differential diagnosis, the femoral hypoplasia–unusual face syndrome (*217*) and the Currarino triad (*310*) should also be considered.

Course, prognosis: Dependent on the severity of the dysplasia and on the quality and consistency of care and multidisciplinary rehabilitation.

Illustrations:
1–3 A 14-year-old girl whose mother had been diabetic for 13 years at the time of the patient's birth. Growth deficiency of 20 cm from the average height for age because of caudal shortening of the trunk. Narrowly spaced ilial wings; abnormal configuration of the lower back and gluteal region (**1b**) with shortened gluteal fold and dimples. Waddling gait with complete bilateral dislocated hips; contracted knee joints; muscle wasting and abundant fat in the lower extremities, the former especially of the calves; absent patellar reflex; sensation in the legs intact. Urinary incontinence (previously also faecal incontinence). Relatively good physical rehabilitation after surgery for club feet and other orthopaedic measures, after surgery for congenital valvular and subvalvular pulmonary stenosis and an atrial septal defect and under paediatric urological care. Very good psychosocial adjustment.

Radiographs (**2 and 3** at 5 years and 6 months and 8 years respectively): absence of the fourth and fifth lumbar vertebrae, all of the sacrum and the coccyx. Ilial wings small and directly apposed dorsally; small heart-shaped pelvis and extremely narrow pelvic outlet. Severe bilateral dysplasia of the hip joints; lateralized capital femoral epiphyses, coxa vara.

References:

Price D L, Dooling E C, Richardson Jr E P: Caudal dysplasia (caudal regression syndrome). *Arch Neurol* 1970, **23**:212.

Amendt P. Goedel E, Amendt U, Becker G: Mißbildungen bei mütterlichem Diabetes mellitus unter besonderer Berücksichtigung des kaudalen Fehlbildungssyndroms. *Zbl Gynäk* 1974, **96**(30):950.

Andrish J, Kalamchi A, MacEwen G D: Sacral agenesis: a clinical evaluation of its management, heredity, and associated anomalies. *Clin Orthopaed* 1979, **139**:52.

Stewart J M, Stoll S: Familial caudal regression anomalad and maternal diabetes. *J Med Genet* 1979, **16**:17; also *ibid* 1980, **17**:57.

Mitnick J, Kramer E *et al*: Radiological case of the month: syndrome of caudal regression... *AJDC* 1982, **136**:637–638.

Fuhrmann K, Reiher H *et al*: Prevention of congenital malformations in infants of insulin-dependent diabetic mothers. *Diabetes Care* 1983, **6**:219–223.

Lausecker M, Stögmann W: Stellen Sie die Diagnose. *Pädiatr Pädol* 1987, **22**:73–77.

Mills J L, Knopp R H *et al*: Lack of relation of increased malformation rates in infants of diabetic mothers to glycemic control during organogenesis. *N Engl J Med* 1988, **318**:671–676.

Bergman M, Newman S A *et al*: Letters: diabetic control and fetal malformations. *N Engl J Med* 1988, **319**:647–649.

Editorial: Congenital abnormalities in infants of diabetic mothers. *Lancet* 1988, **I**:1313–1315.

Duncan P A, Shapiro L R, Klein R M: Sacrococcygeal dysgenesis association. *Am J Med Genet* 1991, **41**:153–161.

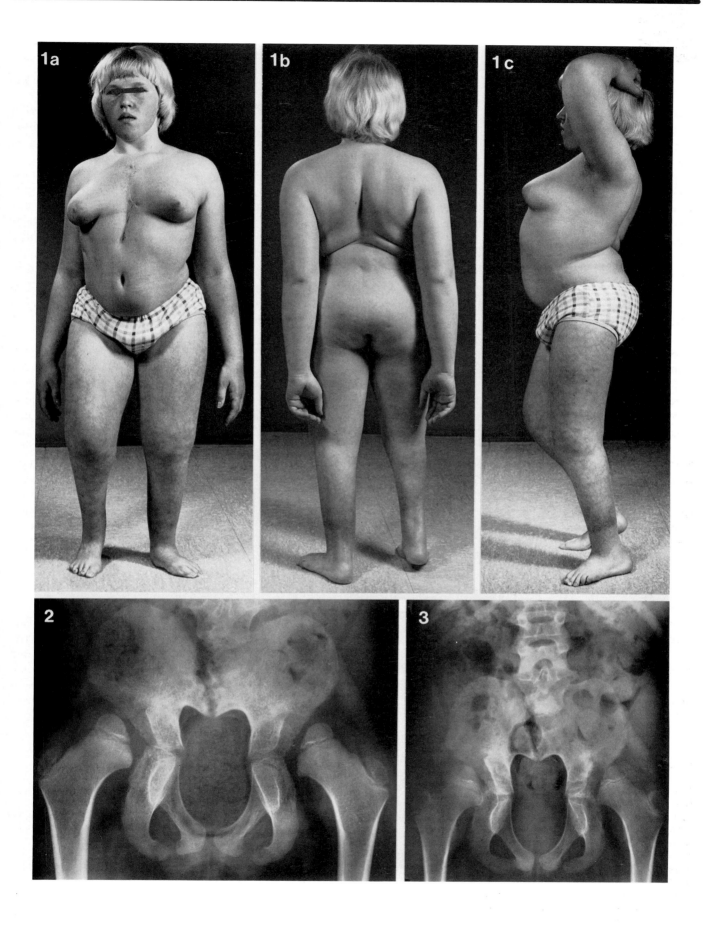

169 **Syndrome of Multiple Benign Ring-Shaped Skin Creases**
(Multiple Ring-Shaped Skin Creases, Michelin Tyre Baby Syndrome)

J.K./H.-R.W

A familial syndrome, manifesting in childhood, with multiple benign ring-shaped contractions of the skin, which are mostly lost in adulthood.

Main signs:
Deep ring-like constrictions of the skin, especially over the extremities, fingers and toes without signs of strangulation or amputation. Less prominent rings on the trunk. No lymphoedema. Nails normal.

Supplementary findings:
Minor anomalies such as medial epicanthus, mongoloid slant of the palpebral fissures, auricular peculiarities, hypertelorism or micrognathia may be present.
The three patients pictured here showed in addition:
• Neuroblastoma, cleft palate.
• Ureterocoeles, cleft palate.
• Complicated febrile seizures.

Manifestation: At birth

Aetiology: Autosomal dominant inheritance. Occurrence both in isolation and in association with malformations.

Frequency: Higher than previously reported, especially in its milder form.

Course, prognosis: The ring-shaped constrictions become less distinct during childhood and are barely demonstrable in the adult.

Differential diagnosis: No relation to amniotic bands (*219*). Reports were published of two patients with diffuse smooth muscle hamartomas; two further patients presented subcutaneous lipomatous naevi; one patient showed a unilateral hemihypertrophy and another had a hemiplegia and microcephaly.
  As dermatomegaly, also known to be symptomatic in skeletal dysplasias, for example, achondroplasia (*130*).

Treatment: None.

Comment: The designation 'Michelin tyre baby syndrome' is a misnomer and should be avoided.

Illustrations:
1a–c A female neonate (6 days old).
2a and b A 4-month-old female infant.
3a A 9-month-old boy.
3b The child's father at age 10 months.

References:
Kunze J, Riehm H: A new genetic disorder: autosomal-dominant multiple ring-shaped skin creases. *Eur J Pediatr* 1982, **138**:310–303.
Niikawa N, Ishikiriyama S, Shikimani T: Letter to the editor: The 'Michelin Tyre Baby' syndrome — an autosomal dominant trait. *Am J Med Genet* 1985, **22**:637–638.
Kunze J: Letter to the Editor: The 'Michelin Tire Baby syndrome': an autosomal-dominant trait. *Am J Med Genet* 1986, **25**:169.
Niikawa N, Ishikiriyama S: Letter to the editor: response to Dr. Kunze. *Am J Med Genet* 1986, **25**:171.
Wiedemann H-R: Letter to the Editor: multiple benign circumferential skin creases on limbs — a congenital anomaly existing from beginning of mankind. *Am J Med Genet* 1987, **28**:225–226.
Glover M T, Malone M, Atherton D J: Michelin-tyre baby syndrome resulting from diffuse smooth muscle hamartoma. *Pediatr Dermatol* 1989, **6**:329–331.
Bass H N, Caldwell S, Brooks B S: Michelin tyre baby syndrome: familial constriction bands during infancy and early childhood in four generations. *Am J Med Genet* 1993, **45**:370–372.
Cohen M M Jr, Gorlin R J, Clark R *et al*: Multiple circumferential skin folds and other anomalies: a problem in syndrome delineation. *Clin Dysmorph* 1993, **2**:39–46.

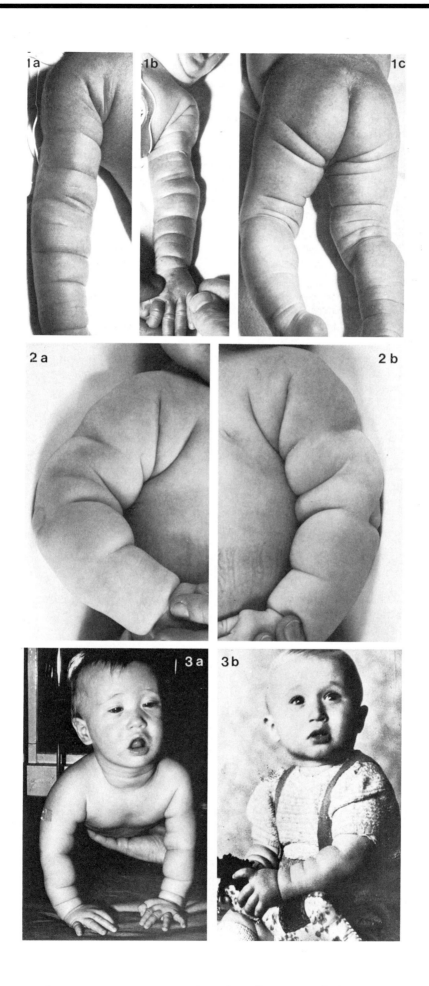

170 Gingival Fibromatosis–Hypertrichosis Syndrome

(Gingival Fibromatosis with Hypertrichosis)

H.-R.W

An hereditary disorder with early manifestation of generalized hypertrichosis and fibromatosis.

Main signs:
- Generalized hypertrichosis, usually with dark hair (even in families with otherwise fair complexions) (**1, 3**).
- Gingival fibromatosis, which more or less covers the teeth, delays eruption, overgrows the crowns and may bring about loss of teeth (**4–6**). In some patients, protrusion of the lips and jaws and other secondary mechanical effects.

Supplementary findings: Epilepsy or mental retardation are often present, especially in the infrequent sporadic cases (possible recessive inheritance).

Manifestation: Development of generalized hypertrichosis in the first 2 years of life; the gingival changes also present in infancy or early childhood.

Aetiology: Hereditary disorder, usually autosomal dominant. Possibly also an autosomal recessive form; heterogeneity is therefore likely.

Frequency: Low.

Prognosis: Favourable with regard to the gingival hyperplasia, assuming adequate treatment.

The prognosis depends on the patient's mental development.

Comment: In a rare type, in which mode of inheritance is uncertain and which cannot be definitely identified before sexual maturity, female carriers develop mammary fibro-adenomatosis with a tendency to malignant degeneration.

Treatment: Very meticulous oral hygiene; gingivectomy; in some patients, extraction of teeth and prosthetic measures. Depilation. Genetic counselling.

Illustrations:

1–4 A boy with typical development of the syndrome; very heavily developed eyebrows, hyperplasia of the eyelashes (three rows), apparent small size of the teeth.

5 and 6 Further demonstration of gingival hyperplasia in two other patients.

References:

Snyder C H: Syndrome of gingival hyperplasia, hirsutism, and convulsions... *J Pediatr* 1965, **67**:499–502.
Witkop C J Jr: Heterogeneity in gingival fibromatosis. *Birth Defects Orig Art Ser* 1971, 7:210.
Winter G B, Simpkiss M J: Hypertrichosis with hereditary gingival hyperplasia. *Arch Dis Child* 1974, **49**:394–399.
Horning G M, Fisher J G *et al*: Gingival fibromatosis with hypertrichosis... *J Periodontol* 1985, **56**:344–347.
Cuestos-Carnero R, Bornancini C A, Hereditary generalized gingival fibromatosis associated with hypertrichosis; report of five cases in one family. *J Oral Maxillofac Surg* 1988, **46**:415–420.
Anavi Y, Lerman P *et al*: Idiopathic familial gingival fibromatosis associated with mental retardation, epilepsy and hypertrichosis. *Dev Med Child Neurol* 1989, **31**:538–542.

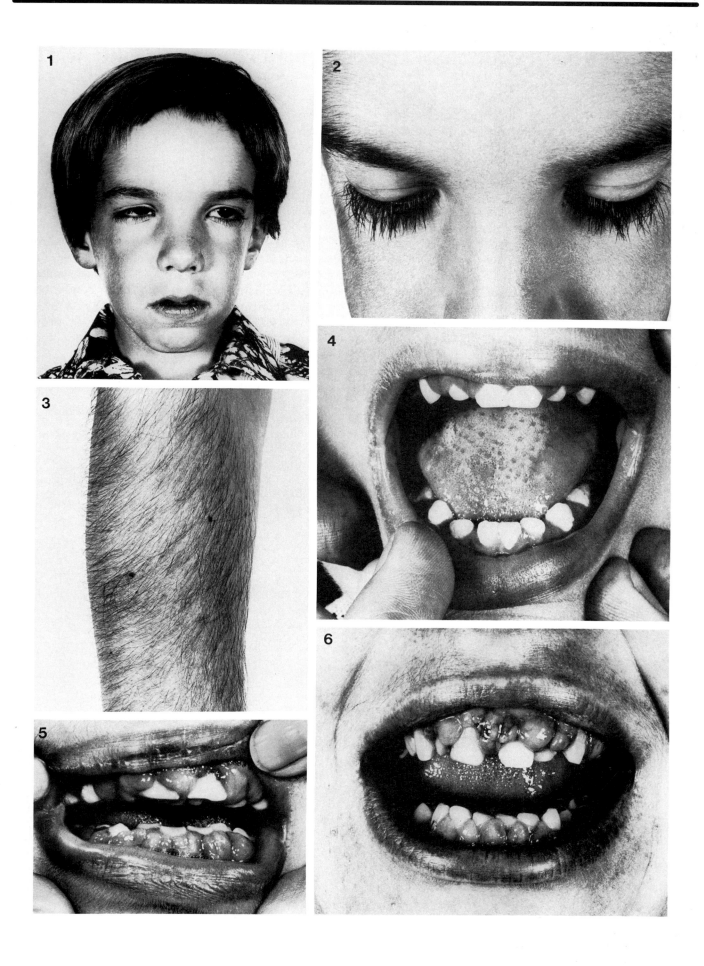

171 Hypertrichosis–Skeletal Dysplasia–Retardation Syndrome with Unusual Facies and Reduced Renal Excretion of Uric Acid

H.-R.W

A clinical picture with congenital hypertrichosis, talipes cavus with claw toes, malpositioning of the thumbs, hip dysplasia, a distinctive facial appearance, mild mental retardation and manifestations of hyperuricaemia beginning in late childhood.

Main signs:
- Congenital, abnormal and increasing hair growth on the face, trunk and limbs (5–9) with premature greying.
- Congenital hollow feet (talipes cavus), claw toes, abnormal positioning of the thumbs (9–13). Brachycephaly. Increasing manifestation of a long neck and long, narrow, protruding thorax with drooping shoulders (1–4, 5, 9, 14, 15).
- Distinctive facial appearance (1–4).
- Mild mental retardation with open, friendly demeanour.
- Gout symptoms starting from the middle of the second decade of life, with hyperuricaemia caused by renal hypo-excretion of uric acid.

Supplementary findings: Coxa valga with subluxation of the hip joints. Neurological examinations all normal.

Manifestation: At birth and thereafter, especially in the case of the gout symptoms.

Aetiology: Unclear, possibly autosomal or X-linked new mutation.

Frequency: Unknown.

Course, prognosis: To date, favourable; the further development of kidney function remains to be seen.

Differential diagnosis: Other hypertrichosis syndromes (e.g. hypertrichosis-gingival fibromatosis syndrome (*170*), Ambras syndrome, Barber–Say syndrome, Gorlin–Chaudhry–Moss syndrome, osteochondrodysplasia with hypertrichosis [Cantú et al. 1982]) and the clinical pictures known in childhood which are associated with hyperuricemia (Lesch–Nyhan syndrome *296* and others).

Treatment: With hyperuricaemia, allopurinol therapy is urgently indicated.

Illustrations:
These concern the same propositus between the ages of 11 months and 19 years.
1–15 from:
Wiedemann H-R, Oldigs H-D, Oppermann, H-C, Oster O: Hirsutism-skeletal dysplasia-mental retardation syndrome with abnormal face and a uric acid metabolism disorder. *Am J Med Genet* 1993, 46:403–409.

References:
Wiedemann H-R, Oldigs H-D, Oppermann H-C, Oster O: Hirsutism-skeletal dysplasia-mental retardation syndrome with abnormal face and a uric acid metabolism disorder. *Am J Med Genet* 1993, 46:403–409.
Oster O, Wiedemann H-R, Duley I A, Simmonds H A, McBride M B: Reduced renal excretion of uric acid in the hirsutism-skeletal dysplasia-mental retardation syndrome (Letter). *Am J Med Genet* 1994, 51:165–167.

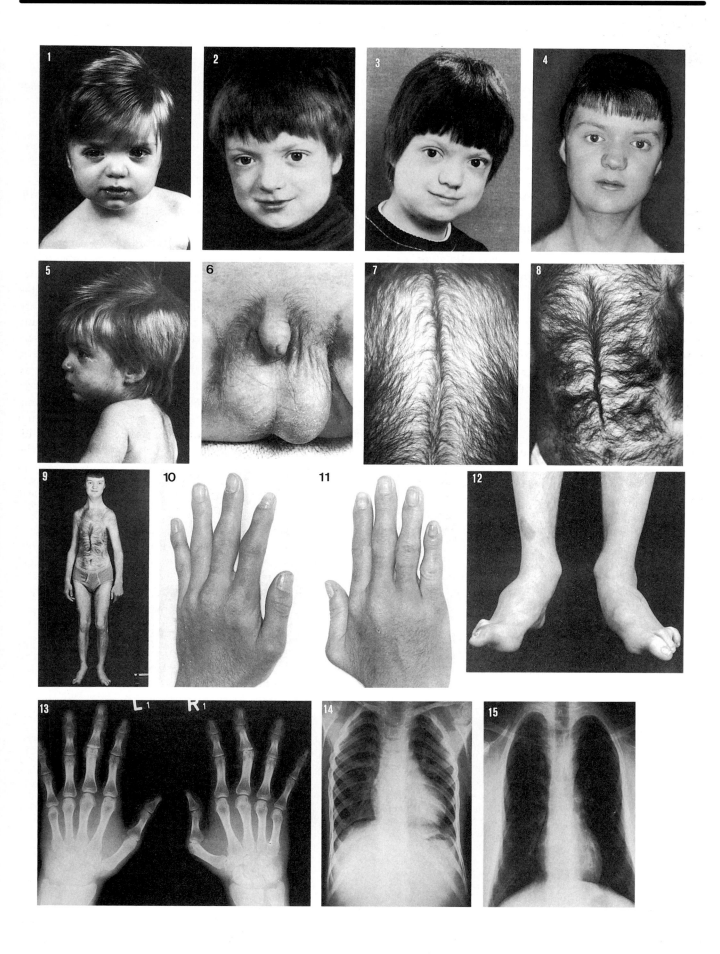

Extensive congenital melanocytic naevus which may be associated with leptomeningeal melanocytosis ('neurocutaneous melanoblastosis').

Main signs:

Skin changes: usually intensive black–brown macular or partially raised and nodular or wartlike, usually with coarse hairs, with bilaterally symmetrical or asymmetrical distribution ('bathing suit', 'bathing trunk', 'cap', 'neck poultice', 'stocking' naevus and so on) with multiple corresponding smaller naevi (**1 and 2**).

Supplementary findings: Development of hydrocephalus or central nervous system seizures or other neurological or psychological features indicate progressive meningocerebral involvement. The presence of an extensive naevus on an extremity impairs its growth.

Manifestation: Hairy naevi present at birth. Although cerebral signs may appear as early as infancy, they generally begin at a pre-school age and occasionally not until much later.

Aetiology: Unclear. Usually sporadic occurrence, familial as an exception (affected family members usually have multiple small naevi only); possibly, multifactorial inheritance. There is possibly a lethal mutation, which survives in the mosaic.

Frequency: Not particularly rare. Up to 1987, there were only about 100 reported patients with neurocutaneous melanosis in the literature; of these, at least 35 with malignant meningeal meningioma.

Course, prognosis, treatment: Central nervous system involvement or its progression may lead to death in infancy or early childhood. (Extensive hairy naevi of the head or neck region are considered to be frequently associated with meningeal melanocytosis, with a consequently less favourable prognosis.) In the region of the skin naevus and the correspondingly affected intracranial area, there is an increased risk of developing a malignant melanoma, which usually presents within the first 5 years of life.

The treatment of choice is complete resection of the entire giant skin naevus (as well as the satellites) with grafting; when not feasible, as is often the case, the most extensive possible excision. Such a procedure may be carried out more successfully after infancy. Definite cosmetic improvement is accomplished by planing (or curettage, followed by planing), although such dermabrasion can probably not markedly decrease the risk of melanoma developing in deeper portions. Considering the associated risk, a hairy naevus requires regular, careful follow-up (preferably with photographic documentation of the course); the patient and sometimes family members require appropriate psychological help and guidance.

Illustrations:

1a–d A newborn with 'bathing trunk' giant hairy naevus and numerous satellite naevi. Relatively large cranium. No pathological growth of the skull or other neurological signs.

2a–c A boy at age 6 years and 6 months. Hairy naevus with satellites. Recent onset of focal seizures.

References:
Voigtländer V, Jung E G: Giant pigmented hairy nevus in two siblings. *Humangenetik* 1974, **24**:79.
Lamas E, Diez Lobato R *et al*: Neurocutaneous melanosis. *Acta Neurochirurgica* 1977, **36**:93.
Solomon L M: The management of congenital melanocytic nevi. *Arch Derm* 1980, **116**:1017.
Hecht F, LaCanne K M, Carroll D B: Inheritance of giant pigmented hairy nevus... *Am J Med Genet* 1981, **9**:177.
Fleissner J, Kleine M, Bonsmann G *et al*: Dermabrasion eines großflächigen kongenitalen Pigmentnävus... *Pädiat Prax* 1982, **26**:505.
Konz B: Problem der angeborenen pigmentierten Nävi. *Pädiat Prax* 1982, **26**:106.
Müller-Holzner E, Weiser G *et al*: Neurokutane Melanose. *Medwelt* 1984, 1184–1187.
Cazzani M, Lampertico P *et al*: La melanosi neurocutanea. *Min Ped* 1987, **39**:43–51.
Drepper H, Hundeiker M: Beurteilung und Behandlung angeborener Pigmentzellnaevi. *Mschr Kinderheilk* 1987, **135**:406–410.
Moss A L H: Congenital 'giant' naevus... new surgical approach. *Br J Plast Surg* 1987, **40**:410.
Schnyder U W, Schneider B V *et al*: Kongenitale Naevuszellnaevi als Melanomprekursoren der Haut. *Mschr Kinderheilk* 1987, **135**:259–264.
Schrudde J, Steffens K: Tierfellnävi... *Pädiat Prax* 1987, **35**:279–286.
Pascual-Castroviejo I: Neurocutaneous melanosis. Chapter 36 in *Neurocutaneous diseases*, ed. by M. R. Gomez. Boston: Butterworth 1987; 329–334.
Krüger M: Behandlung von 'Tierfellnaevi' bei Neugeborenen. *Dtsch med Wschr* 1990, **115**:597–598.
Cremer H: Pigmentierte Hautveränderungen im Kindesalter. *Kongenitale Naevuszellnaevi der kinderarzt* 1992, **23**:1442–1444.
Ruiz-Maldonado R, Tamayo L *et al*: Giant pigmented nevi: clinical, histopathologic and therapeutic considerations. *J Pediatr* 1992, **120**:906–911.
Carroll C B *et al*: Severely atypical... congenital nevus with... satellitosis ..: the problem of congenital melanoma and its simulants. *J Am Acad Dermatol* 1994, **30**:825–828.

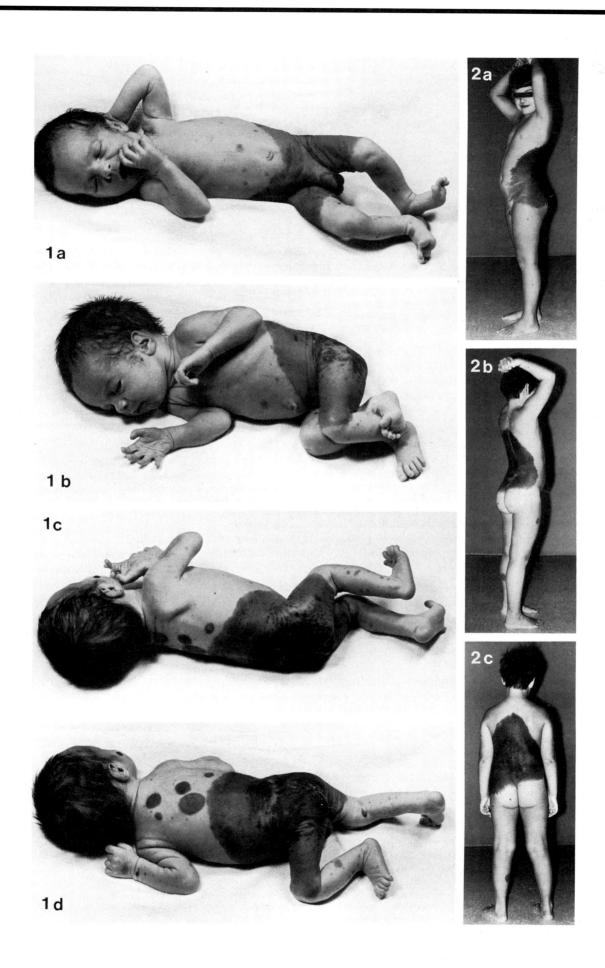

173 Schimmelpenning–Feuerstein–Mims 'Syndrome'

(Linear Sebaceous Naevus 'Syndrome', Epidermal Naevus Syndrome)

H.-R.W

A syndrome of streak-like Jadassohn sebaceous naevus (usually involving the middle of the face), cerebral seizures and mental retardation.

Main signs:
- Sebaceous naevus of Jadassohn; unilateral or bilateral; localized mainly on the head (with focal alopecia), around the ears, on the forehead and temples, often extending to the tip of the nose or to the rest of the face, also possibly elsewhere on the body. Changes varying from narrow and pale to broad, conspicuous stripes. Yellow–brown appearance; greasy, warty consistency (1–3).
- Often additional, widely distributed, pigmented naevi (1 and 2).
- Cerebral seizures, usually in the form of focal epilepsy, of variable severity.
- Very variable mental or psychomotor retardation present in some patients. Frequently behavioural disorder also present.

Supplementary findings: Congenital involvement of one or both eyes in approximately 50% of patients: coloboma of the iris (sometimes involving chorioretina or lid); lipodermoids of the conjunctiva and possibly cornea.

Often markedly asymmetrical development of the two sides of the head and face. Hemimacrocephaly, eye anomalies, dilated ventricles and focal electroencephalogram findings with probably hamartomatous cerebral involvement and atrophy which is, as a rule, ipsilateral to the main naevus involvement.

Frequent excrescences of the oral mucosa and dysodontiasis of variable severity (5).

Possible osteodystrophy with pathological fractures (Milkman phenomenon). Short stature in some patients.

Manifestation: Naevus usually congenital (additional pigmentary anomalies and verrucous changes of the naevus occur later). Cerebral seizures, usually focal, may occur early in infancy or sometimes much later. Mental retardation.

Aetiology: Sporadic occurrence. Probably a lethal mutation that survives in the mosaic.

Frequency: Low; by 1993, only 80 patients reported.

Course, prognosis: Seizures and developmental defects are especially likely when linear sebaceous naevus affects the middle of the face.

The course is very variable, depending on the severity of mental retardation and epilepsy. The former need not be severe; the latter may improve spontaneously or be controlled medically.

The Jadassohn naevus is subject to verrucous hyperplasia in childhood and adolescence and may pose a serious cosmetic problem (1). Difficult dental problems may arise early on (5).

In adulthood, development in the naevus of malignant tumours, for example, basal cell epithelioma, must be anticipated (approximately 15% of patients). In addition, this syndrome may be associated with tumour development (renal hamartoma, nephroblastoma, cystic adenoma of the liver, fibro-angioma, osteoclastic tumours of the jaw in isolated cases).

Differential diagnosis: Encephalocraniocutaneous lipomatosis (*175*), Proteus syndrome (*196*) and other phacomatoses.

Treatment: Symptomatic. Early resection of the naevus as far as possible. Appropriate anticonvulsive medication when indicated. Dental care. Cosmetic attention as needed.

Illustrations:

1–5 A 12-year-old boy, the second child of young, nonconsanguineous parents after a healthy sibling. Congenital Jadassohn naevus in broad stripes bilaterally and asymmetrically on the face, scalp (alopecia), and neck (1 planing); narrow streaks on the abdomen, right leg and foot; spotty hyperpigmentation of the trunk and arms (2). Onset of left focal seizures in the second year; dilated left cerebral ventricle; mental retardation (Hawick IQ 78). Also: neurogenic hemi-atrophy (left-sided for the head and tongue, 1b, 4, 5; below that, right-sided, 2a with dysphagia, abnormal motor function and dysreflexia of the atrophic side. Excrescences of the oral mucosa, numerous pathologic fractures or Looser zones and short stature, below the third percentile. Eyes normal. Father of the patient has a neuromotor disability, one arm covered in pigmental moles and a family history of focal seizure disorders.

References:

Schimmelpenning G W: Klinischer Beitrag zur Symptomatologie der Phakomatosen. *RöFo* 1957, 87:716.
Feuerstein R C, Mims L C: Linear nevus sebaceus with convulsions and mental retardation. *AJDC* 1962, **104**:675.
Schimmelpenning G W: Langjährige Verlaufsuntersuchung... *RöFo* 1983, 139:63.
Grebe T A *et al*: Further delineation of the epidermal nevus syndrome... *Am J Med Genet* 1993, 47:24–30.

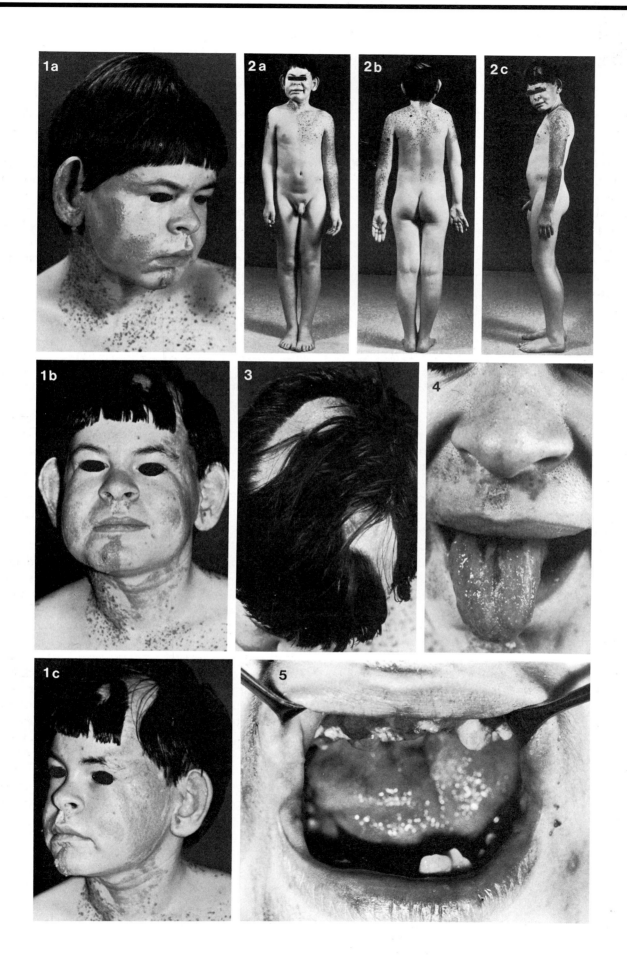

174 Syndrome of Partial Macrosomia, Linear Naevus, Macrocranium with Signs of Cardiac Overload from Intracranial arterio-venous Shunt, Parietal Soft-Tissue Swelling with Alopecia, Psychomotor Retardation and Short Stature

H.-R.W

A syndrome of congenital macrosomia of one lower extremity, linear verrucous naevus on the trunk, macrodolichocephaly with signs of cardiac overload (without evidence of cardiac malformation) from intracranial arterio-venous fistula, biparietal soft-tissue swelling with alopecia, psychomotor retardation and short stature.

Main signs:
- Congenital macrosomia of the left leg (1), from which a cavernous haemangioma of the thigh was removed at 2 years. Excess length over right leg: 2 cm at 3 years, 4 cm at 4 years. Livid discoloration of the left leg with padding-like swelling, especially of the back of the foot. Secondary contractures of the hip and knee. Systolic murmur over the femoral artery but absence of a significant arterio-venous fistula on angiogram.
- Linear hyperpigmented verrucous naevus of the thorax, extending to the mid-line, then continuing downwards (1, 3: note biopsy scar on upper abdomen: epitheliomatous naevus).
- Macrodolichocephaly (53 cm at 2 years and 9 months, 55 cm at 4 years and 9 months) with signs of cardiac overload and cardiomegaly with barrel-shaped chest but without evidence of cardiac malformation. Continuous systolic–diastolic murmur over the cranium. Evidence of an intracranial arterio-venous fistula of the great vein of Galen and dilation of the neighbouring venous sinuses (4).
- Biparietal soft-tissue swelling with alopecia present since the first weeks of life (2). (Biopsy: 'anetoderma'.)
- Physical and psychomotor retardation with muscular dystonia. (No cerebral seizure disorder.)
- Short stature (below the third percentile).

Supplementary findings: High forehead with bossing. Antimongoloid slant of the palpebral fissures, especially the right. High narrow palate; bifid uvula.

Bony protuberance of the lateral rim of the left orbit; on skull radiograph, irregular translucent areas and densities of the parietal cortex.

Oval cystic translucency on the left femur distally.

Slight pareses of the left facial and abducens nerves with strabismus. Ocular fundi hyperpigmented, otherwise normal.

Manifestation: At birth and later.

Aetiology: Uncertain, presumably a genetic basis.

Course: Death of the child at age 5 years from intracranial bleeding.

Comment: The clinical picture of this child suggests the Schimmelpenning–Feuerstein–Mims 'syndrome' (*173*), encephalocraniocutaneous lipomatosis (*175*) or an observation by Goldschmidt *et al*, however, it does not completely correspond to any of these; compare with also syndromes *20* and *225*.

Illustrations:
1–4 A 3-year-old boy, the first child of young, healthy, non-consanguineous parents. Features as described.

References:
Goldschmidt H, Thiede G, Pfeiffer R A *et al*: Hemihypertrophie, Naevus sebaceus, multiple Knochenzysten und zerebroretinale Angiomatose: eine komplexa Phakomatose. *Helv Paediat Acta* 1976, 31:487.

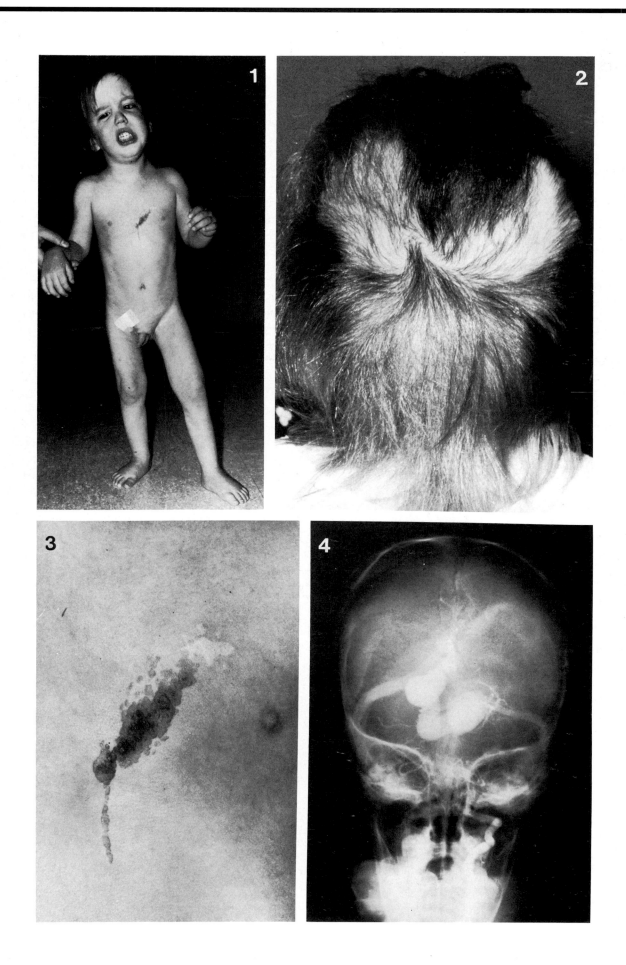

H.-R.W

A clinical picture including macrocephaly, soft-tissue tumours of the head and eyes, cerebral Jacksonian seizures and psychomotor retardation with unilateral porencephalic cysts and cerebral hemiatrophy with lipomatosis.

Main signs:

- Congenital or postnatally manifest macrocrania, which may be clearly asymmetrical and possibly with distinct progression and signs of hydrocephalus (1–5).
- Soft-tissue swellings, small or large, single or multiple, unilateral or bilateral, of the parieto-occipital, frontotemporal, or other parts of the cranial or facial part of the skull; alopecia of the affected area; lipomatous on biopsy (1–5). Bony growths possible (exostoses).
- Possible soft-tissue tumours involving conjunctiva, sclera, cornea or eyelids; lipodermoid on biopsy.
- Focal central nervous system seizures, manifest early.
- Psychomotor retardation of various grades of severity, in some patients with hemispasticity and so on.
- A unilateral porencephalic cyst of variable size communicating with the ventricular system, with ipsilateral atrophy of the brain, can be demonstrated. Autopsy may show fairly extensive intracranial (and possibly intraspinal) lipomatosis, possibly involving the cranial bones.

Supplementary findings: Additional small 'connective tissue naevi', angiofibromas or fibrolipomas possible in the craniofacial area.

Xanthochromia and increased protein in the cerebrospinal fluid in some patients.

Manifestation: At birth and postnatally.

Aetiology: This appears to be the expression of a somatic mosaic (a lethal mutation that survives in the mosaic).

Frequency: Low, barely 20 patients described in the literature.

Course, prognosis: Unfavourable.

Differential diagnosis: Proteus syndrome (196) and Schimmelpenning–Feuerstein–Mims 'syndrome' (173). We consider encephalocraniocutaneous lipomatosis to be a form of Proteus syndrome with more localized, encephalocraniofacial, manifestations. Although there is definite overlap with Schimmelpenning–Feuerstein–Mims 'syndrome', the particular histopathological findings would seem to justify separate classification.

Treatment: Symptomatic.

Illustrations:

1–5 The first child of young, healthy, non-consanguineous parents (**1 and 2** at 4 weeks, **3–5** at 2 years and 6 months). Congenital macrodolichocephaly (41.5 cm) with signs of increasing intracranial pressure, xanthochromia and increased protein in the cerebrospinal fluid. Severe congenital soft-tissue swelling of the left cheek; (hamartoma of the right upper eyelid). Very early focal central nervous system seizures. Psychomotor retardation with signs of cerebral palsy. Ophthalmologically: localized accumulations of chorioretinal pigmentation in the left eye; otherwise normal. Computerized tomography scan showed severe porencephalic dilatation of the left ventricular system. Ventriculo-cardiac shunt. Head circumference at 2 years and 6 months was 62.5 cm; very high forehead. Removal of a lipoma from the left cheek. Death of the child at 3 years and 3 months.

References:

Haberland C, Perou M: Encephalocraniocutaneous lipomatosis. *Arch Neurol* 1970, **22**:144.
Fishman M A, Chang Ch S C, Miller J E: Encephalocraniocutaneous lipomatosis. *Pediatrics* 1978, **61**:580.
Sanchez N P, Rhodes A R, Mandell F *et al*: Encephalocraniocutaneous lipomatosis: a new neurocutaneous syndrome. *Br J Dermatol* 1981, **104**:89.
Schlack H G, Skopnik H: Encephalocraniocutane Lipomatose und lineärer Naevus sebaceus. *Mschr Kinderheilk* 1985, **133**:235–237.
Wiedemann H-R, Burgio G R: Encephalocraniocutaneous lipomatosis and Proteus syndrome. *Am J Med Genet* 1986, **25**:403–404.
Fishman M A: Encephalo-cranio-cutaneous lipomatosis. In: *Neurocutaneous diseases*, ed. by M. R. Gomez. Boston: Butterworth 1987; 349–355.
McCall S, Ramzy M I *et al*: Encephalocraniocutaneous lipomatosis and the Proteus syndrome: distinct entities with overlapping manifestations. *Am J Med Genet* 1992, **43**:662–668.
McMullin G P *et al*: Cranial hemihypertrophy with ipsilateral naevoid streaks, intellectual handicap and epilepsy… *Clin Genet* 1993, **44**:249–253.
Rizzo R, Pavone L *et al*: Encephalocraniocutaneous lipomatosis, Proteus syndrome, and somatic mosaicism. *Am J Med Genet* 1993, **47**:653–655.

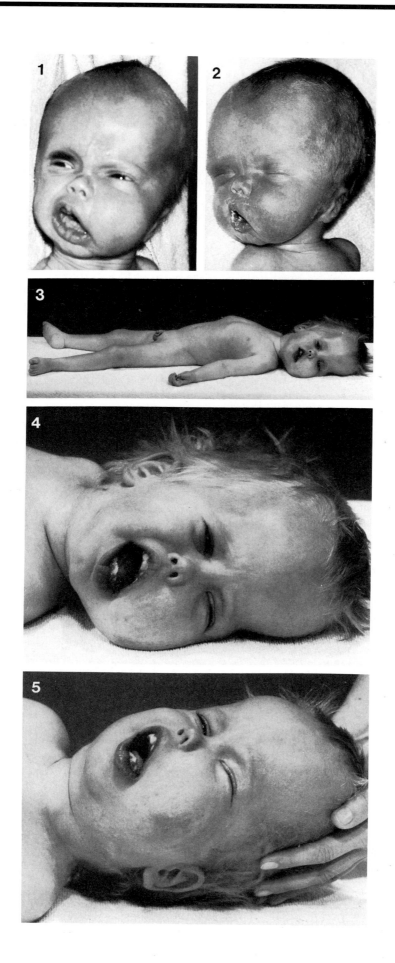

176 McCune–Albright Syndrome

(Albright Syndrome, Weil–Albright Syndrome)

H.-R.W/J.K.

A characteristic syndrome of fibrous dysplasia of the bone, irregular brown hyperpigmentation of the skin and precocious pseudo-puberty (almost exclusively in girls).

Main signs:
- Café au lait or darker-coloured hyperpigmented areas with irregular, sharp map-like borders (**1**), often unilateral along the mid-line, preferentially on the buttocks, thighs, back and neck. (Rarely, these features may be absent.)
- Precocious menarche, followed by premature development of secondary sexual characteristics (in boys, precocious puberty only exceptionally).
- Spontaneous fractures and variable degree of skeletal deformity, usually in the lower extremities, especially the proximal femur, with polyostotic fibrous dysplasia lesions and corresponding radiograph findings (**2**).
- Other autonomous signs of endocrine hyperfunction: hyperthyroidism, hypercortisolaemia (signs of Cushing's syndrome), hypersomatotropism (acromegaly), primary hyperparathyroidism, hyperprolactinaemia, hypophosphataemia.

Supplementary findings: In some cases, accelerated growth in height and skeletal maturity; premature closure of the epiphyses may eventually result in short stature.

Serum calcium and phosphate levels normal; alkaline phosphatase normal or elevated.

Manifestation: Pigmented areas present at birth or shortly thereafter and subsequently grow proportionally. Menarche may even occur in infancy (regular menses usually do not occur until a few years later); further sexual characteristics may develop subsequently. Bony defects manifest mainly during the first decade of life.

Aetiology: Sporadic occurrence. Hypothesis: this clinical picture results from an autosomal dominant lethal gene that can only be expressed phenotypically in mosaic combination with healthy cells. No increased risk for siblings, no transmission to the next generation.

Precocious puberty in girls apparently brought about by gonadotropin-independent oestrogen secretion of the ovaries, which show cystic changes. Mutations have recently been found in the exon 8 of the G_S-alpha gene of affected tissue, which lead to increased G_S protein activity and to an elevation of adenosine cyclic monophosphate. Somatic mutation in early embryogenesis results in the mosaic population of different tissues.

Frequency: Relatively low (up to 1980, approximately 160 reports in the literature).

Course, prognosis: The McCune–Albright syndrome may manifest in early infancy as a hepatobiliary disorder, with cardiac involvement, involvement of other, non-endocrine organs, sudden or early death. The number and extent of bone changes usually progress slowly while the child is growing, as a rule becoming stationary after the second to third decade of life. Life expectancy is normal on the whole (a few patients may develop sarcomas during adolescence). Fractures tend to heal well.

Treatment: Cyproterone acetate, alone or in combination with luteinizing hormone releasing hormone analogues; operative ovarian cystectomy? Avoidance of stress damage, care of pathological fractures and orthopaedic care of skeletal deformities. Attempts at therapeutic application of ionizing radiation contraindicated. Gestagen administration for some patients.

Differential diagnosis: Pseudohypoparathyroidism (*101*) with mutation in the same gene but which leads to decreased activity of the G_S-alpha protein.

Illustrations:

1 A girl aged 13 years and 3 months old: pigmentation anomalies since birth, vaginal bleeding since infancy, secondary characteristics since early childhood. On radiograph: polyostotic fibrous dysplasia with foci in the pelvis and upper leg, left tibia, left scapula, the proximal humeral metaphyses and both temporal bones.

2 Radiograph of the patient. Pelvis oblique and tilted; coxa vara; pathological fracture of the left medial femoral neck; cystic and honeycomb-like changes in the iliosacral region bilaterally, in the region of the left anterior iliac spine and in both proximal femora, the epiphyses being largely spared; cortical thinning of the broadened left diaphysis because of marked cystic expansion.

References:
Grant D B, Martinez, L: The McCune–Albright syndrome without typical skin pigmentation. *Acta Paediatr Scand* 1983, 72:477–478.
Foster C M, Feuillan P *et al*: Ovarian function in girls with McCune–Albright syndrome. *Pediatr Res* 1986, 20:859–863.
Mauras N, Blizzard R M: The McCune–Albright syndrome. *Acta Endocrinol Suppl* 1986, 279:207–217.
Danon M. Crawford J D: The McCune–Albright syndrome. *Erg Inn Med Kinderheilk* 1987, 55:82–115.
Happle R: The McCune–Albright syndrome: a lethal gene surviving by mosaicism. *Clin Genet* 1986, 29:321–324.
Stier B, Ranke M B: Pubertas praecox bei McCune–Albright-Syndrom... *Klin Pädiat* 1987, 199:376–381.
Weinstein L S, Shenker A, Gejman P V *et al*: Activating mutations of the stimulatory G protein in the McCune–Albright syndrome. *N Engl J Med* 1991, 325:1688–1695.
Levine M A: The McCune–Albright syndrome. The whys and wherefores of abnormal signal transduction. *N Engl J Med* 1991, 325:1738–1740.
Shenker A, Weinstein L S *et al*: Severe endocrine and nonendocrine manifestations of the McCune–Albright syndrome associated with activating mutations of stimulatory G protein G_s. *J Pediatr* 1993, 123:509–518.

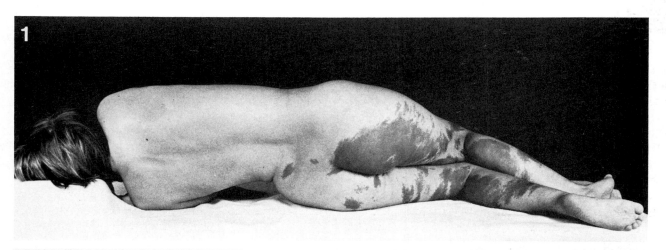

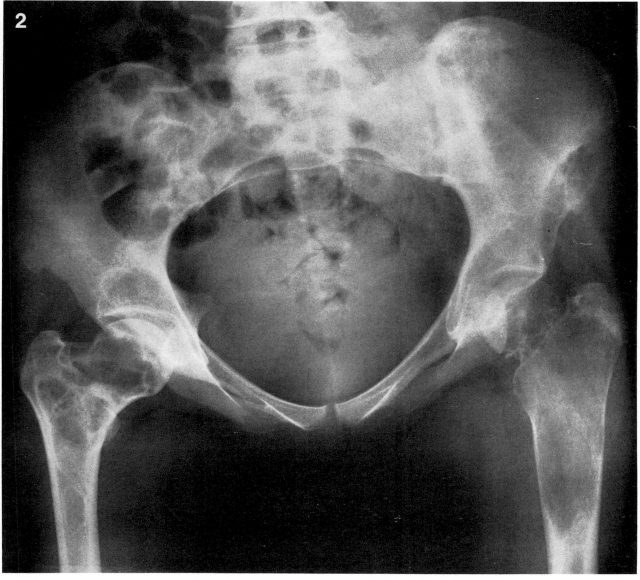

177 Miescher Syndrome

(Bloch–Miescher Syndrome, Mendenhall Syndrome, Rabson–Mendenhall Syndrome)

H.-R.W

A syndrome (closely resembling congenital generalized lipodystrophy) of congenital acanthosis nigricans, hypertrichosis, failure to thrive and short stature, dysmorphism especially of the jaw and oral cavity, insulin-resistant diabetes mellitus and a characteristic general appearance.

Main signs:

- Acanthosis nigricans especially of the neck, axillary, inguinal and genital regions (2–4, 6–8).
- Lanugo-type hypertrichosis of the trunk (5), possibly also of the extremities; overabundant scalp hair in some patients (3, 7).
- Poor physical (and possibly also mental) growth with deficiency of adipose tissue (2), aged appearance (4, 7, 8) and short stature.
- Relatively coarse facial features with prognathism (3, 4, 7, 8), poorly formed, malpositioned teeth (9, 11) and large, relatively low-set ears (7 and 8).

Supplementary findings: High palate, fissured tongue (10); oral mucous membranes coarse, velvety and of milky opacity.

Protruding abdomen, hypertrophic genitals.

Simply formed fingers and toes with thick nails.

Goitre (3 and 4), frequently nodular (hyperplasia of the pineal body).

Highly insulin-resistant diabetes mellitus caused by severely impaired insulin binding capacity.

Manifestation: At birth and in subsequent years; diabetes manifest during childhood or adolescence.

Aetiology: Autosomal recessive disorder. Insulin receptor defect. Gene locus 19p13.3-p.13.2?

Frequency: Very low.

Course, prognosis: Decrease in intensity and extent of the acanthosis nigricans possible after many years. Diabetes relatively benign with minimal tendency to ketosis as likely to occur as death in a keto-acidotic coma during childhood.

Illustrations:

1–11 Siblings with the Miescher syndrome. Latent diabetes mellitus in the father. Both children of short stature. The distinctly more severely affected 13 years and 6 month-old boy has manifest diabetes and nodular goitre; his 11 years and 6 month-old sister, latent diabetes (6, 10, 11: the boy; 9: the girl.)

References:

Miescher G: Zwei Fälle von congenitaler familiärer Akanthosis nigricans, kombiniert mit Diabetes mellitus. *Derm Z* 1921, **32**:276.

Mason H H, Sly G E: Diabetes mellitus: report of a case resistant to insulin... *JAMA* 1937, **108**:2016.

Mendenhall E N: Tumor of pineal body with high insulin resistance. *J Indiana M A* 1950, **43**:32.

Rabson S M, Mendenhall E N: Familial hypertrophy of pineal body... *Am J Clin Pathol* 1956, **26**:283.

Wiedemann H-R, Spranger J, Mogharei M *et al*: Über das Syndrom... und Miescher-Syndrom im Sinne dienzephaler *Syndrome Z Kinderheilk* 1968, **102**:1.

Seip M: Generalized Lipodystrophy. *Ergeb Inn Med Kinderheilk* 1971, **31**:59.

Dumas R, Rolin B, de Paulet P C *et al*: Trois observations de diabète lipoatrophique familial. *Ann Pédiat* 1974, **21**:625.

Barnes N D, Palumbo P J, Hyles A B *et al*: Insulin resistance, skin changes and virilization... *Diabetologia* 1974, **10**:285.

West R J, Lloyd J K, Turner W M L: Familial insulin-resistant diabetes, multiple somatic anomalies... *Arch Dis Child* 1975, **50**:703; also: Holmes J, Tanner M S: Premature eruption and macrodontia associated with insulin resistant diabetes... *Br Dent J* 1976, **141**:280 and West R J, Leonard J V: Familial insulin resistance... *Arch Dis Child* 1980, **55**:619.

Colle M, Doyard P, Chaussain J-L. *et al*: Acanthosis nigricans, hirsutisme et diabète insulino-resistant. *Arch Franç Pédiat* 1979, **36**:518.

Rüdiger H W, Dreyer M *et al*: Familial insulin-resistant diabetes secondary to an affinity defect of the insulin receptor. *Hum Genet* 1983, **64**:407–411.

Dreyer M, Rüdiger H W: Erbliche Rezeptordefekte als Krankheitsursache. *Dtsch Med Wschr* 1986, **111**:465–471.

Moncada V Y, Hedo J A *et al*: Insulinreceptor biosynthesis... from an insulin-resistant patient (Rabson–Mendenhall syndrome)... *Diabetes* 1986, **35**:802–807.

Rittey C D C, Evans T J *et al*: Melatonin state in Mendenhall's syndrome. *Arch Dis Child* 1988, **65**:852–854.

Accili D, Frapier C *et al*: A mutation in the insulin receptor gene... *EMBO J* 1989, **8**:2509–2517.

Kadowaki T, Kadowaki H *et al*: Five mutant alleles of the insulin receptor gene... *J Clin Invest* 1990, **86**:254–264.

Quin J D, Fisher B M *et al*: Acute response to recombinant insulin-like growth factor in a patient with Mendenhall's syndrome. *N Engl J Med* 1990, **323**(20):1425–1426.

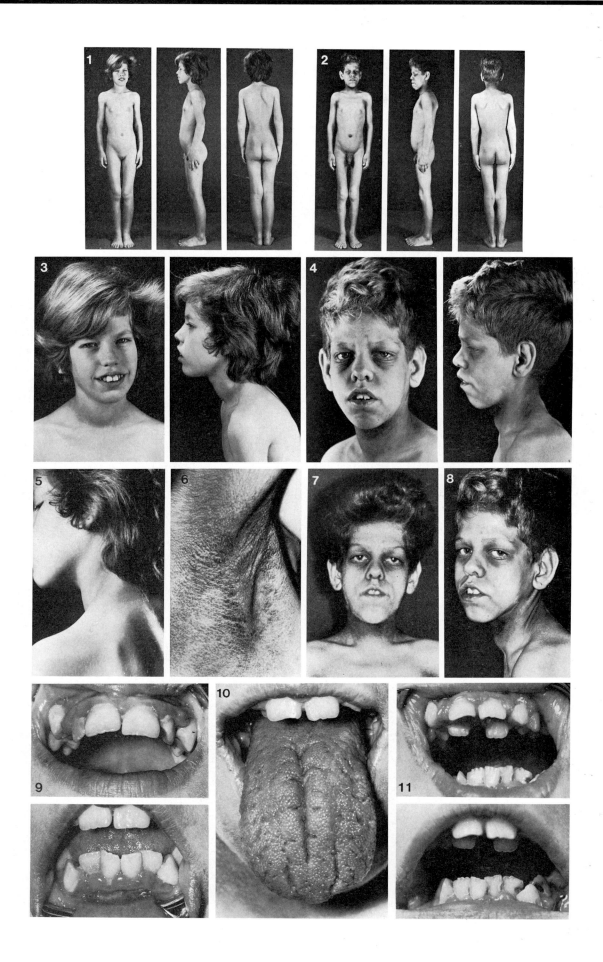

Multiple Lentigines

(LEOPARD Syndrome, Lentiginosis, Lentiginosis-Deafness-Cardiopathy Syndrome)

H.-R.W

A complex hereditary syndrome involving skin, cardiac and other manifestations and with relatively typical facial dysmorphism.

Main signs:
- Multiple lentigines of the skin (dark brown, up to 8 mm diameter), most common on the back of the neck and upper trunk (3–6). Face, scalp, palms, soles and genitalia may also be affected. Mucous membranes not involved.
- Cardiac anomalies (7), usually mild pulmonary stenosis or subaortic stenosis or hypertrophic obstructive cardiomyopathy, with various electrocardiogram changes (e.g. conduction disorders).
- Hypertelorism and 'coarse' facies (2); large ears, pouting lips, prominent lower jaw.

Supplementary findings: Growth and skeletal abnormalities: short stature; possible anomalies of thoracic shape (pectus excavatum or carinatum), winging of the scapula, kyphosis and generalized connective tissue laxity.

Genital dysplasia (cryptorchidism, hypospadias) or delayed puberty. Sensorineural hearing impairment in some patients. Mild mental retardation found in a few patients.

Manifestation: Lentigines present at birth or appear in the first years of life, increasing continuously in number (3 and 4). Hearing impairment may be congenital or of early onset, when present. Cardiac disorder according to severity.

Aetiology: Autosomal dominant disorder. Variable expression. Several sporadic cases.

Frequency: Low (approximately 100 patients reported by 1978).

Course, prognosis: Increasing number of lentigines. Degree of impairment otherwise dependent essentially on the type, development and possible operative correction of the cardiac defect as well as on any hearing or mental impairment; also on the extent of any growth deficiency and delay in sexual maturation.

Differential diagnosis: Von Recklinghausen neurofibromatosis (182). Occasionally, additional single (and rather dark) café au lait spots have been found with the LEOPARD syndrome. Noonan syndrome (105). Peutz–Jeghers syndrome (179).

Comment: The designation LEOPARD syndrome is taken from the initials of the most important signs: lentigines; electrocardiographic conduction defects; ocular hypertelorism; pulmonary stenosis; abnormalities of genitalia; retardation of growth; deafness.

Illustrations:

1–7 An affected child at ages 7 years and 6 months (**1, 3**), 10 (**4**), 11 (**2, 5, 6**) and 12 years (**7**). Note coarsening of the facies (**1 and 2**) and increase in the number of lentigines (**3 and 4**).

Cardiac defect recognized from birth; later demonstrated as marked stenosis of the pulmonary valve along with a left heart anomaly (probably severe subaortic stenosis). Radiograph: markedly enlarged and deformed heart shadow (**7**); Electrocardiogram: pathological right heart pattern with deep Q_3 and extremely high ventricular peaks on the limb leads; extreme right and left ventricular hypertrophy with conduction defect and severe impairment of repolarization. Lentigines have increased continuously since birth. No hearing impairment. Increasing growth deficit (at 7 years and 6 months about 17 cm, and at 12 years and 20 cm below the average for age). Slight mental retardation (attended special school). High, narrow cranium (**2**), epicanthic folds, gothic palate, short neck (**5 and 6**), winging of the scapula, coxa valga. Death because of heart failure in the middle of the second decade of life.

References:

Voron D, Hatfield H, Kalkhoff R: Multiple lentigines syndrome. *Am J Med* 1976, **60**:447.

Sutton S J, Tajik A J *et al*: Hypertrophic obstructive cardiomyopathy and lentiginosis... *Am J Cardiol* 1981, **47**:214–217.

Senn M, Hess O M *et al*: Hypertrophe Kardiomyopathie und Lentiginose. *Schweiz med Wschr* 1984, **114**:838–841.

Hagler D J: Lentiginosis-Deafness-Cardiopathy Syndrome. In: Neurocutaneous diseases. Boston: Butterworth 1987; 80–84.

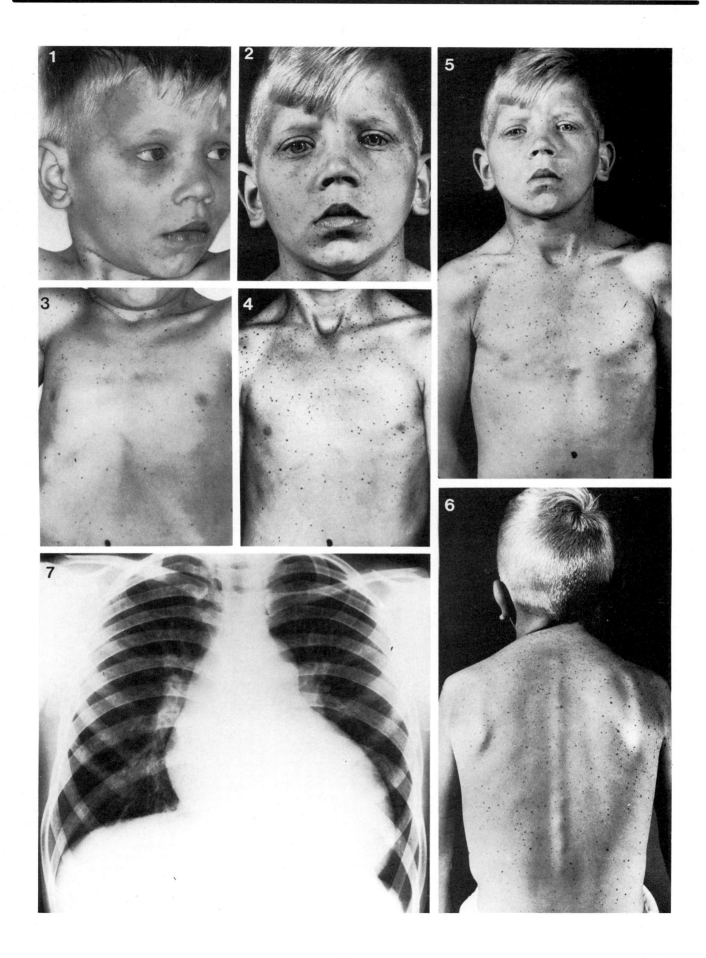

179 Peutz–Jeghers Syndrome

(Mucocutaneous Pigmentation and Intestinal Polyposis Syndrome, Pigment-Spots Polyposis)

J.K./H.-R.W

An autosomal dominant disorder of conspicuous pigmentation, predominantly of the face and oral mucosa, associated with intestinal polyposis.

Main signs:
Dark, brown or bluish grey–black pigmented spots on the skin of the face (especially around the orifices), on the oral mucosa, extremities (including nail beds) and occasionally other areas (1–5).

Supplementary findings: With appropriate studies, usually extensive hamartomatous polyposis of the gastrointestinal tract, especially the jejunum and ileum of 65% an 55%, respectively, and occasionally of the mucosa of the respiratory and urogenital tracts, 1–4 mm in diameter.

Manifestation: The melanin spots may be present at birth, otherwise they appear in early childhood. Manifestations of intestinal polyposis, colicky pain, intestinal bleeding with possible development of anaemia, in some patients recurrent signs of intussusception occur frequently in early childhood. The overall clinical picture is generally not diagnosed until early adulthood.

Aetiology: Autosomal dominant disorder with almost 100% penetrance and decreased expression of the pathological gene. One-third of cases are new mutations.

Frequency: Not particularly low; over 500 patients reported. 1:120 000 liveborn children.

Course, prognosis: The extent of the pigmentation of the oral mucosa does not help predict the extent of visceral polyposis. The pigmented spots of the skin tend to fade after early adulthood. Forty-three per cent of the mortalities are caused by intestinal polyposis (intestinal obstruction, intussusception) and 57% by tumours: gastrointestinal tumours and malignant, extragastro-intestinal tumours such as carcinoma of the pancreas, ductal carcinoma of the breast, adenocarcinoma of the lung, ovarian tumours in 10–15% (granulosa cell tumours with precocious puberty, Brenner tumours, dysgerminomas, cystadenomas, sex cord tumour with annular tubules [SCTAT]), testicular tumours with increased production of aromatase, which leads to gynaecomastia because of increased oestrogen levels.
Possible danger of malignant transformation of the polyps, usually after childhood, with varying familial risks.

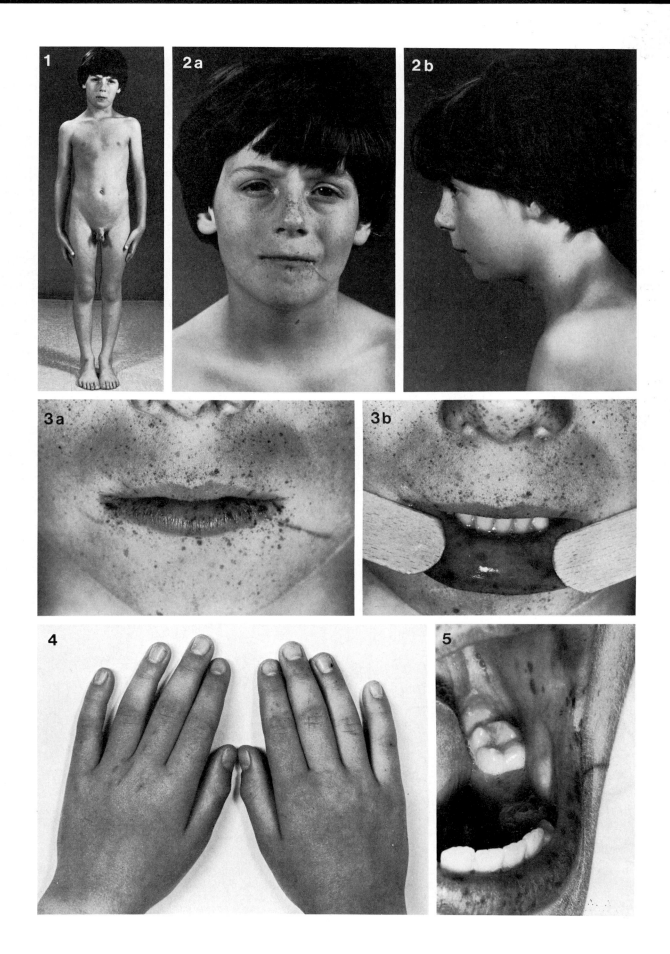

J.K./H.-R.W

Differential diagnosis: Freckles: different distribution and no involvement of the mucous membranes. The latter is also true for the LEOPARD syndrome (*178*). Addison disease: pigmentation of the skin more diffuse or more pronounced in the skin folds (oral mucosa may show similar spots, however). McCune–Albright syndrome (*176*), Gardner syndrome.

Treatment: Intussusception, and so on, may require surgery, resection of polypous segments of the intestine may be necessary.

Regular follow-up. Genetic counselling. Administration of aromatase inhibitors may be indicated.

Illustrations:

Previous page:

1–5 A 9-year-old boy. Pigmented macules noted in the second year of life. Since school age, recurrent signs of early ileus. Also, polyposis demonstrated in the stomach and large intestine. Father of the boy died of ileus secondary to intestinal polyposis; he had allegedly shown no pigmentation anomalies of the skin.

Opposite page:

1 A 5-year-old boy from a large family, with multiple pigmented macules on the face and precious pseudopuberty.
2 Testicular tumour.
3 Large cell calcifying Sertoli-cell tumour; gonadotropin-independent isolated testosterone elevation and elevated aromatase activity.

References:

Jeghers H, McKusick V A, Katz K H: Generalized intestinal polyposis and melanin spots of the oral mucosa, lips and digits. A syndrome of diagnostic significance. *N Engl J Med* 1949, **241**:993.

Klostermann G: *Pigmentfleckenpolypose.* Thieme, Stuttgart 1960.

Long J A Jr, Dreyfuss J R: The Peutz–Jeghers syndrome: a 39 year clinical and radiographic follow-up report. *N Engl J Med* 1977, **297**:1070.

Burdick D, Prior J T: Peutz–Jeghers syndrome... *Cancer* 1982, **50**:2139–2146.

Rasenack U, Caspary W: Das Peutz–Jeghers-Syndrom. *Dtsch med Wschr* 1983, **108**:389–391.

Solh H M, Azoury R S *et al*: Peutz–Jeghers syndrome... *J Pediatr* 1983, **103**:593–595.

Tovar J A, Eizaguirre I *et al*: Peutz–Jeghers syndrome in children... review of the literature. *J Pediatr Surg* 1983, **18**:1–6.

Walecki J K, Hales E D *et al*: Ultrasound contribution to diagnosis of Peutz–Jeghers syndrome... *Pediatr Radiol* 1984, **14**:62–64.

Shields H M: Peutz--eghers-syndrome... *Gastroenterology* 1987, **93**:1135–1141.

Giardiello F M, Welsh S B *et al*: Increased risk of cancer in the Peutz–Jeghers syndrome. *N Engl J Med* 1987, **316**:1511–1514.

Foley T R, McGarrity T J, Abt A B: Peutz–Jeghers syndrome: a clinico-pathologic survey of the 'Harrisburg Family' with a 49-year follow-up. *Gastroenterology* 1988, **95**:535–540.

Coen P, Kulin H *et al*: An aromatase-producing sexcord tumor resulting in prepubertal gynecomastia. *N Engl J Med* 1991, **324**:317–322.

Hizawa K, Iida M *et al*: Cancer in Peutz–Jeghers syndrome. *Cancer* 1993, **72**:2777–2781.

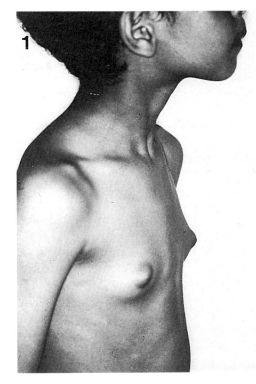

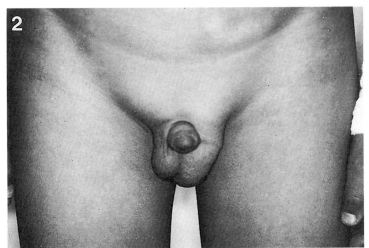

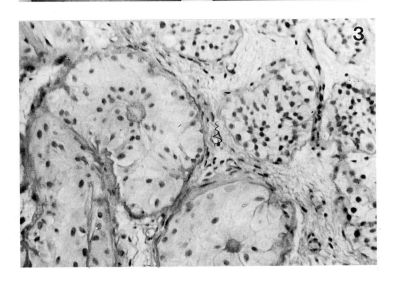

180 Rothmund–Thomson Syndrome
(Congenital Poikiloderma)

H.-R.W

A hereditary disorder of early-onset 'mottling' of the skin frequently combined with development of cataracts, growth deficiency and other anomalies.

Main signs:
- 'Poikiloderma' (mottled skin) as a result of erythema with subsequent patchy atrophy, hyperpigmentation and depigmentation and reticular telangiectasia involving the face, ears, back of the hands, underarms, extensor surfaces of the legs and other areas exposed to light. Photosensitivity. Possibly absence of most of the eyebrows (as a sign of atrophy), involvement of the prolabium, eventual development of spotty hyperkeratoses of the backs of the hands and fingers (1–3).
- Bilateral cataract in some patients.
- Frequently proportional short stature (very variable); 'triangular' face with prominent forehead and low nasal bridge; small hands and feet with brachydactyly.

Supplementary findings: Frequent generalized or partial hypotrichosis; anomalies of nails and teeth.
Cryptorchidism and other signs of hypogonadism.
Skeletal anomalies, especially of the extremities (e.g. hypoplasia or aplasia of the first ray of the upper extremities) in approximately 50% of patients.

Manifestation: Development of skin change in early childhood (from early infancy), of cataracts usually between the second and eighth years of life.

Aetiology: Inherited disorder, autosomal recessive transmission. (Possible uniformity of the syndrome. Possible genetic heterogeneity of cases with and without cataract.) Substantially more frequent in females, up to 75% of observed patients.

Frequency: Low (approximately 100 patients described).

Course, prognosis: Life expectancy normal, unless skin cancer is induced as a result of marked photosensitivity combined with the atrophic skin and hyperkeratoses, which is unusual.

Differential diagnosis: Bloom syndrome (*199*).

Treatment: Symptomatic. Regular ophthalmological, dermatological and oncological surveillance when indicated.
Consistent protection from the sun (sun block).
Genetic counselling.

Illustrations:
1 A 5-year-old girl with typical poikiloderma congenitum.
2 A similarly affected girl aged 4 years 6 months.

References:
Rodermund O-E, Hausmann D: Das Rothmund-Syndrom. *Z Hautkr* 1977, 52:129.
Hall J G, Pagon R A *et al*: Rothmund–Thomson syndrome with severe dwarfism. *AJDC* 1980, **134**:165–169.
Dechenne C, Chantraine J M *et al*: A Rothmund–Thomson case with hypertension. *Clin Genet* 1983, 24:266–272.
Nathanson M, Dandine M *et al*: Syndrome de Rothmund–Thomson avec glaucome. *Ann Pédiatr* 1983, 30:520–525.
Starr D G, McClure J P *et al*: Non-dermatological complications and genetic aspects of the Rothmund–Thomson syndrome. *Clin Genet* 1985, 27:102–104.
Pagon R A: Rothmund–Thomson syndrome. Chapter 12 in: *Neurocutaneous diseases*. M. R. Gomez (ed.). Boston: Butterworth 1987.
Vanscheidt E, Wolff G *et al*: Rothmund–Syndrom oder Thomson–Syndrom... *Mschr Kinderheilk* 1988, **136**:264–269.
Hauschild A, Peschau K *et al*: Rothmund–Thomson Syndrom. *DMW* 1993, **118**:463–466.
Örstavik K H, McFadden N *et al*: Instability of lymphocyte chromosomes in a girl with Rothmund-Thomson syndrome. *J Med Genet* 1994, 31:570–572.

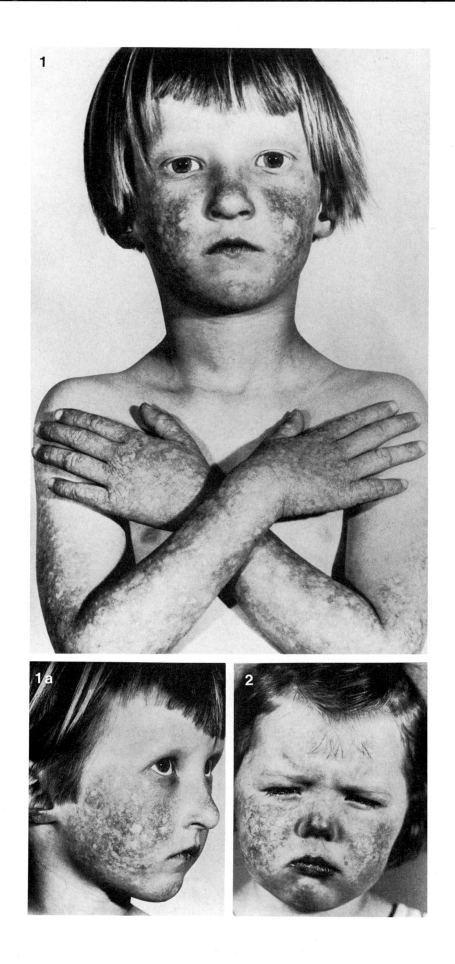

181 Xeroderma Pigmentosum

A hereditary disorder of hypersensitivity to sunlight and photophobia starting early in life, development of pigment anomalies and early development of skin cancer or precancerous lesions.

Main signs:

- Hypersensitivity to sunlight and photophobia (to ultraviolet light) from birth with formation of blisters in over 50% of patients by the 18th month of life.
- Development of hyperpigmentation and depigmentation (**1 and 2**).
- Development of precancerous lesions and of skin cancer in the light-damaged areas (2000-fold increase by the 20th year of life): basal cell carcinomas, squamous cell carcinomas, rarely sarcomas.
- Especially endangered areas are the lips and the eyes (with possible development of keratitis and corneal scars and of malignant growths on the conjunctiva and eyelids).

Manifestation: Photophobia from birth; skin changes from early to mid- infancy.

Aetiology: Hereditary disorder. Usually autosomal recessive inheritance (eight different types, usually endonuclease defects after ultraviolet exposure, excision repair defects, with the same clinical course). A much rarer autosomal dominant type with less severe course, longer life expectancy, ability to reproduce. Gene locus: 1q41-42.

Frequency: Relatively low in Europeans. 1:250 000 in the USA, 1:40 000 in Japan, relatively high in Egypt, Tunisia and in countries with high consanguinity.

Course, prognosis: Unfavourable. Progressive disorder. Some patients develop neurological disorders, mental deterioration, cerebral atrophy, choreo-athetosis, ataxia, spasticity (the minor DNA repair disorders are found in this group). Seventy per cent of patients reach the 40th year of life. Patients in the other groups (with the most marked DNA disorders) do not show neurological signs and live longer.

Differential diagnosis: Cockayne syndrome (*89*), Bloom syndrome (*199*), Rothmund–Thomson syndrome (*180*).

Treatment: As far as possible, avoidance of exposure to sunlight; regular application of a sunscreen lotion (Contralum®); early excision of precancerous lesions. Oral administration of high doses of isotretinoin seems to be effective in preventing skin cancer.
  Genetic counselling of the parents.

Illustrations:

1 and 2 A 5-year-old boy. Development of hypersensitivity to sunlight early in life; appearance of pigmented moles and telangiectases on the face and hands starting in the second year of life. Now all sunlight-exposed areas of the skin are covered with small hyperpigmented and depigmented spots and telangiectases. Up to this age, 10 precancerous lesions. Additional development of numerous haemangiomas and multiple kerato-acanthomas.

References:

Any dermatology textbook.
Maher V M, Rowan L A *et al*: Frequency of UV-induced neoplastic transformation of diploid human fibroblasts is higher in xeroderma pigmentosum cells... *Proc Nat Acad Sci* 1982, **79**:2613–2617.
Welshimer K, Swift M: Congenital malformations and developmental disabilities in... xeroderma pigmentosum families. *Am J Hum Genet* 1982, **34**:781–793.
Imray P, Hockey A *et al*: Sensitivity to ultraviolet radiation in a dominantly inherited form of xeroderma pigmentosum. *J Med Genet* 1986, **23**:72–78.
Robbins J H: Xeroderma pigmentosum. Chapter 10 in: *Neurocutaneous diseases*. M R Gomez (ed.). Boston: Butterworth 1987.
Kraemer K H, DiGiovanna J J *et al*: Prevention of skin cancer in xeroderma pigmentosum with the use of oral isotretinoin. *N Engl J Med* 1988, **318**:1633–1637.
Cleaver J, Kraemer K H: Xeroderma pigmentosum. In: Scriver, C R *et al*. (eds.): *The metabolic basis of inherited disease*, 6th ed. New York: McGraw-Hill 1989; 2949–2973.

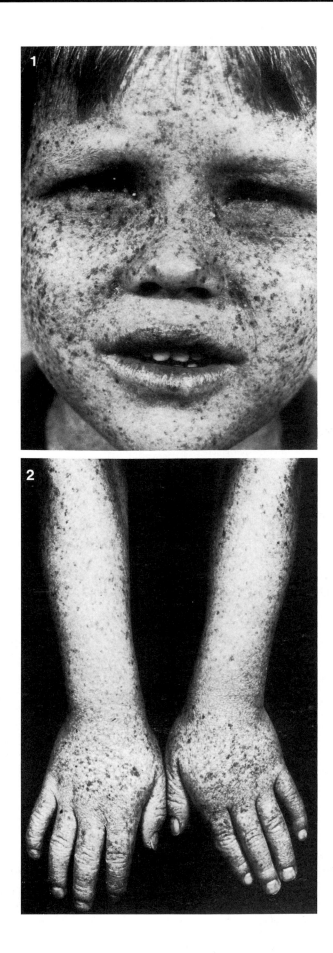

H.-R.W

A characteristic hereditary disorder of multiple café au lait spots, skin tumours, and skeletal, neurological and other signs.

Main signs:
- Variable numbers of café au lait spots, especially on the trunk; also various other pigmentation anomalies (1–9, 12).
- Multiple fibromas or neurofibromas and other dysplastic intracutaneous and subcutaneous growths along the peripheral nerves and other locations (e.g. optic glioma) (11 and 12).
- Frequent neurological or ocular disorders (e.g. caused by nerve compression) (1 and 2).
- Frequent skeletal anomalies: congenital pseudarthrosis of the tibia, club foot, dislocation of the hip; development of kyphoscoliosis; cystic-sclerotic lesions (seen on radiograph) (3, 4, 9). Partial macrosomia in some patients (1, 10).
- Mental retardation in approximately 10%, seizure disorder in approximately 15% of patients.

Supplementary findings: Macrocrania and ocular changes are frequent (neurofibroma of the eyelid, corneal clouding; Lisch nodules of the iris in over 90% of school-age or older patients). Possible precocious puberty or development of pheochromocytoma.

Manifestation: From birth onwards. Initially often only café au lait spots or freckle-like pigmentation, with gradual increase in size and number.

Aetiology: Autosomal dominant disorder with 100% penetrance but very variable expression. Approximately one-half of the cases represent new mutations. Gene locus: 17q11.2.

Frequency: Relatively high. Estimate: one out of 2500–3300 births.

Course, prognosis: In principle, progression can be expected. Blindness, paresis or paralysis, signs of paraplegia, and so on may occur. Possibility of developing dysplastic tumours also on the deep-lying peripheral nerves, on sympathetic nerves, on the spinal roots, cranial nerves or retina, in the brain or intraspinally, on the adrenals, kidneys and other locations. Also danger of later development of malignancy in these sites in over 5% of patients.

Diagnosis: At least six café au lait spots of more than 1 cm diameter can be considered diagnostic of neurofibromatosis. Lisch nodules of the iris (slit lamp) and pigmented moles of the axilla (axillary freckling) are diagnostically valuable.

Differential diagnosis: Multiple lentigenes syndrome (178); perhaps also McCune–Albright syndrome (176). Patients showing signs of classic neurofibromatosis as well as of Noonan syndrome (105) are said to have 'neurofibromatosis-Noonan phenotype'. It is still unclear whether this represents a variant of neurofibromatosis I or is an independent autosomal dominant disorder.

Note: The above applies to the 'classic' (so-called von Recklinghausen, peripheral or type I) form of neurofibromatosis. Additional forms, especially the so-called acoustic or central type, or type II, with the main sign being bilateral acoustic neuromas occurring in the second to third decade of life, show only minimal skin changes, and no Lisch nodules. Type II is at least 100 times less common than type I.

Treatment: Symptomatic. Genetic counselling.

Illustrations:
1 A preschool child from a neurofibromatosis kindred. Clusters of café au lait spots; small tumours of the head and left leg; tumorous macrosomia of the right leg (histologically: neurofibromatosis); intraspinal space-occupying lesion; hypertrophy of the clitoris; congenital dislocation of hips. 2 and 12 A 5-year-old patient, fibroma on the left thigh, multiple smaller tumours, and xanthoma tuberosum. Macrocephaly, ataxia; mild mental retardation. Coxa vara. Neurofibromatosis kindred. 3 A 10-year-old patient: multiple café au lait spots, kyphoscoliosis, mental retardation. 4 A 13-year-old patient: hyperpigmented areas, up to palm size; fibromas; bulbous deformity of the nose; thoracic gibbus; mild mental retardation. 5–8 A 12-year-old patient; short stature, kyphosis, bilateral Lisch nodules; pigmentary anomalies of the fundus. 9 A 5-year-old patient; neurofibromatosis kindred; sacrococcygeal deformity; café au lait spots, short stature, congenital heart defect, hypertelorism, strabismus, prominent optic disc on the left, mental retardation. 10 Left-sided macrodactyly in a 12-year-old patient studded with café au lait spots; hypertelorism, facial asymmetry, fibroma. 11 The back of a woman from a neurofibromatosis kindred.

References:
Flüeler U, Boltshauser E: Iris hamartomata as diagnostic criterion in neurofibromatosis. *Neuropediatrics* 1986, 17:183–185.
Meinecke P: Evidence that the 'Neurofibromatosis-Noonan syndrome' is a variant of von Recklinghausen neurofibromatosis. *Am J Med Genet* 1987, 26:741–745.
Quattrin T, McPherson E *et al*: Vertical transmission of the Neurofibromatosis/Noonan syndrome. *Am J Med Genet* 1987, 26:645–649.
Abuelo D, Meryash D: Neurofibromatosis with fully expressed Noonan syndrome. *Am J Med Genet* 1988, 29:937–941.
DiSimone R E, Berman A T *et al*: The orthopedic manifestations of neurofibromatosis. *Clin Orthopaed* 1988, 230:277–283.
Stambolian D, Zackai E H: Gene location in neurofibromatosis. *Am J Med Genet* 1988, 29:963–965.
Listernick R, Charrow J: Neurofibromatosis type 1 in childhood. *J Pediatr* 1990, 116:845–853.
Valero M C *et al*: Characterization of four mutations in the neurofibromatosis type 1 gene... *Hum Mol Genet* 1994, 3:639–642.

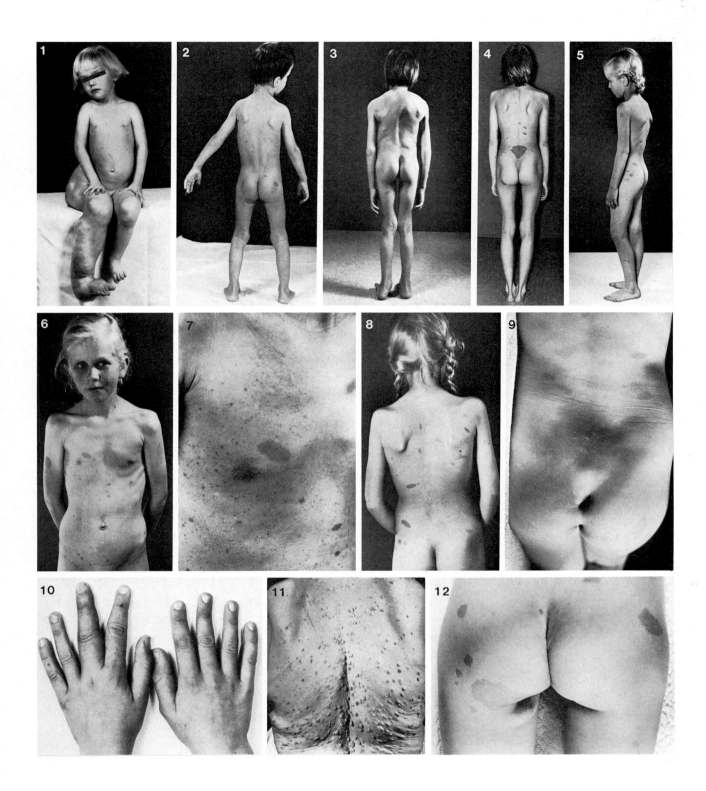

H.-R.W

A complex meso-ectodermal hereditary disorder characterized by focal dermal atrophy with hernias of the adipose tissue, associated with a multitude of possible skeletal, dental, ocular and other anomalies.

Main signs:
- Approximately lentil-sized areas of dermal atrophy in an irregular, in some patients netlike, wormlike or striped or a systematic distribution, together with corresponding larger foci with hernias of adipose tissue (1). Also, pigmentation changes, telangiectases, scars (from congenital skin defects) and possible papillomas (conjunctival, nasal, intra-oral, oesophageal, laryngeal or genito-anal).
- Skeletal anomalies: syndactyly (2 and 3); hypoplasia or aplasia of rays of the fingers and toes (5) in addition to more extensive dysmelia (in extreme cases, cleft hand or foot). Hypoplasia and aplasia also of the truncal skeleton, in some patients leading to kyphoscoliosis and so on.
- Malpositioning and hypoplasia and aplasia of the teeth. Hypoplasia and dysplasia of the nails (2b, 5). Disorders of hair growth (hypotrichosis or local alopecia).
- Possible eye anomalies such as coloboma, aniridia, microphthalmos and others.

Supplementary findings: Microcephaly, cerebral malformations and mental retardation; short stature, asymmetry or hemihypoplasia, ear anomalies and many other developmental defects may occur.

Radiologically, characteristic longitudinal striation of the metaphyses of the long bones and osteoporosis and cystic bone lesions.

Manifestation: Skin changes usually present at birth or developing shortly thereafter from erythematous areas. Papillomas usually develop later.

Aetiology: Genetically determined syndrome with very variable expression; often sporadic cases, usually affecting females. The assumption is of X-linked dominance of the mutated gene, predominantly lethal *in utero* in males. Assumed gene locus Xp22.31.

Frequency: Relatively low; over 200 patients reported up to 1990 (more than 30 of these were boys).

Course, prognosis: Dependent on the type and severity of non-cutaneous involvement.

Differential diagnosis: Mainly the Bloch–Sulzberger syndrome (*187*).

Treatment: Symptomatic (multidisciplinary care may be needed).
Genetic counselling.

Illustrations:
1–5 The second child of healthy, young, non-consanguineous parents. Typical skin changes and additional anomalies much more pronounced on the right side (2, 4: diaphragmatic hernia; 5). Partial syndactyly of the second and third fingers and fifth-finger clinodactyly of the right hand (2b). Aplasia of the 12th rib on the right. Aplasia of two rays of the right foot (5). Radiologically: typical 'osteopathia striata'.

References:
Braun-Falco O, Hofmann C: Das Goltz–Gorlin-Syndrom. *Hautarzt* 1975, **26**:393.
Happle R, Lenz W: Striation of bones in focal dermal hypoplasia.... *Br J Dermatol* 1977, **96**:113.
Fryns J P, Dhondt F, Lindemans L *et al*: Focal dermal hypoplasia (Goltz's syndrome) in a male. *Acta Paed Belg* 1978, **31**:37.
Kunze J, Heyne K, Wiedemann H-R: Diaphragmatic hernia in a female newborn with focal dermal hypoplasia and marked asymmetric malformations (Goltz–Gorlin syndrome). *Eur J Pediatr* 1979, **131**:213–218.
Römke C, Gödde-Salz E, Grote W: Investigations of chromosomal stability in the Gorlin–Goltz syndrome. *Arch Dermatol Res* 1985, **277**:370–372.
Wechsler M A, Papa C M *et al*: Variable expression in focal dermal hypoplasia. *AJDC* 1988, **142**:297–300.
Goltz R W: Focal dermal hypoplasia syndrome; an update. *Arch Dermatol* 1988, **128**:1108–1111.
Gorski J-L: Father-to-daughter transmission of focal dermal hypoplasia... *Am J Med Genet* 1991, **40**:332–337.
Naritomi K *et al*: Combined Goltz and Aicardi syndromes... *Am J Med Genet* 1992, **42**:839–843.
Rodini E S O *et al*: Ectodermal dysplasia, ectrodactyly : nosology of Goltz–Gorlin syndrome versus EEC syndrome. *Am J Med Genet* 1992, **42**:276–280.

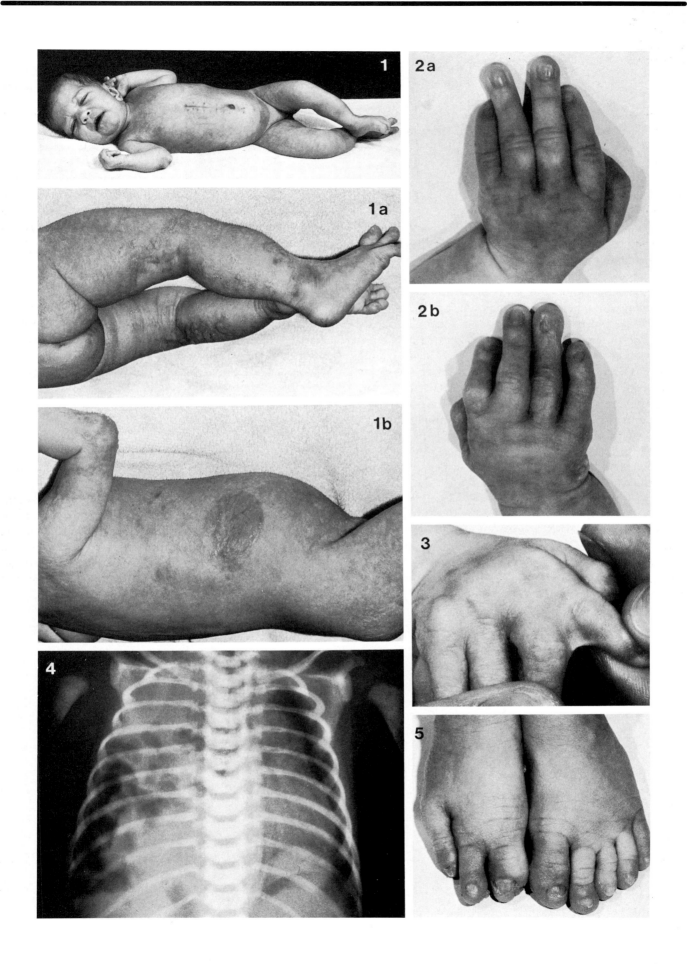

Syndrome of Hemihypoplasia and Symmetrical Localized
Dermal Atrophy of the Hands and Feet

H.-R.W

A clinical picture of congenital general hemihypoplasia, symmetrical foci of atrophied skin and subcutaneous fat on the hands and feet and other anomalies.

Main signs:
- Right-sided hemi-atrophy affecting the entire one-half of the body clinically and radiologically, with marked shortening of the tibia (humerus, radius and ulna each 4–5 mm, femur 6 mm, fibula 7 mm and tibia 11 mm shorter than the opposite side) (**1–4**).
- Atrophy of subcutaneous fatty tissue and overlying skin, which is thin and wrinkled and never showed vesicular or other changes, symmetrically over the extensor surfaces of the wrists and ankles, more pronounced on the right than the left (**3 and 4**). No fat herniation, no telangiectasis.

Skin of the right abdominal region somewhat less pigmented than that of the left; fine, diffuse haemangioma-like changes on the back, more pronounced on the right; one café au lait spot each on the left shoulder, the left elbow and the right upper arm.

Supplementary findings: Flat face with widely spaced eyes, epicanthus. Left supernumerary nipple. Short thumbs bilaterally, deep insertion of the halluces; toes malpositioned and occasionally incurved, more so on the right than the left.

Radiograph: Distinct aortic configuration of the heart. Kidneys normal on pyelogram. Skeletal survey negative for calcium flecks ('stippling') and longitudinal striation of the metaphyses.

Manifestation: At birth.

Aetiology: Not established with certainty.

Course: At age 8 years, height below the second percentile; the right arm now 2 cm shorter and the right leg 5 cm shorter than the left. Small cranium, eyes normal, small triangular mouth, severe malpositioning of the teeth. Widely spaced nipples. Atrophic lesions of the skin and subcutaneous fat unchanged. Faint depigmentations on all extremities. Expressionless face, mental retardation; no seizures or physical handicap. Bone age delayed 3 years in the right hand and 2 years in the left.

Comment: Goltz–Gorlin syndrome (*183*) has to be considered here, however, in addition to other signs, the characteristic fat hernias and striations of the metaphyses on radiograph were not present.

Most likely to be the result of early varicella infection of the embryo (the so-called congenital varicella syndrome), although no evidence at all from the maternal history of a corresponding viral infection.

Illustrations:
1–4 A 7-month-old girl, the second child of healthy parents. Birth after an otherwise unremarkable full-term twin pregnancy, length 48 cm, weight 2800 g and head circumference 34 cm. Slightly retarded motor development, mental development initially considered normal. Measurements (including head circumference) in the low-normal range. Ocular fundi normal; neurological examination normal. Chromosomal analysis normal. Laboratory chemistries and serological examinations normal.

References:
Schlotfeldt-Schäfer I, Schaefer P *et al*: Congenitales Varicellensyndrom. *Mschr Kinderheilk* 1983, **131**:106–108.
König R, Gutjahr P *et al*: Konnatale Varizellen-Embryo-Fetopathie, *Helv Paediat Acta* 1985, **40**:391–398.
Unger-Köppel J, Kilcher P *et al*: Varizellenfetopathie. *Helv Paediat Acta* 1985, **40**:399–404.
Alkalay A L, Pomerance J J *et al*: Fetal varizella syndrome. *J Pediatr* 1987, **111**:320–323.

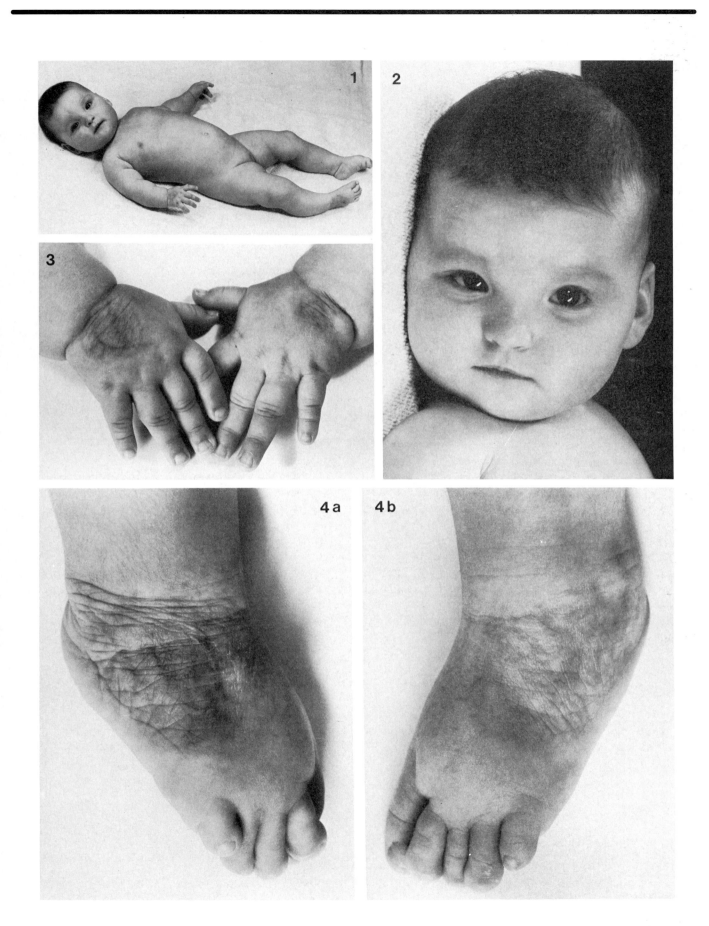

J.K.

A syndrome manifest only in females, with microphthalmia, dermal aplasia and sclerocornea.

Main signs:
- Manifest exclusively in females (one patient with XY-translocation and male phenotype).
- Microphthalmia, bilateral, occasionally unilateral.
- Sclerocornea, bilateral, in some patients asymmetric variation in the severity of clouding. Rarely perforated cornea. No involvement of the cornea observed in three patients.
- Dermal aplasia in the face, cranial region, neck, upper thorax. Distribution corresponds to Blaschko's lines.

Supplementary findings: Other eye anomalies: hypertelorism, blepharophimosis, orbital cysts, opsoclonus-like movements of the eyes, anomalies of the anterior chamber of the eye, coloboma of the iris, pigmentary retinopathy, embryotoxon. Agenesis of the corpus callosum, cerebellar hypoplasia, focal dysplasia of the brain, absent transparent septum, dermoid cysts of the spinal dura mater. Microcephaly. Mental retardation, spasms. Impaired hearing. No voluntary control of the anal sphincter muscle.

Various cardiac defects: atrial septal defect, ventricular septal defect, over-riding aorta, arterio-venous block, arteria lusoria, hypertrophic cardiomyopathy, mitral and tricuspid insufficiency.

Oral-facial anomalies: low-set ears, dysplastic helices, broad nasal bridge, saddle nose, micrognathia, notches in the alveolar ridge, where broad frenula are attached, high palate. Mid-face hypoplasia. Hypodontia. Pre-auricular tags.

Ventrally displaced anus, bicornate uterus, mild hypospadias (a male patient).

Additionally: dysplasia of the nails, simian crease, tapering fingers, proximally placed thumbs. Diaphragmatic hernia.

Manifestation: At birth.

Aetiology: X-linked dominant inheritance with lethality in males. Three patients with X/Y translocation, one of whom has a normal male phenotype. All of the other 12 patients have a deletion in the short arm of the X chromosome: Xp22.2/22.3.

Pathogenesis: Unknown.

Frequency: To date 16 patients, including two mother–daughter cases.

Course, prognosis: Is determined by concomitant malformations. Frequently mental retardation, spasms, delayed motor development, speech delay. Short stature.

Differential diagnosis: Focal Goltz–Gorlin dermal hypoplasia (*183*), Aicardi syndrome (*161*), Delleman syndrome. The MLS syndrome (microphthalmia–linear skin defects syndrome) appears to be identical to the MIDAS syndrome.

Treatment: Symptomatic.

Illustrations:
1a–c 32-year-old mother of the patient in 2a–e: Extremely poor vision with microphthalmia and consecutive ptosis of the upper eyelid. Congenital skin defect, following the course of Blaschko's lines. Early loss of all teeth. Karyotype: 46,XX but SRY-positive.
2a–e A girl aged 30 months with bilateral sclerocornea and microphthalmia, a drainage impairment in the anterior chamber of the eye having led to macrophthalmia, glaucoma and finally spontaneous perforation. Aplasia cutis congenita, ipsilateral and analogous to the mother but considerably more pronounced. Frontal hypodontia (not nursing-bottle syndrome). Microcephaly, mid-face retraction and spastic quadriplegia with agenesis of the corpus callosum. True hermaphroditism with testis on the right and ovotestis on the left side. Hypertrophy of the clitoris and Prader III urogenital sinus with peri-anal fistula.
Use of high-resolution techniques also shows a normal female karyotype but likewise SRY-positive.

References:
Al-Gazali L I, Mueller R F, Caine A *et al*: An XX male and two (X;Y) females with linear skin defects and congenital microphthalmia: a new syndrome at Xp22.3. *J Med Genet* 1988, 25:638–639.
Naritomi K, Izumikawa Y *et al*: Combined Goltz and Aicardi syndromes in a terminal Xp deletion: are they a contiguous gene syndrome? *Am J Med Genet* 1992, 43:839–843.
Lindoe N M, Michels V V, Hoppe D A *et al*: Xp22.3 microdeletion syndrome with microphthalmia, sclerocornea, linear skin defects, and congenital heart defects. *Am J Med Genet* 1992, 44:61–65.
Happle R, Daniels D, Koopman R J J: MIDAS syndrome (microphthalmia, dermal aplasia, and sclerocornea): an X-linked phenotype distinct from Goltz syndrome. *Am J Med Genet* 1993, 47:710–713.
Linsay E A, Grillo A, Ferrero G B *et al*: Microphthalmia with linear skin defects (MLS) syndrome: clinical, cytogenetic, and molecular characterization. *Am J Med Genet* 1994, 49:229–234.
Mücke J, Happle R, Theile H: MIDAS syndrome respectively MLS syndrome (MIM 309801): an autonomous entity rather than a consequence of random ionization of an X-chromosomal gene defect. *Eur J Dermatol* (In press).

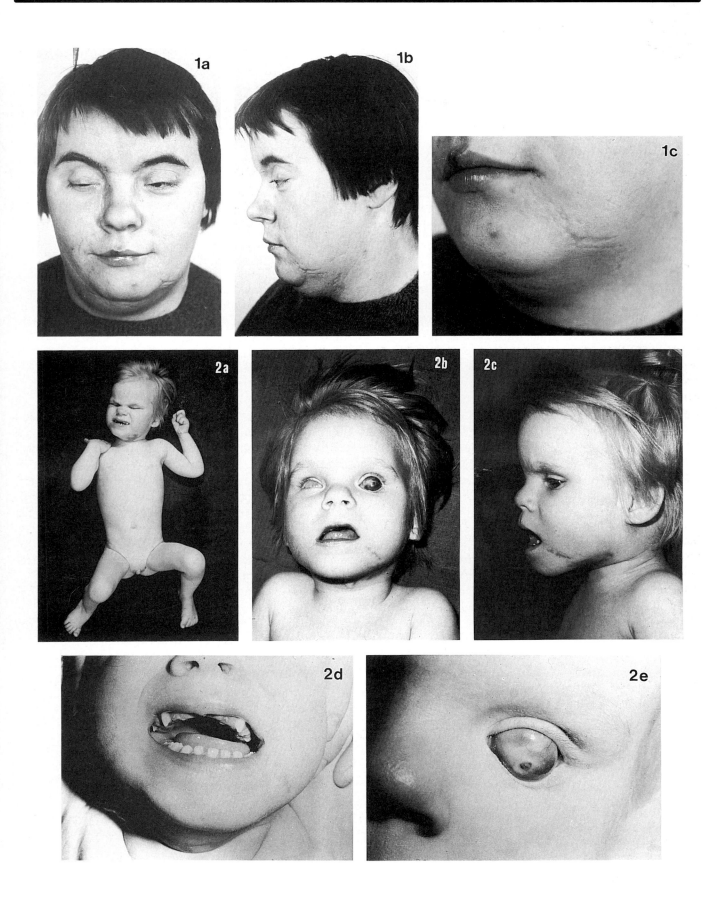

186 Lenz Microphthalmia Syndrome
(Lenz Dysplasia, Lenz Dysmorphogenic Syndrome, Microphthalmia with Associated Anomalies)

J.K.

An inherited, sex-linked clinical picture with microphthalmia, delayed development, microcephaly and finger anomalies.

Main signs:
- Eye anomalies: unilateral or bilateral microphthalmia; anophthalmia; colobomas of the iris, retina and choroid; blepharoptosis; microcornea; strabismus; nystagmus; cataract; myopia; epicanthus medialis; small orbits.
- Facial dysmorphism: high forehead, microcephaly (83%), mongoloid palpebral fissures, asymmetrically large, dysplastic, sometimes protruding ears (macrotia), micrognathia, malpositioning of the teeth, aplasia of the lateral maxillary incisors (65%), diastemata, persistence of the deciduous teeth, high palate.
- Skeletal anomalies: camptodactyly of the second fingers, clinodactyly of the fifth fingers, hypoplastic thumbs, duplication of the thumbs, syndactyly of the fingers and toes (second and third or fourth and fifth), flat feet, 'sandal-gap', valgus and varus malpositioning, narrow shoulders, cylindrical barrel-shaped thorax, hypoplasia of the clavicle, low-set scapula, notched vertebral bodies, kyphosis, scoliosis, cubitus valgus, reduced extension of the hip joints, genu valgum, internal rotation of the knee joints, short stature.

Supplementary findings: Unilateral or bilateral renal agenesis, dysgenesis, hydro-ureter; cryptorchidism, hypospadias; congenital cardiac defect; ileal atresia, anal atresia; umbilical hernia. Impaired hearing. Spastic diplegia. Pterygium colli. Detached retina.
Developmental retardation, mild mental retardation (92%).

Manifestation: At birth, possibly prenatally by ultrasound.

Aetiology: X-linked recessive inheritance. Female carriers show finger anomalies, microcephaly, short stature.

Pathogenesis: Unknown.

Frequency: Twelve published cases up to 1988.

Course, prognosis: Visual impairment. Otherwise dependent on concomitant malformations.

Differential diagnosis: Oculodentodigital dysplasia (240), trisomy 13 (47), Goltz–Gorlin syndrome (183), COFS syndrome (320), microphthalmia-microcephaly syndrome, X-linked, Norrie's syndrome, Waardenburg's recessive anophthalmia.

Treatment: Symptomatic, surgical where indicated.

Illustrations:
Male first twin at age 12 years and 9 months, deaf and blind since birth, bilateral detachment of the retina, delayed psychomotor development, short stature, microcephaly (third percentile).
1a and b Bilateral microphthalmia, small orbits bilaterally. On the right, anterior staphyloma with bulging microcornea, iris anomaly, narrow pupil, mature cataract. On the left, marked corneal clouding. High forehead, macrotia.
1c–e Right and left hands have complete cutaneous syndactyly of the third and fourth fingers, right hand after surgical separation.
1f Partial syndactyly of the second and third toes bilaterally.
2a and b The twin brother's hands with syndactyly of the third and fourth fingers of the left hand.
2c Partial syndactyly of the second and third toes, right. Clinically normal.

References:
Lenz W: Recessiv-geschlechtsgebundene Mikrophthalmie Mit multiplen Mißbildungen. *Z Kinderheilkd* 1955, 77:384–390.
Hoefnagel D, Keenan M E, Allen F H: Heredofamilial bilateral anophthalmia. *Arch Ophthalmol* 1963, 69:760–764.
Herrmann J, Opitz J M: The Lenz microphthalmia syndrome. *Birth Defects Orig Art Ser* 1969, V(2):138–143.
Goldberg M F, McKusick V A: X-linked colobomatous microphthalmos and other congenital anomalies: a disorder resembling Lenz's dysmorphogenetic syndrome. *Am J Opthalmol* 1971, 71:1128–1133.
Dinno N D, Lawwill T *et al*: Bilateral microcornea, coloboma, short stature and other skeletal anomalies — a new hereditary syndrome. *Birth Defects: Orig Art Ser* 1976, XII(6):109–114.
Baraitser M, Winter R M, Taylor D S I: Lenz microphthalmia — a case report. *Clin Genet* 1982, 22:99–101.
Siber M: X-linked recessive microencephaly, microphthalmia with corneal opacities, spastic quadriplegia, hypospadias and cryptorchidism. *Clin Genet* 1984, 26:453–456.
Graham C A, McLeary B G *et al*: Linkage analysis in a family with X-linked anophthalmos. *J Med Genet* 1988, 25:643.
Traboulsi E I, Lenz W, Gonzales-Ramos M, Siegel J, Macrae W G, Maumenee I H: The lenz microphthalmia syndrome. *Am J Ophthalmol* 1988, 105:40–45.
Warburg M: X-linked cataract and X-linked microphthalmos: how many deletion families? *Am J Med Genet* 1989, 34:451–453.

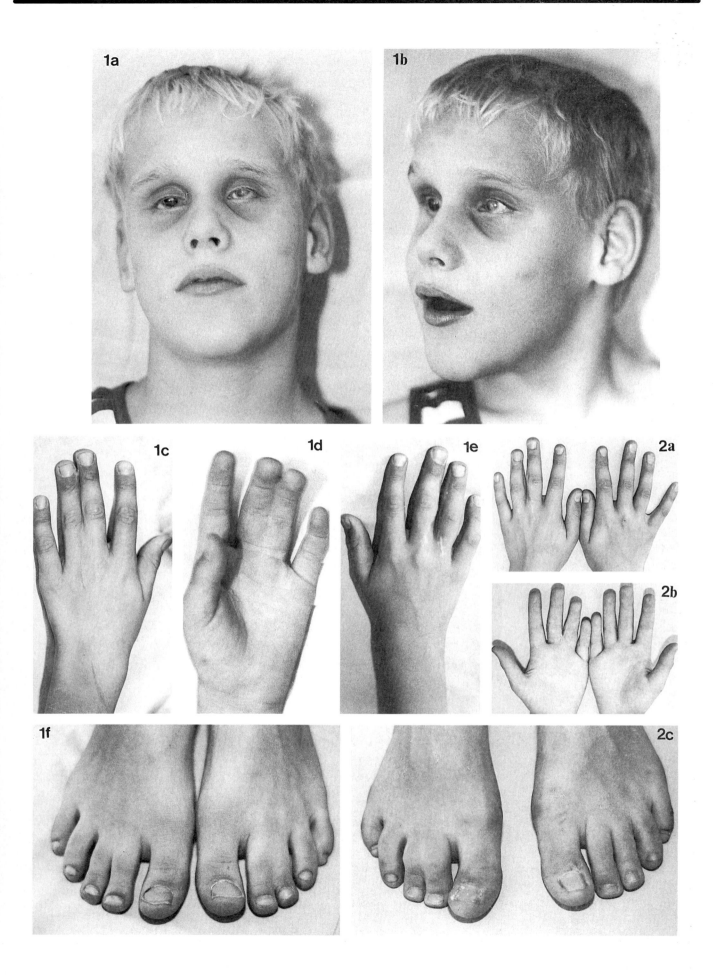

187 Incontinentia Pigmenti
(Block–Sulzberger Syndrome)

H.-R.W

A hereditary dermatosis–herpetiform dermatitis, patchy or verrucous hyperkeratosis and streaky hyperpigmentation, with anomalies of the dentition, central nervous system and eyes.

Main signs:
• Skin manifestations can be divided into three stages:
I Papules, vesicles and pustules on an erythematous base, frequently linear distribution, usually sparing the face, present at birth or appearing during the first months of life, persisting or taking an intermittent course for several months (1), occasionally for years.
II Somewhat macular or verrucous pigmented hyperkeratoses following the lesions in stage I, also usually lasting several months (2 and 3), occasionally years.
III Dirty-brown, streaky, garland-like distribution of hyperpigmentation, frequently symmetrical, preferentially affecting the lateral trunk, axillae, groin and thighs (3–6).
 The stages occur consecutively with overlap. Stage III may occur on previously normal skin, usually healing completely by the third decade of life, occasionally with residual depigmentation.
• Dental anomalies almost always present (delayed eruption, malformed teeth, hypodontia). Focal alopecia common; nail deformities less common.

Supplementary findings: In approximately 30% of patients, eye anomalies (strabismus, cataract, pseudoglioma and others) and central nervous system disorders (spastic quadriplegia, seizure disorder, mental retardation and others), microcephaly.
 In stage I, up to 50% blood eosinophils; eosinophilic granulocytes in the vesicles.

Manifestation: Stage I, at birth and in early infancy. Stage II, principally in the second to sixth week and stage III in the 12th to 26th week of life.

Aetiology: The prevailing view is of an X-linked dominant disorder. The mutated gene is usually lethal *in utero* for males, so that girls are affected almost exclusively (approximately 97%). Gene loci: Xp11 (sporadic type); Xp28 (familial form).

Frequency: Approximately 1:40 000 girls. Over 650 patients, 16 of them male, became known in the past 50 years.

Course, prognosis: In the absence of severe neurological impairment, life expectancy normal.

Differential diagnosis: Goltz–Gorlin syndrome (*183*), Ito syndrome (*188*), among others.

Treatment: None known, even for the skin disorder.
 Genetic counselling; prenatal diagnosis by means of DNA analysis.

Illustrations:
1 Patient 1 at age 2 weeks; male infant but with Klinefelter syndrome (XXY sex chromosomes). Tooth buds present. Neurologically normal.
2 and 3 Patient 2 at ages 2 months and 16 months. Hypodontia. Seizure disorder since the seventh week of life. Normal intelligence.
4 Patient 3 at age 19 months, normal psychological development up to that point. Delayed dentition, hypodontia.
5 and 6 Patient 4 at 12 years. Malformed teeth, microdontia. Seizure disorder since the fourth week of life, right-sided spastic hemiparesis.

References:
Kunze J, Frenzl U H *et al*: Klinefelter's syndrome and incontinentia pigmenti… *Hum Genet* 1977, 35:237–240.
Hohenauer L, Wilk F: Incontinentia pigmenti. *Pädiat Prax* 1977/78, 19:417.
Korting G W, Bechtold M: Alternierende Manifestationsäquivalente der Incontinentia pigmenti in 2 Generationen. *Med Welt* 1980, 31:759.
Kurczynski T W, Berns J S *et al*: Studies of a family with incontinentia pigmenti variably expressed in both sexes. *J Med Genet* 1982, 19:447–451.
Lenz W, Ullrich E, Witkowski R *et al*: Halbseitige Incontinentia pigmenti… *Pädiat Pädol* 1982, 17:187.
Hecht F, Hecht B K: The half chromatid mutation model and bidirectional mutation in incontinentia pigmenti. *Clin Genet* 1983, 24:177–179.
Sommer A, Liu P H: Incontinentia pigmenti in a father and his daughter. *Am J Med Genet* 1984, 17:655–659.
Avrahami E, Harel S *et al*: Computed tomographic demonstration of brain changes in incontinentia pigmenti. *AJDC* 1985, 139:373–374.
Brien J E, Feingold M: Incontinentia pigmenti; a longitudinal study. *AJDC* 1985, 139:711–712.
Hodgson S V, Neville B *et al*: Two cases of X/autosome translocation in females with incontinentia pigmenti. *Hum Genet* 1985, 71:231–234.
Larsen R, Ashwal S *et al*: Incontinentia pigmenti: association with anterior horn cell degeneration. Neurology 37, 446-450 (1987).
Rosman, P: Incontinentia pigmenti. Chapter 32 in: *Neurocutaneous diseases*, M R Gomez (ed.). Boston: Butterworth 1987.
Sefiani A, Sinnett D *et al*: Linkage studies do not confirm the cytogenetic location of incontinentia pigmenti on Xp 11. *Hum Genet* 1988, 80:282–286.
Smahi A *et al*: The gene for the familial form of incontinentia pigmenti (IP$_2$) maps to the distal part of Xq28. *Hum Mol Genet* 1994, 3:273–278.

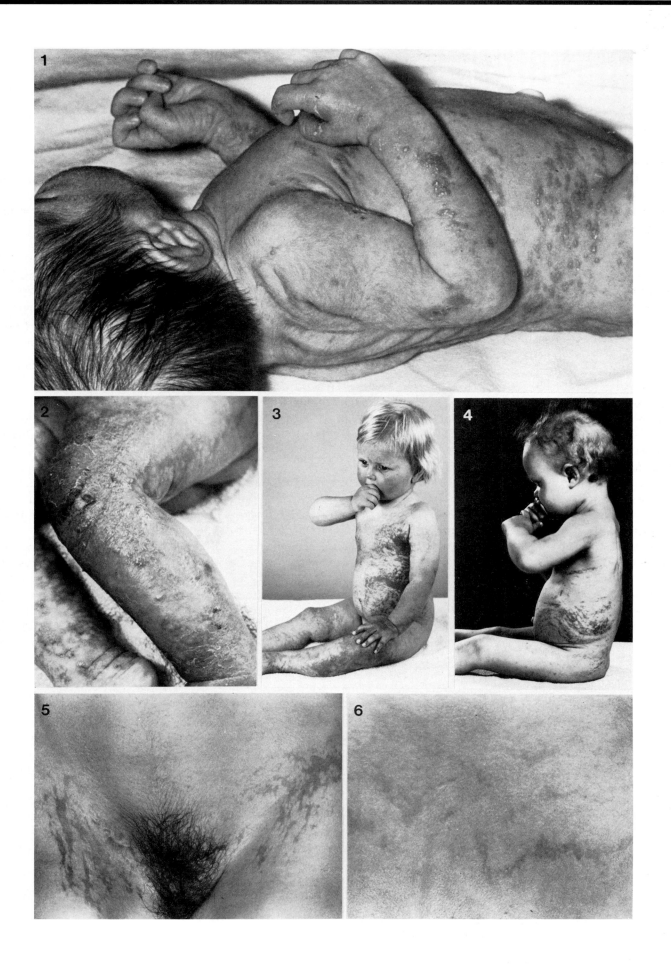

188 Hypomelanosis of Ito
(Ito Syndrome; Incontinentia Pigmenti Achromians)

H.-R.W

A neurocutaneous 'syndrome' of streaky, patchy or spray-like depigmentation of the skin, frequently associated with other diverse anomalies.

Main signs:
- Systemic leukoderma, with bizarre, usually symmetrical (but occasionally unilateral) depigmented streaks, patches, whorls or sprays. The changes usually follow Blaschko's lines (1–3), occurring most commonly on the trunk (not crossing the mid-line), less frequently on the face; in the extremities, with a predominantly axial course and on the flexor surfaces. Apart from the hypopigmentation and occasional hyperkeratosis follicularis, the skin is unremarkable. No preceding or accompanying vesico-bullous or verrucous changes.
- Associated noncutaneous anomalies in approximately 50% of the patients. Especially central nervous system seizures or seizure disorders; gross motor and psychomotor retardation; ophthalmological findings (strabismus, myopia, changes of the fundus and others); dyscrania (e.g. macrocrania).

Supplementary findings: Hypertelorism, anomalies of the external ears, 'coarse' facies, sometimes with hypertrichosis; high or cleft palate possible. Hamartomatous growths on the upper and lower incisors.

Legs possibly of unequal lengths or other asymmetries, scoliosis, hip dysplasia and other skeletal anomalies.

Manifestation: Birth or early to late infancy. Obviously, the changes appear lighter and more marked in people with a dark complexion than in those with fair skin (in doubtful cases, examine under a Wood's lamp). During early childhood the depigmented areas may at least give the impression of spreading.

Aetiology: Almost exclusively sporadic occurrence. Not an entity. Genetic heterogeneity. Various chromosomal defects have been described. Sex ratio males:females 1:2.5. For affected males, somatic mosaicism for an autosomal dominant gene defect that is lethal for the ectoderm and its derivatives has been suggested; this would imply no risk for the offspring of affected males. For affected females, X-linked dominant inheritance has been assumed; gene locus Xp11.21.

Frequency: Considered low; approximately 180 patients reported by 1992.

Course, prognosis: Dependent on the presence and severity of associated anomalies.
The depigmented skin areas may darken with time.

Differential diagnosis: Bloch–Sulzberger syndrome (187), which has been described as the 'negative' of Ito syndrome. However, 'incontinentia pigmenti' hyperpigmentation is the residual of an inflammatory process (with a different histological picture and genetics).

Treatment: Symptomatic. Genetic counselling.

Illustrations:
1–3 A 5-year-old boy with typical Ito syndrome. Depigmentation noted in the first year of life, which subsequently increased in size and area. In early infancy, abnormal growth of skull (hydrocephalus); insertion of a shunt. A focal seizure disorder starting in infancy, eventually well controlled. Tapetoretinal degeneration with poor visual acuity; strabismus, nystagmus. Hearing normal. Delayed motor, good intellectual development.
Sturdy, stocky body build; dark complexion. No hyperpigmented lesions. Follicular hyperkeratoses of the arms and back. Foci of alopecia on the top of the head; mild hypertrichosis of the face and back. Macrocranium; computerized tomography scan now normal. Impaired motor coordination, right more than left; electroencephalogram still with focal changes. IQ (for language) 112. Slight mongoloid slant of the palpebral fissures, epicanthi, high palate, malpositioning of the teeth and long, narrow, peg-like front teeth. Short, broad neck with low nuchal hairline. Increased dorsal kyphosis and compensatory lumbar lordosis. Elevation of the right gluteal fold, hypoplasia of the right gluteal region. Loose excessive tissue in the left flank. Scrotum palmatum (surgically corrected); small penis with true phimosis. Small hands with abnormally abductable thumbs; small feet with syndactyly.

References:
Moss C, Burn J: Genetic counseling in hypomelanosis of Ito... review. *Clin Genet* 1988, **34**:109–115.
Ritter C L *et al*: Chromosome mosaicism in hypomelanosis of Ito. *Am J Med Genet* 1990, **35**:14–17.
Koiffmann C P *et al*: Incontinentia pigmenti achromians... localization at Xp11. *Am J Med Genet* 1993, **46**:529–533.
Gordon N: Hypomelanosis of Ito... *Dev Med Child Neurol* 1994, **36**:271–274.
Rott H-D *et al*: Klinik und Genetik des Ito-Syndroms. *Mschr Kinderheilk* 1994, **142**:396–401.

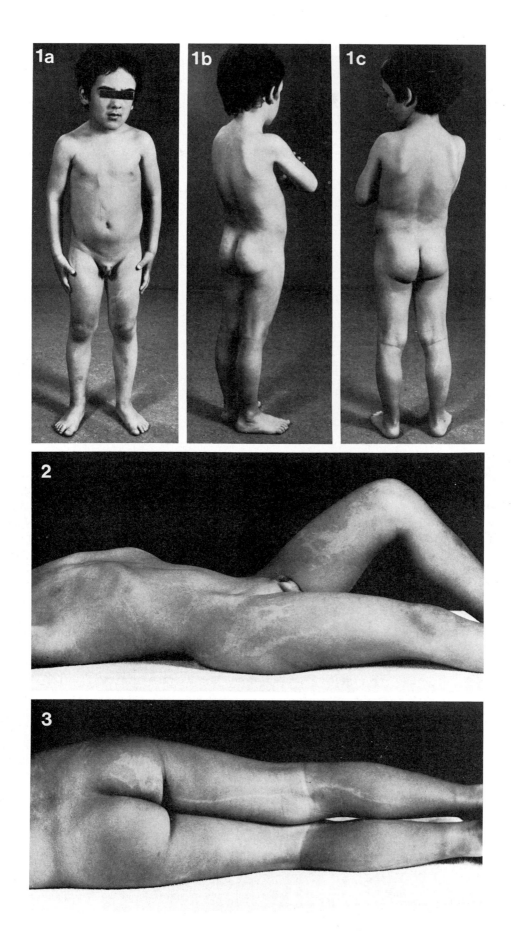

387

H.-R.W

A characteristic hereditary disorder comprising skin changes, mental retardation and epileptic manifestations.

Main signs:
• Skin changes:
Varying numbers of 'white spots': irregular but sharply outlined leaf or lancet-shaped areas of depigmentation 0.5–3.0 cm in diameter on the trunk and extremities (1).
Butterfly-like yellow–red nodular paranasal rash also on the cheeks and chin (so-called adenoma sebaceum, Pringle type; 2–6).
Possible fibro-epitheliomas, shagreen patch (lumbosacral, also facial), subungal or periungual angiofibromas (8a and 8b).
• Mental retardation, frequent and often severe.
• Seizure disorder (initially very often as jacknife of salaam spasms, then possibly grand mal or any of the other forms). Possible spastic pareses.

Supplementary findings: Occasionally, tumours of the lids or nodules of the conjunctiva. Frequent mushroom or mulberry-like nodules in the optic disc or elsewhere in the fundus ('white spots').
Not infrequently, pit-like enamel defects of the teeth, depigmented tufts of hair.
Often renal tumours and cysts (usually bilaterally [9]; often angiomyolipomas) and rhabdomyomas of the heart.
Tumour-like nodules of the cerebral cortex, ventricular or subependymal hamartomas (7), possibly leading to obstructive hydrocephalus, malignant degeneration, and so on, with strong tendency to calcify.

Manifestation: White spots usually the first cutaneous abnormality, often from birth (seen in the first years of life in up to 90% of patients, less frequently later). Usually early onset of seizures (first 2 years of life). 'Adenoma sebaceum' rarely in infancy, usually not until later (2–6).

Aetiology: Autosomal dominant disorder, variable expression, incomplete penetrance. Often a new mutation. Gene loci 9q34 and 16p13.

Frequency: Not low; estimated 1:20 000 to 1:40 000.

Course, prognosis: Essentially progressive. The mental status, in some patients normal, may deteriorate at any time (whereas seizures are more readily controlled or decrease with increasing age). Death (in status epilepticus from cardiac rhabdomyoma or as a result of renal tumours) not infrequently before adulthood.

Diagnosis: Jacknife of salaam spasms and white spots in an infant should suggest tuberous sclerosis. In light-skinned individuals, a Wood's lamp may be needed to identify white spots. Intracranial foci can now be detected more easily and earlier by computerized tomography and nuclear magnetic resonance scan. Also in potential gene carriers. (In rare cases, computerized tomography scan of the parents negative but further offspring affected, suggesting reduced penetrance.) Prenatal detection of cerebral foci.

Treatment: Symptomatic (possibly including cosmetic skin surgery). Genetic counselling.

Illustrations:
1, 5, 6, 8a A child at ages 10 and 12 years. Multiple white spots on the trunk, increasing adenoma sebaceum, periungual fibroma of the hallux. Fine macular skin depigmentation and fibromatous plaques. Increased intracranial pressure, unilateral exophthalmos, diplopia and facial paresis; intracranial calcification; space-occupying lesion in one kidney.
2, 8b A 4-year-old boy with primary Pringle naevus, subungual fibroma, white spots, macrocephaly, choreoathetosis.
3 A 3-year-old patient with distinct Pringle naevus, white spots, hamartoma in the nasal meatus; macrocephaly, markedly decreased visual acuity, tumours of the fundus.
4, 9 A 7 year and 6 month-old patient, microcephaly, secondarily increased intracranial pressure; palpable kidney tumours, possible cardiac involvement.
7 Pneumo-encephalogram of a 7-year-old patient with white spots, Pringle naevus, shagreen patch and fundal involvement; lateral indentation of the right lateral ventricle.
Mental retardation and a history of epilepsy in all five children (in three patients, beginning with infantile spasms).

References:
Flinter F A, Neville B G R: Examining the parents of children with tuberous sclerosis. *Lancet* 1986, II:1167.
McLaurin R L, Towbin R R: Tuberous sclerosis: diagnostic and surgical considerations. *Pediatr Neurosci* 1986, **12**:43–48.
Gomez M R: Tuberous sclerosis. In: Neurocutaneous diseases. Boston: Butterworth 1987, 30–52.
Terwey B, Doose H: Tuberous sclerosis: magnetic imaging of the brain. *Neuropediatrics* 1987, **18**:67–69.
Narla L D, Slovis T L *et al*: The renal lesions of tuberosclerosis... screening with sonography and computerized tomography. *Pediatr Radiol* 1988, **18**:205–209.
Janssen L A *et al*: Genetic heterogeneity in tuberous sclerosis. *Genomics* 1990, 8:237–242.
Neumann H P H, Kandt R S: Klinik und Genetik der tuberösen Sklerose. *Dtsch Med Wschr* 1993, **118**:1577–1583.
Green A J *et al*: Loss of heterozygosity on chromosome 16p13.3 in hamartomas from tuberous sclerosis patients. *Nature Genet* 1994, **6**:193–196.
Povey S, Burley M W *et al*: Two loci for tuberous sclerosis: one on 9q34 and one on 16p13. *Ann Hum Genet* 1994, **58/2**:107–129.

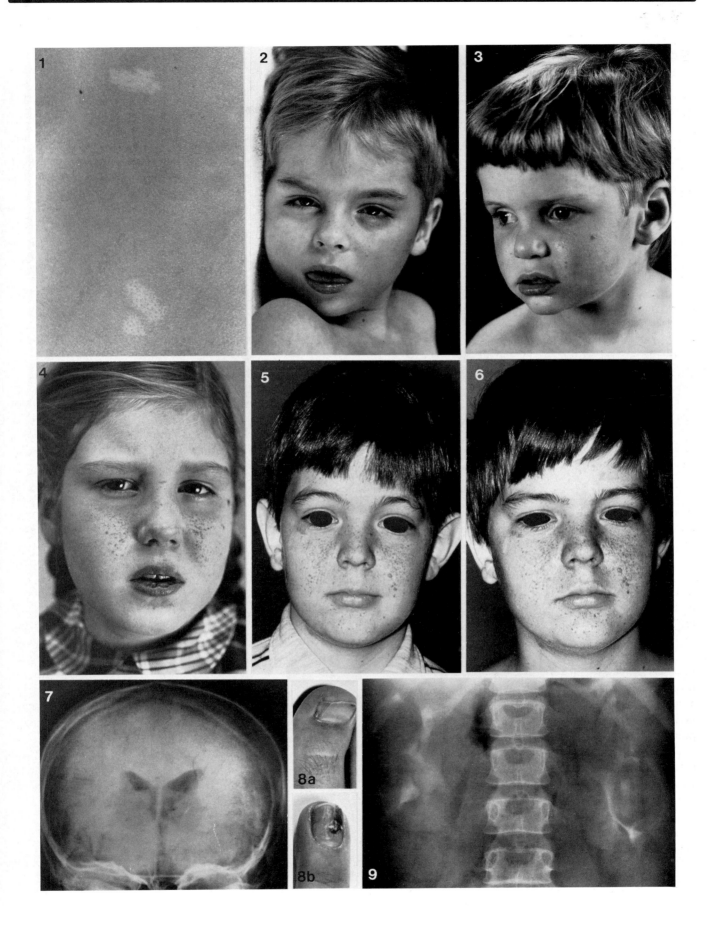

H.-R.W

Syndrome of facial anomalies, partial albinism and possible deafness.

Main signs:
Lateral displacement of the inner corners of the eyes ('dystopia canthorum' resulting in short palpebral fissures; **2 and 3**) and of the lacrimal ducts, both in type I only; broad, high nasal root and bridge (**1–3**); eyebrows pronounced medially, possible synophrys; strands of white hair above the mid-forehead (**1, 4**) and other signs of partial albinism; in some patients, congenital sensorineural hearing impairment (apparently much more frequent with type II, without dystopia canthorum; frequently bilateral and severe; altogether in approximately 40% or more of patients).
The facial appearance may be distinctive.

Supplementary findings: Apart from a white forelock, partial albinism may be manifest as: pale blue colouring, heterochromia, of the iris, depigmented areas of skin; pigment-free strands of hair elsewhere on the head or pigmentation anomalies of the retina.
A relatively small cranium, thick heavy scalp hair with low anterior hairline, relative hypoplasia of the alae nasi, protrusion of the lower jaw and full lower lip may be present. Furthermore, hyperopia, Marcus–Gunn ptosis; cleft lip and palate, occasionally combined with Hirschsprung disease (in types I and II); relatively short stature, diverse skeletal anomalies of the upper extremities (this sign apparently in a further variant or type). Occasional mental retardation.

Manifestation: At birth (for the malformations including hearing impairment). The white forelock may be present at birth and darken later on. Also, possible premature greying or whitening of the scalp hair, either generalized or localized.

Aetiology: Inherited disorder. Heterogeneity. Mode of transmission for both types autosomal dominant with considerably variable penetrance and expression. High paternal age favours new mutations. Type I gene locus: 2q35; type II: possibly 3p12-p14.1.

Frequency: Estimate for the Netherlands of 1:42 000 individuals and of 4% of patients with congenital deafness (1951); the latter figure approximately the same for Thuringia (Germany) (1965); more than 1300 reported patients by 1977.

Prognosis: Normal life expectancy. Crucial to the prognosis is whether a hearing impairment is present, whether unilateral or bilateral, how severe and whether or not it is progressive.

Diagnosis: From appearance (especially type I) and details of clinical findings, including audiogram. Early diagnosis is important so that hearing can be evaluated and treatment started if impairment present (to avoid possible deaf-mutism and incorrect diagnosis of mental retardation).

Treatment: Symptomatic and as above. Genetic counselling.

Illustrations:
1 A 9-year-old girl and her mother, both with Waardenburg syndrome (probably type II). Note the striking facies in the child, with broad, coarsely formed nose, high nasal bridge, and white forelock (the forelock being more pronounced in the mother and her similarly affected twin sister). Further findings in the child: low anterior hairline and very thick hair; bluish sclerae; macular depigmentation of the trunk; increased lanugo hair on the back; small cranium; somewhat short stature; kyphoscoliosis; asymmetry of the thorax and slight coxa valga; high palate and caries; hyperopia; mild mental retardation; audiogram normal so far; normal female karyotype.
2–4 Two sisters, 3 years and 4 months and 2 years and 3 months old, with type I Waardenburg syndrome. Typical facies in both (distinct telecanthus, distance between the inner canthi 42 and 37 mm, characteristically formed nose with prominent bridge and broad, flat tip, synophrys; **2 and 3**) but white forelock, which both girls showed at birth, no longer present (**4:** the younger sister as a newborn). Right-sided severe and moderately severe sensorineural hearing impairment in both children; the younger also showing heterochromia of the iris (right blue, left green). The father of the girls and his mother both show the syndrome (white forelock, heterochromia of the iris), as does her mother and the father's younger sister and both of her children (typical facies, telecanthus, median white forelock).

References:
Ahrendts H: Das Waardenburg-Syndrom... *Z Kinderheilk* 1965, **93**:295.
De Haas E B H *et al*: Waardenburg's Syndrome. *Doc Ophthalmol* 1966, **21**:239.
Meinecke P: Das Waardenburg-Syndrom Typ I. *Klin Pädiat* 1982, **194**:112.
Meire F *et al*: Waardenburg syndrome, Hirschsprung megacolon, and Marcus Gunn ptosis. *Am J Med Genet* 1987, **27**:683–686.
da-Silva E O: Waardenburg I syndrome... *Am J Med Genet* 1991, **40**:65–74.
Ishikiriyama S: Gene for Waardenburg syndrome type I... *Am J Med Genet* 1993, **46**:608.
Lindhout D: Waardenburg syndrome and neural tube defects. *Am J Med Genet* 1994, **50**:387.
Hughes A E *et al*: A gene for Waardenburg syndrome type 2... at chromosome 3p12-p14.1. *Nature Genet* 1994, **7**:509–512.

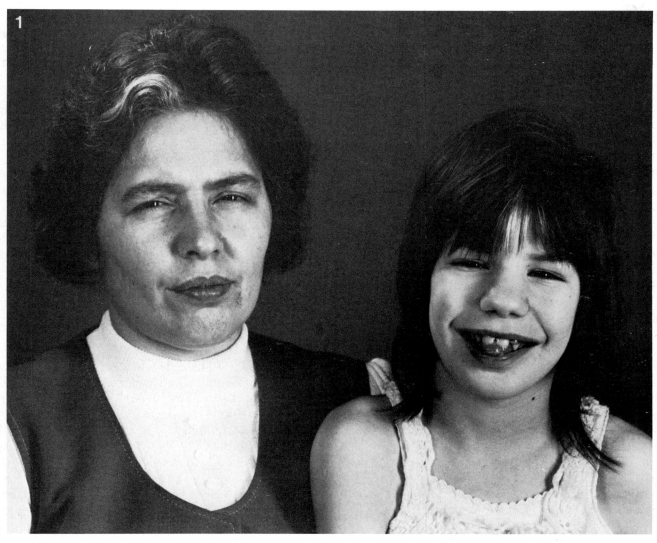

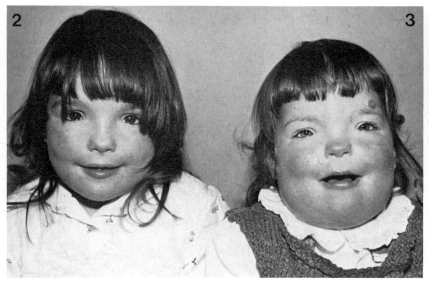

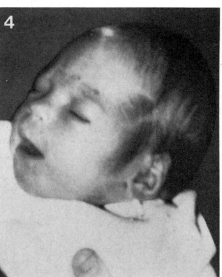

191 Piebaldness

J.K.

A genetically determined, congenital, patchy localized hypopigmentation of the skin, found mostly on the ventral surfaces of the head and trunk.

Main signs:
- Circumscribed areas of skin devoid of pigmentation on the ventral surfaces of the head and trunk. White forelock; absent pigmentation medially of the eyebrows, eyelids, eyelashes, nose and chin. Occasional pigmentation anomalies of the chest, abdomen and ventral region of the arms and legs. Hands, wrists, feet, ankles, occipital region, back of the neck and back are normally pigmented.
- Hyperpigmented borders between the pigmented and unpigmented zones.

Supplementary findings: Islands of pigmentation within the hypopigmented areas; occasionally hypopigmentation of the gingiva, heterochromia of the iris. Histologically, melanocytes absent but Langerhans cells present.

Manifestation: At birth or shortly thereafter.

Aetiology: Incomplete migration of the melanocytes from the neural crest to the ventral midline or disorder of differentiation of ventrally lying melanocytes. Autosomal dominant inheritance. Gene locus: 4q12-13.

Frequency: Described worldwide, especially in the African population.

Course, prognosis: Normal life expectancy. No increased morbidity or mortality.

Treatment: Cosmetic.

Differential diagnosis: No clear clinical differentiation from Waardenburg syndromes I and II (*190*), sometimes possible based on history. Vitiligo (begins peripherally, progresses intermittently, and occurs anywhere on the body).

Illustrations:
1 Healthy 25-year-old, white forelock since birth.
2a–c Diabetic 13-year-old with depigmentation of the forehead, extending to the left eyebrow, to the eyelid and eyelashes; also in the lateral eyebrow region and in front of the left ear (N.B. sides reversed in the pictures). Isolated islands of pigment. Remainder of skin normal.

References:
Jahr H M, McIntyre M S: Piebaldness, or familial white skin spotting (partial albinism). *Am J Dis Child* 1954, **88**:481–484.
Comings D E, Odland G F: Partial albinism. *JAMA* 1966, **195**:510–523.
Taylor D R: Piebaldism. *Br J Dermatol* 1976, **95**:43–44.
Bonevandi J J, Baran R, Breton A *et al*: Piebaldism. Clinical, pathological and ultrastructural study of three cases. *Am J Dermatol Venerol* 1978, **105**:67–72.
Hultén M A, Honeyman M M, Mayne A J *et al*: Homozygosity in piebald trait. *J Med Genet* 1987, **24**:568–571.
Kaplan P, Chaderévian J-P de: Piebaldism-Waardenburg syndrome… *Am J Med Genet* 1988, **31**:679–688.
Küster W: Piebaldismus. *Der Hautarzt* 1987, **38**:481–483.
Yamamoto Y, Nishimoto H, Ikemoto S: Interstitial deletion of the proximal long arm of chromosome 4 associated with father-child incompatibility within the Gc-system: probable reduced gene dosage effect and partial piebald trait. *Am J Med Genet* 1989, **32**:520–523.
Winship I, Young K *et al*: Piebaldism: an autonomous autosomal dominant entity. *Clin Genet* 1991, **39**:330–337.

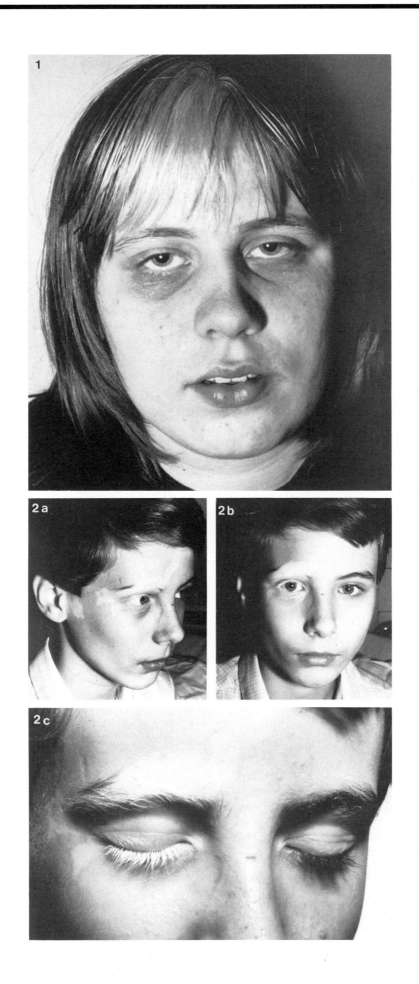

H.-R.W

The 'classic' form of albinism with total absence of pigment from all of the skin and hair and from the eyes and absent pigment formation in the tyrosinase test.

Main signs:

- Generalized absence of visible pigment in the skin and hair (**1–4**). No tanning of the skin. Absence of pigmented naevi and freckles. White hair.
- Total pigment deficiency of the eyes. Unpigmented fundus, 'red pupils', translucent irides, appearing blue to grey–blue in oblique light. Marked nystagmus, pronounced photophobia and poor vision. Absence of binocular vision.
- No pigment formation by hair roots incubated in L-tyrosine solution.

Supplementary findings: Possible additional anomalies of the eyes.

Manifestation: At birth.

Aetiology: Hereditary defect with autosomal recessive inheritance; gene locus 11q14-q21.

Frequency: Approximately 1:20 000 (1–2% of all individuals are heterozygotes for albinism).

Course, prognosis: No change of the pigment deficiency, nor improvement in visual acuity during the course of life. Average life expectancy probably somewhat shortened by increased risk of accidents because of poor vision and increased disposition to develop skin cancer.

Differential diagnosis: Tyrosinase-positive oculocutaneous albinism (*193*) and other forms of albinism.

Treatment: Avoidance of exposure to sunlight (clothing, sun-ray filter cream). Tinted spectacles or contact lenses. Genetic counselling.

Illustrations:

1–3 Two individuals with this form of albinism.
4 Two affected brothers with their healthy sister.

References:

Witkop C J Jr *et al*: Oculocutaneous albinism. In: Nyhan, W L (ed.): *Heritable disorders of amino acid metabolism*. New York: Wiley 1974.
Witkop C J Jr, Jay B *et al*: Optic and otic neurologic abnormalities in oculocutaneous and ocular albinism. *Birth Defects Orig Art Ser* 1982, 18(6): 299–318.
Dorp D B van, Delleman J W *et al*: Oculocutaneous albinism and anterior chamber cleavage malformations. *Clin Genet* 1984, 26:440–444.
King R A: Albinism. Chapter 35 in: *Neurocutaneous diseases*. M R Gomez (ed.). Boston: Butterworth 1987.
Taylor W O G: Prenatal diagnosis in albinism. *Lancet* 1987 I:1307–1308.
Dorp D B van: Albinism, or the NOACH syndrome. *Clin Genet* 1987, 31:228–242.
Barton D E *et al*: Human tyrosinase gene, mapped to chromosome 11(q14-q21)... *Genomics* 1988, 3:17–24.
Giebel L B *et al*: Organization and nucleotide sequences of the human tyrosinase gene... *Genomics* 1991, 9:435–445.

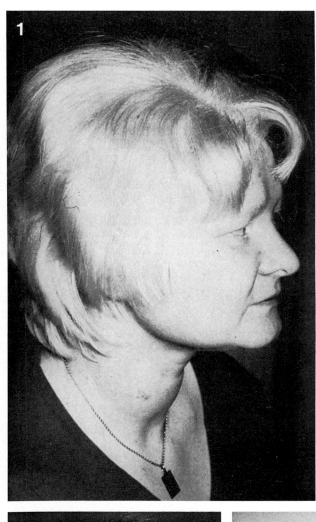

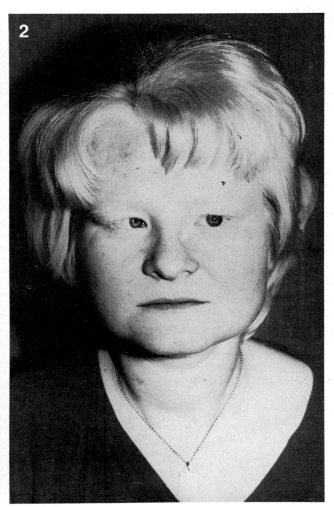

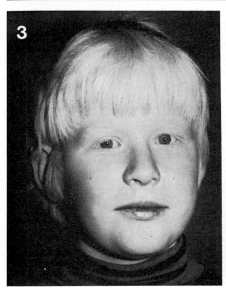

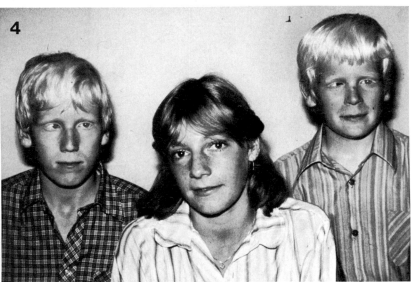

Oculocutaneous Albinism (Tyrosinase Positive Type)

('Albinism Type II')

H.-R.W

Oculocutaneous albinism with decreased pigment in all of the skin, the hair and the eyes and evidence of pigment formation in the tyrosinase test.

Main signs:
- Generalized decrease of pigment of all skin and hair (**1 and 2**). The degree of pigment deficiency depends on age (and race) and the clinical picture of this form varies from that of 'classic' albinism (*192*) to that of a normal pale complexion. Pigmented naevi and freckles may be present.
- Pigment deficiency of the eyes. Unpigmented fundus and 'red pupils' in early childhood (possibly with some improvement later). Translucent irides. Distinct nystagmus and photophobia (but both less severe than in 'classic' albinism). Poor vision. Absence of binocular vision.
- Pigment formation by hair roots incubated in L-tyrosine solution.

Supplementary findings: Possible additional eye anomalies.

Manifestation: At birth.

Aetiology: Hereditary defect with autosomal recessive inheritance; gene locus: 15q11-q13.

Frequency: Approximately 1:20 000 (in American blacks approximately 1:15 000, in Ibos approximately 1:1000).

Course, prognosis: Increasing pigmentation over the years with corresponding darkening and changing of eye and hair colour (in some cases to light brown) and improvement of vision.

However, average life expectancy probably somewhat shortened as a result of increased risk of accidents because of poor vision and increased disposition to develop skin cancer.

Differential diagnosis: Oculocutaneous albinism, tyrosinase negative type (*192*) and other forms of albinism.

Treatment: Avoidance of exposure to sunlight (clothing, sun-ray filter cream). Tinted spectacles or contact lenses. Genetic counselling.

Illustrations:
1 Affected siblings.
2 Dark-complexioned parents and their affected child.

References:
Witkop C J Jr *et al*: Oculocutaneous albinism. In: Nyhan W L, (ed.): *Heritable disorders of amino acid metabolism.* New York: Wiley 1974.
King R A: Albinism. Chapter 35 in: Gomez M R, (ed.) *Neurocutaneous diseases.* Boston: Butterworth 1987.
Taylor W O G: Prenatal diagnosis in albinism. *Lancet* 1987, **I**:1307–1308.
Dorp D B van: Albinism, or the NOACH syndrome. *Clin Genet* 1987, **31**:228–242.
Kedda M A *et al*: The tyrosinase-positive oculocutaneous albinism gene shows locus homogeneity on chromosome 15q11-q13... *Am J Hum Genet* 1994, **54**:1078–1084.
Lee S T *et al*: Mutations of the P gene in oculocutaneous albinism... *N Engl J Med* 1994, **330**:529–534.

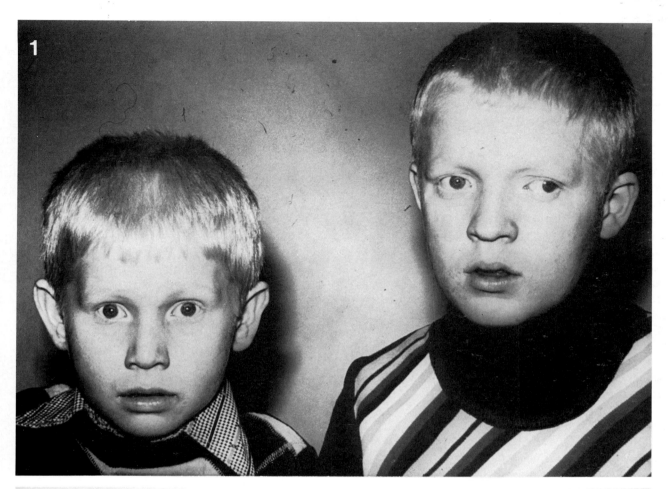

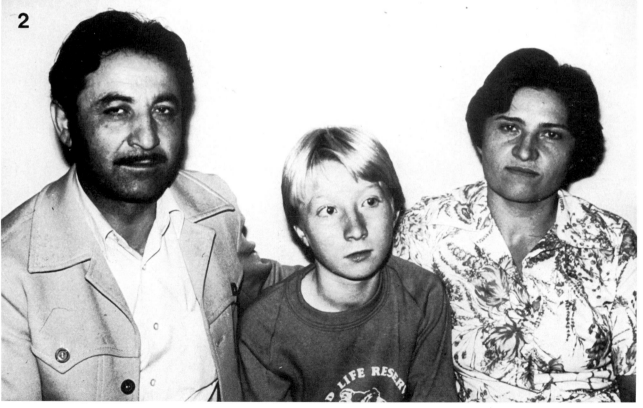

J.K.

An autosomal recessive syndrome of the neural crest, with albinism, black lock, cell migration disorder of the neurons of the gut and deafness.

Main signs:
- Oculocutaneous albinism.
- Persistence of black strands of hair.
- Sensorineural deafness.
- Total aganglionosis of the large intestine, total absence of neurocytes and nerve fibres from the entire small intestine.

Supplementary findings: 'Large for dates' baby, high haematocrit, polycythaemia, absence of peristalsis, vomiting.

Manifestation: At birth.

Aetiology: Based on the large number of affected siblings, autosomal recessive inheritance is assumed.

Pathogenesis: Disorder of the neural crest, which is the origin of the ganglia of the autonomic nervous system, the ganglia of the cranial nerves and also of the vestibulocochlear nerve, the vagus nerve, the paravertebral ganglia of the sympathetic trunk, the prevertebral ganglia of the thorax and abdomen (cardiac, coeliac and inferior and superior mesenteric ganglia), the parasympathetic or intramural ganglia inside the intestines (myenteric or submucosal plexus) and the chromaffin cells of the paraganglia. Also derived from the neural crest are the melanoblasts.

Course, prognosis: Lethal; no intestinal absorption in the absence of peristalsis.

Differential diagnosis: Albinism of the Hermelin phenotype. Waardenburg syndrome with Hirschsprung disease.

Treatment: Possible intestinal transplantation

Illustrations:
1a and b Overweight, mature newborn with albinism and unilateral black strands of hair, occipitotemporally on the right side. Deafness was diagnosed on the basis of auditory evoked potentials.
1c Radiograph contrast imaging with the entire small and large intestine resembling a 'rigid tube'.
1d Absence of all nerve plexuses in the ileum.
1e Colonic aganglionosis.

References:
O'Doherty N J, Gorlin R J: The ermine phenotype: pigmentary-hearing loss heterogeneity. *Am J Med Genet* 1988, 30:945–952.
Badner J A, Chakravarti A: Waardenburg syndrome and Hirschsprung disease: evidence for pleiotropic effects of a single dominant gene. *Am J Med Genet* 1990, 35:100–104.
Groß A, Kunze J, Stoltenburg-Didinger G, Grimmer I, Maier R F, Obladen M: A new syndrome: an autosomal-recessive neural crest syndrome with albinism, black lock, cell migration disorder of the neurons of the gut and deafness — ABCD syndrome. *Am J Med Genet* 1995, 56:322–326.

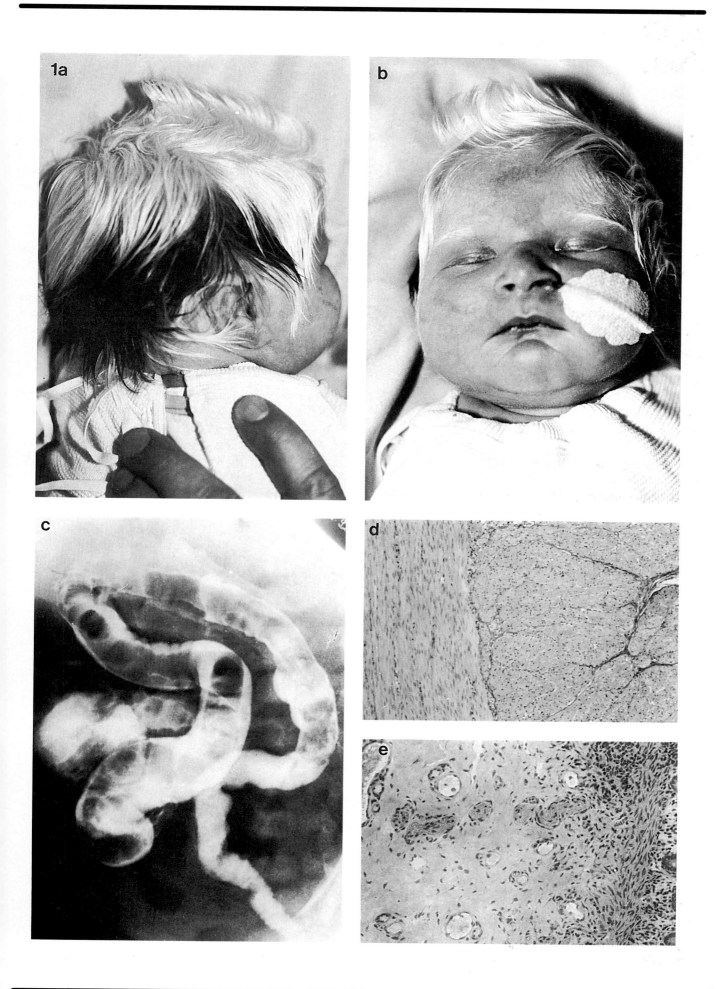

J.K.

A syndrome of oculocutaneous albinism, frequent bacterial infections and large lysosomal granules in the granulocytes.

Main signs:
- Fair skin, fair hair with silvery sheen (compare with the parents in picture), light-coloured iris, photophobia, nystagmus.
- Recurrent bacterial infections, especially of the upper and lower respiratory tract and skin (50–90%). Less frequently, infections of the gastro-intestinal tract, ears and urinary tract.
- Giant azure-blue granules in all granulocytes, accounting for a maximum of 5% of the cells.
- Anaemia in 80% of all affected individuals.

Supplementary findings: Leukopaenia, giant granules also in marrow cells, impaired phagocytosis, generalized bleeding tendency, epistaxis, intestinal bleeding, thrombocytopaenia in over 50%, prolonged bleeding time.

Neurological complications: ataxia, susceptibility to muscle fatigue, tendon hyporeflexia, reduced velocity of nerve conduction, pathological electromyogram, seizures; mental retardation in 10–15%, two-thirds of whom come from consanguineous marriages.

Manifestation: At birth and into the first months of life. Possible prenatal diagnosis.

Aetiology: Autosomal recessive inheritance. Approximately 10 published cases from 15 countries and four continents.

Pathogenesis: Impaired function of the neutrophils in the cell membrane as a result of colonization by giant granules, impaired chemotaxis and intracellular bacterial killing.

Course, prognosis: Sixty per cent of the patients die by 4 years of age showing the following clinical signs: hepatosplenomegaly, lymphadenopathy, pancytopaenia, meningiosis. Fewer than 10% survived until 20 years of age.

Treatment: Vitamin C, antibiotics, steroids, cytostatics, bone marrow transplantation.

Illustrations:
1 A 20-month-old female infant with silver-grey hair (parents dark-haired), hepatosplenomegaly and sepsis.
2 Characteristic giant granules in a granulocyte.

References:
Blume R S, Wolff S M: The Chediak–Higashi syndrome: studies in four patients and a review of the literature. *Medicine* 1972, **51**:247–280.
Barak Y, Nir E: Chediak–Higashi syndrome. *Am J Pediatr Hematol Oncol* 1987, 9:42–55.
Kahraman M M, Prieur D J: Chediak–Higashi syndrome: prenatal diagnosis by fetal blood examination in the feline model of the disease. *Am J Med Genet* 1989, 32:325–329.
Diukman R, Tanigawara S, Cowan M J, Golbus M S: Prenatal diagnosis of Chediak–Higashi syndrome. *Prenat Diagn* 1992, **12**:877–885.
Anderson L L, Paller A S, Malpass D, Schmidt M L, Berger T G: Chediak–Higashi syndrome in a black child. *Pediatr Dermatol* 1992, 9:31–34.
Belohradsky B H, Laminger B: Das Chédiak–Higashi-Syndrom. In: *Ergebnisse der Inneren Medizin und Kinderheilkunde.* Vol. 60. Berlin, Heidelberg, New York: Springer, 1992, 151–240.

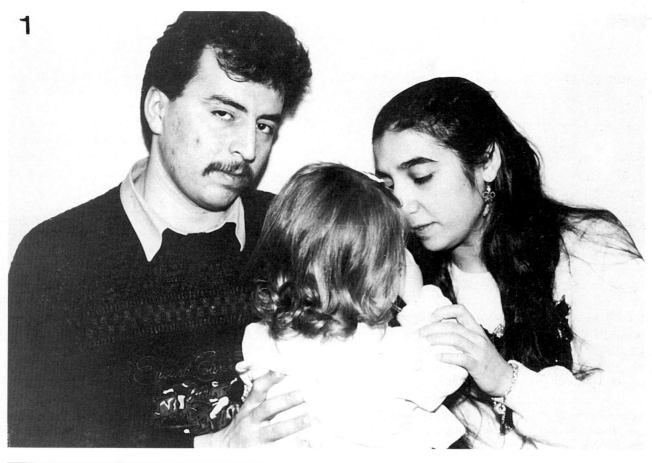

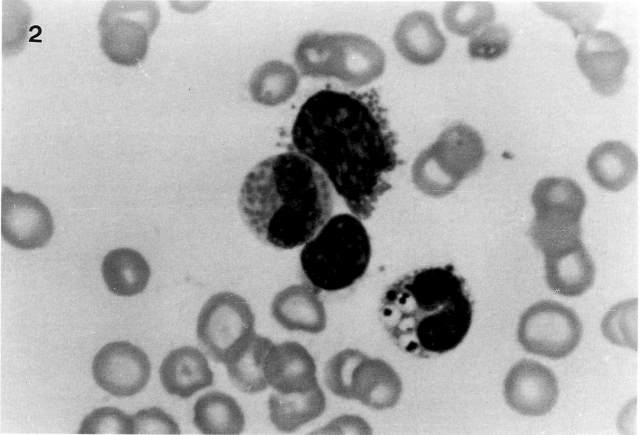

H.-R.W

An almost exclusively sporadically observed 'Proteus-like' polymorphic and variable dysplasia syndrome of the phakomatosis and hamartosis type, partly present at birth and partly later in childhood.

Main signs:
- Partial, perhaps bizarre macrosomia involving the hands and feet (including metacarpals or metatarsals) (1–3).
- Hemiatrophy, partial or complete (1).
- Cranial anomalies: macrocrania with prominent forehead, cranial asymmetry, *Buckelschädel* ('bumpy' skull) caused by hyperostoses and exostoses (the latter also possibly in the auditory canal, alveolar process and other locations).
- Other anomalies of growth: sometimes generalized 'gigantism' with or without accelerated ossification but also growth deficiency; abnormal length of the trunk and neck caused by 'megaspondylodysplasia', which may lead to a 'gazelle-neck' appearance. Distension of the ribs.
  Frequent development of progressive kyphoscoliosis.
- Pigmented and non-pigmented naevi, usually widespread, often generalized and sometimes with raised, rough, papillomatous surfaces (1). Vascular naevi and venectasia also possible.
- Subcutaneous tumours: lipomas, lymphomas and haemangiomas or correspondingly 'mixed' tumours, especially on the trunk, in the axillae, on the flanks (1). Intra-abdominal development of tumours not infrequent, sometimes with protrusion of the abdominal wall, intestinal obstruction and so on.
- Soft-tissue hypertrophy involving the soles and possibly also the palms, especially caused by lipomatous deposits, naevus-like and possibly gyriform ('moccasin soles'). Also hypertrophy of the genitals.

Supplementary findings: Possible atrophy of subcutaneous adipose tissue and muscle atrophy of variable severity; joint disorders.
  Dysplasia of the external ears in some patients; anomalies of the eyes (ptosis, strabismus, epibulbar and chorioretinal hamartomas), the palate and the dentition. Occasional cysts of the lung, anomalies of the heart and the urinary organs and tract. According to experience to date, mental impairment is the exception but may be severe when present, occasionally with central nervous system seizures.

Manifestation: At birth and later. The latter is true especially for subcutaneous tumours but also for the appearance of naevi, exostoses, elongation of the neck, scoliosis and 'moccasin soles'.

Aetiology: Mosaicism for a somatic mutation (with lethal effect in the non-mosaic state) is presumed. For practical purposes, there should be no risk of recurrence.

Frequency: Not particularly low. Since publication of the syndrome in 1983, dozens of other patients have been reported and a not insignificant number of fairly similar cases were found in the older literature.

Course, prognosis: Very uncertain. Possible progression for years of excessive growth of fingers or toes, of soft-tissue hypertrophy or constant new manifestation of hamartomatous tumours but standstill also possible, even spontaneous regression, for example, of soft-tissue tumours. Intra-abdominal tumours may become dangerous, auditory canals may become closed by bony growths and the appearance of diverse semimalignant or malignant growths in different locations must be anticipated. There are adults who become independent (albeit sometimes after numerous operations) but equally patients who die in early childhood. Crucial, of course, is whether cerebral function is impaired.

Differential diagnosis: Bilateral macrosomia of fingers and toes, 'gazelle neck', soft-tissue tumours of the trunk and 'moccasin soles' (or corresponding naevi elsewhere) are so unusual that they can be considered diagnostic within the framework of the complete clinical picture. Incomplete or weak manifestations of this syndrome may not be infrequent and could cause diagnostic difficulties.
  For the purposes of differential diagnosis, consider the following: the Klippel–Trenaunay (*198*) and possibly the Sturge–Weber (*197*) syndromes; furthermore, the Maffucci syndrome (*233*), von Recklinghausen disease (*182*) and the Schimmelpenning–Feuerstein–Mims syndrome (*173*). For encephalocraniocutaneous lipomatosis, see syndrome *175*.

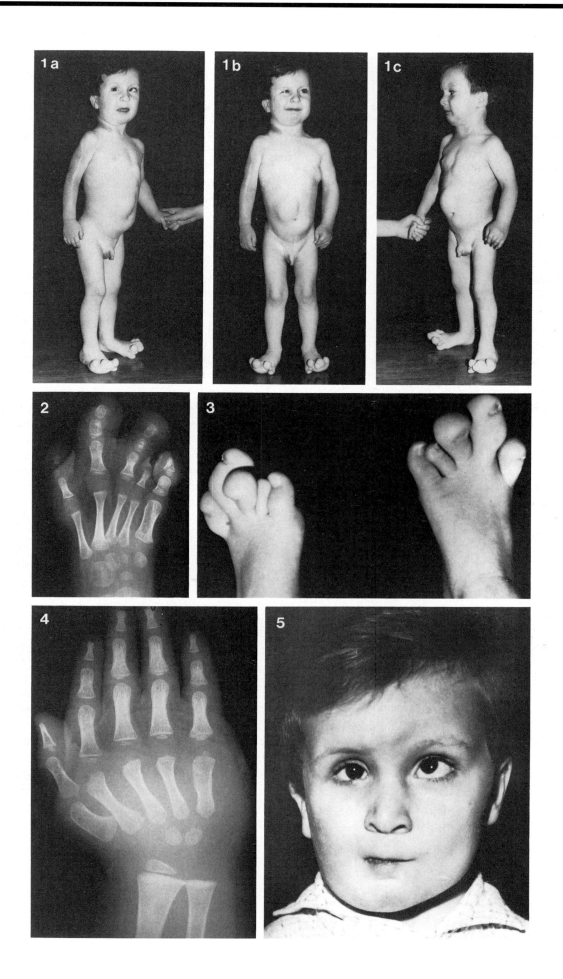

H.-R.W

Treatment: Symptomatic. Amputation of severely over-sized rays of the hands and feet may be indicated in consultation with a hand surgeon. Otherwise, restraint with operative measures is advised because wound-healing impairment or triggering of a local increase of excess growth cannot be ruled out.

Psychological guidance. Genetic counselling for the parents.

Illustrations:

Previous page:

1–5 A 2-year-old, the first of four children of young, healthy, non-consanguineous parents. Congenital, mostly symmetrical macrosomia of the third, the fifth and, especially, the fourth toes bilaterally. Considerably more marked development of the left side of the face, the left arm and, especially, the left forearm with a short, stubby left hand. Over a great part of the right side of the throat, the right half of the trunk and the right arm, epidermal naevoid dysplasia of the skin (grey–brown discolouration of variable intensity with a mostly coarse, rough surface) with sharp medial borders, also on right side of the penis and scrotum. Within this pigmented naevus, several thin streaks of normal skin on the right arm. Subcutaneous 'tumours', some congenital, some appearing in early childhood: venous angioma on the right of the neck,

lumpy swellings on the soles of both feet and on the left thenar and hypothenar eminences. Soft, mobile cystic lymphangiomas (or lymphohaemangiomas; lipomatous components could not be ruled out) on both sides of the chest, in the left epigastric and right para-umbilical areas. Asymmetric macrocranium (51 cm) with two bony protuberances on the forehead. Low-set, dysplastic right ear. Considerable left amblyopia with ipsilateral convergent strabismus. Normal height and mental development.

Opposite page:

1–6 A 4-year-old boy, the second child of healthy, non-consanguineous parents. Congenital asymmetric macrosomia of fingers II–IV bilaterally and of the feet and toes (I–V left, III–V right). Hemihypertrophy of the whole left side of the body. Extensive left-sided epidermal naevoid dysplasia. Lipomas and lipolymphohaemangiomas on both sides of the upper trunk. 'Moccasin soles', similar but less severe soft-tissue hypertrophy of the palms. Asymmetric *Buckelschädel* ('bumpy' skull). Convergent strabismus. General 'gigantism' (greater than 98%); incipient development of 'gazelle-neck' appearance. Normal mental development for age.

7 A severely affected older boy, the first child of healthy, non-consanguineous parents.

References:

Wiedemann H-R, Burgio G R *et al*: The Proteus syndrome. *Eur J Pediatr* 1983, **140**:5–12.

Burgio G R, Wiedemann H-R: Further and new details on the Proteus syndrome. *Eur J Pediatr* 1984, **143**:71–73.

Gorlin R J: Proteus syndrome. *J Clin Dysmorphol* 1984, **2**:8–9.

Lezama D B, Buyse M L: The Proteus syndrome. The emergence of an entity. *J Clin Dysmorphol* 1984, **2**:10–13.

Costa T, Fitch N *et al*: Proteus syndrome... *Pediatrics* 1985, **76**:984–989.

Mücke J, Willgerodt H *et al*: Variability in the Proteus syndrome... *Eur J Pediatr* 1985, **143**:320–323.

Azouz E M, Costa T *et al*: Radiologic findings in the Proteus syndrome. *Pediatr Radiol* 1987, **17**:481–485.

Clark R D, Donnai D *et al*: Proteus syndrome: an expanded phenotype. *Am J Med Genet* 1987, **27**:99–117.

Cremin B J, Viljoen D L *et al*: The Proteus syndrome... *Pediatr Radiol* 1987, **17**:486–488.

Malamitsi-Puchner A, Kitsiou S *et al*: Severe Proteus syndrome... *Am J Med Genet* 1987, **27**:119–125.

Viljoen D L, Nelson M M *et al*: Proteus syndrome in Southern Africa... *Am J Med Genet* 1987, **27**:87–89.

Burke J P *et al*: Proteus syndrome: ocular complications. *J Pediatr Ophthalmol* 1988, **25**:99–102.

Viljoen D L *et al*: Cutaneous manifestations of the Proteus syndrome. *Pediatr Dermatol* 1988, **5**:14–21.

Samlaska C P *et al*: Proteus syndrome. *Arch Dermatol* 1989, **125**:1109–1114.

Beluffi G *et al*: Pelvic lipomatosis in the Proteus syndrome... (Letter). *Eur J Pediatr* 1990, **149**:866.

Benichou *et al*: Le syndropme de Proteus. *Arch Fr Pédiatr* 1990, **47**:441–444.

Frydman M *et al*: Ambiguous genitalia in the Proteus syndrome. *Am J Med Genet* 1990, **36**:511–512.

Hotamisligil G: Proteus syndrome and hamartoses with overgrowth. *Dysmorphol Clin Genet* 1990, **4**:87–102.

Malamitsi-Puchner A *et al*: Proteus syndrome: course of a severe case. *Am J Med Genet* 1990, **35**:283–285.

Goodship J *et al*: Transmission of Proteus syndrome from father to son? *J Med Genet* 1991, **28**:781–785.

Demetriades D *et al*: Proteus syndrome: musculoskeletal manifestations and management... *J Pediatr Orthopaed* 1992, **12**:106–113.

Brinkmann H: Das Proteus-Syndrom. *Pädiat Prax* 1993, **45**:347–357.

Cohen M M Jr: Proteus syndrome: clinical evidence for somatic mosaicism and selective review. *Am J Med Genet* 1993, **47**:645–652.

Krüger G *et al*: Transmission of Proteus syndrome from mother to son? (Letter). *Am J Med Genet* 1993, **45**:117–118.

Ram S P: Neonatal Proteus syndrome (Letter). *Am J Med Genet* 1993, **47**:303.

Shaw C *et al*: Proteus syndrome with cardiomyopathy and a myocardial mass. *Am J Med Genet* 1993, **46**:145–148.

Skovby F *et al*: Compromise of the spinal canal in Proteus syndrome. *Am J Med Genet* 1993, **47**:656–659.

Griffiths P D, Welch R J *et al*: The radiological features of hemimegalencephaly including... Proteus syndrome. *Neuropediatrics* 1994, **25**:140–144.

Rudolph G *et al*: Growth hormone (GH), insulin-like growth factors... in a child with Proteus syndrome. *Am J Med Genet* 1994, **50**:204–210.

Smeets E et al: Regional Proteus syndrome and somatic mosaicism. *Am J Med Genet* 1994, **51**:29–31.

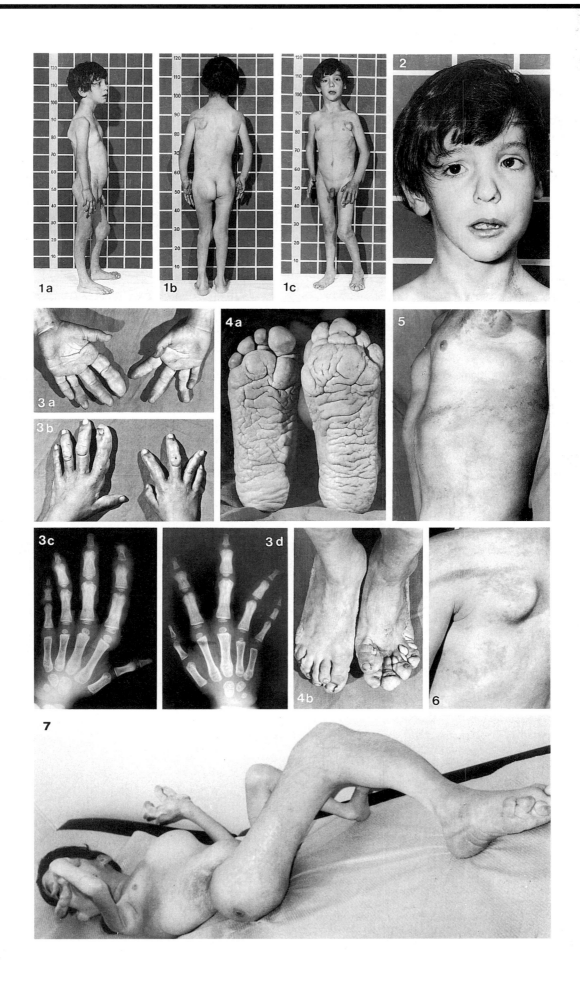

197 Sturge–Weber Syndrome

(Cerebrocutaneous Angiomatosis Syndrome, Angiomatosis Encephalofacialis)

H.-R.W

A characteristic syndrome of macular haemangiomas especially of the face, signs of cerebral foci (caused by ipsilateral meningeal angiomas) and usually mental retardation.

Main signs:
- Port-wine colour naevus flammeus of the face and head, varying in extent, preferentially of the trigeminal area, mostly unilateral, often sharply outlined medially (possibly with corresponding involvement of the oral mucosa), less frequently bilateral and sometimes involving the body (1–5)
- Focal or generalized cerebral seizures. Spastic hemiparesis (contralateral to the side of the angioma). Secondary mental impairment, of varying severity.

Supplementary findings: In almost 50% of patients, angiomatous changes of the ipsilateral choroid, possibly resulting in congenital glaucoma (buphthalmos) (7). Possible hemianopia contralateral to the facial angioma.

Macrocephaly. Skull radiograph: garland-like, double-contoured calcifications, varying in extent, especially over the posterior parietal and occipital regions on the side of the haemangioma (6, 8).

Occasionally, markedly asymmetrical development of the cranium.

Manifestation: Naevus flammeus usually present at birth. Possible congenital glaucoma (7). First signs of epileptic activity, spastic hemiparesis and mental impairment usually in infancy. Calcifications within the cerebral cortex usually not demonstrable on a routine skull radiograph until the latter half of early childhood; demonstration of increased density possible much earlier by means of computerized tomography scan.

Aetiology: In spite of almost invariable sporadic occurrence, inherited factors are probably of causal significance; this could be the manifestation of a lethal gene in the mosaic.

Frequency: Not particularly low: it is estimated that there is one case of the fully expressed syndrome out of 230000 of the general population.

Course, prognosis: Epileptic seizures often very difficult to control. Occurrence also of mildly affected patients with fewer signs, some with undiminished intelligence.

Although the intensity of the colour of the angiomas tends to decrease with increasing age, the affected area of skin usually tends to become thicker and coarser.

Treatment: Prompt surgery for glaucoma when indicated; otherwise, conservative in principle. A neurosurgical procedure, possibly even hemispherectomy, should only be considered for patients with very widespread intracranial changes and for whom consistent appropriate anti-epileptic treatment is ineffective in preventing relentless progressive intellectual and psychological deterioration. More recently, laser therapy has been recommended for the naevus flammeus; in older children the naevus can be cosmetically covered with cosmetic products.

Illustrations:

1 Patient 1 at birth. Congenital glaucoma on the right, seizures since birth; early development of left-sided spasticity and of retardation; intracranial calcifications demonstrable since age 18 months.

2, 7 Patient 2 at birth (2). Glaucoma and buphthalmos on the left (7) with subsequent need for enucleation; right-sided focal findings on electroencephalogram, left-sided seizures.

3–6, 8 Patients 3, 4, and 5 (boys aged 6 years, 9 years and 6 months and 14 years) all mentally retarded and epileptic; hemiparesis in patients 3 and 4; foci of calcification in patient 4 (6, 8) and also patient 5, who was operated on for glaucoma at age 3 months.

References:

Any textbook on neurology, paediatrics or internal surgery.

Noe J, Barsky S *et al*: Portwine stains and the response to argon laser therapy... *Plast Reconstr Surg* 1980, **65**:130–136.

Enjolras O, Riche M C *et al*: Facial portwine stains and Sturge–Weber syndrome. *Pediatrics* 1985, **76**:48–51.

Fritsch G. Sacher M *et al*: Klinik und Verlauf des Sturge–Weber Syndroms im Kindesalter. *Mschr Kinderheilk* 1986, **134**:242–245.

Garden J M, Tan O T *et al*: The pulsed dye laser: its use at 577 nm wavelength. *J Dermatol Surg Oncol* 1987, **13**:134–138.

Gomez M R, Bebin E M: Sturge–Weber syndrome. In: *Neurocutaneous diseases*. Boston: Butterworth 1987, 356–367.

Hall J G: Somatic mosaicism: observation related to clinical genetics. *Am J Hum Genet* 1988, **43**:355–356.

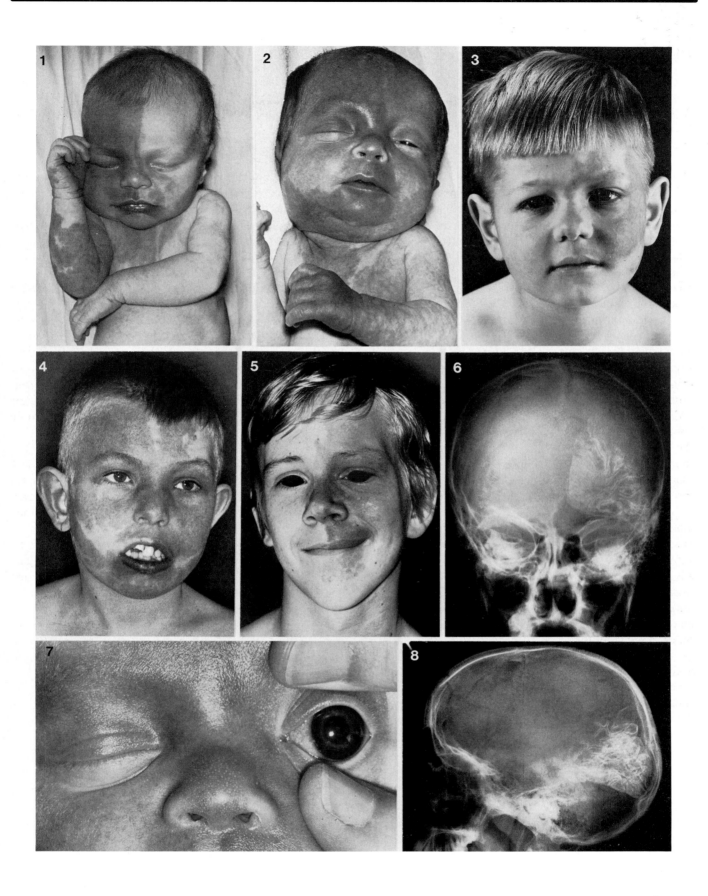

(Angio-Osteohypertrophy; Naevus Varicosus Osteohypertrophicus Syndrome)

H.-R.W

A dysplasia syndrome with localized, frequently dispro-portionate, macrosomia, naevi and varicosities on the affected side.

Main signs:

- As a rule, one extremity is completely or partially affect-ed, the lower ones much more frequently than the upper.
- Flat haemangiomas of the skin (naevus flammeus), bright red to dark violet, varying in extent, solitary or multiple, irregularly contoured and when located on the trunk, not necessarily sharply outlined at the mid-line. (1, 3, 4a, 6).
- Partial macrosomia involving all tissues, usually in the region of the vascular naevus (1, 3, 4) but also occa-sionally contralaterally (6 and 7), which is frequently also disproportionate.
- Venous angiomas; varices may be readily apparent (5) or only detectable by ultrasound, on radiograph (phle-boliths) or by venous angiography (lymphangiectasis exclusively by lymphangiography).

Supplementary findings: Local anomalies of hair, sweat-ing and so on.

Frequent secondary osteo-articular changes (4).

Numerous other anomalies may or may not occur, for example, remotely situated vascular dysplasias, macrocra-nia, hemimegalencephaly, changes involving the skin, skeleton, eyes, oral cavity, urinary tract and so on.

Thus, a highly variable clinical picture.

Manifestation: At birth and later. Vascular naevi usually congenital but postnatal appearance and expansion possi-ble. Variably rapid onset and progression of macrosomic development; skeletal involvement radiologically demon-strable only with time. Varicosities usually not clinically identifiable in young children.

Aetiology: The great majority of cases are sporadic; there is probably a lethal mutation, which survives in the mosa-ic. In exceptional cases, an autosomal dominant pleiotropic gene with relatively low penetrance may be responsible or an autosomal recessive gene.

Frequency: Not particularly low (well over 1000 patients described).

Course, prognosis: At first often distinct progression of development of the macrosomia and handicap; after the child stops growing, the changes may remain stationary. Possible late complication: leg ulcers with tendency for poor healing.

Diagnosis: Venous angiography to rule out an obstruc-tion; dysplasia or aplasia of deep leg veins may be found. In some patients, arteriography to rule out an arterio-venous fistula. Possible lymphangiography. The studies can be done once the child has reached an appropriate age.

Prenatal diagnosis by ultrasound in isolated cases.

Differential diagnosis: In some cases, Sturge–Weber syn-drome (197), von Recklinghausen neurofibromatosis (182), F P Weber syndrome (225), Proteus syndrome (196).

Treatment: Symptomatic (compression, positioning and so on). Orthopaedic care, conservative and operative. In some patients, removal of a section causing venous steno-sis. NB: procedures on superficial varices contraindicat-ed.

Illustrations:

1–3 A patient at 3 and 14 months. Macrosomia of the right leg and generalized, mild hemihypertrophy. Flat hae-mangioma on the right, in part sharply bordered at the mid-line, in part extending onto the left side. Scoliosis.

4 and 5 A 3-year-old patient with an irregular flat hae-mangioma, varicosities and excessive growth of the left leg (tilted pelvis, scoliosis), especially of second and third toes.

6 A patient aged 21 months: angioma especially of the right leg (and the left half of the trunk) with macrosomia of the left leg.

7 Lower extremity of an infant: macular vascular naevus on the right, disproportionate macrosomia on the left.

References:

Weber J: Der umschriebene Riesenwuchs, Typ Parkes Weber (Beitrag zur Diskussion des Klippel–Trenaunay-Weber-Syndroms). *Fortschr Röntgenstr* 1970, 113:734.

Servelle M: Klippel and Trenaunay's syndrome: 768 operated cases. *Ann Surg* 1985, 201:365–373.

Stickler G B: Klippel–Trenaunay syndrome. In: *Neurocutaneous diseases.* Gomez M R. (ed.). Boston: Butterworth 1987, 368–375.

Mahmoud S F, El-Benhawi M O *et al*: Klippel–Trenaunay syndrome. *J Am Acad Dermatol* 1988, 18(5/2):1170–1172.

Aelvoet G E *et al*: Genetic aspects of the Klippel–Trenaunay syndrome. *Br J Dermatol* 1992, 126:603–607.

Cristaldi A, Vigevano F *et al*: Hemimegalencephaly, hemihypertrophy and vascular lesions. *Eur J Pediatr* 1994, 154:134–137.

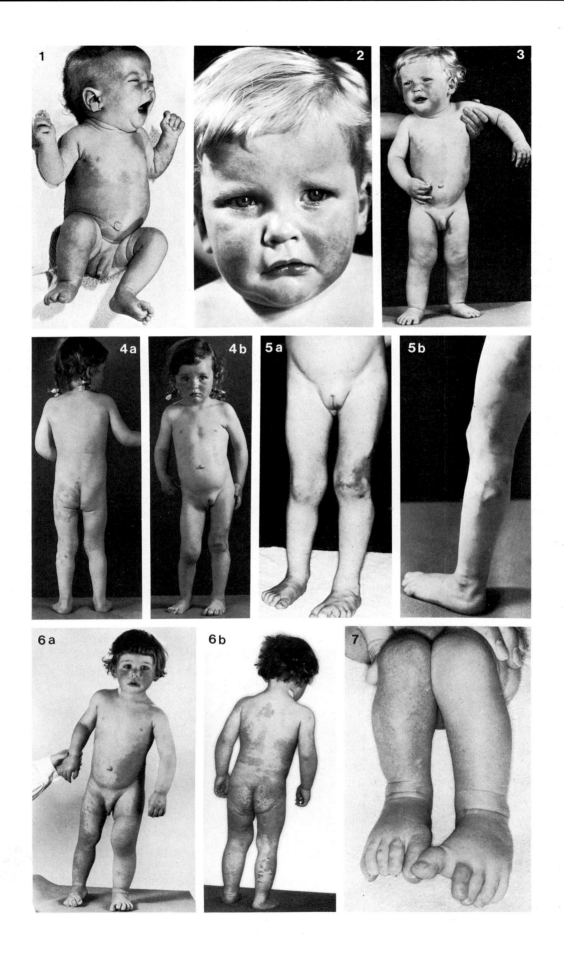

H.-R.W
E. Passarge
J.K.

A recessive hereditary syndrome of primordial growth deficiency, telangiectatic erythema and tendency to malignant tumours.

Main signs:
- Marked prenatal and postnatal growth deficiency (average birth weight of males 2100 g, of females 1850 g; adult height up to 150 cm), with a distinctly slender body build (**1**).
- Telangiectatic erythema (not obligatory), more marked after exposure to sun, more commonly in a butterfly distribution on the face, also on the dorsal surfaces of the forearms. Sometimes blistering and scarring of the lips and lower eyelids. Skin changes more pronounced in males than in females (**1–3**).
- Long, narrow face with prominent nose; hypoplastic zygoma region; micrognathia; sometimes microcephaly (**1 and 2**).

Supplementary findings: Small testes, probable infertility in males (reports of three women with normal children).

Frequent infections, especially when younger.

Tendency in the younger age group to develop malignant tumours, especially leukaemia and lymphoma and later adenocarcinomas.

Chromosome instability with typical chromosome breaks and rate of sister chromatid exchange increased to approximately 50–60% but not in heterozygotes.

Manifestation: At birth, however, erythema usually appears during the first summer after birth.

Aetiology: Autosomal recessive disorder without any indication of genetic heterogeneity. The preponderance of males probably explained by easier diagnosis because of more marked skin involvement. In a few patients, demonstration of a DNA ligase I defect, which is not, however, regarded as the decisive defect. Gene localized distally on the long arm of chromosome 15 (15q26.1).

Frequency: Low (Ashkenazim particularly affected); since first described in 1954, over 130 patients have been reported.

Prognosis: Dubious. Early malignant tumours have occurred in approximately 25% of the patients to date. The rate is probably much higher, as the average age of living patients in 1987 was low, at 18.9 years, and so far all patients over 30 years have developed tumours (carcinomas, lymphomas, leukaemia, Hodgkin's disease; only three Wilms' tumours to date).

Differential diagnosis: Rothmund–Thomson syndrome (*180*); in Bloom syndrome the reticular pigmentation of poikiloderma is not present, growth deficiency tends to be more distinct and the shape of the face is different. Russell–Silver syndrome (*82*).

Treatment: Regular check-ups for cancer, restricted exposure to sun, genetic counselling.

In case of further pregnancies, prenatal diagnosis (ultrasound, amniocentesis and chromosomal analysis).

NB: Extremely low tolerance of chemotherapy.

Illustrations:

1–3 A patient at ages 7 years and 11 months (**1**) and 8 years and 6 months (**2 and 3**). Birth measurements 2020 g and 45.5 cm. Moderately retarded development in early childhood. Erythema appeared in the first summer of life. Frequent infections during the first year of life.

Body measurements at 7 years: height 116 cm (third to 10th percentile), weight 16.3 kg (less than third percentile) and head circumference 47.1 cm (third percentile).

Typical chromosomal findings.

References:

Thomas P: Das Bloom-Syndrom. *Pädiatr Prax* 1980/81, **24**:283.
Mulcahy M T, French M: Pregnancy in Bloom's syndrome. *Clin Genet* 1981, **19**:156.
Vanderschueren-Lodeweyckx M, Fryns J-P *et al*: Bloom's syndrome. *AJDC* 1984, 138:812–816.
Cahn J Y H, Becker F F *et al*: Altered DNA ligase I activity in Bloom's syndrome cells. *Nature* 1987, **325**:357–359.
Cairney A E L, Andrew M *et al*: Wilms tumor in three patients with Bloom syndrome. *J Pediatr* 1987, **11**:414–416.
Takemiya M, Shiraishi S *et al*: Bloom's syndrome with... multiple cancers... *Clin Genet* 1987, **31**:35–44.
Willis A E, Lindahl T: DNA ligase I deficiency in Bloom's syndrome. *Nature* 1987, **325**:355–357.
Kerekhove C W Van, Ceuppens J L *et al*: Bloom's syndrome... immunologic abnormalities of four patients. *AJDC* 1988, **142**:1089–1093.
German J, Passarge E: Bloom's syndrome. XII report from the registry for 1987. *Clin Genet* 1988, **35**:57–69.
Passarge E: Bloom's syndrome: the German experience. *Ann Génét* 1991, **34**:179–197.
German J: Bloom syndrome: a mendelian prototype of somatic mutational disease. *Medicine* 1993, **72**:393–406.

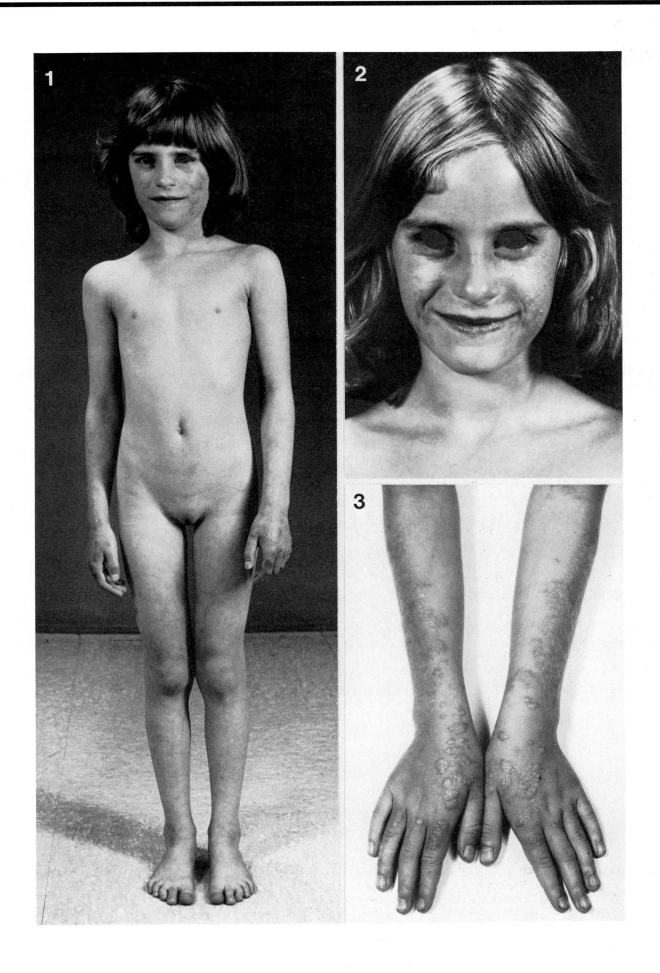

200 Congenital Telangiectatic Cutis Marmorata

(Van Lohuizen Syndrome)

J.K.

Main signs:
- Marble-like mottling of the newborn's skin both in cold conditions and at normal temperature (e.g. warm bed), spread over the entire body. Red to blue, reticular pattern, garland-like. In 50% of newborns, the mottling disappears after they have been brought back into the warm. Mostly observed in premature children.
- A persistent type of cutis marmorata presents over the whole body or segmentally, occasionally with incrusted ulcerations, regardless of the ambient temperature.

Supplementary findings: In the event of persistence, also consider hypothermia, sepsis or hypothyroidism.

The persistent forms are associated with mental retardation, central nervous system malformations, spina bifida, glaucoma, clouding of the cornea, cleft lip, cleft palate, cardiac defect, skeletal anomalies.

Additionally: Sturge–Weber syndrome with hemiparesis, macrocephaly, hemifacial hypertrophy and hypertrophy and hypoplasia of the extremities.

Manifestation: At birth.

Aetiology: Unknown.

Pathogenesis: Defective innervation of the cutaneous vessels in response to thermal stimuli. Dilation of the capillaries and small veins, atrophy of the skin.

Course, prognosis: With thermal dependence, the findings persist for a few months only and are then fully reversible. With the permanent forms, dependent on the primary disease or alternatively the associated signs.

Differential diagnosis: Adams–Oliver Syndrome (*215*), thyroid dysfunction, Brachmann–De Lange Syndrome (*98*), Trisomy 18 (*48*).

Treatment: Warmth. For the persistent forms, unknown.

Illustrations:

1a–c Male newborn, 3 days old, with partially encrusted ulcerations.
2a–c Female infant, 5 weeks old, neurologically unusual, microcephalic. In both patients, the symptoms are independent of temperature.

References:

Fahrig H: Zur Cutis marmorata telangiectatica congenita (Phlebectasia congenita) und ihren Beziehungen zu fakultativ mit Naevi teleangiectatici kombinierten Mißbildungen. *Zeitschr Kinderheilkd* 1986, 102:179–192.
South D A, Jacobs A H: Cutis marmorata teleangiectatica congenita. *J Pediatr* 1978, 93:944–949.
Kurczynski T W: Hereditary cutis marmorata telangiectatica congenita. *Pediatrics* 1982, 70:52–53.
Powell S T, Daniel W P Sr: Cutis marmorata telangiectatica congenita: report of nine cases and a review of the literature. *Cutis* 1984, 34:305–312.
Börnsdottir U S, Laxdal T, Björnsson J: Cutis marmorata telangiectatica congenita with terminal transverse limb defects. *Acta Paediatr Scand* 1988, 77:780–782.
Pehr K, Moroz B: Cutis marmorata telangiectatica congenita: long-term follow-up, review of the literature, and report of a case in conjunction with congenital hypothyroidism. *Pediatr Dermatol* 1993, 10:6–11.

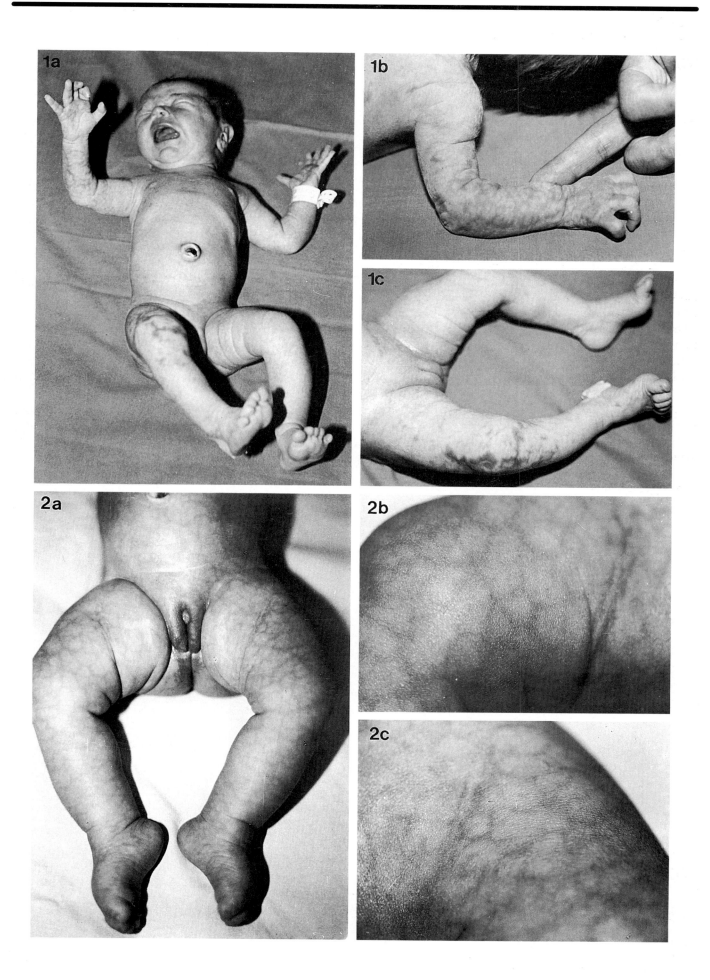

Kasabach–Merritt Syndrome

J.K.

A sequence resulting from large haemangiomas with thrombocytopaenia and haemorrhagia

Main signs:
- Large haemangiomas with rapid growth.
- Thrombocytopaenia.
- Bleeding, petechiae, ecchymoses, hypofibrinogenaemia. Consumption coagulopathy.

Supplementary findings: Hypoprothrombinaemia. Visceral haemangiomas. Congestive heart failure.

Manifestation: From birth up to an advanced age. Usually around the fifth week of life.

Aetiology: Local vascular dysplasia.

Pathogenesis: Consumption coagulopathy.

Course, prognosis: Twenty per cent mortality among treated patients by 5 weeks of age.

Treatment: Steroids, laser treatment, splenectomy.

Illustrations:
1 Female infant, age 6 months, with severe thrombocytopaenia.
2 Two months later, after treatment (laser).
3 Male infant, age 2 months.
4 Age 6 months (4 months after laser treatment).

References:
David T J, Evans D I K, Stevens, R F: Hemangioma with thrombocytopenia (Kasabach–Merritt syndrome). *Arch Dis Child* 1983, **58**:1022–1023.
Larsen E C, Zinkham W H, Eggleston J C, Zitelli B J: Kasabach–Merritt syndrome: therapeutic considerations. *Pediatrics* 1987, **79**:971–980.
Özsoylu S, Irken G, Gürgey A: High dose intravenous methylprednisolone for Kasabach–Merritt syndrome. *Eur J Pediatr* 1989, **148**:403–405.

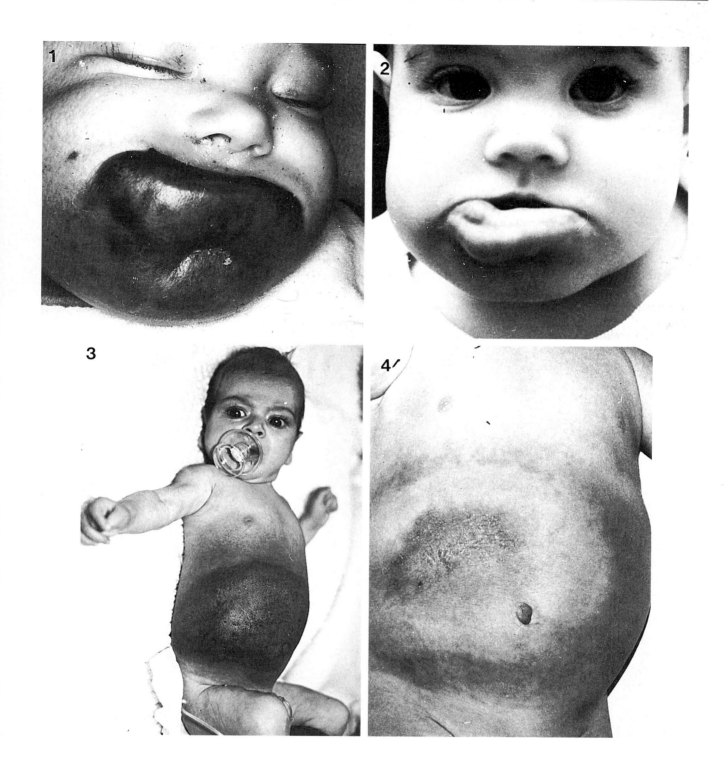

202 Simple Joint Hyperextensibility Syndrome

(Familial Simple Joint Laxity/Hypermobility Syndrome)

J.K.

A familial hyperextensibility of all joints without further unusual phenotypic features.

Main signs:
Generalized hyperextensibility of the joints, seldom dislocation of joints.

Supplementary findings: Only occasional further problems involving the connective tissue, such as inguinal hernia and so on. Subluxation, malformation of the vertebral column, pes planus, mitral valve prolapse, distortions.

Manifestation: At birth.

Aetiology: Autosomal dominant inheritance with high penetrance. Basic defect unknown.

Frequency: Not rare, inasmuch as the spectrum blends smoothly into the normal. Great intrafamilial variability.

Course, prognosis: As a rule, no complications.

Differential diagnosis: Ehlers–Danlos syndrome types III and VII (*203*), familial joint instability syndrome with joint dislocations ('congenital or acquired dislocation of the hip'), Marfan syndrome (*76*), osteogenesis imperfecta (*204, 205*), Larsen syndrome (*230*).

Treatment: None.

Illustrations:
A 24-year-old patient.

References:
Beighton P H, Horan F T: Dominant inheritance in familial generalized articular hypermobility. *J Bone Joint Surg* 1970, **52B**:145–147.
Horton W A, Collins D L, DeSmet A A *et al*: Familial joint instability syndrome. *Am J Med Genet* 1980, **6**:221–228.
Child A, Symmons D, Light N *et al*: Joint hypermobility syndrome: an inherited collagen disorder? *J Med Genet* 1984, **21**:138.
Beighton P *et al*: International nosology of heritable disorders of connective tissue, Berlin 1986. *Am J Med Genet* 1988, **29**:581–594.

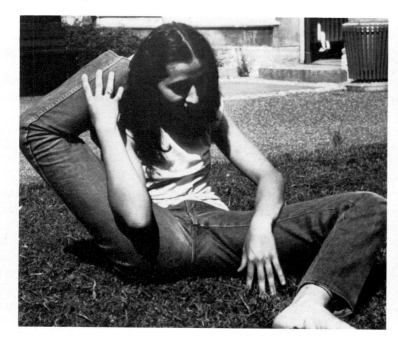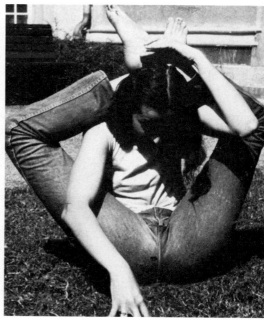

H.-R.W/ J.K.

A group of diseases with connective-tissue weakness characterized by hyperelastic skin, hypermobility of the joints, tissue fragility, eye changes and bleeding diathesis.

Main signs:

- Hyperelastic, velvety, in childhood strikingly white, very fragile skin, with characteristic 'fish mouth' gaping after trauma. When injured, slow to heal, leaving a cigarette paper-like scar, for example, on the forehead. Development of so-called molluscoid pseudotumours on exposed areas, for example, knees, elbows, shins (3–5). Ears very elastic and pliable. Blood vessels easily damaged, thus skin and soft-tissue haemorrhages, which may calcify. Calcification of frequently occurring subcutaneous fatty cysts also.
- Hypermobility of the joints (2, 6–8) with danger of dislocation, instability and bleeding into the joints. Kyphoscoliosis (1). Spondylolisthesis; pes planus (2).
- Epicanthus, blue sclera, strabismus; myopia; ectopic lenses, retinal detachment and bulbar tears after light trauma.

Supplementary findings: Raynaud's phenomenon. Inguinal hernias, incisional hernias, diaphragmatic hernias.

Occasionally, short stature.

Rapid physical fatigability.

Diverticula and perforations of the gastro-intestinal tract in some patients.

Haemorrhages from any possible site; dissecting aneurysms; heavy bleeding after dental extractions (frequent periodontitis, early loss of teeth). Rumpel–Leede sign often positive. Varicosities.

Possible demonstration of specific enzyme defects for certain types.

Pregnancy signifies a high risk for the affected mother because of further slackening of the connective tissue and heavy post partum bleeding; also for the affected child, because of the risk of premature rupture of the dysplastic foetal membranes and subsequent premature birth.

Manifestation: At birth. The diagnosis is usually made later.

Aetiology: A heterogeneous group of collagen-synthesis disorders: type I (gravis) and II (mitis) with 80% of all patients, type III (hypermobile type = 10%), IV (vascular = 4%), type V corresponds to type II, VI (ocular scolistic type), VII (arthrochalasis multiplex congenita), VIII (periodontitis type), IX (vacant), X (fibronectin abnormality type), XI (vacant). Autosomal dominant transmission of types I–III and VIII, autosomal dominant and recessive transmission of types IV and VII, X-linked recessive transmission of type V and autosomal recessive transmission of type VI.

Frequency: Relatively low. 1:150 000.

Course, prognosis: Average life expectancy reduced because of the possible complications (e.g. in type IV approximately 25% mortality during pregnancy because of rupture of uterine or intestinal vessels). The other types have normal life expectancy.

Treatment: Avoidance of trauma. Surgery only if unavoidable. As sutures do not hold well, tissue clamps preferable. Caution with angiography.

Very thorough biochemical and genetic analysis and genetic counselling. Prenatal diagnosis sometimes possible, for example, with type IV.

Illustrations:

1–8 A girl at age 12 years, probably affected with autosomal recessive type VI. Myopia, keratoconus.

References:

McKusick V A: Multiple forms of the Ehlers–Danlos syndrome. *Arch Surg* 1974, **109**:475.

McEntyre R L, Raffensperger J G: Surgical complications of Ehlers–Danlos syndrome in children. *J Pediatr Surg* 1977, **12**:531.

Byers P H, Holbrook K A *et al*: Ehlers–Danlos syndrome. In: *Principles and practice of medical genetics*. A E Emery, D L Rimoin (eds.). Edinburgh: Churchill Livingstone 1983, 836-850.

Kozlova S I, Prytkov A N *et al*: Presumed homozygous Ehlers–Danlos syndrome type I... *Am J Med Genet* 1984, **18**:763–767.

Sartoris D J, Luzzatti L *et al*: Type IX Ehlers–Danlos syndrome. *Radiology* 1984, **152**:665–670.

Sulh H M B, Steinmann B *et al*: Ehlers–Danlos syndrome type IV D... *Clin Genet* 1984, **25**:278–287.

Beighton P, Curtis D: X-linked Ehlers–Danlos syndrome type V... *Clin Genet* 1985, **27**:472–478.

Tsipouras P, Byers P H *et al*: Ehlers–Danlos syndrome type IV... *Hum Genet* 1986, **74**:41–46.

Rizzo R, Contri M B *et al*: Familial Ehler–Danlos syndrome type II... *Pediatr Dermatol* 1987, **4**:197–204.

Pope R M, Narcisi P *et al*: Clinical presentations of Ehlers–Danlos syndrome type IV. *Arch Dis Child* 1988, **63**:1016–1025.

Editorial: Type III collagen deficiency. *Lancet* 1989, **I**:197–198.

Beighton P *et al*: International nosology of heritable disorders of connective tissue, Berlin 1986. *Am J Med Genet* 1988, **29**:581–594.

Hausser I, Anton-Lamprecht I: Differential ultrastructural aberrations of collagen fibrils in Ehlers–Danlos syndrome types I-IV as a means of diagnostics and classification. *Hum Genet* 1994, **93**:394–407.

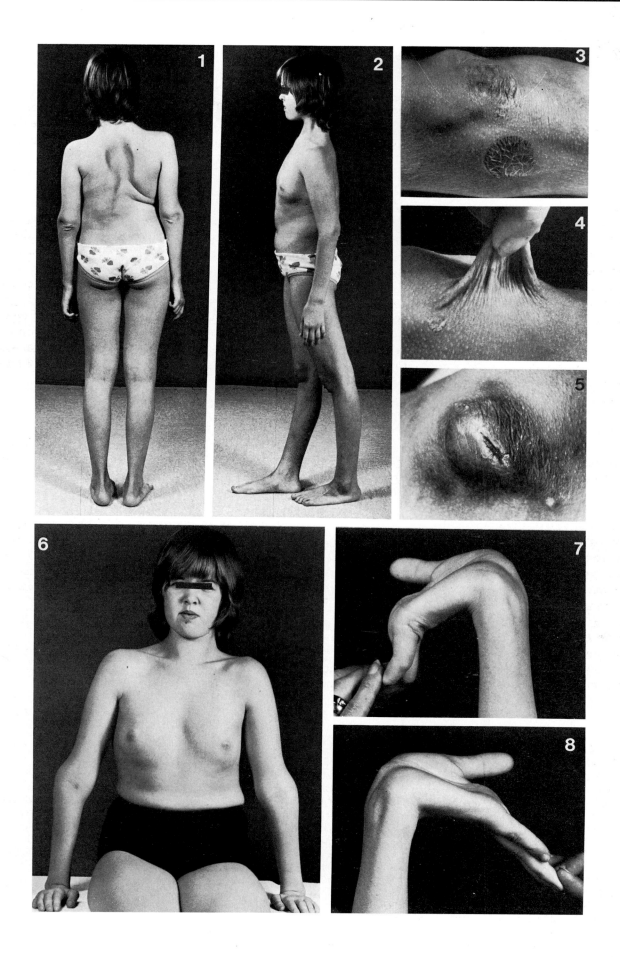

419

A clinically and genetically heterogeneous hereditary disease of various collagen defects with bone fractures, blue sclerae and otosclerosis. Types II A, B, and C and type III are always present at birth and have a poor prognosis. Here: the most common clinical picture in newborns (types II and III).

Main signs:

- Congenitally abnormal proportions because of abnormally short, fractured, compressed, 'pseudomicromelic', bowed extremities, some possibly with pseudarthrosis, a trunk of approximately normal length (often with multiple broken ribs, 'beaded ribs'), large head with membranous calvaria ('rubber skull'), and usually normal hands and feet (**1**).
- Radiologically: thick, short, fractured, bowed shafts of the long bones, especially the legs ('accordion femora'), often with signs of prenatal callus formation; platyspondylisis; little calcification of the skull; generalized osteoporosis (**2–4**). Additionally: multiple wormian bones of the cranial vault, pseudarthrosis, heart-shaped abdomen, cystic changes of the epiphyses and metaphyses (usually type III) and kyphoscoliosis (type III).

Supplementary findings: Frequent exophthalmos, low nasal bridge, small nose.

Blue sclerae; lax ligaments, possible inguinal hernias; muscular hypotonia.

Often hypertrichosis (lanugo hair).

Manifestation: At birth.

Aetiology: Type II A has autosomal dominant transmission; type II B autosomal dominant (?) and autosomal recessive; type II C autosomal recessive; type III is genetically heterogeneous but predominantly autosomal recessive.

Frequency: Type II = 1.6:100 000.

Diagnosis: Type II is always lethal. Type III A: telescopically shortened long bones, multiple fractures of the ribs, blue sclerae. Type II B: severely bowed femora, shortening only after a few days as a result of new fractures, fractures of the ribs only in isolated cases, blue sclerae. Type II C: thin, bowed, metaphyseally distended long bones with few fractures but numerous fractures of the ribs and blue sclerae. Type III: thin, severely bowed long bones, scarcely any fractures of the ribs and blue–white sclerae.

Course, prognosis: Very unfavourable; death often perinatally, otherwise in early infancy. High incidence of fractures with type III up to the 10th year of life, deformities of the lower extremities, later disproportionate short stature. In adulthood, wheelchair.

Differential diagnosis: There are further forms of osteogenesis imperfecta with variable congenital manifestations (types IV A and B). These show variable but as a whole less severe clinical pictures, better prognosis for survival; autosomal dominant inheritance.

Treatment: Symptomatic. Genetic counselling. In case of further pregnancy, prenatal diagnosis with ultrasound.

Illustrations: **1** and **2** (NB: A separate skull radiograph added.) A 4-day-old newborn with caput membranaceum, blue sclerae, right-sided inguinal hernia, lanugo hypertrichosis. Death at 17 days (subarachnoid bleeding, pulmonary bleeding). **3** and **4** radiographs of a further child, in the second month of life (serial rib fractures).

References:

Sillence D O, Senn A, Danks D M: Genetic heterogeneity in osteogenesis imperfecta. *J Med Genet* 1979, **16**:101.

Sillence D O, Rimoin D L, Danks D M: Clinical variability in osteogenesis imperfecta... *Birth Defects Orig Art Ser* 1979, XV5B:113.

Spranger J, Cremin B, Beighton P: Osteogenesis imperfecta congenita... *Pediatr Radiol* 1982, **12**:21.

Shapiro J E, Phillips J A, Byers P H et al: Prenatal diagnosis of lethal perinatal osteogenesis imperfecta... *J Pediatr* 1982, **100**:127.

Gillerot Y, Druart J M et al: Lethal perinatal type II... in a family with a dominantly inherited type I. *Eur J Pediatr* 1983, **141**:119–122.

Byers P H, Bonadio J F et al: Osteogenesis imperfecta: update... *Am J Med Genet* 1984, **17**:429–435.

Maroteaux P, Cohen-Salal L: L'ostéogènese imparfaite létale. *Ann Génét* 1984, **27**:11–15.

Sillence D O, Barlow K K et al: Osteogenesis imperfecta type II delineation of the phenotype with reference to genetic heterogeneity. *Am J Med Genet* 1984, **17**:407–423.

Spranger J: Osteogenesis imperfecta: a pasture for splitters and lumpers. *Am J Med Genet* 1984, **17**:425–428.

Maroteaux P, Frézal J et al: Les formes anténatales de l'ostéogenèse imparfaite. *Arch Fr Pédiat* 1986, **43**:235–241.

Sillence D O, Barlow K K et al: Osteogenesis imperfecta type III... *Am J Med Genet* 1986, **23**:821–826.

Stöss H, Pontz B F et al: Heterogeneity of osteogenesis imperfecta... *Eur J Pediatr* 1986, **145**:34–39.

Ternes M L, Pontz B F: Kinder mit Osteogenesis imperfecta. *Der Kinderarzt* 1987, **16**:769–774.

Thompson E M, Young J D et al: Recurrence risk and prognosis in severe sporadic osteogenesis imperfecta. *J Med Genet* 1987, **24**:390–405.

Young J D, Thompson E M et al: Osteogenesis imperfecta type IIA: evidence for dominant inheritance. *J Med Genet* 1987, **24**:386–389.

Byers P H, Tsipouras P et al: Perinatal lethal osteogenesis imperfecta (OI type II)... *Am J Hum Genet* 1988, **42**:237–248.

Williams E M, Nicholls A C et al: Phenotypical features... osteogenesis imperfecta. *Clin Genet* 1989, **35**:181–190.

Superti-Furga A, Pistone F et al: Clinical variability of osteogenesis imperfecta linked to COL I A2 and associated with a structural defect in the type I collagen molecule. *J Med Genet* 1989, **26**:358–362.

Vetter U, Brenner R, Teller W M, Wörsdorfer O: Osteogenesis imperfecta, Neue Gesichtspunkte zu Grundlagen, Klinik und Therapie. *Klin Pädiat* 1989, **201**:359–368.

Lynch J R, Ogilvie D et al: Prenatal diagnosis of osteogenesis imperfecta by identification of the concordant collagen 1 allele. *J Med Genet* 1991, **28**:145–150.

Constantine G, McCormack J Jr, McHugo J, Fowlie A: Prenatal diagnosis of severe osteogenesis imperfecta. *Prenat Diagn* 1991, II:103–110.

Brenner R E, Schiller B et al: Osteogenesis imperfecta in Kindheit und Adoleszenz. *Monatsschr Kinderheilkd* 1993, **141**:940–945.

Osteogenesis imperfecta — 4th International Conference, 9-12.9.1990. *Am J Med Genet* 1993, **45**:139–283.

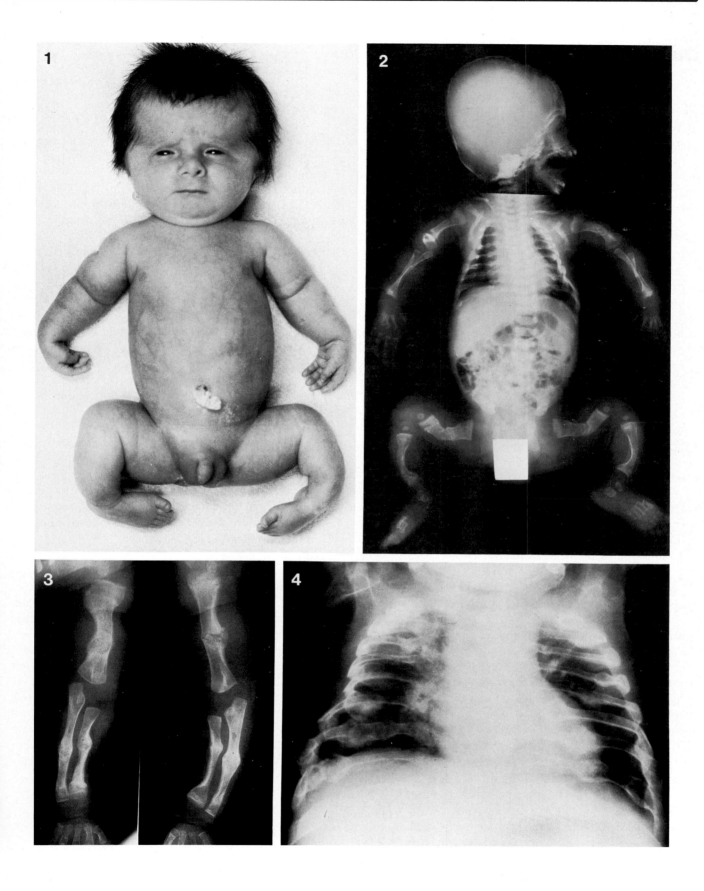

J.K./H.-R.W

Hereditary disorders with abnormal fragility of bones (frequently with secondary deformities of extremities, spine and thorax), small face with bulging forehead and temples, frequently short stature, laxity of joint capsules and ligaments, blue or, less frequently, blue–white sclerae, hypoplasia of dentin and enamel in some patients and hearing impairment (possibly with late onset).

Main signs:
- Increased fragility of bones (commonly called 'brittle-bone disease'), often especially of the proximal extremities, with frequent secondary deformities of the limbs, spine and thorax and correspondingly reduced height (1–3, 6).
- Small 'triangular' face below a relatively large calvaria; bulging forehead and temples (1 and 2).
- Blue sclerae (not infrequently, also tympanic membrane); possible dentinogenesis imperfecta with increased disposition to caries and possible otosclerotic hearing impairment.
- Laxity of joint capsules and ligaments, possible tendency to dislocate. Tendency to develop hernias. Genu valgus. Pes planus.

Thin, translucent skin, possible bleeding diathesis. Formation of broad, hypertrophic scars.

Supplementary findings: Radiologically, mineral-deficient, narrow, frequently bowed, long (tubular) bones with thin cortices (4–6) and flat or biconcave transparent vertebral bodies; delayed ossification of the calvaria with a wormian bone mosaic-like picture.

In some patients, marginal corneal clouding (embryotoxon, with blue sclerae), farsightedness or other eye anomalies.

Manifestations: During childhood; occasionally at birth. Hearing impairment possibly not until adulthood.

Aetiology: This is a group of hereditary disorders, of which at least four show autosomal dominant transmission (types I A, B; IV A, B) with variable expression. Often caused by new mutations. Good prognosis for the first two types, variable for the latter two. Delineation of further types can be expected. Gene locus of type IV (collagen, type I, alpha I and II): 7q21.3-q22.1.

Frequency: Approximately 1:25 000.

Diagnosis: Type I A has blue sclerae but no dentinogenesis imperfecta. Type I B likewise has blue sclerae, with dentinogenesis imperfecta. Type IV A has blue–white sclerae without dentinogenesis imperfecta. Type IV B has blue–white sclerae with dentinogenesis imperfecta but nearly every patient has his or her 'own' disease.

Course, prognosis: Dependent on the severity of the clinical picture. With early presentation, increased mortality; but after survival of the first half of infancy, usually good life expectancy. As a rule, decrease in bone fragility after puberty.

For the most part, good healing of fractures but development of pseudarthroses not unusual. High tendency to fracture up to the 10th year of life with type IV, hyperplastic callus formation, later disproportionate short stature; three-quarters of all adult patients require wheelchairs.

Treatment: Multidisciplinary. Attempts at modification with medication are still in the experimental stage. Conservative and operative treatment of fractures and deformities, avoiding long immobilization as far as possible. Caesarean section may be indicated with pregnancies. Conservative and operative methods to improve hearing for otosclerotic hearing impairments.

Genetic counselling.

Illustrations:

1 An 18-month-old patient with typically shaped head, blue sclerae, bowing and shortening of the extremities (subsequent successful osteotomies).

2, 4, 5 A patient, age 5 years and 6 months, with 'triangular' face, pseudarthroses of the right tibia and left humerus, short stature.

3–6 A girl, aged 13 years and 6 months, severely deformed after extremely numerous fractures (recently, a decrease in the tendency to breaks); asymmetric thorax, extreme lumbar lordosis, scoliosis and gibbus of the thoracic spine with 'fish vertebrae'; normal hands and feet.

References:

Paterson C R, McAllion S *et al*: Heterogeneity of osteogenesis imperfecta type I. *J Med Genet* 1983, **20**:203–205.

Paterson C R, McAllion S *et al*: Osteogenesis imperfecta after the menopause. *N Engl J Med* 1984, **310**:1694–1696.

Spranger J: Osteogenesis imperfecta: a pasture for splitters and lumpers. *Am J Med Genet* 1984, **17**:425–428.

Beighton P, Winship I *et al*: The ocular form of osteogenesis imperfecta: a new autosomal recessive syndrome. *Clin Genet* 1985, **28**:69–75.

Stefan L S, Wright J M *et al*: Osteogenesis imperfecta... *Am J Med Genet* 1985, **21**:257–269.

Shea-Landry G, Cole D E C: Psychosocial aspects of osteogenesis imperfecta. *CMAJ* 1986, **135**:977–981.

Wenstrup R J, Hunter A G W *et al*: Osteogenesis imperfecta type IV... *Hum Genet* 1986, **74**:47–53.

Paterson C R, McAllion S *et al*: Clinical and radiological features of osteogenesis imperfecta type IV A. *Acta Paediatr Scand* 1987, **76**:548–552.

Tsipouras P, Schwartz R C *et al*: Prenatal prediction of osteogenesis imperfecta... type IV... *J Med Genet* 1987, **24**:406–409.

Levin L S, Young R J *et al*: Osteogenesis imperfecta type I... *Am J Med Genet* 1988, **31**:921–932.

Ternes M L, Pontz B F: Kinder mit Osteogenesis imperfecta. *Der Kinderarzt* 1988, **19**:769–774.

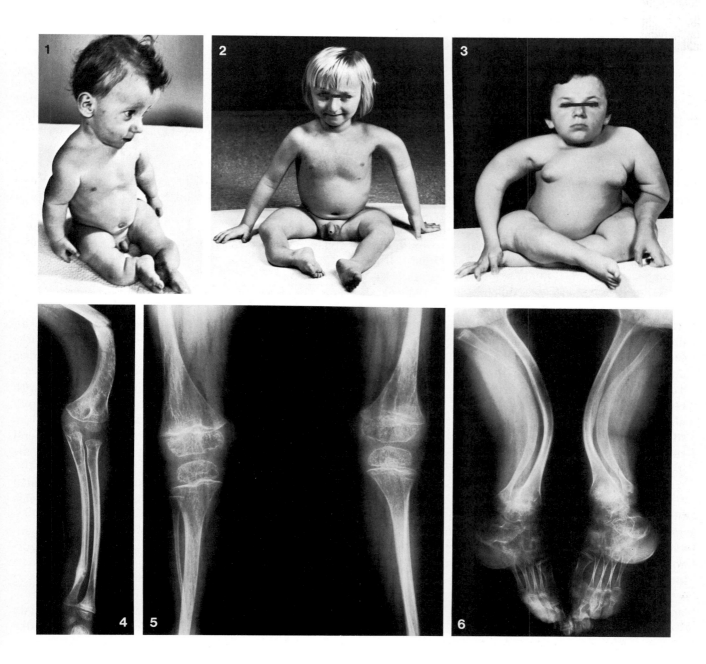

H.-R.W

A fairly extensive and characteristic malformation sequence caused by maternal ingestion of thalidomide during early pregnancy.

Main signs:
- Hypogenesis and agenesis of the extremities of all grades of severity. Ranges from minimal expression such as hypoplasia of the thumb or thenar eminence (or excessive growth in the form of triphalangeal thumb), to hypoplasia or aplasia of the radius, to intercalary phocomelia with absence of the marginal radial rays, to amelia. Similar but less frequent involvement of the legs. In extreme cases, tetra-'phocomelia' or tetra-amelia (**1 and 2**).
- Malformations of the head region: ear abnormalities, microtia to anotia, frequently combined with deafness or with defects of the seventh, also of the third, fourth and sixth cranial nerves, occasionally with malformation of the labyrinths. Malformations of the eyes: epiphora, coloboma, microphthalmos. Dental anomalies (**2, 6**).
- Malformation of internal organs, especially of the heart, the great vessels and the lungs, the kidneys and the urogenital tract, the biliary tract and the gastro-intestinal tract (oesophageal, duodenal–intestinal or anal atresia).

Supplementary findings: Frequently broad, flat nasal bridge and nose; pronounced naevus flammeus of the mid-face area varying in extent (occasionally also isolated 'moustache' distribution) (**1–5**).
  Intelligence normal as a rule.

Manifestation: At birth.

Aetiology: Maternal ingestion of substances containing thalidomide (alpha-phthalimidoglutarimide), 34–50 days after the last menstrual period or between 25–27 and 44 days after conception.

Frequency: Between 1958 and 1963, thousands of children were born with thalidomide embryopathy in Europe, Australia, America and Japan.

Course, prognosis: High rate of early mortality. Further prognosis dependent on the extent of the individual defects and success of surgical correction.

Differential diagnosis: Holt–Oram syndrome (*248*), tetraphocomelia-cleft palate syndrome (*207*), Fanconi anaemia syndrome (and conditions in its differential diagnosis) (*249*).

Treatment: Comprehensive rehabilitation.

Illustrations:
1–6 Children with thalidomide embryopathy, born between 1958 and 1962.
1 Neonate with bilateral 'phocomelia', each hand with three three-segmented fingers, naevus flammeus of the entire medial region of the face; kidney malformations; cardiac anomaly.
2 A 4-week-old infant. Hypoplasia of the radius with wrist-drop and absence of the first ray bilaterally; proximal radio-ulnar synostoses. Severe bilateral abnormalities of the ears with aplasia of the auditory canal. Peripheral paresis of the facial nerve. Capillary haemangioma of the face. Cardiac anomaly.
3–5 Three children with non-specific but so-called thalidomide facies; in 5 only the suggestion of a 'moustache' haemangioma remaining.
3 Neonate with radial aplasia and absence of the marginal rays; dislocated left hip; dysplasia of the right hip; possible cardiac anomaly.
4 A 3-month-old girl with 'phocomelia' and absence of the first ray bilaterally; possible cardiac defect.
5 A 2-year-old boy with radial aplasia or intercalary hemimelia bilaterally and absence of the marginal radial rays.
6 An 11 year-old, mentally normal girl. Severe bilateral abnormalities of the ears, hypoplastic external auditory canal on the left only. Severe hearing impairment. Disturbance of balance. Paresis of the right facial nerve; also paralysis of lateral conjugate gaze bilaterally. Left side of the face flatter than the right. Congenital facial capillary haemangioma, which has receded. Maternal intake of thalidomide preparation on the 27th day after conception.

References:
Wiedemann H-R: Klinische Bemerkungen zur pharmakogenen Teratogenese. In: *Teratogenesis*. Basle: Schwabe, 1964.
Willert H-G, Henkel, H-L: *Klinik und Pathologie der Dysmelie*. Berlin, Heidelberg, New York. Springer 1969.
Burgio G R: The thalidomide disaster briefly revisited. *Eur J Pediatr* 1981, **136**:229.
Lenz W: Thalidomide embryopathy in Germany, 1959–1961. In: *Prevention of physical and mental congenital defects, part C: basic and medical science, education and future strategies*. New York: Alan Liss, 1985.
Newman C G H: Teratogen update: clinical aspects of thalidomide embryopathy — a continuing preoccupation. *Teratology* 1985, **32**:133–144.
Fraser F C: Thalidomide retrospective: what did we learn? *Teratology* 1988, **38**:201–202.
Lenz W: A short history of thalidomide embryopathy. *Teratology* 1988, **38**:203–215.

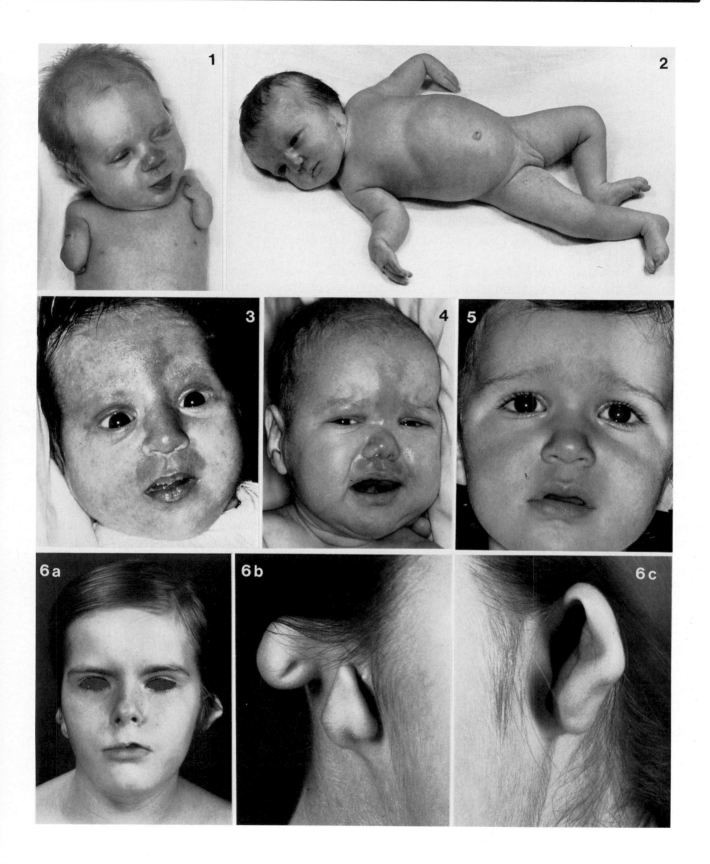

207 Roberts Syndrome

(Tetraphocomelia–Cleft Palate Syndrome; Pseudothalidomide Syndrome; SC Syndrome)

H.-R.W

An autosomal recessive syndrome of tetraphocomelia, primordial growth deficiency, cleft lip and palate and mental retardation.

Main signs:
- Tetraphocomelia caused by absence or shortening of the long bones of the extremities (1–6); usually reduction of the rays of the fingers and occasionally toes to four or less. Syndactyly and fusion of metacarpals and metatarsals (5 and 6).
- Usually bilateral cleft lip and palate (1 and 2); cleft palate alone or high palate also possible.
- Mental retardation.

Supplementary findings: Primordial growth deficiency. Hypertelorism, hypoplastic alae nasi (4). Haemangioma of the face; fine, thin, silver–blond hair.

Penis or clitoris relatively large; cryptorchidism; anomalies of the uterus and vagina. Possible horseshoe kidneys, polycystic kidneys.

Possible encephalocoele, hydrocephalus.

Divided centromere region in C-banded metaphase chromosomal preparations.

Manifestation: At birth.

Aetiology: Monogenic disorder, autosomal recessive with very variable expression.

Frequency: Very low; between first description in 1829 and now, little more than 100 patients described.

Prognosis: Approximately 50% of patients are stillborn or die within the first weeks of life, frequently of pneumonia.

Differential diagnosis: Thalidomide syndrome (206), Baller–Gerold syndrome (208).

Treatment: Operative correction of clefts and orthopaedic care as indicated.

After birth of an index patient, prenatal diagnosis in subsequent pregnancies (ultrasound; chromosomal analysis, premature separation of the centromeres is suggestive of this syndrome).

Illustrations:

1 A 16-month-old, the second child of young, healthy, non-consanguineous parents after a healthy girl. The proband was followed by two similarly affected foetuses (pregnancies terminated) and a further healthy child.

2 A male newborn: typical appearance with 'phocomelia' and bilateral cleft lip and palate; cytogenetically, 'fissured centromeres'.

3 and 4 A child, aged 4 years and 6 months, only 64 cm tall, head circumference 46 cm. Mental retardation. Dermoid cyst of the anterior neck region; cleft palate.

5 and 6 Radiographs of the child in **3 and 4** at 2 days and 4 years and 6 months, respectively. Absent radii, shortened ulnae, fusion of metacarpals I, II, III, IV and V bilaterally; high, narrow pelvis with rudimentary ischial rami; the only long bone present in the legs is probably the tibia; fusion of metatarsals IV and V; the bone age corresponds to that of a girl aged 2 years and 6 months.

References:

Freeman M V R, Williams W W, Schimke R N, Temtamy, S A, Vachier E, German J: The Roberts syndrome. *Clin Genet* 1974, 5:1–16.
Grosse F-R, Pandel C, Wiedemann H-R: The Tetraphocomelia–Cleft Palate Syndrome. *Humangenetik* 1975, 28:353.
Herrmann J, Opitz J M: The SC phocomelia and the Roberts syndrome: nosologic aspects. *Eur J Pediatr* 1977, 125:117.
Quazi Q H, Kassner E G, Masakawa *et al*: The SC phocomelia syndrome: report of two cases with cytogenetic abnormality. *Am J Med Genet* 1979, 4:231.
Fryns H, Goddeeris P, Moerman F *et al*: The tetraphocomelia–cleft palate syndrome in identical twins. *Hum Genet* 1980, 53:279.
Leonard P, Rendle-Short J, Skardoon L: Robert's-SC phocomelia syndrome with cytogenetic findings. *Hum Genet* 1982, 60:379.
Pfeiffer R A, Zwerner H: Das Roberts-Syndrom. *Mschr Kinderheilk* 1982, 130:296.
Zergollern L, Hitrec V: Four siblings with Robert's syndrome. *Clin Genet* 1982, 21:1.
Römke C, Froster-Iskenius U, Heyne K *et al*: Roberts syndrome and SC phocomelia. A single genetic entity. *Clin Genet* 1987, 31:170–177.
Robins D B, Ladda R L *et al*: Prenatal detection of Roberts-SC phocomelia syndrome. *Am J Med Genet* 1989, 32:390–394.
Holmes-Siedle M *et al*: A sibship with Roberts-SC phocomelia syndrome. *Am J Med Genet* 1990, 37:18–22.
Huson S M *et al*: The Baller–Gerold syndrome... overlap with Roberts syndrome. *J Med Genet* 1990, 27:371–375.
Maserati E *et al*: Roberts syndrome... *Ann Génét* 1991, 34:239–246.
Van den Berg D J, Francke J: Roberts syndrome: a review... *Am J Med Genet* 1993, 47:1104–1123.
Satar M *et al*: Roberts-SC phocomelia syndrome... *Clin Genet* 1994, 45:107–108.
Sinha A K, Verma R S *et al*: Clinical heterogeneity of skeletal dysplasia in Roberts syndrome... *Hum Heredity* 1994, 44:121–126.

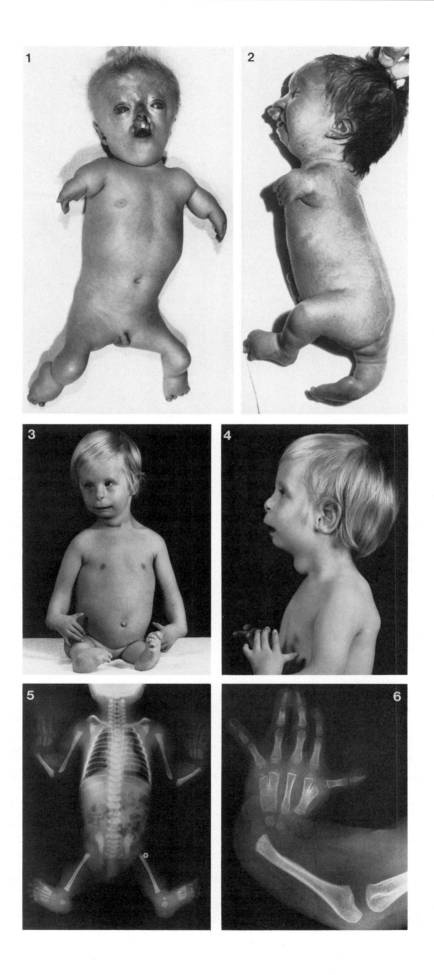

208 Baller–Gerold Syndrome
(Craniosynostosis–Radial Aplasia Syndromes)

J.K.

A genetically determined growth deficiency syndrome with premature craniosynostosis and radial ray defects.

Main signs:

- Premature craniosynostosis involving various sutures (in 80% of patients, affecting the coronal sutures, either in isolation or in combination with synostosis of the lambdoid, sagittal or metopic sutures). Depending on the type of synostosis, oxycephaly, plagiocephaly, clover-leaf deformities.
- Radial ray defects, generally symmetrical but combinations of unilateral radial aplasia and contralateral radial hypoplasia are not unusual. Ulna usually short and bowed. Associated deformities of the hand: oligodactyly with unilateral/bilateral aplasia or hypoplasia of the thumb; the metacarpals and carpals are fused, hypoplastic or absent. Club hand. Postaxially, bowed ulna and fifth-finger clinodactyly not unusual.

Supplementary findings:

- Facial dysmorphism: epicanthus medialis, hypertelorism, prominent nasal bridge, low-set ears with dysplastic helices, micrognathia, prognathia, cleft palate, bifid uvula, choanal stenosis.
- Small-for-dates babies, secondary growth deficiency.
- Skeletal anomalies: lordosis, anomalies of the vertebral bodies (double vertebrae, flattened vertebrae), limited mobility of the shoulder, elbow and knee joints, fused ribs, abdominal anomalies.
- Cardiac anomalies: ventricular septal defect, patent ductus arteriosus tetralogy of Fallot, valvular aortic stenosis.
- Renal anomalies: pelvic kidney, renal ectopy, unilateral agenesis, hydronephrosis, rectovaginal fistula.
- Anal anomalies: ventrally displaced anus, cutaneous anal stenosis, perineal fistula.
- Neurological signs: psychomotor retardation rare; secondary as a result of premature synostosis. Polymicrogyria. Thin, absent/hypoplastic corpus callosum, hypoplastic rhinencephalon. Hydrocephalus.

Congenital deafness. Seizures.
- Intelligence generally normal, 30% of patients are retarded.

Manifestation: Prenatal and postnatal.

Aetiology: Autosomal recessive inheritance with 1:1 sex ratio. Intrafamilial variability.

Pathogenesis: Unknown.

Frequency: Between the first report and 1993, 22 patients were reported.

Course, prognosis: In isolated cases, sudden death in early infancy between the second and sixth months of life. Rarely mental and motor retardation. Usually normal intelligence.

Differential diagnosis: TAR syndrome (*209*), Roberts syndrome (*207*), Holt–Oram syndrome (*248*), Fanconi anaemia (*249*).

Treatment: Prenatal diagnosis by ultrasound. Neurosurgical intervention. Orthopaedic measures.

Illustrations:

1 Age 3 years and 7 months, short stature (80 cm). 1a–e Oxycephalic plagiocephalus (NB: premature closure of the right coronal suture), broad forehead, hypertelorism, epicanthus, small nose, long indistinct philtrum, narrow upper lip, mild micrognathia. 1a–c and h Club hands bilaterally, aplasia of the thumb, fifth fingers with only two phalanges. Condition after bilateral club foot operation. 1f and g Bilateral radial aplasia, right ulna radially bowed, left ulna severely bowed and shortened with cystic changes.

1c, d, h from: H Reichenbach, D Hörmann, H Theile. Ein weiterer Fall mit Baller–Gerold-Syndrom. *Kinderärztl Prax* 1993, **61**:161–167.

References:

Boudreaux J M, Colon M A, Lorusso G D, Parro E A, Pelias M Z: Baller–Gerold syndrome: an 11th case of craniosynostosis and radial aplasia. *Am J Med Genet* 1990, 37:447–450.
Galea P, Tolmie J L: Normal growth and development in a child with Baller–Gerold syndrome (craniosynostosis and radial aplasia). *J Med Genet* 1990, 27:784–787.
Huson S M, Rodgers C S, Hall C M, Winter R M: The Baller–Gerold syndrome: phenotypic and cytogenetic overlap with Roberts syndrome. *J Med Genet* 1990, 27:371–375.
Lewis M E S, Rosenbaum P L, Paes B A: Baller–Gerold syndrome associated with congenital hydrocephalus. *Am J Med Genet* 1991, 40:307–310.
van Maldergem L, Verloes A, Lejeune L, Gillerot Y: The Baller–Gerold syndrome. *J Med Genet* 1992, 29:266–268.
Dallapiccola B, Zelante L, Mingarelli R, Pellegrino M, Bertozzi V: Baller–Gerold syndrome: case report and clinical and radiological review. *Am J Med Genet* 1992, **42**:365–368.
Lin A L, McPherson E, Nwokoro N A, Clemens M, Losken H W, Mulvihill J J: Further delineation of the Baller–Gerold syndrome. *Am J Med Genet* 1993, 45:519–524.
Nwokoro N A, Jaffe R, Barmada M: Baller–Gerold syndrome: a post mortem examination. *Am J Med Genet* 1993, 47:1233.
Reichenbach H, Hörmann D, Theile H: Ein weiterer Fall mit Baller–Gerold-Syndrom (Craniosynostosis-Radial Aplasia Syndrome) - Überblick und neue Gesichtspunkte bei einem seltenen Syndrom. *Kinderärztl Praxis* 1993, **61**:161–167.
Ramos-Fuentes F J, Nicholson L, Scott Jr C I: Phenotypic variability in the Baller–Gerold syndrome: report of a mildly affected patient and review of the literature. *Eur J Pediatr* 1994, 15:483–487.

428

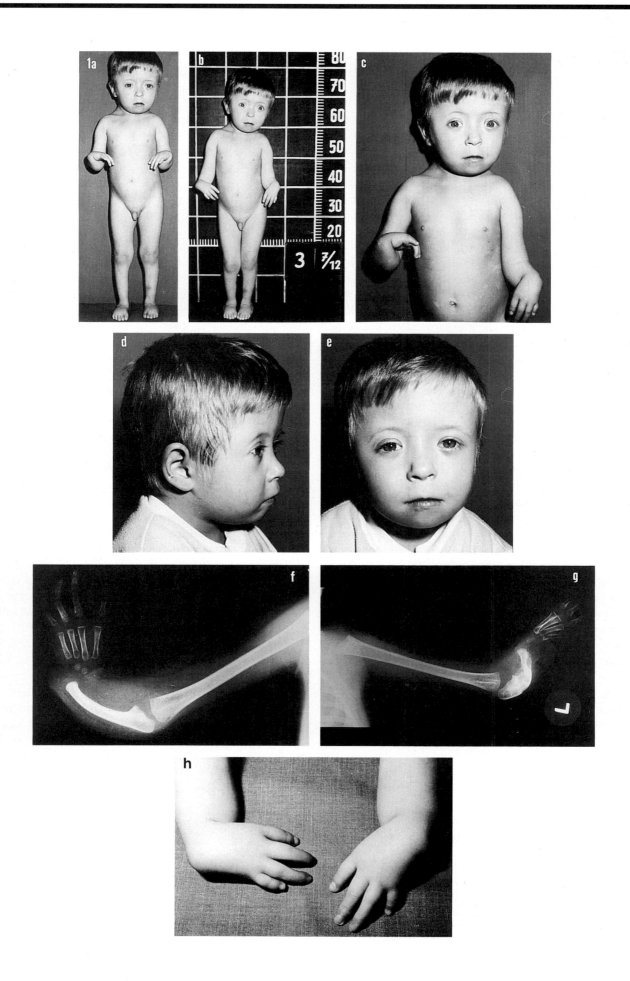

429

H.-R.W

A syndrome of bilateral radial aplasia with retention of the thumbs, thrombocytopaenia and other anomalies.

Main signs:
- Bilateral aplasia of the radius with radial wrist-drop, thumbs always present (**1–6**). Frequently also hypoplasia of the humerus, aplasia in isolated cases ('phocomelia').
- Thrombocytopaenia, fluctuating and often severe, with megakaryocytopaenia and, particularly during the first few months of life, frequent life-threatening episodes of bleeding or bleeding tendency (including cerebral haemorrhages).

The platelet deficiency is episodic and possibly exacerbated by allergy to cow's milk, intercurrent infections and so on. Anaemia caused by bleeding and especially haemolysis are also possible in infancy. Often pronounced eosinophilia. Leukocytosis. Also frequent leukoemoid reactions (possibly with hepatosplenomegaly) in infancy.
- Cardiac defect in approximately one-third of patients (atrial septal defect, tetralogy of Fallot).
- Short stature (at or below the 10th percentile).

Supplementary findings: Allergy to cow's milk not unusual, precipitating abrupt fall in platelet count and haemolysis; episodes of diarrhoea with vomiting and dehydration during the first year of life.

Other skeletal anomalies not infrequent: hypoplasia of the lower jaw and midface with depressed nasal bridge (**1 and 2**). Hypoplasia of the shoulder girdle, ribs or vertebral column. Hip dysplasia; limited movement at the knees, dislocation of the patellae; internal rotation of the tibiae; genu varum; club feet.

Exceptionally, also severe reduction defects of the lower extremities.

Possible extensive capillary haemangioma on the face, including 'moustache' location (**2**). Cutis laxa in the nuchal area (**2**); oedema of the dorsum of the feet.

Radiologically, distinct hypoplasia and bowing of the ulnae possible (**5 and 6**), and occasionally aplasia; hypoplasia involving wrists and fingers; hook formation on the lateral ends of the clavicles and other signs.

Manifestation: At birth.

Aetiology: Genetically determined syndrome. Severity of skeletal, haematological and cardiac anomalies varies within and among families. The assumption of autosomal recessive inheritance does not fit all observed patients; possible different mutations at the same gene locus.

Frequency:
Low; estimated at 1:500 000 to 1:1 million newborns; by 1988, more than 100 published observations.

Course, prognosis: Tendency for platelet count to improve (normal values in adulthood). If the child survives the first year of life, during which mortality is very high, life expectancy is probably almost normal. Mental development dependent on the occurrence of intracranial haemorrhages during the first 2 years of life.

Differential diagnosis: Aase syndrome (*247*), Holt–Oram syndrome (*248*), Fanconi anaemia (*249*), thalidomide embryopathy (*206*), pseudo-thalidomide syndrome (*207*), trisomy 18 (*48*).

Treatment: Intensive haematological support (platelet or whole-blood transfusions). Conservative orthopaedic care. Withdrawal of cow's-milk protein from the diet in some patients. Operative repair of cardiac defect if indicated.

As far as possible, prevention of infection and avoidance of operative procedures and other stress during the first year of life to safeguard against life-threatening episodes of thrombocytopaenia and bleeding. Later, possible orthopaedic treatment (e.g. to correct malpositioned knees). Genetic counselling. Prenatal diagnosis by ultrasound for further pregnancies. Patients diagnosed prenatally should be delivered by caesarean section.

Illustrations:
1–6 A newborn, the first child of young, healthy parents. Fully expressed syndrome; thrombocytopaenia, hypereosinophilia, anaemia. Hypoplasia of the distal humeri and of the shoulder girdles; bilateral hip dysplasia, mild talipes calcaneus; clinodactyly of both little fingers (5 and 6). Pronounced allergy to cow's milk, exposure being followed by diarrhoea, vomiting and decreased weight and platelet count, making a cow's milk-free diet mandatory. Persistent depressed nasal bridge; development of pronounced bowed legs.

References:
Ward R E, Bixler D *et al*: Parent to child transmission of the thrombocytopenia absent radius (TAR) syndrome. *Am J Med Genet Suppl* 1986, 2:207–214.
Giuffré L, Cammarata M *et al*: Two new cases of... TAR syndrome... *Klin Pädiat* 1988, **200**:10–14.
Marec B Le, Odent S *et al*: Genetic counseling in a case of TAR... *Clin Genet* 1988, **34**:104–108.
Lipson A: Radial ray defects and associated anomalies; unique nature of the radial deficiencies and facial dysmorphism in the TAR syndrome (Letter). *Clin Genet* 1990, **37**:78–79.

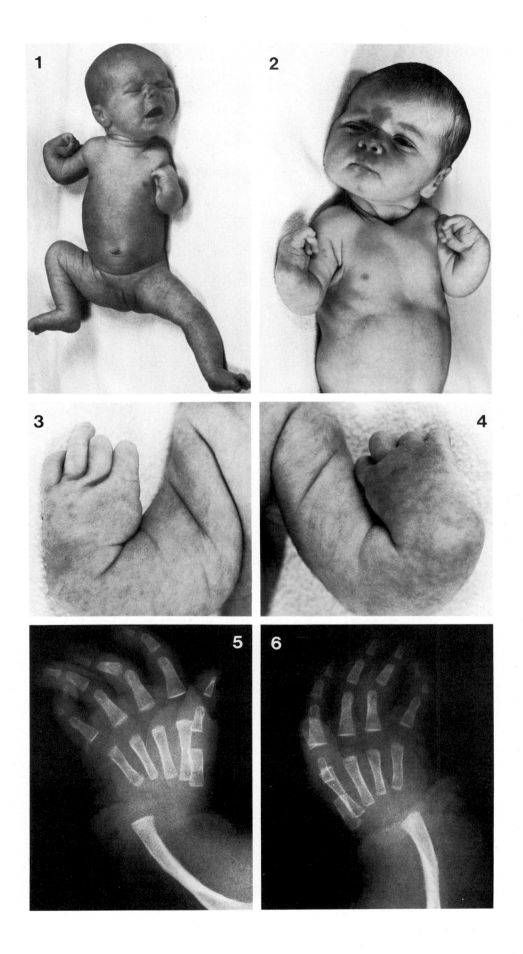

Syndrome of Deafness, Radial Hypoplasia and Psychomotor Retardation

H.-R.W

A syndrome of congenital deafness and marked psychomotor retardation in combination with mild bilateral hypoplasia of the radius and other anomalies.

Main signs:
- Congenital bilateral deafness.
- Mild bilateral hypoplasia of the radius with radial abduction of the hands, hypoplasia of the thenar musculature and of the thumbs (left side more severely affected radiologically and clinically) (**1, 7–9**).
- Considerable mental and motor retardation (still unable to stand without support at almost 2 years old) (**1–3**).

Supplementary findings: High, short cranium with broad forehead (**1, 3**). Low-set, prominent, dysplastic ears (**4–6**). Hypoplasia of the first ribs.
Slightly retarded ossification of the bones of the hand.
Ocular fundi normal; heart normal; intravenous pyelogram normal; blood count, including thrombocytes, normal.

Manifestation: At birth.

Aetiology: Unknown.

Diagnosis, differential diagnosis: The clinical picture described here does not appear to be one of the many recognized syndromes with either hearing impairment or radial hypoplasia.

Treatment: Symptomatic.

Illustrations:
1–9 The proband at almost 2 years of age. The first child of young, healthy parents. Consanguinity status not known. No family history of hearing impairment.
Pregnancy unremarkable, birth at term. Normal development of height and weight.

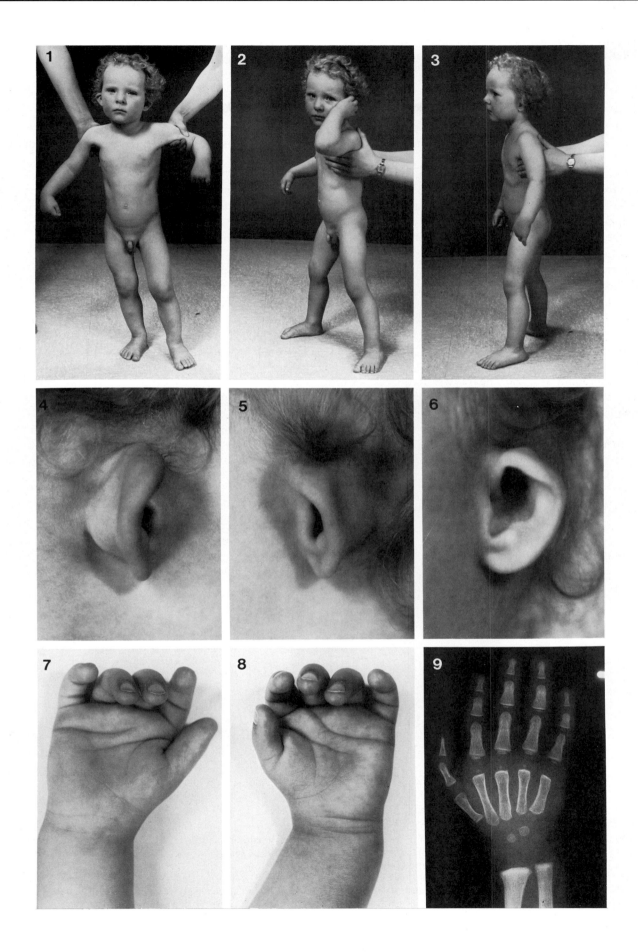

211 Lacrimo-Auriculo-Dento-Digital Syndrome

(LADD Syndrome)

H.-R.W

A syndrome of hypoplasia, aplasia or atresia involving the lacrimal system, ear anomalies and hearing impairment, aplasia or atresia within the salivary system and anomalies of teeth and fingers.

Main signs:

- Epiphora or deficiency of tears as a result of atresia, hypoplasia or aplasia of the lacrimal apparatus (e.g. absence of the lacrimal puncta, atresia of the tear ducts, aplasia of the lacrimal glands).
- Malformed external ears; possible hearing impairment (different types).
- Dryness of the mouth with eating difficulties because of hypoplasia or aplasia of the large salivary glands or absence of the duct openings.
- Possibly hypoplasia or aplasia of the teeth or other anomalies of dentition.
- Diverse anomalies of the fingers (less frequently of the toes), usually of the pre-axial rays (e.g. hypoplasia of the thumbs, bifid thumb).

Supplementary findings: Irritation of ocular and oral mucous membranes; possible candidiasis. Early development of dental caries, possibly severe and leading to total loss of teeth. Additional renal anomalies optional. Mild facial anomalies (form of the nose, mid-face hypoplasia 1–4).

Manifestation: Infancy and later.

Aetiology: Autosomal dominant disorder with very variable expression.

Frequency: Low; to date only 15 patients that appear certain.

Course, prognosis: No decrease in life expectancy providing kidneys are normal. Early recognition important because of possible hearing impairment and for the early institution of oral hygiene.

Diagnosis, differential diagnosis: In spite of unremarkable facial outline, hypoplasia or aplasia of the parotids may be present (computerized tomography scan, scintiscan). Hypohydrotic ectodermal dysplasia (258), oculo-dento-osseous dysplasia (240), the EEC syndrome (218) and several other clinical pictures can be easily ruled out. Nevertheless, there is discussion over whether the LADD syndrome could perhaps represent a mild expression of the gene responsible for the EEC syndrome.

Treatment: Ophthalmological surgical measures (e.g. for stenosis or atresia of the nasolacrimal ducts). Hearing and speech aids may be indicated. Intensive oral hygiene and dental care.

Illustrations:

1–4 A boy, aged 2 years and 6 months, with LADD: deficient tears, anomalies of the external ears, dental decay (3) with deficient salivation. Note also the short neck and form of the nose; in addition, short stature (third percentile).

References:

Wiedemann H-R, Drescher J: LADD syndrome: report of new cases and review of the clinical spectrum. *Eur J Pediatr* 1986, **144**:579–582.
Calabro A *et al*: Lacrimo-auriculo-dento-digital (LADD) syndrome. *Eur J Pediatr* 1987, **146**:536–537.
Hennekam R C M: LADD syndrome: a distinct entity? *Eur J Pediatr* 1987, **146**:94–95.
Milunsky J M *et al*: Agenesis or hypoplasia of major salivary and lacrimal glands. *Am J Med Genet* 1990, 37:371–374.
Roodhooft A M *et al*: Lacrimo-auriculo-dento-digital (LADD) syndrome with renal and foot anomalies. *Clin Genet* 1990, 38:228–232.
Wiedemann H-R: Agenesis or hypoplasia of major salivary and lacrimal glands. *Am J Med Genet* 1991, 41:269.
Bamforth J S, Kaurah P: Lacrimo-auriculo-dento-digital syndrome: evidence for lower limb involvement and severe congenital renal anomalies. *Am J Med Genet* 1992, **43**:932–937.
Lacombe D *et al*: Split hand/split foot deformity and LADD syndrome in a family: overlap between the EEC and LADD syndromes. *J Med Genet* 1992, **30**:700–703.

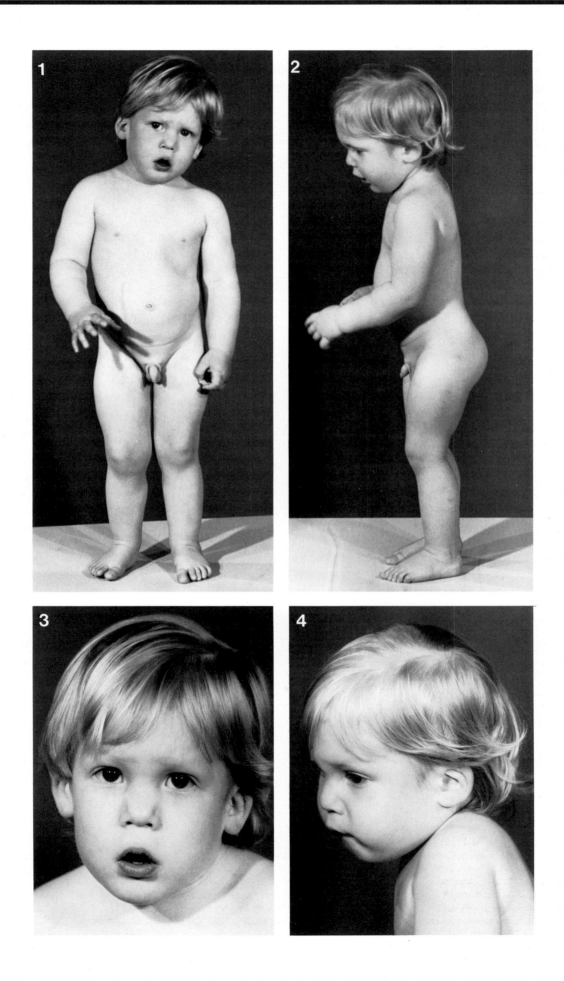

212 Oro-Acral Malformation Complex

(Aglossia-Adactyly Syndrome, Ankyloglossia Superior Syndrome, Glossopalatine Ankylosis Syndrome, Hanhart Syndrome, Hypoglossia-Hypodactyly Syndrome, Oro-Acral Syndrome, Oromandibular-Limb Hypogenesis Syndrome)

H.-R.W/J.K.

A spectrum of malformations of the oral cavity region and reduction anomalies of the extremities.

Main signs:
- Microglossia to aglossia; possible cleft lip or palate.
- Adhesion of the tongue to the upper jaw; fibrous bands between the upper and lower jaws, also (rarely) bony adhesions; micrognathia (**1–3**).
- Transverse reduction anomalies of the extremities, ranging from stump-like hands and feet to upper arm and upper leg stumps. Symmetry or pronounced right–left and upper–lower asymmetry (**1, 3**).
- Syndactyly, symbrachydactyly.

Supplementary findings: Low birth weight (average of 21 patients was 2572 g). Cranial nerve palsies (see Möbius sequence, *280*). Absence of the dental germs. Exceptionally, mental retardation.
(Possible situs inversus, splenogonadal fusion, anal atresia.)

Manifestation: At birth.

Aetiology: Unknown. Developmental field defect. No increased risk of recurrence.

Frequency: Low; approximately 80 patients reported up to 1985.

Course, prognosis: Good, except for the danger of aspiration as a result of oral malformations. Speech development amazingly good, even with aglossia, with the exception of 'tongue–teeth consonants'. Full development of the mandible is not unusual.

Treatment: Surgery for oral malformations. Prostheses.

Differential diagnosis: Möbius sequence (*280*), in which cranial nerve palsy is always present, whereas malformations of the extremities are rare except for frequent club feet. Whenever malformations of the extremities of the type described here are associated with micrognathia, oro-acral malformation complex should be considered. Poland sequence (*220*).

Comment: This spectrum includes the mentioned 'syndromes', some of which were previously regarded as independent entities.

Illustrations:
1–3 Two newborns. Note the extreme micrognathia in **2** (same patient as in **1**). Unfortunately, clinical records on these children were not available, so that the oral anomalies are not known.

References:
Hermann J, Pallister P D, Gilbert E F *et al*: Nosologic studies in the Hanhart and the Möbius syndrome. *Eur J Pediatr* 1976, **122**:19.
Grosse F-R, Wiedemann H-R: Syndromes with reduction and surplus anomalies of the hand. *Birth Defects Orig Art Ser XIII* 1977, 1:301.
Johnson G F, Robinow M: Aglossia-adactylia. *Radiology* 1978, **128**:127.
Schmitt K, Fries R *et al*: Das oro-akrale Syndrom. *Mschr Kinderheilk* 1981, **129**:245–247.
Pauli R M, Greenlaw A: Limb deficiency and splenogonadal fusion. *Am J Med Genet* 1982, **13**:81–89.
Bökesoy I, Aksüyek C *et al*: Oromandibular limb hypogenesis/Hanhart's syndrome... *Clin Genet* 1983, **24**:47–49.
Ikeda T, Ohdo S *et al*: Syndromes associated with microglossia and ectrodactyly... *Cong Anom* 1983, **23**:195–205.
Sekhar C *et al*: Hanhart's syndrome with... temporal bone findings. *Ann Otol Rhinol Laryng* 1987, **96**:309–314.
Gillerot Y *et al*: Hypoglossia-hypodactyly syndrome with hydrocephalus... *J Med Genet* 1991, **28**:490–491.

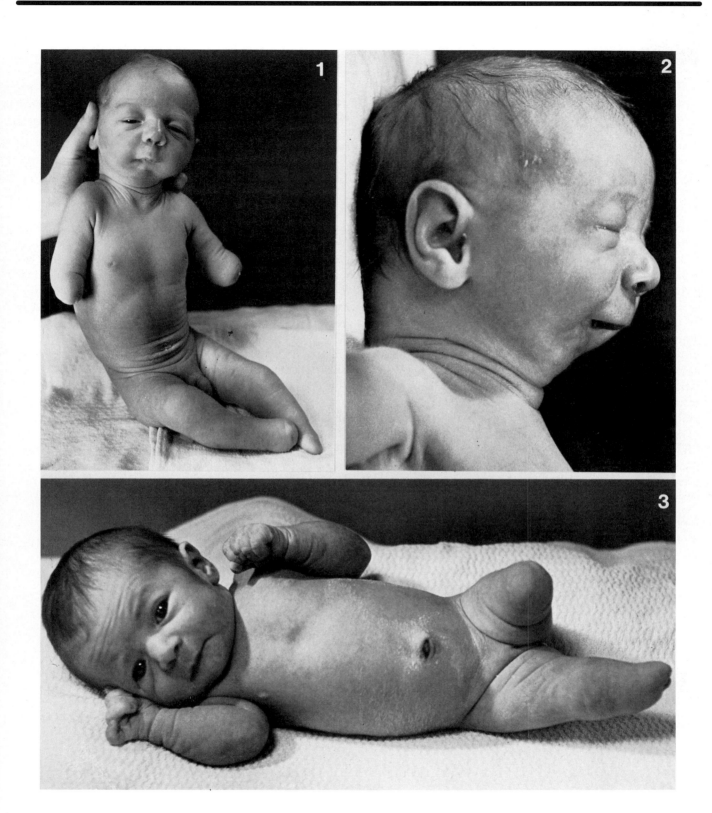

213 Syndrome of Symmetrical Tetraperomelia with Anal Atresia, Microphallus with Hypospadias and Accessory Lacrimal Puncta

H.-R.W

A malformation complex comprising symmetrical peromelia of the upper and lower extremities associated with multiple other internal and external anomalies.

Main signs:

- Symmetrical peromelia of the arms directly below the elbows (with congenital lateral scars) and of the legs just below the knees (1–3, 7, 8).
- Anal atresia. Hypoplasia of the external genitalia (6) with glandular hypospadias; bilateral undescended testes.
- Bilateral dislocated hips.
- Accessory lacrimal puncta (below the lower lacrimal puncta 4) with occasional secretion.

Supplementary findings: Mild micrognathia (present at birth) (1–3); tongue, oral mucosa and palate unremarkable. However, hypoplasia of the left processus muscularis mandibulae and (at 2 years and 6 months) absence of the germs of the first and second left lower deciduous molars.

Dissimilar auricles with pre-auricular pit on the left (5).

Bilateral cervical ribs. Right convex lumbar scoliosis. Asacria. Marked bilateral hydronephrosis and hydroureter; dystopia of the bladder superiorly and laterally; multiple diverticula of the urinary bladder.

Normal mental development for age.

Manifestation: At birth.

Aetiology: Unknown.

Course, prognosis: With appropriate physical rehabilitation, favourable.

Comment: The clinical picture of this child is close to that of the oro-acral or Hanhart syndrome (*212*). Whether it can be classified under that 'syndrome' or, in view of atypically minimal oral manifestations, atypically symmetrical limb defects, the 'extended spectrum' and other peculiarities, whether it is a separate entity cannot be resolved at this time.

Treatment: Symptomatic: surgery for anal atresia; treatment of the hip; prostheses; orthodontic dental care; appropriate handicap aids.

Illustration:

1–6 The proband at 5 years and 6 months. The second child of young, healthy, non-consanguineous parents (first and third-born children healthy). Birth after an unremarkable pregnancy, 3 weeks before term at 2500 g. No problems with early care.

7 and 8 Radiographs taken at 2 years.

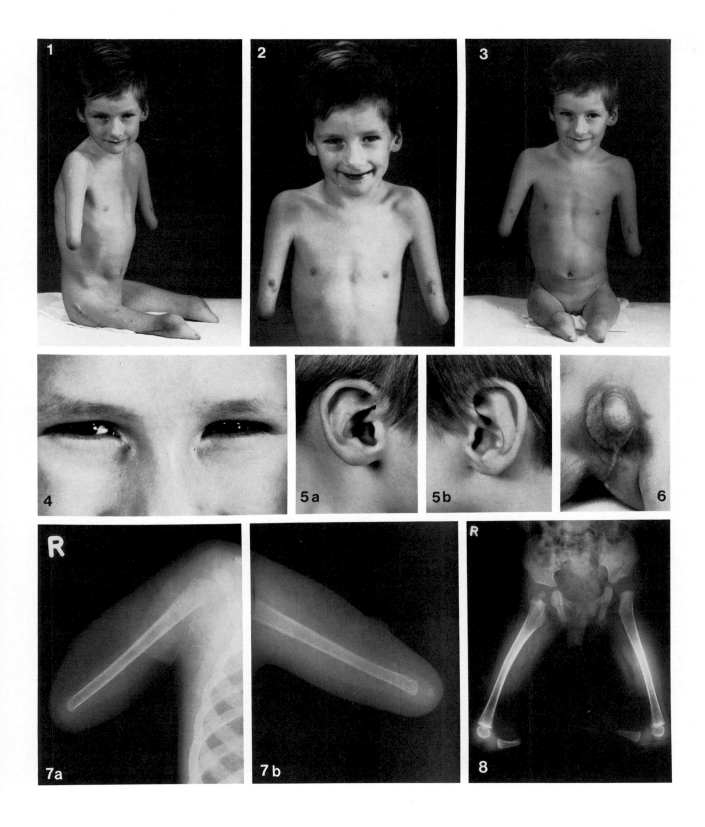

J.K.

The combination of hypertelorism and hypospadias, predominantly in males.

Main signs:
- Hypertelorism.
- Hypospadias.
- Cranial asymmetry (plagiocephalus).
- Mental retardation (in approximately 50%).

Supplementary findings: Strabismus, cryptorchidism, cardiac defect, cleft lip and palate, urinary tract anomalies. Prominent nasal bridge, dysplasia of the ears, multiple naevi flammei, epicanthus medialis, hernias. Additionally: agenesis or hypoplasia of the corpus callosum, cerebellar worm aplasia, cortical atrophy, obstructive hydrocephalus, Dandy–Walker anomaly.

Manifestation: Soon after birth.

Aetiology: X-linked or autosomal dominant inheritance.

Pathogenesis: Mid-line defect.

Frequency: Unknown.

Course, prognosis: Dependent on the severity of mental retardation. Mental retardation unknown in females.

Differential diagnosis: G syndrome, Greig's hypertelorism, frontonasal dysplasia (23).

Treatment: Symptomatic surgery.

Illustrations:
1 Father with hypertelorism and telecanthus, youngest son with hypertelorism, older son normal.
2 Condition after surgical correction of hypospadias.
3 A further son, 17 days old, interpupillary distance 4.5 cm.
4 Hypospadia glandis.
A further son died aged 7 days from holoprosencephaly, arhinencephaly, microcephaly, pachygyria, hypotelorism, micropenis, hypospadias.

References:
Funderburk S J, Stewart R: The G and BBB sydromes: case presentations, genetics and nosology. *Am J Med Genet* 1978, **2**:131–144.
Cordero J F, Holmes L B: Phenotypic overlap of the BBB and G syndromes. *Am J Med Genet* 1978, **2**:145–152.
Stoll C, Geraudel A, Berland H, Roth M-P, Dott B: Male-to male transmission of the hypertelorism-hypospadias (BBB) syndrome. *Am J Med Genet* 1985, **20**:221–225.
Sedano H O, Gorlin R J: Opitz oculo-genital-laryngeal syndrome (Opitz BBB/G compound syndrome). *Am J Med Genet* 1988, **30**:847–849.
Neri G, Cappa M: The Opitz syndrome. *Am J Med Genet* 1988, **30**:851.
Hogdall C, Siegel-Bartelt J, Toi A, Ritchie S: Prenatal diagnosis of Opitz (BBB) syndrome in the second trimester by ultrasound detection of hypospadias and hypertelorism. *Prenat Diagn* 1989, **9**:783–793.
Krause M, Meinecke P, Krins M, Grote W: Das Hypertelorismus-Hypospadie-(BBB)-Syndrom. *Monatsschr Kinderheilkd* 1991, **138**:31–33.
Guion-Almeida M L, Richieri-Costa A: CNS midlines anomalies in the Opitz G/BBB syndrome: report on 12 Brazilian patients. *Am J Med Genet* 1992, **43**:918–928.
MacDonald M R, Schaefer G B, Olney A H, Tamayo M, Frias J L. Brain magnetic resonance imaging findings in the Opitz G/BBB syndrome: extension of the spectrum of midline brain anomalies. *Am J Med Genet* 1993, **46**:706–711.

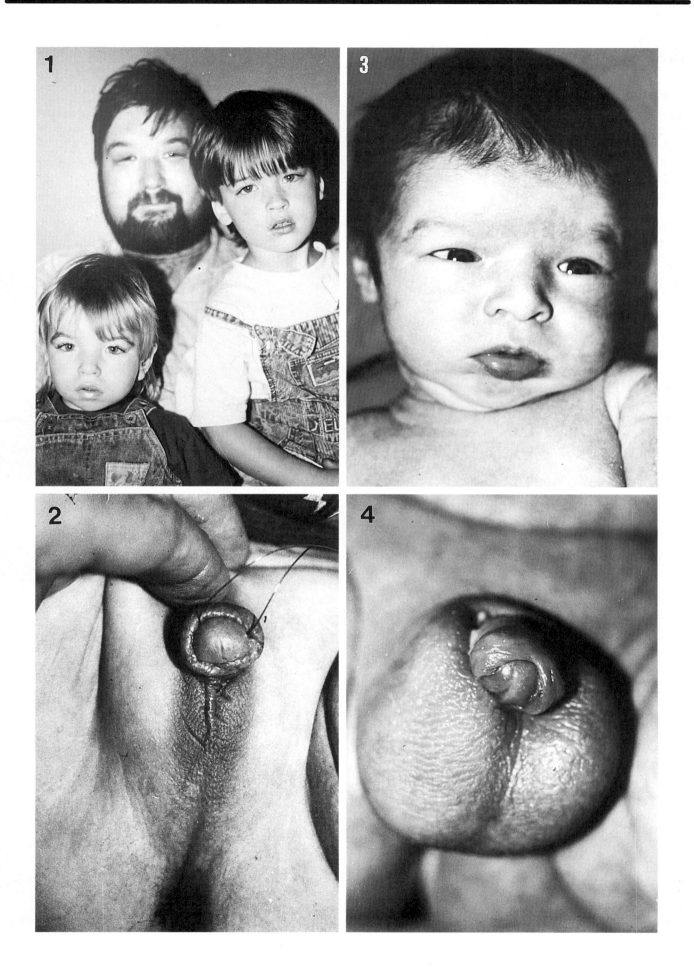

J.K.

A combination of terminal transverse defects with scalp and skull defects.

Main signs:
- Congenital scalp defects around the vertex; 2.5 mm x 5 mm to 7 cm x 9 cm, sometimes ulcerating.
- In isolated cases, underlying osseous skull defects. Rarely acrania.
- Terminal reduction defects of one or more extremities, affecting the lower extremities more severely than the upper extremities: aphalangia, adactyly, acheiria, transverse hemimelia.

Supplementary findings: Telangiectatic cutis marmorata, markedly dilated and tortuous cranial veins. Rarely: postaxial polydactyly, cardiac defect, cleft lip, club feet, cryptorchidism, microcephaly, epilepsy, retardation, arhinencephaly, hydrocephalus, renal anomalies.

Manifestation: Prenatal and at birth.

Aetiology: Sporadic occurrence in 50% of the patients observed. Genetic heterogeneity: primarily autosomal dominant inheritance with complete penetrance and variable expression. Approximately 100 patients reported.

Pathogenesis: Developmental defect resulting from vascular disruption.

Course, prognosis: Normal life expectancy, normal intelligence. Impaired functions of affected limbs. Spontaneous healing of the scalp defect in the first months of life.

Differential diagnosis: Oro-acral syndrome (*212*), amniotic constriction grooves (*219*), syndrome of multiple benign ring-shaped skin creases (*169*), trisomy 13 (*47*), aplasia cutis congenita.

Treatment: In some patients, grafting of the scalp defect. Surgical and prosthetic repair of the extremities.

Illustrations:

1a–c Twin, female, 1 year old; cicatrized aplasia cutis, partial aphalangia. Second twin clinically normal.
2a–c Female newborn, partial aphalangia, occipital aplasia cutis.
2d–f Age 1 year, cicatrization of the aplasia cutis.

References:

Küster W, Lenz W, Kääriäinen H, Majewski F: Congenital scalp defects with distal limb anomalies (Adams–Oliver syndrome): report of ten cases and review of the literature. *Am J Med Genet* 1988, **31**:99–115.
Sybert V P: Congenital scalp defects with distal limb anomalies (Adams–Oliver syndrome — McK 10030): further suggestion of autosomal-recessive inheritance. *Am J Med Genet* 1989, **32**:266–267.
Jaeggi E, Kind C, Morger R: Congenital scalp and skull defects with terminal transverse limb anomalies (Adams–Oliver syndrome): report of three additional cases. *Eur J Pediatr* 1990, **149**:565–566.
Der Kaloustian V M, Hoyme H E, Hogg H, Entin M A, Guttmacher A E: Possible common pathogenetic mechanisms for Poland sequence and Adams–Oliver syndrome. *Am J Med Genet* 1991, **38**:69–73.
David A, Rozé J-C, Melon-David V: Adams–Oliver syndrome associated with congenital heart defect: not a coincidence. *Am J Med Genet* 1991, **40**:126–127.
Whitley C B, Gorlin R J: Adams–Oliver syndrome revisited. *Am J Med Genet* 1991, **40**:319–326.
Chitayat D, Meunier C, Hodkinson K A, Robb L, Azouz M: Acrania: a manifestation of the Adams–Oliver syndrome. *Am J Med Genet* 1992, **44**:562–566.
Bamforth J-S, Kaurah P, Ferreira P: Adams–Oliver syndrome: a family with extreme variability in clinical expression. *Am J Med Genet* 1994, **49**:393–396.

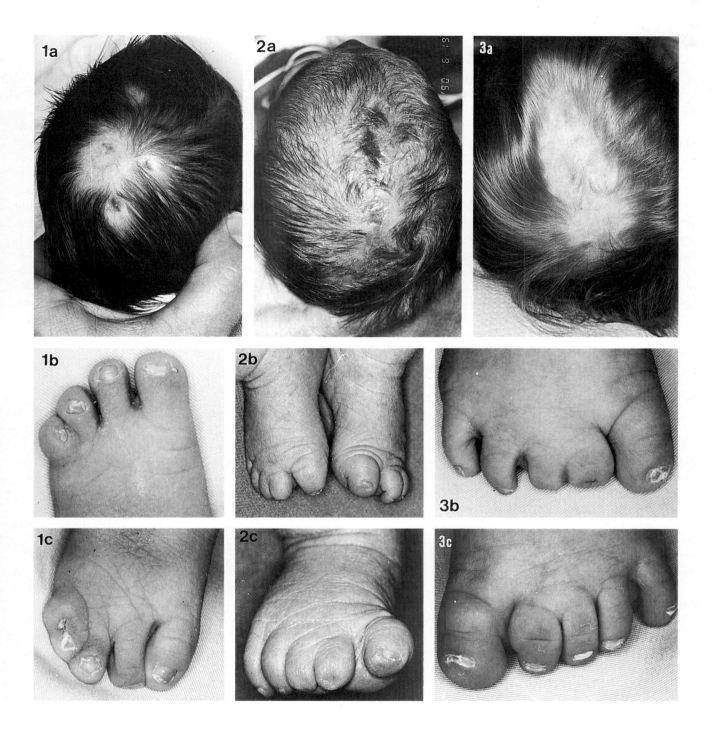

A usually asymmetrically occurring combination of femoral and fibular defects with contralateral malformation of the ulna (FFU Complex).

Main signs: Divided into four clinical groups:
I: in 44.4% of all patients only one extremity is affected; II: two extremities affected in 33.6%; III: three affected in 11.2%; IV: four extremities affected in 10.8%. The upper extremities are more frequently affected than the lower. In groups I and II the upper extremities are relatively infrequently affected compared with the lower extremities. In group III, the lower extremities are more frequently affected than the upper. All malformations are preferentially unilateral right. The right arm is most frequently affected, the left leg least frequently. In group II, there is a trend towards bilaterality.

- Most frequent defects of the upper extremities: ulnar malformation including humero-radial synostoses and absence of the ulnar rays (258 out of 491), peromelia of the humerus (96 out of 491) and amelia (46 out of 491).
- Most frequent defects of the lower extremities: fibular defects (hypoplasia, aplasia, malformations or absence of the fibular rays: 215 out of 491), the femoral defect (hypoplasia or aplasia, proximal defect) (152 out of 491), amelia (six out of 491).

In each of the four groups, peromelia of the humerus is twice as more frequent than amelia and the ulnar defect is three times more frequent than peromelia. No patients with amelia have been observed in groups I and II, however, the fibular defect is more frequent than the femoral defect. In groups III and IV, on the other hand, femoral and fibular defects are equally common.

Supplementary findings: Patients with only one malformed extremity usually show an ulnar defect of upper extremity or a fibular defect of the lower. The most common combination in patients with more than one affected extremity is a fibular defect together with defects of the fibular rays (142 out of 491).

Simultaneous femoral, fibular and ulnar defects were only observed in 21 out of 491 patients, femur–fibula combinations in 94 out of 491, fibula–ulna malformations in 30 out of 491 and femur–ulna combinations in 33 out of 491. The predominance of the right side has been confirmed repeatedly.

The right-sided ulnar defect is found 48 times in combination with contralateral defects of the finger rays, and right-side finger defects are found with the left-side ulnar defect in 50 patients.

Manifestation: Prenatal and postnatal.

Aetiology: These malformations have been described in the literature for centuries. Out of 491 patients, 302 were male and 170 female. Sex ratio 1.9:F, rising to 2.5 with three affected extremities and normalizing at 1.08 with four affected extremities. The 491 patients had 275 siblings and there was only one family with two affected individuals.

All cases are sporadic and none of the following precipitating factors has been observed: paternal-age effect, monogenic inheritance, chromosomal abnormalities, increased incidence in consanguineous marriages, combination of malformations of primary syndromes, geographic or temporal clustering, exogenous noxae (rays, infections, medicaments, maternal diabetes mellitus and so on). In monozygotic twins, occurrence is always discordant.

Frequency: Many hundreds of patients have been observed worldwide. General prevalence of deformed extremities 5–10:10 000.

Course, prognosis: Normal intelligence. No internal malformations. Normal life expectancy.

Treatment: Orthopaedic measures; any appropriate handicap aids.

Differential diagnosis: Ectrodactyly, oro-acral syndrome (*212*), postaxial acrofacial dysostosis (*238*), Roberts syndrome (*207*), focal dermal hypoplasia (*183*).

Illustrations:
1–6 A female newborn. **1** Shortening of the right thigh, malformations of the right foot and left hand.
2 Asymmetry of the ilial wings; no acetabulum on the right; hypoplasia of the caudal portion of the os ilium; severe hypoplasia of the right femur; ipsilateral tibial hypoplasia and absence of the fibula.
3a and b The left hand with complete cutaneous syndactyly of rays I and II, partial syndactyly of rays II and III, normal ray IV and absent ray V.
6a and b Corresponding radiographs: Only three rays in the metacarpal region; the broad ray in the middle may represent a fusion of rays II and III, to which the partially fused proximal phalanges of rays II and III are adjoined; ray V is absent.
4 and 5 The child's right foot: absence of both fibular marginal rays.

References:
Lenz W, Feldmann U: Unilateral and asymmetric limb defects in man: delineation of the femur–fibula–ulna complex. *Birth Defects Orig Art Ser Vol XIII* 1977, **1**:269–285.
Zlotogora J, Rosenmann E, Menashe M *et al*: The femur, fibula, ulna (FFU) complex in siblings. *Clin Genet* 1983, **24**:449–452.
van den Anker J N, van Vught E E *et al*: Severe limb abnormalities: analysis of a cluster of five cases born during a period of 45 days. *Am J Med Genet* 1993, **45**:659–667.
Lenz W, Zygulska M, Horst J: FFU complex; an analysis of 491 cases. *Hum Genet* 1993, **91**:347–356.

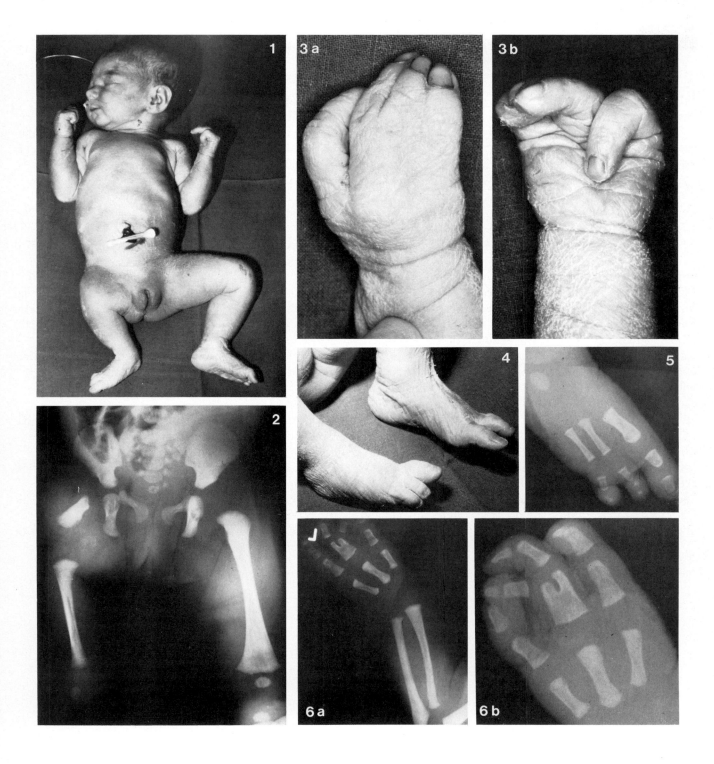

217 Femoral Hypoplasia: Unusual Facies Syndrome
(Femoral–Facial Syndrome)

J.K.

Bilateral femoral hypoplasia with characteristic facial signs.

Main signs:
- Facial dysmorphism: short nose with hypoplastic alae nasi (65%), dysplastic ears (45%), flat philtrum and narrow upper lip (65%), micrognathia (80%).
- Cleft palate (80%).
- Short femur caused by bilateral femoral hypoplasia. Secondary growth deficiency.

Supplementary findings: Infrequently cleft lip and palate. Involvement of the upper extremities and shoulder girdle in three-quarters of all patients: shortening of the humerus, limited mobility of the shoulder and elbow joints. Sprengel's deformity. Syndactyly of the toes. Cardiac defect in 20%, including: ventricular septal defect, pulmonary stenosis. Inguinal hernias. Urogenital anomalies in 60%: absent or hypoplastic labia, cryptorchidism, hypoplastic penis, polycystic kidneys, renal aplasia.

On radiographs: hypoplasia and aplasia of femora and fibulae and acetabula. Vertebral anomalies in 35% (scoliosis, hemivertebrae, spina bifida occulta, sacral segmentation defect). Anomalies of the ribs. Hypoplastic abdomen. Radio-humeral and radio-ulnar synostoses. Club feet. Duplication of the first toe, rarely polydactyly or aplasia.

Manifestation: *In utero* and postnatal.

Aetiology: One in three patients are the children of diabetic mothers. However, two out of every three patients are sporadic occurrences. Autosomal dominant inheritance very rare. Barely 100 patients known to date.

Pathogenesis: Unknown.

Course, prognosis: Normal intelligence, no reduction of life expectancy.

Differential diagnosis: Femoral hypoplasia without facial dysmorphism, FFU complex (*216*), caudal dysplasia (*168*), diabetic embryopathy (*299*), Currarino triad (*310*).

Treatment: Orthopaedic measures. Further surgical intervention according to signs.

Illustrations:
1a, d, e A 6-week-old with short nose and anteverted nostrils, hypoplastic alae nasi and micrognathia. Remaining pictures at age 8 days.
1b and c Characteristic femoral dimples, fixed abduction of the femur.
1f Labial hypoplasia, short stubby femora in fixed dislocation.
1g Dislocated heads of femora, hypoplastic roofs of acetabulum, bowed hypoplastic femora. Fracture right?

References:
Johnson J P, Carey J C, Gooch W M, Petersen J, Beattie J F: Femoral hypoplasia — unusual facies syndrome in infants of diabetic mothers. *J Pediatr* 1983, **102**:866–872.
Burck U, Riebel T, Held K R, Stockenius M: Bilateral femoral dysgenesis with micrognathia, cleft palate, anomalies of the spine and pelvis and foot deformities. *Helv Paediat Acta* 1981, **36**:473–482.
Lampert R P: Dominant inheritance of femoral hypoplasia — unusual facies syndrome. *Clin Genet* 1980, **17**:255–258.
Baraitser M, Reardon W, Oley C, Fixsen J: Femoral hypoplasia unusual facies syndrome with preaxial polydactyly. *Clin Dysmorphol* 1994, **3**:40–45.
Bau C H D, Ribeiro C A, Ribeiro A A, Flores R Z: Bilateral femoral hypoplasia associated with Rokitansky sequence: another example of a mesodermal malformation spectrum? *Am J Med Genet* 1994, **49**:205–206.
Hitti J F, Glasberg S S *et al*: Bilateral femoral hypoplasia and maternal diabetes mellitus: case report and review of the literature. *Pediatr Pathol* 1994, **14**:567–574.

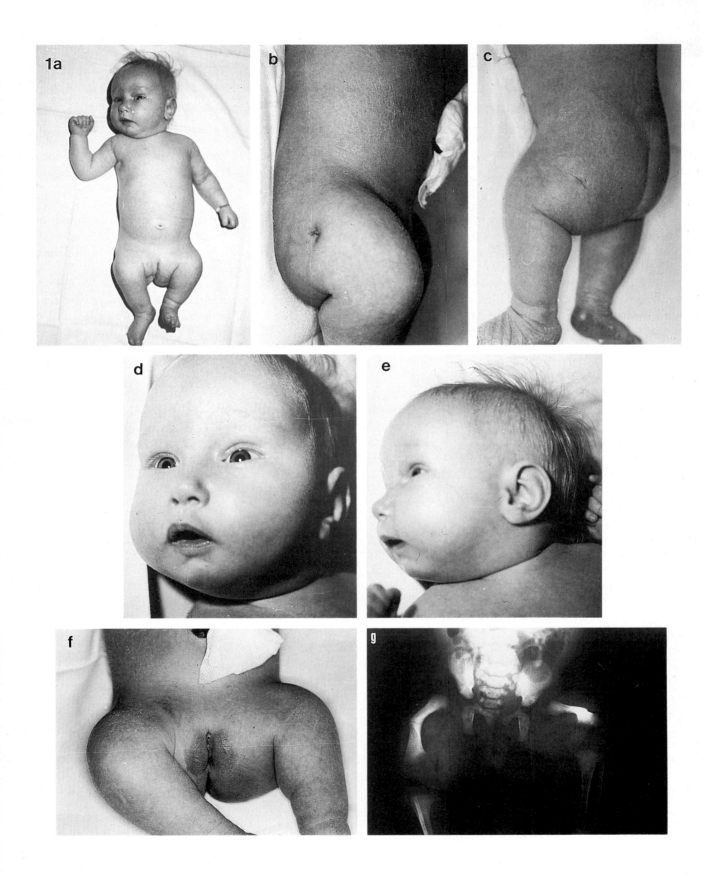

'EEC' Syndrome

(Ectrodactyly-Ectodermal Dysplasia-Clefting Syndrome)

H.-R.W

A syndrome comprising ectrodactyly of the hands and feet (usually clefts), signs of ectodermal dysplasia and facial clefts (usually of the lips).

Main signs:
- Variably severe anomalies of the midportion of the hands and feet, ranging from syndactyly to clefting of the hands and feet (usually present) (**1, 3–5**).
- Cleft lip, palate or both. High palate, hypoplastic maxilla.
- Sparse, thin, light-coloured scalp hair; sparse eyebrows and eyelashes (**2b**). Thin, light, dry and possibly hyperkeratotic skin; inability to sweat. Possible mamillary hypoplasia, nail anomalies, small pigmented naevi.
- Stenosis or atresia of the nasolacrimal canals, blepharitis, keratoconjunctivitis (possible dacryocystitis, corneal scars), blepharophimosis, photophobia (**2b**).
- Dysodontiasis (small carious teeth with hypoplastic enamel; also, missing teeth). Possible xerostomia.

Supplementary findings: Conductive hearing impairment may be a feature, also (not infrequently) anomalies of the kidneys, urinary tract and genitalia.

Mental development usually normal, however, retardation, sometimes with microcephaly, occasionally reported. Diabetes insipidus and hypogonadism.

Manifestations: At birth.

Aetiology: Genetically determined syndrome. Frequently sporadic occurrence, probably a result of new mutations. Autosomal dominant inheritance with reduced penetrance and variable expression (no one sign is obligatory). Heterogeneity or multiple alleles are possible. Basic defect unknown.

Frequency: Low (approximately 150 patients in the literature).

Course, prognosis: Dependent on the severity of the features and on the success of efforts toward 'rehabilitation' and social integration.

Diagnosis, differential diagnosis: In case of doubt, other syndromes in which facial clefts may occur (and perhaps also the LADD syndrome, *211*) should be considered.

Treatment: Early correction of stenosis of the nasolacrimal canals; continuous ophthalmologic care for this problem may be very important in some patients. In addition, care by an orthopaedic surgeon, oral surgeon and orthodontist. A wig may be beneficial.
  Genetic counselling.

Illustrations:
1–6 A patient at age 10 weeks (**2a, 4b, 5**), 3 years (**1, 2b, 3a, 3b, 4a, 6**) and 4 years (**3c**). Psychomotor retardation, microcephaly. High palate, mild mamillary hypoplasia, left renal agenesis and right hydronephrosis, cryptorchidism.
3 The left hand.
4 The right hand.
5 The feet.
  In addition to the familiar signs of EEC, the child shows the following: bilateral microphthalmos with coloboma of the iris, the choroid membrane, the retina and the optic nerve (**2a**); bifid clavicle on the right (**6**); ventricular septal defect with pulmonary hypertension. Height below the third percentile.

References:
Gehler J, Grosse R: Fehlbildungs-Syndrom mit Spalthänden-Spaltfüßen, Iriskolobom, Nierenagenesie und Ventrikelseptumdefekt. *Klin Pädiat* 1972, 184:389.
Pashayan H M *et al*: The EEC syndrome. *Birth Defects* 1974, 10:105–127.
Schmidt R, Nitowsky H M: Split hand and foot deformity... (EEC). *Hum Genet* 1977, 39:15–25.
Mücke J, Sandig K-R: Zur Expressivität des EEC-Syndroms. *Kinderärztl Praxis* 1980, 48:198–203.
Predine-Hug F, Merrer M le *et al*: Dysplasie ectodermique et ectrodactylie familiale. *Arch Fr Pédiatr* 1984, 41:49–50.
Küster W, Majewski F *et al*: EEC syndrome without ectrodactyly? *Clin Genet* 1985, 28:130–135.
London R, Heredia R M *et al*: Urinary tract involvement in EEC syndrome. *AJDC* 1985, 139:1191–1193.
Knudtson J, Aarskog D: Growth hormone deficiency associated with the ectrodactyly-ectodermal dysplasia-clefting syndrome and isolated absent septum pellucidum. *Pediatrics* 1987, 79:410–412.
Majewski F, Küster W: EEC syndrome sine sine? *Clin Genet* 1988, 33:69–72.
Rollnick B R, Hoo J J: Genitourinary anomalies are a component manifestation in the... (EEC) syndrome. *Am J Med Genet* 1988, 29:131–136.
Rodini E S O *et al*: EEC syndrome... *Am J Med Genet* 1990, 37:42–53.
Aguinaldo C *et al*: Urinary tract involvement in EEC syndrome... *Am J Med Genet* 1992, 44:803–806.
Lacombe D *et al*: Split hand/split foot deformity and LADD syndrome in a family... *J Med Genet* 1992, 30:700–703.
Kuna J M *et al*: EEC syndrome with diabetes insipidus and hypogonadism. *Eur J Pediatr* 1994, 153:300.

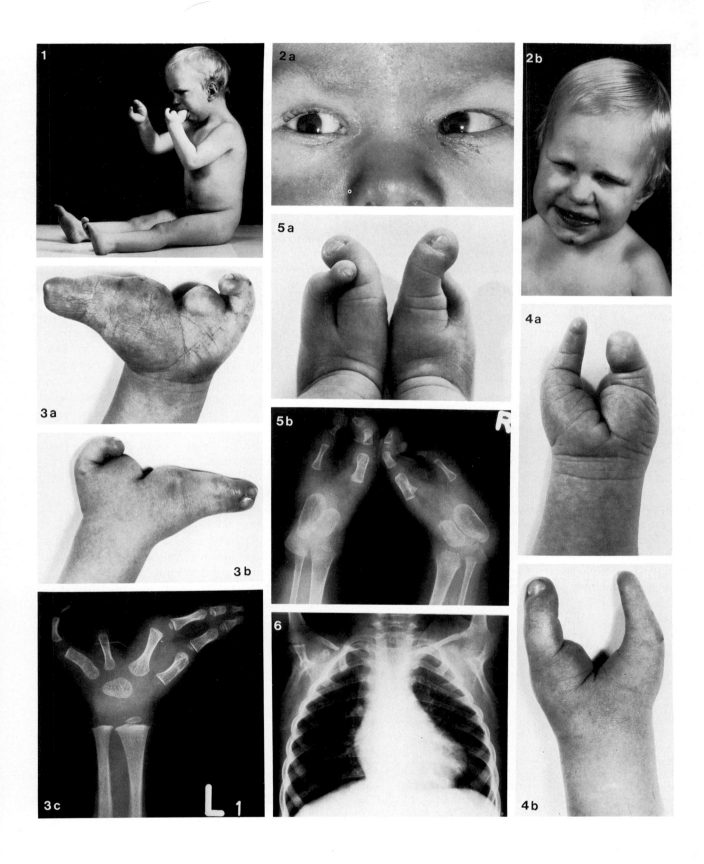

219 Amniotic Constriction Grooves

(ABS: Amniotic Band Sequence; ADAM Complex: Amniotic Deformity, Adhesions, Mutilations; Amniotic Band Disruption Complex or Sequence; Amniotic Bands; Amniotic Constriction Bands; Congenital Amputations; Early Amnion Rupture Sequence; Ring Constrictions; Streeter Anomaly or Dysplasia)

H.-R.W/ J.K.

A syndrome of usually multiple malformations resulting from grooves, constrictions and adhesions caused by amniotic bands *in utero*.

Main signs:
- Circular grooves mainly involving the extremities usually with swelling, hypoplasia or even amputation of the distal structures (**3, 5, 6**).
- Peripheral syndactyly, frequently with grooves from the amniotic bands encircling the fused rays (**2**). Adhesions of the cranium to the placenta. Defects of the cranium with or without herniation of the brain or other brain anomalies (**1, 4**).
- Cleft lip and palate (or its individual components) or facial clefts, which frequently do not correspond to temporal physiological intra-uterine development (**1, 4**).
- Clefts and adhesions of the eyelids; microphthalmos or anophthalmos. Anomalies of the nose and auricles (**1, 4**).
- Ectopia cordis, abdominal clefts, focal skin defects (**4**).
- Not infrequently, evidence of residual amnion in the grooves (**2, 5, 6**).

The anomalies may occur alone or in varied combinations, depending on the timing of amniotic rupture.

Supplementary findings: Scoliosis, dislocated hips, club feet and club hands are regarded as the results of the above-mentioned malformations. Very rarely, 'birth' of an amputated limb.
Occurrence also of associated malformations that are not aetiologically related (e.g. holoprosencephaly).

Manifestation: At birth.

Aetiology: Controversial. The prevailing theory is that fibrous strands that are formed after amniotic rupture cause the anomalies by constriction and adhesion. Almost always sporadic occurrence; practically no risk of recurrence. Familial occurrence as an exception (genetic factors here?).

Frequency: Approximately 1:3000 newborns.

Course, prognosis: Decreased life expectancy only for patients with brain malformations or deep facial clefts.

Differential diagnosis: The multiple deep, benign transverse grooves of the skin, especially of the extremities, that occur in some individuals as an autosomal dominant trait (*169*) should not be confused with those of the amniotic band syndrome. The same holds true for the congenital scalp defects occurring with amniotic band-like changes of the extremities; Adams–Oliver syndrome (*215*).

Treatment: Symptomatic (possibly plastic surgery, prostheses). Genetic counselling. Prenatal diagnosis by ultrasound in some patients.

Illustrations:
1–3 Case 1 on the first day of life; death on the second day because of respiratory insufficiency. Dysplasia of the left pinna, internal hydrocephalus, left club foot.
4–6 Case 2 at age 5 days. Death at 3 months from pneumonia. Aplasia of the corpus callosum.
In both cases, pregnancy unremarkable.

References:
Keller H, Neuhäuser G, Durkin-Stamm, M. V. *et al*: 'ADAM complex' (Amniotic Deformity, Adhesions, Mutilations) — a pattern of craniofacial and limb defects. *Am J Med Genet* 1978, 2:81.
Higgenbottom M C, Jones K L, Hall B D *et al*: The amniotic band disruption complex: timing of amniotic rupture and variable spectra of consequent defects. *J Pediatr* 1979, 85:544.
Etches P C, Stewart A R *et al*: Familial congenital amputations. *J Pediatr* 1982, 101:448–449.
Lubinsky M, Sujansky E *et al*: Familial amniotic bands. *Am J Med Genet* 1983, 14:81–87.
Donnenfeld A E, Dunn L K: Discordant amniotic band sequence in monozygotic twins. *Am J Med Genet* 1985, 20:685–694.
Hunter A G W, Carpenter B F: Implications of malformations not due to amniotic bands in the amniotic band sequence. *Am J Med Genet* 1986, 24:691–700.
Küster W, Lenz W *et al*: Congenital scalp defects with distal limb anomalies (Adams–Oliver syndrome)... *Am J Med Genet* 1988, 31:99–115.
Garza A, Cordero J F *et al*: Epidemiology of the early amnion rupture spectrum of defects. *AJDC* 1988, 142:541–544.
Bamforth J S: Amniotic band sequence: Streeter's hypothesis reexamined. *Am J Med Genet* 1992, 44:280–287.
Van Allen M I *et al*: Constriction bands and limb reduction defects... *Am J Med Genet* 1992, 44:598–604.
Czeizel A E *et al*: Study of isolated apparent amniogenic limb deficiency... *Am J Med Genet* 1993, 46:372–378.
Froster U G *et al*: Amniotic band sequence and limb defects... *Am J Med Genet* 1993, 46:497–500.

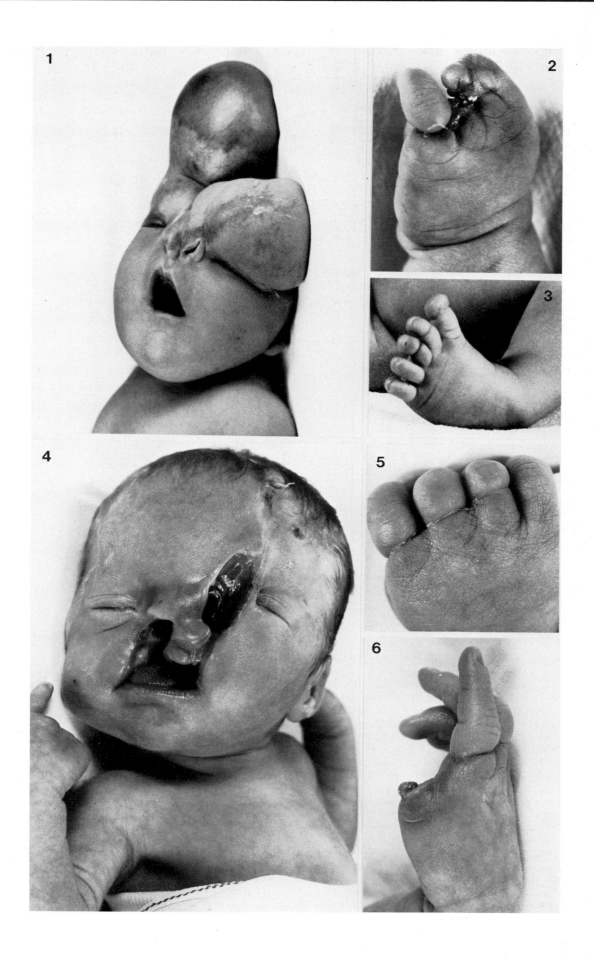

H.-R.W/ J.K.

Unilateral aplasia of the pectoral muscle and ipsilateral hand anomalies.

Main signs:
- Aplasia of pectoralis major muscle (usually only the sternocostal portion) and also pectoralis minor, with frequent hypoplasia and occasionally aplasia of the ipsilateral mamilla and mamillary gland (1). Not infrequently, flattening of the ipsilateral thoracic skeleton; rarely bony defects.
- Ipsilateral anomalies of the upper extremity, mainly in the form of symbrachydactyly but also with absent rays, ankylosis of finger joints, hypoplasia of the forearm and very rarely of the upper arm (2–6).

Supplementary findings: Very occasionally, ipsilateral hypoplasia of the kidneys and hemivertebrae, growth hormone deficiency, Goldenhar 'syndrome', ventral fissures of the chest and abdominal walls with herniation of the viscera.
Defect on the right side in 75% of patients.
Sex ratio (boys:girls) 3:1 to 4:1.

Manifestation: At birth.

Aetiology: Sporadic occurrence in the great majority of patients; autosomal dominant inheritance has been assumed in occasional patients. No increased risk of recurrence for the affected family when neither parent is affected. Developmental field defect. Presumed to be a disruption sequence resulting from embryonal interruption of the subclavian artery.

Frequency: Approximately one out of 30 000 of the general population. Over 500 patients reported by 1985.

Course, prognosis: Normal life expectancy.

Differential diagnosis: The Poland anomaly may occur as part of the Möbius sequence (280): observed 12 times up to 1982.

Treatment: Plastic surgery may be indicated. Genetic counselling.

Illustrations:
1–3, 6 Patient 1: Symbrachydactyly, rudimentary index finger.
4 Patient 2: aplasia of first to fourth fingers on the right, rudimentary fifth finger, ipsilateral absence of pectoralis major muscle.
5 Patient 3: symbrachydactyly on the right with hypoplastic middle phalanges, short right arm, aplasia of the right pectoralis major muscle.

References:
Ireland D C R, Takayama N, Flatt A E: Poland's syndrome. A review of forty-three cases. *J Bone Jt Surg* 1976, 58(A):52.
Sujansky E, Riccardi V M, Matthew A L: The familial occurrence of Poland syndrome. *Birth Defects Orig Art Ser* 1977, 13(3A):117.
Castilla E E, Paz J E, Orioli I M: Pectoralis major muscle defect and Poland complex. *Am J Med Genet* 1979, 4:263.
Parker D L, Mitchell P R, Holmes G L: Poland-Möbius syndrome. *J Med Genet* 1981, 18:317.
David T J: Familial Poland anomaly. *J Med Genet* 1982, 19:293–296.
Hegde H R, Shokeir M H K: Posterior shoulder girdle abnormalities with absence of pectoralis major muscle. *Am J Med Genet* 1982, 13:285–293.
Hester T R, Bostwick J: Poland's syndrome: correction with latissimus muscle transposition. *Plast Reconstr Surg* 1982, 69:226–233.
König R, Lenz W: Pektoralis-Handdefekte. *Z Orthopaed* 1983, 121:244–254.
Lowry R B, Bouvet J-P: Familial Poland anomaly. *J Med Genet* 1983, 20:152–154.
Oppolzer A, Sacher M: Poland-Syndrom. *Klin Pädiat* 1983, 185:135–137.
Bosch-Banyeras J M, Zusanabar A *et al*: Poland-Möbius syndrome... *J Med Genet* 1984, 21:70–71.
Gausewitz S H, Meals R A *et al*: Severe limb deficiency in Poland's syndrome. *Clin Orthopaed* 1984, 185:9–13.
David T J, Winter R M: Familial absence of the pectoralis major, serratus anterior, and latissimus dorsi muscles. *J Med Genet* 1985, 22:390–392.
Bavinck J N B, Weaver D D: Subclavian artery supply disruption sequency... *Am J Med Genet* 1986, 23:903–918.
Esquembre C, Ferris J *at al*: Poland syndrome and leukaemia. *Eur J Pediatr* 1987, 146:444.
McGivillray B C, Lawry R B: Poland syndrome in British Columbia: incidence and reproductive experience of affected persons. *Am J Med Genet* 1977, 1:65–74.
Larizza D, Maghnie M: Poland's anomaly associated with growth hormone deficiency. *J Med Genet* 1990, 27:53–55.
Rojas-Martinez A, Garcia-Cruz D *et al*: Poland-Moebius syndrome in a boy and Poland syndrome in his mother. *Clin Genet* 1991, 40:225–228.
Cobben J M, van Essen A J *et al*: A boy with Poland anomaly and facio-auriculo-vertebral dysplasia. *Clin Genet* 1992, 41:105–107.
Bamforth J S, Fabian C *et al*: Poland anomaly with a limb body wall disruption defect: case report and review. *Am J Med Genet* 1992, 43:780–784.
Stewart F J, Nevin N C: Poland anomaly with a limb body wall defect. *Am J Med Genet* 1993, 46:350.
Kabra M, Suri M *et al*: Poland anomaly with unusual associated anomalies: case report of an apparent disorganization defect. *Am J Med Genet* 1994, 52:402–405.

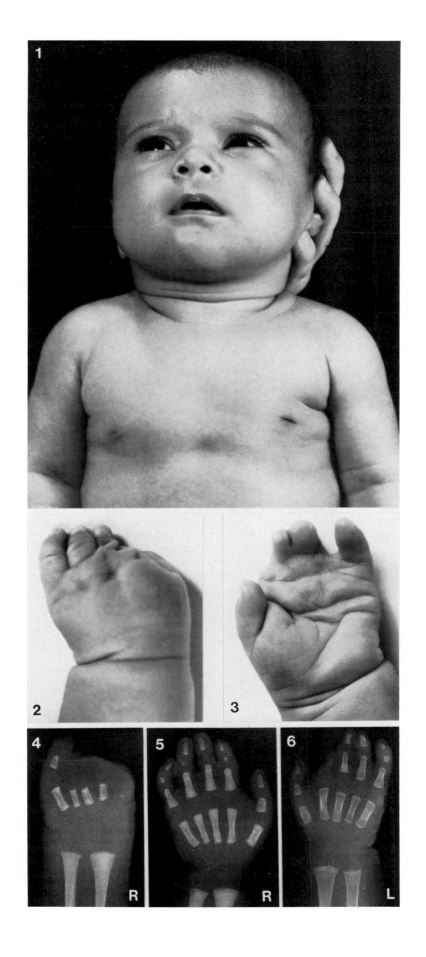

221 Tibial Aplasia or Hypoplasia with Cleft Hand and Cleft Foot

H.-R.W

A relatively rare, autosomal dominant anomaly of extreme variability.

Main signs:
- Ectrodactyly (in approximately 75% of observed familial patients).
- Tibial defects of different grades of severity (in up to 60%); club feet.
- Ulnar defects, variously manifest (in approximately 12%).
- Femoral defects of varied severity (in approximately 8%); bifurcation of the distal end of the femur, among other anomalies.

Supplementary findings: Contractures of the knee joints, occasionally absent patellae, hypoplasia of the halluces, polydactyly, malformation of the external ears.

Manifestation: At birth.

Aetiology: Although heterogeneity cannot be excluded with certainty, an autosomal dominant gene with extraordinarily variable expression, decreased penetrance, and low 'specificity' appears likely.

The variability of expression of anomalies extends from cleft hands and feet (monodactyly in severely affected patients) through bilateral tibial aplasia and contractures of the knee joints to mere syndactyly of two fingers or even only hypoplasia of one or both halluces.

Frequency: Relatively low; up to 1985 only 30 sporadic patients were known and perhaps the same number of families with affected members.

Course, prognosis: Dependent on the degree of expression. As mental development and internal organs are unaffected, the outlook for even severely affected patients is relatively favourable, providing they receive the best treatment possible.

Diagnosis, differential diagnosis: Tibial aplasia or hypoplasia with pre-axial polydactyly (222).

Treatment: Orthopaedic care and appropriate handicap aids. Genetic counselling. Prenatal diagnosis by ultrasound for some patients.

Illustrations:
1–3 A male newborn with right-sided cleft hand (**1 and 2**) and ipsilateral tibial aplasia, shortening of the lower leg, and club foot with toe anomalies. Sporadic case.
4 and 5 A female newborn, the first child of a similarly affected father, with bilateral cleft hand (with a postminimus on the left hand). Bilateral tibial aplasia with club feet. Hypoplasia of the right foot with tibial deviation of the hallux, complete cutaneous syndactyly of the third and fourth toes, absence of the second and a somewhat enlarged fifth toe. On the left, a broadened hallux, absence of the second and third toes.

References:
Lenz W: Genetische Ursachen von Fehlbildungen beim Menschen. *Verh Dtsch Ges Path* 1982, 66:16–24.
Majewski F, Küster W, ter Haar B *et al*: Aplasia of tibia with split-hand/split-foot deformity. Report of six families with 35 cases and considerations about variability and penetrance. *Hum Genet* 1985, 70:136–147.
Richieri-Costa A, Ferrareto I, Masiero D *et al*: Tibial hemimelia: report on 37 new cases, clinical and genetic considerations. *Am J Med Genet* 1987, 27:867–884.
Richieri-Costa A, Brunoni D, Filho J L *et al*: Tibial aplasia-ectrodactyly as variant expression of the Gollop-Wolfgang complex: report of a Brazilian family. *Am J Med Genet* 1987, 28:971–980.
Sener R N, Isikan E *et al*: Bilateral split-hand with bilateral tibial aplasia. *Pediatr Radiol* 1989, 19:258–260.
Sener R N, Sayli B S *et al*: Tetra-oligodactyly with bilateral aplasia and hypoplasia of long bones of upper and lower limbs: a variable manifestation of the syndrome of ectrodactyly with tibial aplasia. *Pediatr Radiol* 1990, 21:57–61.

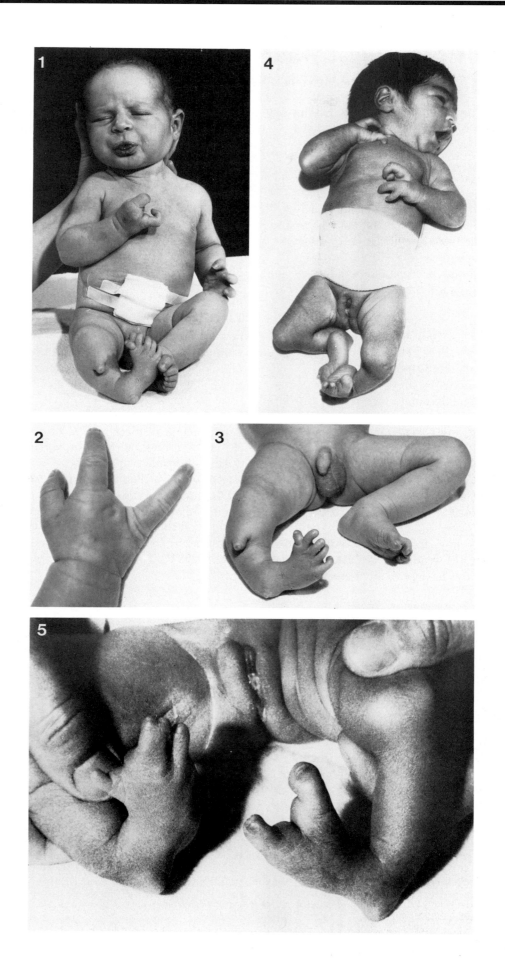

222

Tibial Aplasia or Hypoplasia with Pre-axial Polydactyly and Triphalangeal 'Thumbs'

(Werner Syndrome; Eaton–McKusick Syndrome)

H.-R.W

A relatively rare autosomal dominant anomaly with very variable expression.

Main signs:
- Absence or hypoplasia of the tibiae bilaterally.
- Bõwed and thickened fibulae.
- Club feet with pre-axial octadactyly or nonodactyly.
- Five to six-fingered hands without thumbs; the first ray is not opposable, the thenar musculature is absent.

Supplementary findings: Occasional syndactyly and camptodactyly of fingers and toes. The first metacarpal is long and has a distal epiphysis.

Rarely, also postaxial polydactyly of the hands. Radio-ulnar synostosis in isolated patients.

Manifestation: At birth.

Aetiology: An autosomal dominant gene is responsible for the anomaly, which affects the two sexes equally frequently and equally severely. Penetrance usually high but occasionally reduced and (rarely) even absent. Variable expression. The variability extends from the full picture, through pre-axial polydactyly of the feet without tibial defect, to a unilateral five-fingered (thumbless) hand without tibial hypoplasia.

Frequency: Relatively low; maybe 10 sporadic patients and 12 families with the syndrome are known to date, however, numerous cases have probably remained unpublished.

Course, prognosis: Dependent on the degree manifest but even when fully manifest, relatively favourable with 'rehabilitation'.

Diagnosis, differential diagnosis: Syndrome *223*. In addition, tibial aplasia or hypoplasia with cleft hand (*221*).

Treatment: Orthopaedic care and appropriate handicap aids. Genetic counselling. In future pregnancy or pregnancy in an affected individual, prenatal diagnosis with ultrasound.

Illustrations:

1–3 A 5-month-old boy, the first child of young, healthy, non-consanguineous parents. No patellae palpable; skin retracted over the knee joints. Shortened lower legs with radiologically bowed and thickened fibulae and absent tibiae. Club feet. Bilaterally, six metatarsals and eight toes; of these, three pre-axial supernumerary; the hypoplastic first toe is syndactylous with the second toe. A triphalangeal finger instead of a thumb bilaterally; on the left, five rays, on the right, six plus an additional pre-axial rudimentary appendage. On the right, bony syndactyly of rays III and IV with V-shaped forking, up to 80% cutaneous syndactyly; rays IV and V show complete cutaneous syndactyly. In addition, camptodactyly of rays I and II on the right, III and IV on the left.

Internal organs of the child unremarkable but somewhat large testes (3–4 ml). Short penis. Epicanthus.

References:

Werner P: Über einen seltenen Fall von Zwergwuchs. *Arch Gynäkol* 1915, **104**:278–300.

Eaton G O, McKusick V A: A seemingly unique polydactyly-syndactyly syndrome in four persons in three generations. *Birth Defects Orig Art Ser* 1969,**V(3)**:221–225.

Lamb S W, Wynne-Davies R, Whitmore J M: Five-fingered hand associated with partial or complete tibial absence and pre-axial polydactyly. *J Bone Jt Surg* 1983, **65(B)**:60–63.

Canún S, Lomeli R M, Martínez R *et al*: Absent tibia, triphalangeal thumbs and polydactyly: description of a family and prenatal diagnosis. *Clin Genet* 1984, **25**:182–186.

Canún S: Absent tibiae, triphalangeal thumbs, polydactyly and non-penetrance. *Clin Genet* 1986, **29**:347.

Cordeiro I, Santos H, Maroteaux P: Congenital absence of the tibiae and thumbs with polydactyly. A rare genetic disease (Werner's syndrome). *Ann Génét* 1986, **29**:275–277.

Majewski F: *Persönliche Mitteilungen* 1986.

Richieri-Costa A, de Miranda E *et al*: Autosomal dominant tibial hemimelia-polysyndactyly-triphalangeal thumbs syndrome... *Am J Med Genet* 1990, **36**:1–6.

Vargas F R, Pontes R L *et al*: Absent tibiae - polydactyly - triphalangeal thumbs... *Am J Med Genet* 1995, **55**:261–264.

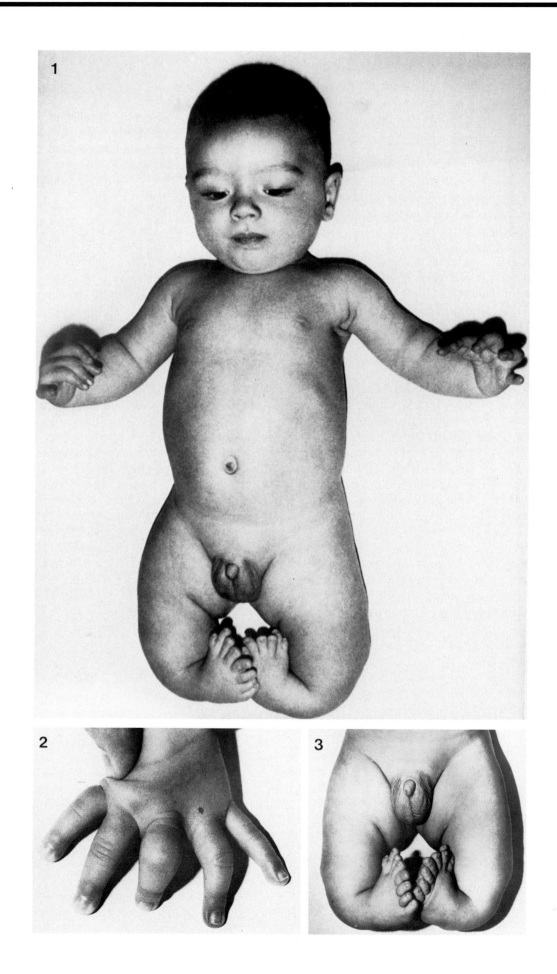

223 A Rare Syndrome of Dysplastic Extremities, Polydactyly, Dyscrania

H.-R.W

A syndrome of partial tibial defect, pre-axial polydactyly, generalized micromelia and macrotrigonocephaly.

Main signs:

- Unilateral partial tibial defect (**1a, 2, 5**). Ipsilateral pre-axial polydactyly (clinically, nonodactyly, **3**; radiologically, octadactyly). Generalized micromelia (**1**).
- Macrotrigonocephaly with prominent medial ridge of the forehead (**1a**). Low nasal bridge. Initially slight antimongoloid slant of the palpebral fissures. Bluish sclerae.
- Short neck. Thickset trunk with low-lying umbilicus (**1a**). Dislocation of the left hip, limited extension of the left knee joint. Dislocation of the right knee joint.

Supplementary findings: Normal hands and fingers.

Left inguinal hernia, left cryptorchidism, undescended testicle on the right. Muscular hypotonia.

On radiograph: large cranium with relatively small facial part of the skull; convex curvature of the base of the skull; delayed closure of the fontanelles (anterior fontanelle still open at age 3 years).

High, narrow pelvis with vertically aligned ischia. Dislocation of the left hip, dysplasia of the right. Strikingly narrow femora, with the left shorter than the right. Half-moon-shaped, dysplastic, shortened tibia on the right; short, crudely formed, dislocated fibula. Short left tibia with relatively elongated fibula. Seven metatarsals on the right. The four toes on the fibular side correspond to four three-membered toes; two additional three-membered toes pre-axially (and the rudimentary third pre-axial toe also later showed three bony phalanges); abnormally broad proximal phalanx of the hallux, duplicated second pha-

lanx (clinically: double nail). Duplication of the right talus was also recognizable later.

Bilateral ureteral dilation and blunting without evidence of gross renal malformation.

Manifestation: At birth.

Aetiology: Genetic basis likely. Mother macrocephalic with flat orbits and mild exophthalmos (very marked facial resemblance of the proband to his mother); the mother's grandfather had a congenital malformation of the right foot, perhaps with shortening because he 'limped' (further medical details unavailable).

Course, prognosis: Favourable, with 'rehabilitation'.

Comment: The typical picture of the tibial defect and the accompanying formation of seven metatarsals and pre-axial polydactyly is presented here within the framework of a clinical picture of generalized dysplasia, which we have been unable, despite overlaps with other syndromes, to identify as a previously described syndrome. Not Werner syndrome (*222*).

Illustrations:

1–5 The child discussed here, at age 3 months. The boy is the second child of young, healthy parents (first child healthy); no parental consanguinity. Birth at term with normal weight but length (47 cm) below average.

Head circumference: at 5 months, 44.5 cm; at 2 years and 6 months, 52.5 cm; at 5 years, 54 cm. Mental development normal for age.

References:
Wiedemann H-R, Opitz J M: Unilateral partial tibia defect... *Am J Med Genet* 1983, **14**:467–471.

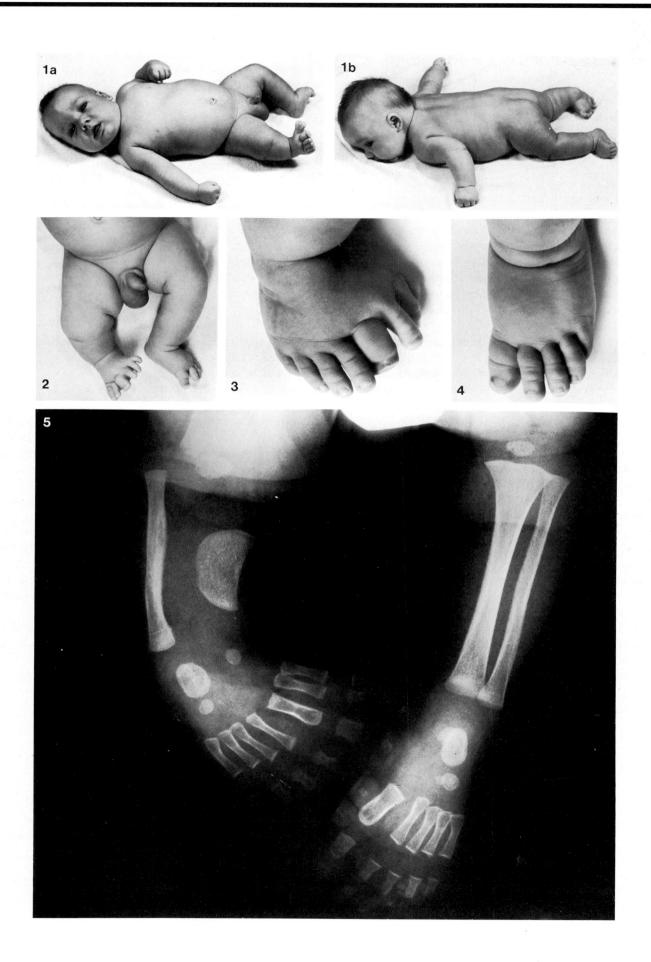

(Trevor Disease, 'Tarsomegaly')

H.-R.W

Osteochondromatous outgrowth and overgrowth usually at one but possibly several joints of a lower extremity, with consequent disability, deformity and possibly pain.

Main signs:
- Usually unilateral swelling (more frequently medially than laterally) or limited movement at an ankle or knee joint. Occasionally, other joints, such as the hip or wrist, are involved. In addition, deformity of the affected joint in the form of pes valgo-planus or equinus, genu valgum or varum or occasionally unequal length of the legs, usually caused by shortening rather than to lengthening of the affected extremity (1–4). Pain usually occurs later, particularly in the ankle region.
- Radiologically, usually evidence of accelerated development of the ossification centre in the affected area and of an irregular, frequently multicentric opacity adjacent to the affected epiphysis or to the affected carpal or tarsal bone (5), later fusing with it and giving the appearance of irregular enlargement or of a protuberance (5, 7).

Supplementary findings: The dysplasia principally affects epiphyses of tarsal bones, only exceptionally is the analogous region of an upper extremity affected instead (even more rarely, the sternum or clavicles). Usually localized medially, less frequently laterally, involvement of the whole epiphysis is an exception (5 and 6). Not infrequently, several epiphyses in one extremity are affected. Involvement of more than one limb very unusual; systemic involvement has been reported only in isolated cases.

Manifestation: The disorder is usually discovered sometime during childhood (or later), exceptionally in the first year of life or even at birth. Beware misdiagnosis as a malignant process.

Aetiology: Unclear; possible somatic mutation. Sporadic occurrence; boys:girls is approximately 3:1.
(The formal pathogenesis involves asymmetrical cartilaginous overgrowth and extension of one or several epiphyses or of a carpal or tarsal bone with subsequent endochondral ossification.)

Frequency: Low; up to 1985, approximately 140 observations in the literature.

Course, prognosis: Good with early and adequate orthopaedic care. The process ends after the child has stopped growing.

Differential diagnosis: Enchondromatosis (233), metachondromatosis, carpotarsal osteochondromatosis (Maroteaux), multiple cartilaginous exostoses (231) and chondrodysplasia punctata (123–126).

Treatment: Prompt orthopaedic care of a conservative or, if indicated, operative nature.

Illustrations:
1–7 The first child of young, healthy, non-consanguineous parents. Contractures of all large joints of the right lower limb noted at birth and increasing overgrowth of the extremity after the second month of life.
1–4 The severely physically handicapped boy as a 3 year old; the left lateral malleolus is also enlarged and lower than normal; limited pronation and supination of both hands and limited movement of the fingers bilaterally.
5 Overgrowth of the right pelvis and proximal femur with epiphyseal dysplasia from age 10 months.
6 and 7 Similar coarse changes in the right knee and foot ('tarsomegaly' with severe deformity of the talus) at age 3 years.
  Milder epiphyseal changes in the left lower extremity and subtle changes in both of the upper extremities, as in a systemic disorder.

References:
Kettelkamp D B, Campbell C J, Benfiglio M: Dysplasia epiphysealis hemimelica. A report of fifteen cases, *J Bone Jt Surg* 48(A):746.
Spranger J W, Langer Jr L O, Wiedemann H-R: *Bone dysplasias. An atlas of constitutional disorders of skeletal development.* Stuttgart and Philadephia: G Fischer and W B Saunders; 1974.
Fasting O J, Bjerkreim I: Dysplasia epiphysealis hemimelica. *Acta Orthopaed Scand* 1976, 47:217.
Carlson D H, Wilkinson R H: Variability of unilateral epiphyseal dysplasia. *Radiology* 1979, 133:369.
Wiedemann H-R, Mann M, Spreter v Kreudenstein P: Dysplasia epiphysealis hemimelica. *Eur J Pediatr* 1981, **136**:311.
Lamesch A J: Dysplasia epiphysealis hemimelica of the carpal bones. *J Bone Jt Surg* 1983, 65(A):398–400.
Azouz E M, Slomic A M *et al*: The variable manifestations of dysplasia epiphysealis hemimelica. *Pediatr Radiol* 1985, 15:44–49.
Hoeffel J C, Capron F *et al*: Dysplasia epiphysealis hemimelica of the ulna. *Eur J Pediatr* 1986, **145**:450.
Hinkel G K, Rupprecht E: Hemihypertrophie als Leitsymptom einer Dysplasia epiphysealis hemimelica. *Klin Pädiatr* 1989, **201**:58–62.
Maroteaux P *et al*: Dominant carpotarsal osteochondromatosis. *J Med Genet* 1993, 30:704–706.
Kotzot D *et al*: Dysplasia epiphysealis hemimelica mit atypischer Lokalisation an der Brust. *Mschr Kinderheilk* 1994, 142:189–191.

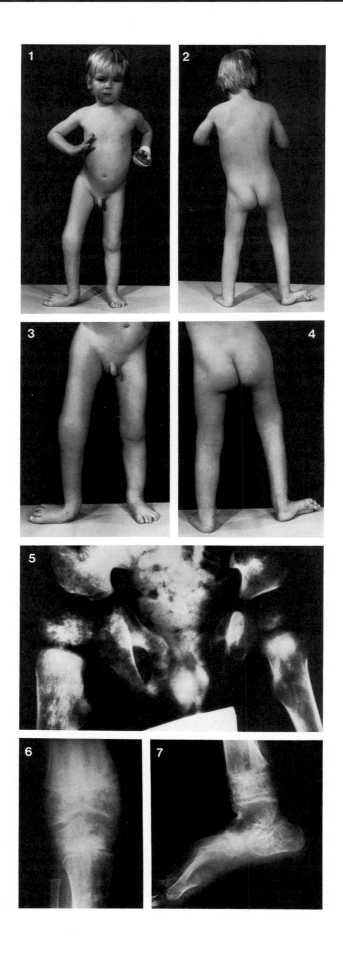

225 F.P. Weber 'Syndrome'
(Angiomatous Dysplasia F. P. Weber Type; Partially Macrosomic Limb with a Haemodynamically Significant Arterio-venous Fistula)

H.-R.W/ J.K.

A dysplasia syndrome comprising partial macrosomia, usually proportional in itself and usually of a lower extremity, caused by haemodynamically active, usually multiple, congenital arterio-venous (A-V) fistulas.

Main signs:
- Partial macrosomia of an extremity or part of a limb. As a rule, a lower extremity is affected and the enlarged region usually remains more or less proportional (1–4).
- Evidence of an A-V shunt: dilation of arteries and veins; prominent vascular pulsations, continuing into the veins, vascular thrills and hyperthermic skin.
- Arteriographic evidence of congenital A-V fistulas, usually multiple, in soft tissue or bone.

Supplementary findings: Large A-V shunts lead to signs of cardiac overload and possibly to severe cardiac failure, with no signs of cardiac malformation.

Possibly secondary osteo-articular changes such as tilted pelvis, scoliosis and so on.

Naevus flammeus may occur over the affected region or in other areas.

Manifestation: In childhood.

Aetiology: Unexplained. Genetic factors may be assumed. Usually sporadic occurrence. Compare with Klippel–Trenaunay syndrome (198).

Frequency: Relatively low.

Course, prognosis: Tendency to continue to progress after the child has stopped growing. The affected extremity and the patient's life may be seriously threatened.

Diagnosis: Careful angiographic analysis essential.

Differential diagnosis: Simple partial macrosomia without vascular malformations (309). Klippel–Trenaunay syndrome (198), which may be extremely difficult to differentiate, if, in fact, this is a different entity (opinions vary).

Treatment: Urgent measures to decrease the shunt volume by vascular surgery, if possible. If unsuccessful or impossible, amputation may need to be considered as a last resort.

Illustrations:
1–4 A 10-year-old girl with 'gigantism' of the entire right lower extremity, especially of the lower leg and foot. Equinus position of the foot, flexion contracture of the knee, tilted pelvis and scoliosis. No naevus flammeus of the skin. Hyperthermia of the affected leg. Dilated veins, pulsations. Multiple A-V fistulas on angiogram.

References:
Weber F P: Angioma formation in connection with hypertrophy of limbs and hemihypertrophy. *Br J Derm* 1907, **19**:231–235.
Vollmar J: Zur Geschichte und Terminologie der Syndrome nach F. P. Weber und Klippel–Trenaunay. *VASA* 1974, 3:231.
Vollmar J: Die Chirurgie kongenitaler arteriovenöser Fisteln der Gliedmaßen. In: *Arteriovenöse Fisteln - Dilatierende Arteriopathien.* J F Vollmar, F P Nobbe (ed). Stuttgart: thieme, 1976:66
Leipner N, Janson R *et al*: Angiomatöse Dysplasie (Typ F. P. Weber). *Fortschr Röntgenstr* 1982, **137**:73–77.
Leipner N, Lackner K *et al*: Röntgenbefunde bei einer angiomatösen Dysplasie (Typ Weber). *Fortschr Röntgenstr* 1985, **142**:571–573.

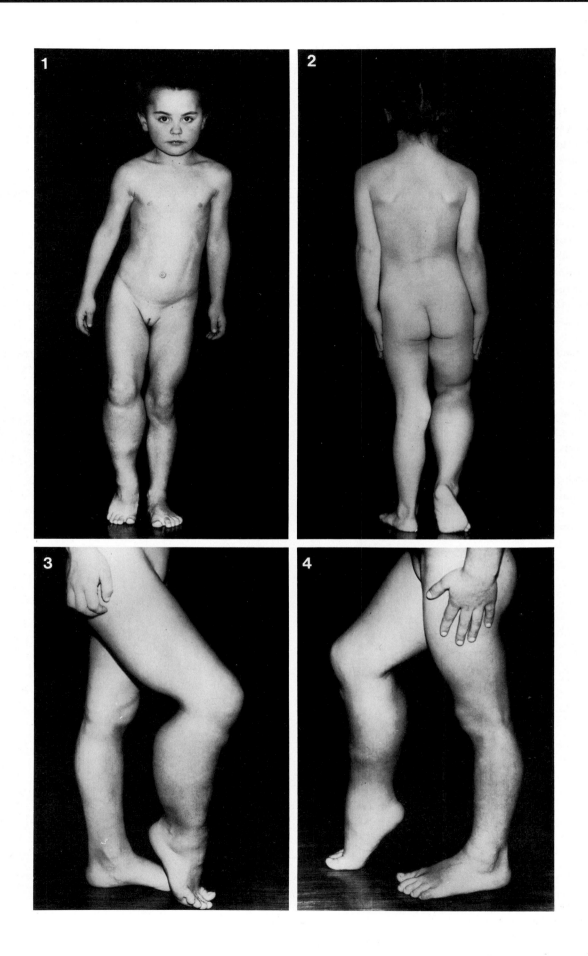

H.-R.W

A sporadically occurring 'classic' clinical picture of congenital non-progressive joint contractures (because of impaired muscle development) with characteristic positioning of the extremities and round face.

Main signs:
- Multiple congenital contractures (with taut connective and adipose tissue replacing muscle) and typical positioning of the extremities: usually, shoulders internally rotated; elbows in extension; wrists flexed; usually severe talipes equinovarus (**1**, **4**). Knee and hip joint contractures in various positions; fingers flexed.
- Frequent absence of normal flexion creases over the joints; presence of abnormal skin dimples or of soft-tissue folds in the joint regions (**3–5**).
- Typical round face with capillary angioma in the upper midline and micrognathia (**2**).
- Normal intelligence.

Supplementary findings: Although usually all extremities are fairly symmetrically affected, in some patients, contractions may occur mainly in the legs and, even less frequently, mainly in the arms. Hypoplasia of the fingers, hypoplasia of the labia or scrotum, cryptorchidism and other anomalies possible.

History of decreased foetal movements during pregnancy; breech presentation frequent.

Manifestation: At birth.

Aetiology: Unknown. Sporadic occurrence. No monozygotic twin concordance.

Frequency: Not particularly low.

Course, prognosis: Delayed motor development because of limitation of movements. Otherwise dependent on the severity of the disorder and on the quality and intensity of treatment.

Differential diagnosis: Other causes of arthrogryposis (also syndrome *78*).

Treatment: Intensive physiotherapy and multiple orthopaedic measures are required and not infrequently orthopaedic surgery. Genetic counselling.

Illustrations:
1–5 A newborn with arthrogryposis.

References:
Hall J G, Reed S D *et al*: Amyoplasia: a common, sporadic condition with congenital contractures. *Am J Med Genet* 1983, **15**:571–590.
Hall J G, Reed S D *et al*: Amyoplasia: twinning... *Am J Med Genet* 1983, **15**:591–599.
Hageman G, Ippel E P F *et al*: The diagnostic mangagement of newborns with congenital contractures: a nosologic study of 75 cases. *Am J Med Genet* 1988, **30**:883–904.
Vuopala K, Leisti J *et al*: Lethal arthrogryposis in Finland... study of 83 cases... *Neuropediatrics* 1994, **25**:308–315.

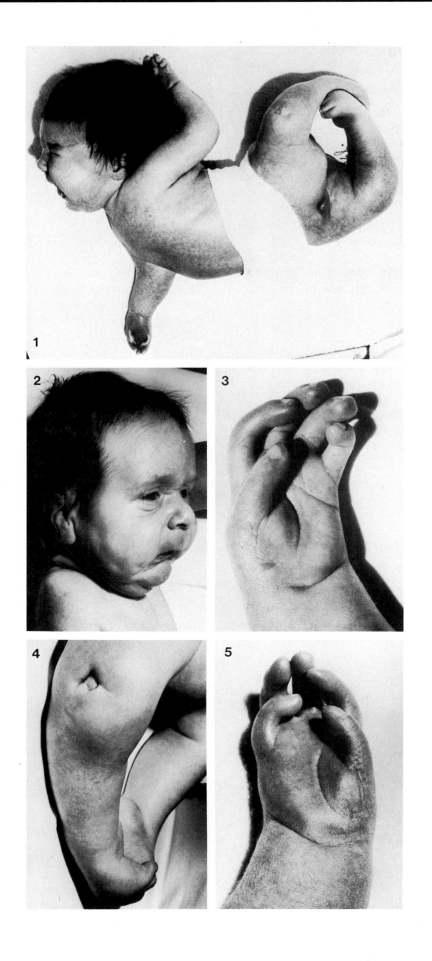

J.K.

Congenital contractures of the joints, primarily the fingers, with malpositioning of the feet.

Main signs:
- Flexion contractures of the fingers with overlapping fingers 'as in trisomy 18' (in 98%). In adulthood, ulnar deviation in the metacarpophalangeal joints.
- Involvement of the feet in 88%: equinovarus position or calcaneovalgus deformity.

Supplementary findings: Dislocation of the hips, fixation of the elbow and knee joints. Absence of the interphalangeal flexion creases.

Manifestation: At birth.

Aetiology: Autosomal dominant inheritance with variable expression. Possible prenatal diagnosis.

Pathogenesis: Incorrectly attached, hypoplastic or absent tendons. Fibrosis or atrophy of the muscles.

Course, prognosis: Regular physiotherapy and surgical intervention should prevent secondary atrophy.

Differential diagnosis: Trisomy 18 (*48*), Pena–Shokeir phenotype (*319*), Freeman–Sheldon syndrome (*27*), otopalatodigital syndrome type II (*229*), Gordon syndrome (*228*).

Treatment: Physical and orthopaedic measures.

Illustrations:
1a–c Female patient aged 28 years, flexion contractures of the hands, ulnar deviation of the fingers, mild cutaneous syndactyly, absence of the interphalangeal flexion creases, club foot (surgically corrected on several occasions).
2a The 29-year-old father of **2b and c:** with camptodactyly and ulnar deviation of the fingers in the region of the metacarpophalangeal joint.
2b and c The 2-month-old daughter of **2a** with typical flexion of the fingers 'as in trisomy 18'.

References:

Hall J G, Reed S D, Greene G: The distal arthrogryposes: delineation of new entities — review and nosologic discussion. *Am J Med Genet* 1982, 11:185–239.
Barty B J, Cubberly D, Morris C, Carey J: Prenatal diagnosis of distal arthrogryposis. *Am J Med Genet* 1988, 29:501–510.
Bui T-H, Lindholm H, Demir N, Thomassen P: Prenatal diagnosis of distal arthrogryposis type I by ultrasonography. *Prenat Diagn* 1992, 12:1047–1053.

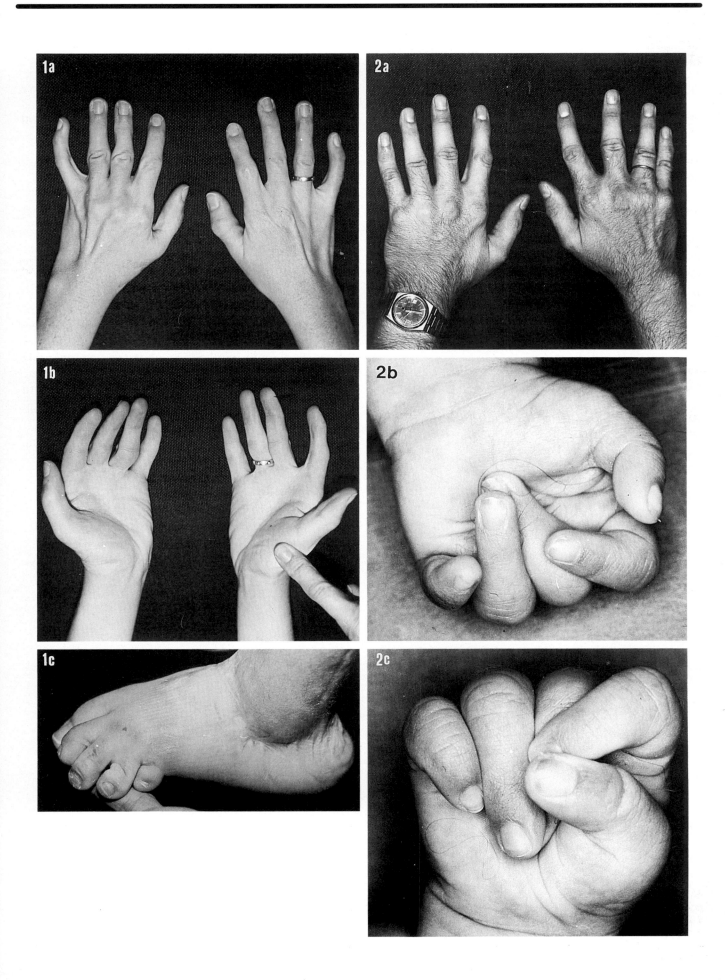

228 Distal Arthrogryposis Type II A
(Gordon Syndrome)

J.K.

A familial syndrome with camptodactyly, club feet and cleft palate.

Main signs:
- Camptodactyly in 90% of all patients.
- Club feet in 75%.
- Cleft palate in 30%, high palate.

Supplementary findings: Mild cutaneous interdigital syndactyly, absence of the interphalangeal creases, contracture of the large joints, muscular hypoplasia. Scoliosis, pectus excavatum, short stature. Undescended testes. Normal intelligence.

Manifestation: At birth.

Aetiology: Autosomal dominant inheritance with incomplete penetrance and reduced expression in females.

Pathogenesis: Unknown.

Frequency: Six families have been reported to date with 51 affected individuals.

Course, prognosis: Good with regard to intelligence and life expectancy.

Differential diagnosis: Distal arthrogryposis type I (227), Tel-Hashomer camptodactyly.

Treatment: Orthopaedic measures. Speech therapy after cleft palate operation.

Illustrations:

1a and b A 6-week-old male, large eyes, ptosis, depressed nasal bridge, small nose, anteverted nostrils, narrow upper prolabium, indistinct philtrum, retrognathia, microstomia, short neck (cleft palate);

1c and d Camptodactyly of fingers II–V, proximally situated thumb, bilateral simian creases;

1e Club feet encased in plaster bilaterally.

References:

Gordon H, Davies D, Berman M: Camptodactyly, cleft palate, and club foot. A syndrome showing the autosomal-dominant pattern of inheritance. *J Med Genet* 1969, **6**:266–274.

Halal F, Fraser F C: Camptodactyly, cleft palate, and club foot (the Gordon syndrome). *J Med Genet* 1979, **16**:149–150.

Say B, Barber D H, Thompson R C, Leichtman L G: The Gordon syndrome. *J Med Genet* 1980, **17**:405.

Robinow M, Johnson G F: The Gordon syndrome: autosomal dominant cleft palate, camptodactyly, and club feet. *Am J Med Genet* 1981, **9**:139–146.

Hall J G, Reed S D, Greene G: The distal arthrogryposes: delineation of new entities — review and nosologic discussion. *Am J Med Genet* 1982, **11**:185–239.

Ican D M, Belengeanu V, Maximilian C, Fryns J P: Distal arthrogryposis with autosomal dominant inheritances and reduced penetrance in females: the Gordon syndrome. *Clin Genet* 1993, **43**:300–302.

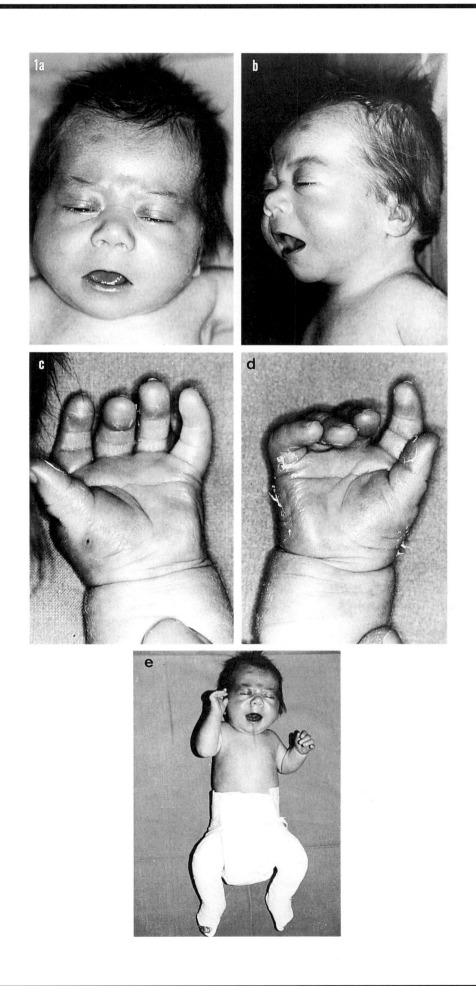

J.K.

A syndrome with signs and symptoms similar to those of trisomy 18 (cranio-oro-digital syndrome).

Main signs:
- At birth, large open anterior fontanelle with wide cranial sutures, wormian bones, ossification defects, prominent forehead.
- Cleft palate, microstomia, micrognathia.
- Facial dysmorphism (as in trisomy 18): hypertelorism, low-set ears, antimongoloid slant of the palpebral fissures, flat nasal bridge, micrognathia.
- Overlapping fingers (as in trisomy 18) because of flexion contractures and camptodactyly, short thumbs, broad halluces.

Supplementary findings: Short metacarpals, especially of the first finger, broad proximal phalanges II–IV of the hands, clinodactyly of the second and fourth fingers, partial syndactyly, short feet, metatarsals I, II and V absent or short, proximal phalanges of the first and fifth toes short or absent. Distal phalanges of the halluces short or absent. Anterior bowing of the tibia and fibula, hypoplastic fibula, curvature of the arms, dislocation, subluxation of the elbow and wrist. Flat vertebral bodies. Flat acetabula. Short, deformed ribs.

Manifestation: At birth.

Aetiology: X-linked semidominant inheritance, hitherto manifest only in males. The maternal carriers present a clinical picture of mild dysmorphism: prominent forehead, antimongoloid slant of the palpebral fissures, flat nose, hypertelorism, low-set ears, hypoplastic mandibles, flat abdomen, conductive hearing disorder, high palate, cleft uvula, cleft palate.

Pathogenesis: Unknown.

Course, prognosis: Severe mental retardation, however, normal intelligence has also been observed.

Diagnosis, differential diagnosis: Pena–Shokeir phenotype (*319*), Freeman-Sheldon syndrome (*27*), distal arthrogryposis I (*227*), trisomy 18 (*48*), Melnick–Needles syndrome (*18*).

Treatment: Surgical repair of the cleft palate. Symptomatic treatment.

Illustrations:
1–6 10 years old, kyphosis of the thoracic region of the vertebral column, contractures of the large and small joints, broad thumbs, antimongoloid slant of the palpebral fissures, bulging forehead. Pectus carinatum. Anterior bowing of the lower leg (1–3).

References:
Brewster T G, Lachmann R S, Kushner D C, Holmed L B, Isler R J, Rimoin D L: Oto-palato-digital syndrome, type II — an X-linked skeletal dysplasia. *Am J Med Genet* 1985, **20**:249–254.
Ogata T, Matsuo N, Nishimura G, Hajikano H: Oto-palato-digital syndrome, type II: evidence for defective intramembranous ossification. *Am J Med Genet* 1990, **36**:226–231.
Stratton R F, Bluestone D L: Oto-palato-digital syndrome II with X-linked cerebellar hypoplasia/hydrocephalus. *Am J Med Genet* 1991, **41**:169–172.
Hoar D I, Field L L, Beards F, Hoganson G, Rollnick B, Hoo J J: Tentative assignment of gene for oto-palato-digital syndrome to distal Xq(Xq26-28). *Am J Med Genet* 1992, **42**:170–172.
Holder S E, Winter R M: Otopalatodigital syndrome type II. *J Med Genet* 1993, **30**:310–313.
Preis S, Kemperdinck H, Majewski F: Oto-palato-digital syndrome type II in two unrelated boys. *Clin Genet* 1994, **45**:154–161.

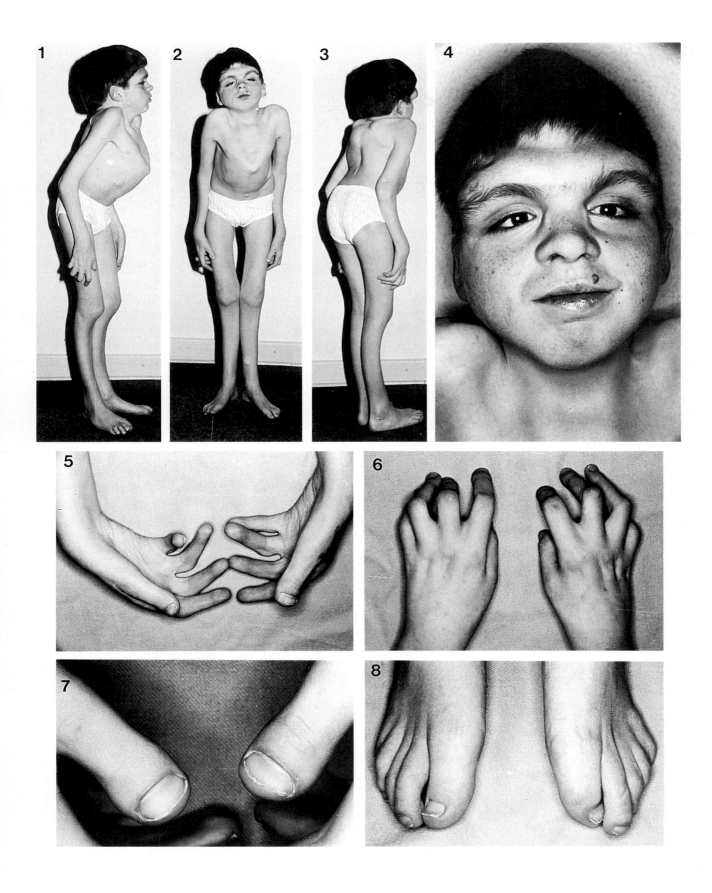

H.-R.W

A characteristic syndrome with multiple congenital joint dislocations, facial dysmorphism and anomalies of the hands, fingers and feet.

Main signs:
- Dislocations especially of the hips, knees and elbows (**1**, **3**). Flat, rectangular face with depressed nasal bridge, prominent forehead and hypertelorism (**2, 3, 5**).
- 'Spatula-like' thumbs and, in general, cylindrically shaped fingers with broad ends and short nails (**4**). Short arms. Talipes equinovarus or equinovalgus with torsion of the anterior part of the foot (**3**).

Supplementary findings: Cleft palate in approximately 50% of patients. Frequent development of progressive curvature of the spine. Decreased adult height.

On radiograph, distal phalanx of the thumb triangular; further distal phalanges short and broad, shortened metacarpals (especially II), accessory ossification centres in the wrist bones and an accessory ossification centre in the calcaneus. Frequent segmentation anomalies especially in the upper spine.

Possible cardiovascular anomalies, for example, aortic lesions.

Manifestation: At birth.

Aetiology: Monogenic disorder; heterogeneity; clinically, an autosomal dominant and a more severe autosomal recessive form, which to date cannot be differentiated with certainty. More girls than boys affected. Basic defect unknown, probable collagen defect.

Frequency: Relatively low, although it is likely that many patients are not recognized; well over 100 reports in the literature.

Course, prognosis: Respiration may be impaired in early infancy because of softness of thoracic cartilage, especially in the laryngotracheal airway (and especially in the recessive form?). Variable, frequently severe physical disability because of the dislocations. In the absence of appropriate measures to prevent severe deformity of the vertebral column, danger of developing spinal cord compression.

As a rule, mental development within normal limits.

Differential diagnosis: Precise differentiation from the otopalatodigital syndrome (*14, 229*) is often difficult. Numerous dislocated joints, including the knee joint, multiple carpal ossicles and an additional ossification centre in the calcaneus would suggest Larsen syndrome. The two syndromes may be closely associated genetically.

Ehlers–Danlos syndrome (*203*), the Marfan syndrome (*76*) and arthrogryposis (*226–228*) are easily excluded by their characteristic features.

Diastrophic dysplasia (131) should be considered.

Treatment: Early application of various orthopaedic measures (for the feet and hips and the particularly problematic severe knee dislocations; careful observation of the vertebral column and so on and comprehensive, continuous, multidisciplinary care for the physical handicaps.

Genetic counselling. Ultrasonographic prenatal diagnosis should be feasible (dislocations).

Illustrations:
1 A characteristically affected newborn; severe genu recurvatum.
2–5 A typically affected 6-year-old boy. Height, when supported by orthopaedic appliances, at the third percentile. Kyphoscoliosis; two cervicothoracic cleft vertebrae; 13 pairs of ribs. Slight pectus excavatum. Bifid uvula.

References:
Spranger J W, Langer Jr L O, Wiedemann H-R: *Bone dysplasias. An atlas of constitutional disorders of skeletal development.* Stuttgart and Philadephia: G Fischer and W B Saunders; 1974.
Micheli L J, Hall J E, Watts H G: Spinal instability in Larsen's syndrome. *J Bone Joint Surg* 1976, **58A**:562.
Galanski M, Statz A: Radiologische Befunde beim Larsen-Syndrom. *Fortschr Röntgenstr* 1978, **128**:534.
Kiel E A, Frias J L, Victorica B E: Cardiovascular manifestations in the Larsen syndrome. *Pediatrics* 1983, **71**:942–946.
Stanley D, Seymour N: The Larsen syndrome occurring in four generations of one family. *Int Orthopaed* 1985, 8:267–272.
Stanley C S et al: Mixed hearing loss in Larsen syndrome. *Clin Genet* 1988, **33**:395–398.
Mostello D et al: Recurrence and prenatal diagnosis of lethal Larsen syndrome. *J Hum Genet* 1989, **45A**:56.
Pierquin G et al: Two unrelated children... with the phenotype of the Larsen syndrome. *Hum Genet* 1991, **87**:587–591.

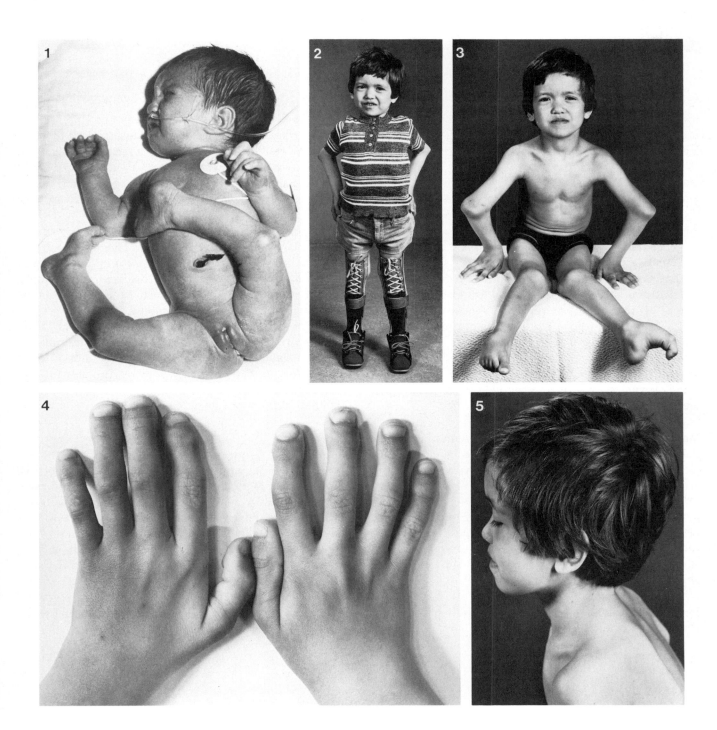

H.-R.W

A hereditary syndrome, which is very characteristic in its severe form, with variable numbers of bony outgrowths and protuberances, usually at the ends of the long bones, resulting in deformity and limited movement of the extremities.

Main signs:
- Multiple bony excrescences (covered by hyaline cartilage) especially on the ends of the long bones (**1b, 2, 3**), usually in the knee region but also often on the ribs, the medial edges of the scapulae, the iliac crest and other areas.
- Secondary deformities of the long bones such as shortening and bowing; most frequently of the ulna, with shortening of the forearm (**1a and 1b**) and ulnar deviation of the hand; radio-ulnar synostosis in some patients. Also shortening of the fibula, tibiofibular synostosis, genu valgum or pes valgus.

Supplementary findings: Possible moderate short stature.
Radiographs show exostoses in addition to those which are palpable.

Manifestation: Variable; usually early childhood and into the first decade of life. (The exostoses originating in the metaphyseal areas move to the diaphyses as the child grows.)

Aetiology: Autosomal dominant disorder with complete penetrance in males, incomplete in females. Definite sporadic cases should be considered as new mutations.
There seems to be genetic heterogeneity with gene loci on chromosomes 11 and 19.

Frequency: Not low (by 1964 over 1000 patients had been reported in the literature).

Course, prognosis: During adolescence, slowing of growth of the exostoses (with occasional exceptions); after puberty, no further growth of excrescences. Impaired function because of resulting disproportion of parts of the skeleton and possibly also impairment from pressure on the tendons, vessels or nerves. Neoplastic degeneration of the exostoses possible in adulthood (approximately 10% of patients).

Differential diagnosis: The Langer–Giedion syndrome (*232*) should not be difficult to rule out. Some newly described syndromes should be considered, for example, exostoses combined with anetodermia and brachydactyly; exostoses associated with hypochondroplasia.

Treatment: Surgery for patients with markedly impaired function (e.g. to prevent dislocation of a radial head) with excision of exostoses together with osteotomies for suspected development of malignancy.
Regular follow-up. Genetic counselling.

Illustrations:
1a and 1b A 6-year-old boy with deformity of the left forearm, typical radiograph findings (bowing of the radius, which alone articulates with the wrist and especially of the ulna, which is markedly shortened with distal exostoses), bilateral pes valgus and multiple further palpable or radiologically demonstrable exostoses.
2 Large, sharply demarcated exostosis originating from the proximal humeral metaphysis in a 7-year-old boy with multiple bony excrescences.
3 Radiograph of the right knee of a boy aged 3 years and 6 months, with exostoses on all long bones and on several ribs, one scapula and the hands and feet.

References:
Spranger J W, Langer Jr L O, Wiedemann H-R: *Bone dysplasias. An atlas of constitutional disorders of skeletal development.* Stuttgart and Philadephia: G Fischer and W B Saunders; 1974.
Ochsner P E: Zum Problem der neoplastischen Entartung bei multiplen kartilaginären Exostosen. *Z Orthopäd* 1978, **116**:369.
Shapiro F, Simon S, Glimcher M J: Hereditary multiple exostoses. *J Bone Jt Surg Ser A* 1979, **61/6**:815.
Gordon S L, Buchanan J R *et al*: Hereditary multiple exostoses... *J Med Genet* 1981, **18**:428–430.
Finidori G, Allard de Grandmaison P. *et al*: Anomalies de la croissance osseuse de la maladie exostosante. *Ann Pédiatr* 1983, **30**:657–662.
Hudson T M, Chew F S *et al*: Scintigraphy of benign exostoses... *AJR* 1983, **140**:581–586.
Dominguez R, Young L W *et al*: Multiple exostotic hypochondroplasia... *Pediatr Radiol* 1984, **14**:356–359.
Fogel G R, McElfresh E *et al*: Management of deformities of the forearm in multiple hereditary osteochondromas. *J Bone Jt Surg* 1984, **66A**:670–680.
Mollica F, Li Volti S *et al*: Exostoses, anetodermia, brachydactyly. *Am J Med Genet* 1984, **19**:665–667.
Hall J G, Wilson R X *et al*: Familial multiple exostoses — no chromosome 8 deletion observed. *Am J Med Genet* 1985, **22**:639–640.
Pritchett J W: Lengthening the ulna in patients with hereditary multiple exostoses. *J Bone Jt Surg* 1986, **68B**:561–565.
Hennekam R C M: Hereditary multiple exostoses. *J Med Genet* 1991, **28**:262–266.
Cook A *et al*: Genetic heterogeneity in... hereditary multiple exostoses. *Am J Hum Genet* 1993, **53**:71–79.
Wu Y-Q *et al*: Assignment of a second locus for multiple exostoses to... chromosome 11. *Hum Mol Genet* 1994, **3**:167–171.
Le Merrer M *et al*: A gene for hereditary multiple exostoses maps to chromosome 19p. *Hum Mol Genet* 1994, **3**:717–722.

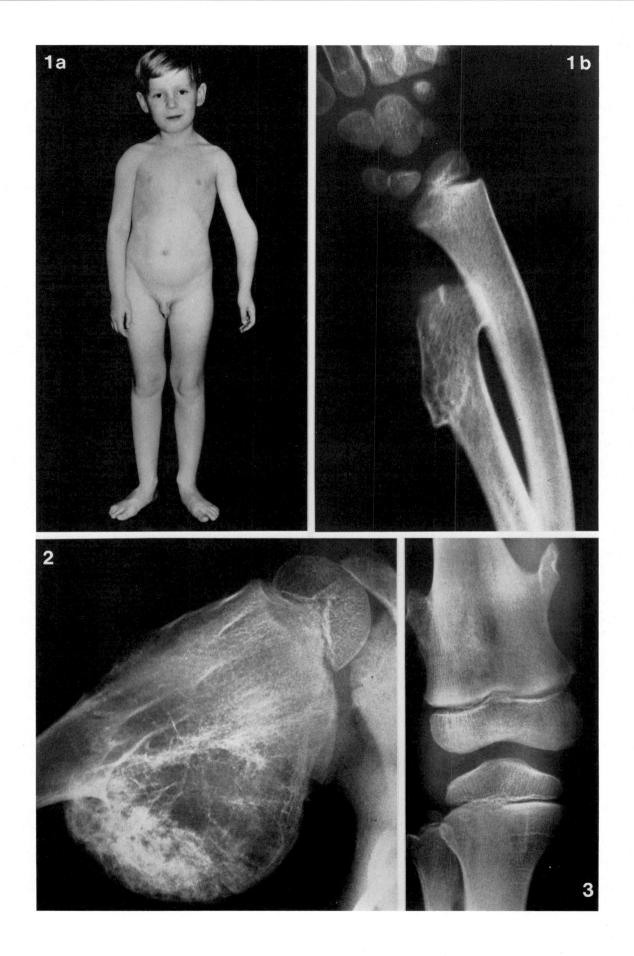

232 Langer–Giedion Syndrome
(Giedion–Langer Syndrome, Trichorhinophalangeal Dysplasia Type II, Syndrome of Acrodysplasia with Exostoses)

H-R.W

A malformation–retardation syndrome of short stature, unusual facies, sparse, fragile scalp hair, multiple exostoses, mild microcephaly and mental retardation.

Main signs:
- Typical facial dysmorphism: large, prominent, poorly differentiated ears; broad, upward-slanting eyebrows; deep-set eyes; bulbous nose with a broad septum and simple alae; long philtrum; long, narrow upper lip; high palate; malocclusion; receding chin (**1**).
- Short stature. Mild microcephaly and mild to moderate mental retardation.
- Fine scalp hair (**1**).
- Early features include flaccid or loose, wrinkled skin and muscular hypotonia.
- Later, maculopapular pigmented naevi especially on the upper half of the body.
- Multiple cartilaginous exostoses of the long tubular bones (also possibly on the short tubular bones, the shoulder blades, ribs and pelvis). Radiographs show cone-shaped epiphyses of the hands and feet (**2**).

Supplementary findings: Optic defects, sensorineural hearing impairment and delayed speech development may occur. Also, winged scapulae and generalized hyperextensibility of the joints, Perthes-like dysplasia of the femoral head and increased tendency to fractures; clinobrachydactyly, abnormal nails.

In early childhood, possible failure to thrive, increased susceptibility to infections.

Manifestation: At birth and in early childhood. Radiologically, the characteristic combination of exostoses with cone-shaped epiphyses usually becomes apparent by the age of 3–4 years.

Aetiology: Initially, all reported cases were sporadic, with both sexes affected; only subsequently was there a case report of transmission from father to daughter. Thus, autosomal dominant inheritance, possibly with new mutations in the majority of previously published observations.

Clearly affected is the long arm of chromosome 8 (8q24.11-q24.13).

Frequency: Very low (up to 1986, only approximately 50 reports in the literature).

Course, prognosis: The loose, wrinkled skin tends to improve in infancy; the susceptibility to infections disappears by about school age. The extent to which the patient is handicapped depends principally on the severity of mental and hearing impairments, then on the exostoses and their effect on joint mobility and local growth. General health and life expectancy are not necessarily reduced.

Differential diagnosis: In multiple cartilaginous exostoses (*231*) only exostoses and possible short stature are seen. In trichorhinophalangeal dysplasia type I (*239*): absence of exostoses and no microcephalic mental retardation, short stature, or other features.

Treatment: Symptomatic. Genetic counselling.

Illustrations:

1a and b A 15-year-old with the typical syndrome but unimpaired mental development. Exostoses at both ends of the long bones toward the end of the first year of life. Head circumference 48.5 cm; height (133.5 cm) below the third percentile. Delayed speech development; considerable hearing impairment (first noted at 4 years old). Normal sexual development.

2a and b Radiographs of the same child at different ages.

References:

Spranger J W, Langer Jr L O, Wiedemann H-R: *Bone dysplasias. An atlas of constitutional disorders of skeletal development.* Stuttgart and Philadephia: G Fischer and W B Saunders; 1974.

Oorthuys J W E, Beemer F A: The Langer–Giedion syndrome or trichorhino-phalangeal syndrome, type II. *Eur J Pediatr* 1979, **132**:55.

Bühler E M, Bühler U K, Stalder G R *et al*: Chromosome deletion and multiple cartilaginous exostoses. *Eur J Pediatr* 1980, **133**:163.

Zabel B U, Baumann W A: Langer–Giedion syndrome with interstitial 8q-deletion. *Am J Med Genet* 1982, **11**:353.

Fryns J P, Heremans G *et al*: Langer–Giedion syndrome and deletion of the long arm of chromosome 8... *Hum Genet* 1983, **64**:194–195.

Bühler E M, Malik N J: The tricho-rhino-phalangeal syndrome(s)... *Am J Med Genet* 1984, **19**:113–119.

Brenholz P *et al*: Dominant inheritance of the Langer–Giedion syndrome (Abstract). *Am J Hum Genet* 1989, **45**(Suppl)A:41.

Lüdecke H-J *et al*: Molecular definition of the shortest region of deletion overlap in the Langer–Giedion syndrome. *Am J Hum Genet* 1991, **49**:1197–1206.

Parris J M *et al*: Molecular analysis... in patients with Langer–Giedion syndrome. *Genomics* 1991, **11**:54–61.

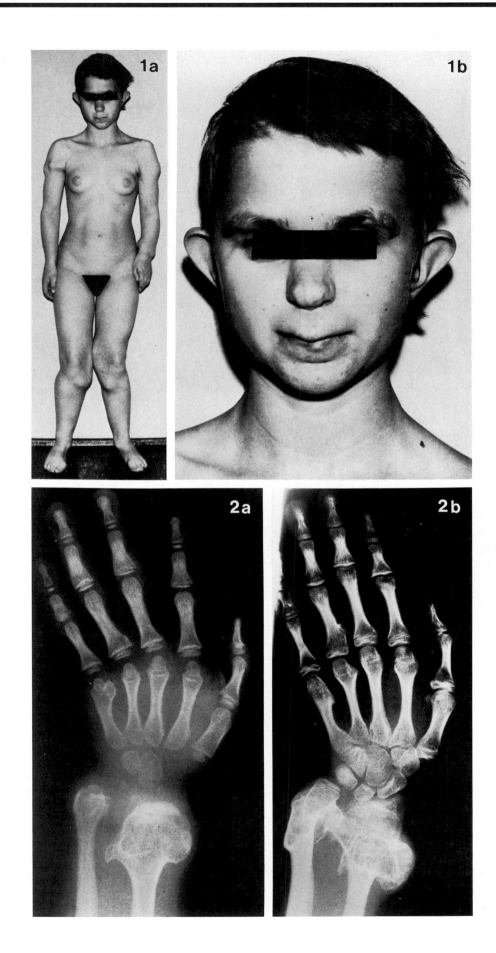

233 Ollier–Type Enchondromatosis

(Dyschondroplasia; Multiple Enchondromas, Ollier Type; Ollier's Disease; Osteochondromatosis)

H.-R.W

A syndrome of firm, localized, asymmetrical swellings of the fingers or toes combined with asymmetrical shortening of the extremities.

Main signs:
- Tautly elastic, firm, indolent, rounded swellings or outgrowths continuous with the bone on one or more fingers or toes (**1 and 2**).
- Shortening and possibly bowing of parts of the extremities, most frequently the forearm or lower leg. (**1, 4**).
- Marked asymmetry of the swellings (unilateral involvement possible).

Supplementary findings: Possible secondary impairment of mobility of one or several joints; occasional compression effects.

Occasional 'spontaneous' fracture in an affected area.

On radiograph, characteristic ovoid, pyramid-shaped and linear translucent defects in the metaphyses of affected long bones and in flat bones (with sparing of the calvarium and vertebral bodies); often considerable swelling and cortical thinning of the affected area (**3 and 4**).

Manifestation: Usually after the second year of life.

Aetiology: Not known (somatic mutation?). Isolated reports of familial occurrence are viewed sceptically. Sporadic occurrence. No increased risk of recurrence for the affected family.

Frequency: Relatively low.

Course, prognosis: Guarded. Further lesions may appear and grow until sexual maturity; impairment of growth and mobility of all or part of the extremities may be substantial and thus cause considerable handicap. As a rule, no new lesions after adolescence; rather, replacement of old lesions by bony substance. Malignant degeneration of enchondromas may occur in adulthood (perhaps in 5% of patients); renewed growth of a lesion should suggest this possibility.

Comment: Multiple enchondromas combined with multiple cavernous haemangiomas (tending to form pheboliths) and capillary haemangiomas in the same area represent a special form, the so-called Maffucci syndrome. This is associated with a high risk of degeneration (approximately 15%).

For the purposes of differential diagnosis, several recently delineated special forms with anomalies (of variable severity) of the vertebral bodies and other peculiarities should be considered.

Treatment: Surgical resection for patients with marked impairment of function, considerable disfigurement or suspected malignant transformation. Orthopaedic management of leg-length discrepancy (either surgical or conservative).

Illustrations:

1–4 A boy, aged 6 years and 6 months, normal psychological development; endochondromatosis since the third year of life. Only unilateral involvement. Left extremities, especially the leg, shorter than the right. Secondary tilting of the pelvis. Considerable impairment and disfiguration of the left hand. Carpal bones, radius, humerus, ilium, os pubis, tarsal bones and toes also show enchondromatous changes.

References:

Spranger J W, Langer Jr L O, Wiedemann H-R: *Bone dysplasias. An atlas of constitutional disorders of skeletal development.* Stuttgart and Philadephia: G Fischer and W B Saunders; 1974.

Shapiro F: Ollier's disease. *J Bone Jt Surg* 1982, **64A**:95.

Sun T-C, Swee R G *et al*: Chondrosarcoma in Maffucci's syndrome. *J Bone Jt Surg* 1985, **67A**:1214–1219.

Blauth W, Sönnichsen S: Enchondromatosen der Hand. *Z Orthop* 1986, **124**:165–172.

Urist M R: A 37-year follow-up evaluation of multiple-stage femur and tibia lengthening in dyschondroplasia... with a net gain of 23.3 centimeters. *Clin Orthopaed Rel Res* 1989, **242**:137.

Menger H, Kruse K, Spranger J: Spondyloenchondrodysplasia. *J Med Genet* 1989, **26**:93–99.

Raupp P, Kemperdick H: Neonatal radiological aspect of enchondromatosis... *Pediatr Radiol* 1990, **20**:337–338.

Le Merrer M *et al*: Genochondromatosis. *J Med Genet* 1991, **28**:485–489.

Freisinger P *et al*: Dysspondyloenchondromatosis. *Am J Med Genet* 1993, **45**:460–464.

Kozlowski K, Brostrom K *et al*: Dysspondyloenchondromatosis in the newborn. *Pediatr Radiol* 1994, **24**:311–315.

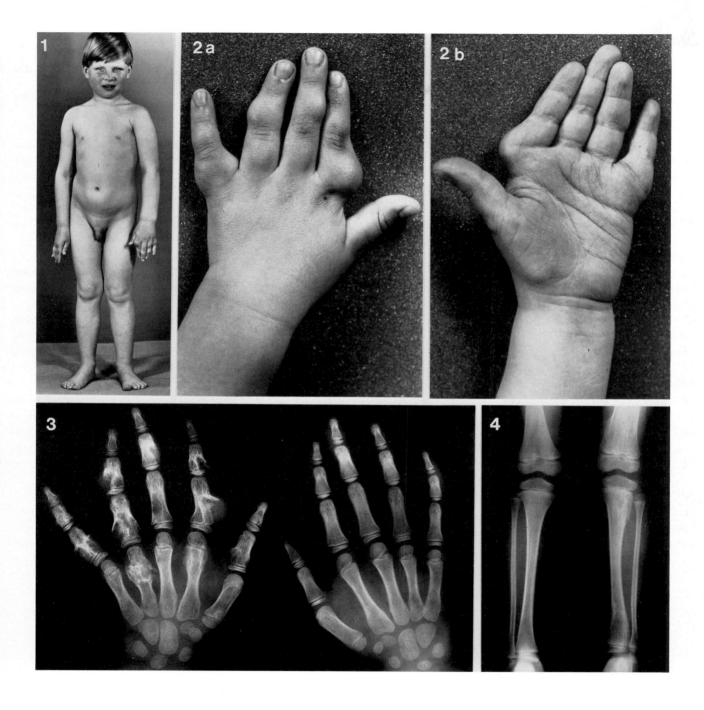

J.K.

An autosomal recessive syndrome with Apert-like spoon hands (syndactyly) and dysphalangism of the toes but an otherwise unremarkable phenotype.

Main signs:
- Almost complete syndactyly of all fingers but occasionally only partial syndactyly. Fixation of the metacarpophalangeal and interphalangeal joints in flexion.
- Dysphalangism of the toes, occasionally syndactyly.
- On radiograph, synostosis of the metacarpals, occasionally radio-ulnar synostosis.

Supplementary findings: Occasionally, shortened forearms with radio-ulnar, carpal and tarsal synostoses. Otherwise unremarkable phenotype, normal intelligence.

Manifestation: At birth.

Aetiology: Autosomal recessive disorder.

Frequency: Maybe 20 patients have been reported to date; of these, sibling observations in five different families.

Course, prognosis: Normal life expectancy.

Treatment: Microsurgery.

Differential diagnosis: Apert syndrome (9); polysyndactyly with brachymetacarpia, Bonola type (235).

Illustrations:
1a–c A 7-year-old male; total syndactyly bilaterally, flexion and extension restricted, pronation and supination impossible. Symmetrical syndactyly of the third and fourth toes.
2a–d The 4-year-old brother of **1**: hands identical, club hand, second and third toes close together. Radiograph: radio-ulnar synostoses, differentiated first metacarpal, remaining metacarpals undifferentiated.

References:
Cenani A, Lenz W: Totale Syndaktylie und totale radioulnare Synostose bei zwei Brüdern. Ein Beitrag zur Genetik der Syndaktylien. *Z Kinderheilk* 1976, **101**:181–190.
Drohm D, Lenz W, Yang T S: Totale Syndaktylie mit mesomeler Armverkürzung, radioulnären und metacarpalen Synostosen und Disorganisation der Phalangen ('Cenani-Syndaktylie'). *Klin Pädiatr* 1976, **188**:359–365.
Varma I C, Joseph R, Bhargava S *et al*: Split-hand and split-foot deformity inherited as an autosomal recessive trait. *Clin Genet* 1976, **9**:8–14.
Dodinval P: Oligodactyly and multiple synostoses of the extremities: two cases in sibs. A variant of Cenani-Lenz syndactyly. *Hum Genet* 1979, **48**:183–189.
Pfeiffer R A, Meisel-Stosiek M: Present nosology of the Cenani–Lenz type of syndactyly. *Clin Genet* 1982, **21**:74–79.

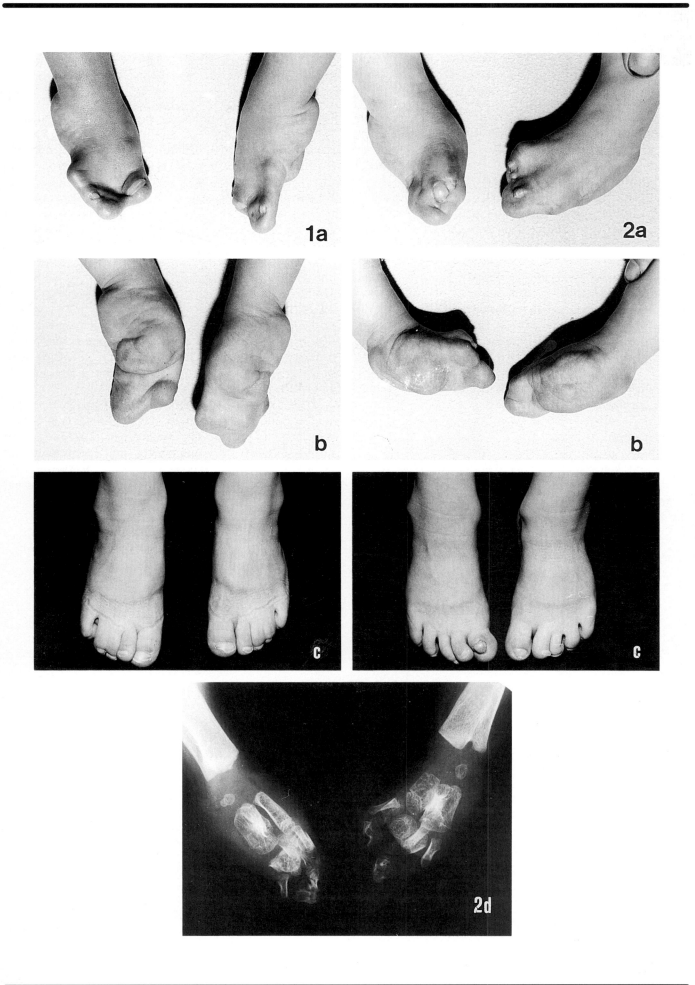

J.K.

A familial type of polysyndactyly with short thumbs, metacarpals and middle phalanges and analogous malformations of the feet.

Main signs:
- Short, stubby, projecting thumbs,
- Short, stubby metacarpals, sometimes deformed.
- Polysyndactyly of all fingers or of fingers III–V (**6**) or III and IV, fusion of the distal phalanges with short middle phalanges.
- Mild cutaneous syndactyly of the toes, hypoplasia of the toes, dysphalangism.

Radiologically, long slender proximal phalanges of the fingers, bony syndactyly. 11 and 12 carpal bones. Short, stubby metatarsals, absent middle phalanges of the toes, supernumerary toes.

Supplementary findings: Normal height, exceptional dexterity, normal intelligence.

Manifestation: At birth.

Aetiology: Autosomal recessive inheritance.

Frequency: Five patients reported to date, one concerning siblings (male and female) from a consanguineous marriage.

Course, prognosis: Normal life expectancy.

Diagnosis, differential diagnosis: Cenani–Lenz syndactyly (*234*); syndactyly type IV (Haas type).

Treatment: The dexterity of the patients when fastening buttons, writing, sewing, and so on is so impressive that a specialist hand surgeon should be consulted on the question of early surgery.

Illustrations:
1 A 15-year-old boy.
2 His 20-year-old sister.
1c–f The patient's hands; on the right: first, second and fifth fingers single; third and fourth fingers syndactylous; tripartite nail; on the left: corresponding situation with syndactyly of third and fourth fingers but only one nail.
1g Dysphalangism of the feet.
2c–f Similar changes in the sister: first finger, one phalangeal bone present; second and fifth fingers, two phalangeal bones present; the syndactylous third and fourth fingers show the same numbers of nails on the right and the left hands respectively as those of the brother.
Radiograph: no radio-ulnar synostoses; 11 and 12 carpal bones.

References:
Kunze J, Lenz W, Sugiura Y, Yang T-S: Polysyndaktylie mit Brachymetacarpie (Typ Bonola). *Klin Pädiatr* 1992, **204**:43–47.

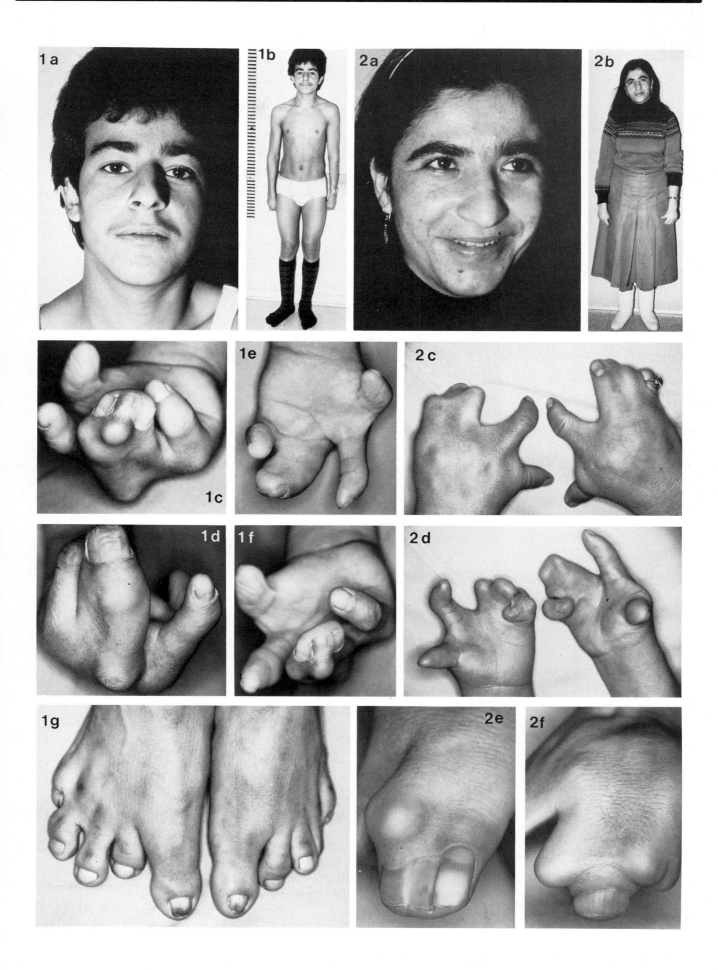

H.-R.W/ J.K.

A syndrome of polydactyly and syndactyly of the hands and feet with an unusually shaped skull.

Main signs:
- Broad thumbs and halluces or pre-axial polydactyly of the feet and (occasionally) the hands and postaxial polydactyly of the hands, less frequently also of the feet. Usually significant syndactyly of the second to fourth (fifth) fingers and of various toes (**3–6**).
- Macrocephaly and brachycephaly with high, prominent forehead with a median ridge (**1 and 2**). Broad nasal bridge, hypertelorism, possible slight antimongoloid slant of the palpebral fissures and wide nares (**2**).

Supplementary findings: Radiological picture of the thumbs and halluces varies from minor abnormalities of shape to complete duplication of the ray.

Manifestation: At birth.

Aetiology: Autosomal dominant hereditary defect with complete penetrance but variable expression. Gene localized to the short arm of chromosome 7 (7p13).

Frequency: Low (at least 100 patients reported to date).

Course, prognosis: Favourable.

Diagnosis, differential diagnosis: Differentiation from Carpenter syndrome (*11*) should not be difficult. The acrocallosal syndrome (Schinzel) shows agenesis of the corpus callosum (cranial ultrasound useful), psychomotor retardation and autosomal recessive inheritance as differentiating features.

Treatment: Surgical correction of the extremities should be started sufficiently early, at a time determined with the hand surgeon and suited to the individual.
Genetic counselling.

Illustrations:
1 A 4-month-old boy.
2 His twin brother.
3, 5 Polysyndactyly (clinically and radiologically) of the right hand of the boy in **1**.
4 The right forefoot of the same boy.
6 Unusually severe polysyndactyly of the right foot of the twin in **2**.

References:
Hootnick D, Holmes L B: Familial polysyndaktyly and craniofacial anomalies. *Clin Genet* 1972, 3:124.
Fryns J P, van Noyen G, van den Berghe H: The Greig polysyndactyly craniofacial dysmorphism syndrome. *Eur J Pediatr* 1981, 136:217.
Chudley A E, Houston C S: The Greig cephalopolysyndactyly syndrome… *Am J Med Genet* 1982, 13:269–276.
Fryns J P: Le syndrome de Greig… *J Génét Hum* 1982, 30(Suppl)5:403–408.
Baraitser M, Winter R M et al: Greig cephalopolysyndactyly: report of 13 affected individuals… *Clin Genet* 1983, 24:257–265.
Tommerup N, Nielsen F: A familial reciprocal translocation t(3;7)(p 21.1;p13) associated with the Greig… syndrome. *Am J Med Genet* 1983, 16:313–321.
Gollop T R, Fontes L R: The Greig cephalopolysyndactyly syndrome… *Am J Med Genet* 1985, 22:59–68.
Kunze J, Kaufmann H J: Greig cephalopolysyndactyly syndrome. *Helv Paediatr Acta* 1985, 40:489–495.
Legius E, Fryns J P et al: Schinzel acrocallosal syndrome: a variant example of the Greig syndrome? *Ann Génét* 1985, 28:239–240.
Brueton L, Huson S M et al: Chromosomal localisation of a developmental gene in man… *Am J Med Genet* 1988, 31:799–804.
Philip N, Apicella N et al: The acrocallosal syndrome. *Eur J Pediatr* 1988, 147:206–208.
Krüger G, Götz J et al: Greig syndrome in a large kindred due to reciprocal chromosome translocation t(6;7)(q27;p13). *Am J Med Genet* 1989, 32:411–416.
Pettigrew A L, Greenberg F et al: Greig syndrome…; confirmation of the localisation… to 7p13. *Hum Genet* 1991, 87:452–456.
Fryns J P, de Waele P et al: Apparent Greig cephalopolysyndactyly and sinus node disease. *Am J Med Genet* 1993, 45:38–40.
Vortkamp A, Gessler M et al: Isolation of a yeast artificial chromosome… (GCPS) gene region. *Genomics* 1994, 22:563–569.

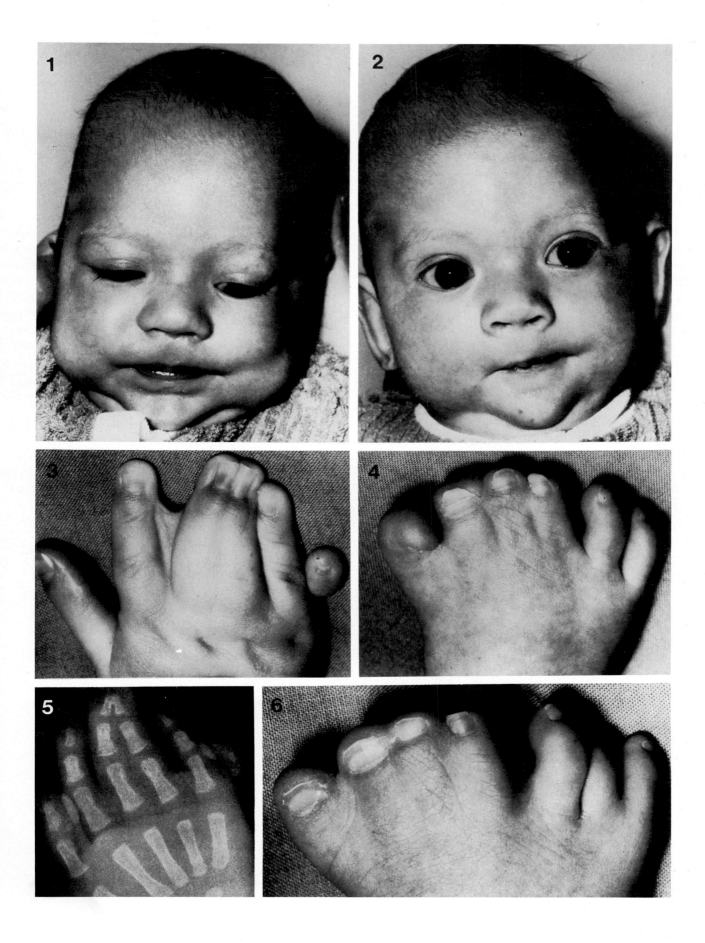

237 Orofaciodigital Syndrome Type II

(OFD Syndrome II, Mohr Syndrome)

H.-R.W

A hereditary disorder occurring in both sexes and comprising bilateral postaxial polydactyly of the hands, polysyndactyly of the halluces, lobulation of the tongue, hyperplastic frenula and unusual facies.

Main signs:
- Postaxial and sometimes also pre-axial polydactyly of the hands, as well as brachydactyly, syndactyly and clinodactyly (**1**).
- Duplication of the halluces; possibly also postaxial polydactyly of the feet (**2**).
- Clefting or lobulation of the tongue (into two or more lobes) with nodules at the base of the lobular clefts; hyperplastic oral frenula.
- Unusual facies: hypertelorism or telecanthus; broad nasal bridge and broad nasal tip, which may show a median groove; possible median cleft of the upper lip; mandibular and maxillary hypoplasia; central incisors frequently absent; high palate or cleft palate.

Supplementary findings: Radiographs of the feet show broad, short (or possibly duplicated) first metatarsal, cuneiform and navicular bones.

Possible conductive hearing impairment with malformation of the incus. Mental development normal as a rule. Occasionally, brain malformations, short stature.

Manifestation: At birth.

Aetiology: Autosomal recessive disorder.

Frequency: Low.

Course, prognosis: Usually normal life expectancy.

Differential diagnosis: Orofaciodigital syndrome I only occurs in females (X-chromosomal dominant inheritance); for differentiating characteristics see syndrome 36.

Treatment: Surgical correction of clefts and hypertrophic frenula; early evaluation of hearing with treatment when indicated; orthodontic and dental care; removal of supernumerary halluces and correction of the hands for some patients.

Genetic counselling.

Illustrations:

1 and 2 A girl with Mohr syndrome, the second child of healthy parents. Broad nasal bridge, median notch of the upper lip, cleft tip of the tongue with small fibromas bilaterally; high palate, notched alveolar ridges and thick frenula. Polydactyly of the hands and feet with duplication of the rays of the halluces.

References:

Pfeiffer R A, Majewski F, Mannkopf H: Das Syndrom von Mohr und Claussen. *Klin Pädiatr* 1972, **184**:224.
Levy E P, Fletcher B D, Fraser C: Mohr syndrome with subclinical expression of the bifid great toe. *Am J Dis Child* 1974, **128**:531.
Annerén G, Arvidson B *et al*: Oro-facio-digital syndromes I and II... *Clin Genet* 1984, **26**:178–186.
Baraitser M: The orofaciodigital (OFD) syndromes. *J Med Genet* 1986, **23**:116–119.
Silengo M C, Bell G L *et al*: Oro-facio-digital syndrome II... *Clin Genet* 1987, **31**:331–336.
Reardon W, Harbord M G *et al*: Central nervous system malformations in Mohr's syndrome. *J Med Genet* 1989, **26**:659–663.
Toriello H V: Heterogeneity and variability in the oral-facial-digital syndromes. *Am J Med Genet Suppl* 1988, **4**:149–159.
Annerén G, Gustavson K-H *et al*: Abnormalities of the cerebellum in oro-facio-digital syndrome II (Mohr syndrome). *Clin Genet* 1990, **38**:69–73.

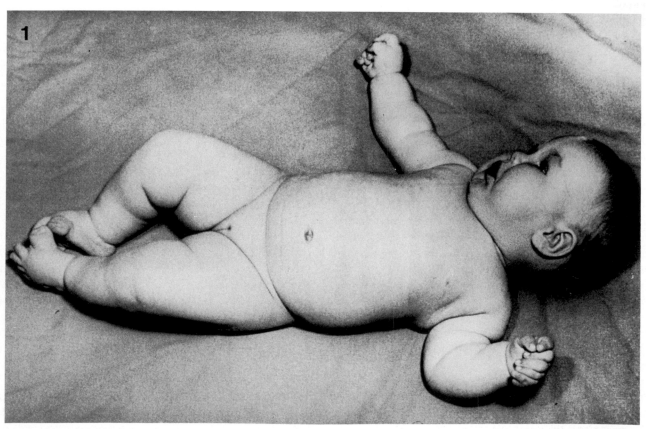

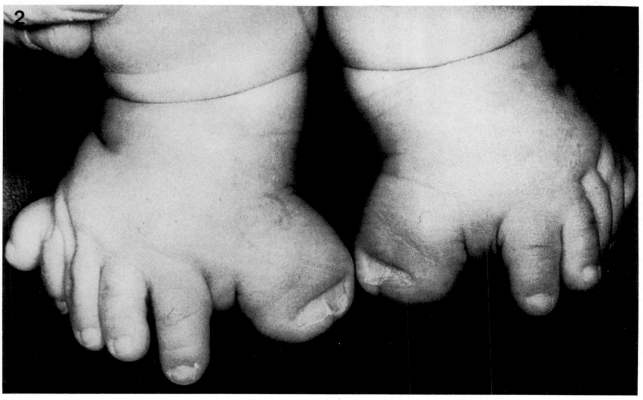

238 Acrofacial Dysostosis of the Predominantly Postaxial Type

(Acrofacial Dysostosis, Genée-Wiedemann Type; Genée-Wiedemann Syndrome; 'Miller Syndrome'; Postaxial Acrofacial Dysostosis Syndrome [POADS])

H.-R.W
P. Meinecke

A hereditary mandibulofacial dysostosis with hypoplasia of the extremities, especially oligodactyly caused by absence of the fifth rays of the upper extremities.

Main signs:
- Bilateral absence (or rudimentary appendage in isolated cases) of the fifth fingers and toes with abnormally short forearms (particularly the ulnae) and a tendency to club-hand position with ulnar deviation (1–4, 6–7).
- Malar and mandibular hypoplasia; frequent cleft palate or lip; deformity of the external ears (5); anomalies of the eyelids (short palpebral fissures with antimongoloid slant; usually distinct lateral coloboma of the lower lids; deficient eyelashes; inability to close the eyes completely and in some patients characteristically large-appearing eyes).

Supplementary findings: Accessory nipples frequently found.

Psychomotor retardation in a few patients.

Besides the absence of the fifth ray, radiographs show carpal anomalies and possibly radio-ulnar synostosis. In some patients, there may be various other clinical or radiological skeletal anomalies, ranging from pre-axial limb defects to 'phocomelia' and involvement of the scapular bones, thoracic cage and the pelvic girdle or even of the internal organs (heart, genitalia).

Possible conjunctivitis, inflammation of the middle ear; possible hearing impairment.

Manifestation: At birth.

Aetiology: Sporadic occurrence in most patients. Autosomal recessive and, less frequently, autosomal dominant inheritance. Heterogeneity. Polytopic field defect during blastogenesis.

Frequency: Low (approximately 40 documented observations to date).

Differential diagnosis: Nager's acrofacial dysostosis (29) could be said to present an 'opposite clinical picture', with marked pre-axial involvement of the extremities. Mandibulofacial dysostosis, as in the Treacher–Collins syndrome (28), corresponds only with regard to facial signs. A series of other mandibulofacial and acrofacial dysostoses, some of which result in early death, still await a more precise delineation (see *Opitz et al*, 1993, for an overview).

Treatment: Symptomatic. Initially, attention to possible problems with breathing and drinking. Closure of clefts. Orthopaedic or limb surgery, cosmetic surgery or orthodontic correction may be indicated. Early assessment of hearing. Speech therapy when indicated. Genetic counselling. Prenatal diagnosis.

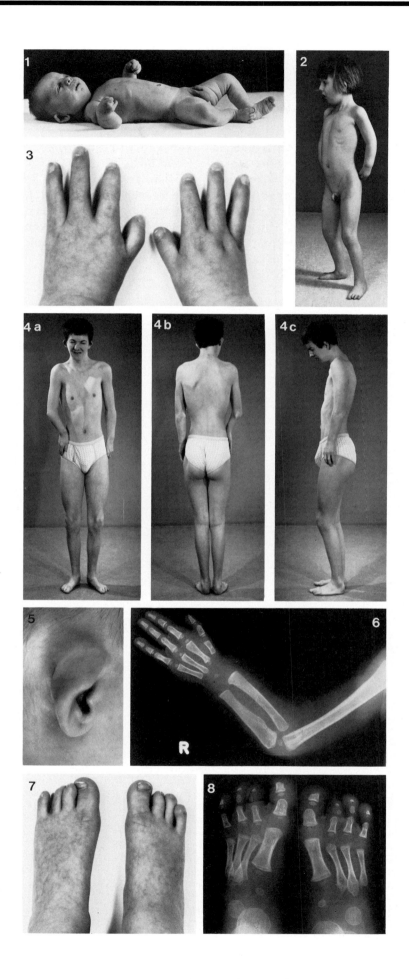

H.-R.W
P. Meinecke

Illustrations:

Previous page:

1–8 The same patient as an infant (**1, 5**), at 3 years (**6, 8**), at 4 years and 6 months (**2, 3, 7**) and at 15 years (**4a–c**). Brachycephaly. Eyelid anomalies with notching of the lateral lower lids; incomplete closure of the eyelids, large-appearing eyes. Cleft palate, micrognathia. Congenital heart defect (ventricular septal defect). Cryptorchidism. Pes planus. Mental retardation. Radiologically (**6, 8**), apart from aplasia of the fifth ray, hypoplasia of the ulna with proximal broadening; delayed ossification; anomalies of the bones of the hand and foot.

Opposite page:

1–4 A 13-year-old boy.

5 and 6 His 19-year-old sister.

2 Micrognathia and malar and mandibular hypoplasia (**5 and 6**), blepharophimosis, cleft palate; in the girl, also lateral ectropion of the lower eyelid. Hypoplastic, biphalangeal fifth finger, proximally displaced thumbs and aplasia of the fifth toe (all bilaterally). Normal mental development.

References:

Genée E: Une forme extensive de dysostose mandibulofaciale. *J Génét Hum* 1969, 17:45–52.

Wiedemann H-R: Mißbildungs-Retardierungs-Syndrom mit Fehlen des 5. Strahls an Händen und Füßen, Gaumenspalte, dysplastischen Ohren und Augenlidern und radioulnarer Synostose. *Klin Pädiatr* 1973, 185:181–186.

Miller M, Fineman R, Smith D: Postaxial acrofacial dysostosis syndrome. *J Pediatr* 1979, 95:970–975.

Lewin S O, Opitz J M: Fibular A/hypoplasia: review and documentation of the fibular developmental field. *Am J Med Genet Suppl* 1986, 2:215.

Donnai D, Hughes H E, Winter R M: Postaxial acrofacial dysostosis (Miller) syndrome: *J Med Genet* 1987, 24:422.

Meinecke P, Wiedemann H-R: Robin sequence and oligodactyly in mother and son... *Am J Med Genet* 1987, 27:953.

Opitz J M, Stickler G B: The Genée-Wiedemann syndrome... *Am J Med Genet* 1987, 27:971.

Hauss-Albert H, Passarge E: Postaxial acrofacial dysostosis syndrome... *Am J Med Genet* 1988, 31:701–703.

Chrzanowska K H, Fryns J P *et al*: Phenotype variability in... acrofacial dysostosis syndrome... *Clin Genet* 1989, 35:157–160.

Le Merrer M *et al*: Acrofacial dysostoses. *Am J Med Genet* 1989, 33:318–322.

Richieri-Costa A *et al*: Postaxial acrofacial dysostosis... *Am J Med Genet* 1989, 33:477–479.

Robinow M *et al*: Genée-Wiedemann syndrome in a family (Letter). *Am J Med Genet* 1990, 37:293.

Ogilvy-Stuart A L *et al*: Miller syndrome... *J Med Genet* 1991, 28:695–700.

Giannotti A *et al*: Familial postaxial acrofacial dysostosis syndrome. *J Med Genet* 1992, 29:752.

Pereira S C S.*et al*: Postaxial acrofacial dysostosis... *Am J Med Genet* 1992, 44:274–279.

Chrzanowska K *et al*: Miller postaxial acro-facial dysostosis... (Letter). *Clin Genet* 1993, 43:270.

Opitz J M *et al*: Acrofacial dysostoses: review... *Am J Med Genet* 1993, 47:660–678.

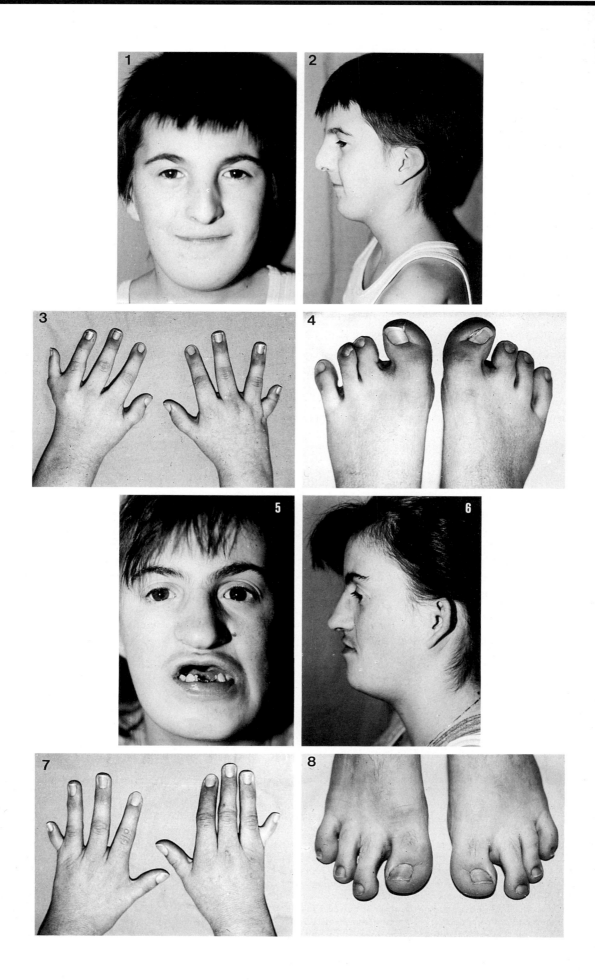

H.-R.W

A syndrome of unusual facies, sparse, brittle scalp hair, clinical and radiological abnormalities of the hands and, not infrequently, short stature.

Main signs:

- Facial dysmorphism with 'bulbous' or 'pear-shaped' nose, large and sometimes prominent ears, long broad philtrum and thin upper lip. Eyebrows poorly developed laterally (1).
- Sparse, fine, brittle and usually light-coloured scalp hair (1).
- Short hands and feet with finger deformities caused by broadening of the proximal interphalangeal joints and sometimes deviation of the phalangeal axis, with little or no limitation of movement. Thumbs and halluces short and broad (2 and 3). 'Cone-shaped' epiphyses on radiograph; shortening of some metacarpals and metatarsals (5 and 6).

Supplementary findings: Not infrequently, moderately short stature.

Soft, brittle fingernails and toenails. Possible dysodontiasis.

Perthes-type dysplasia of the head of the femur, kyphosis, scoliosis, winged scapulae, thoracic deformity and cardiovascular anomalies may occur.

Manifestation: Facial characteristics and sparse hair growth may be apparent from birth but as a rule the children are first brought to medical attention later in childhood because of 'swellings' over the proximal interphalangeal joints.

Aetiology: Autosomal dominant inheritance with variable penetrance and very variable expression. Apparently there is also an autosomal recessive form. Thus, presumably, heterogeneity. Presumed gene locus 8q24.12.

Frequency: Low; up to 1985 approximately 200 patients had been reported in the literature.

Course, prognosis: Normal life expectancy. The osteo-articular changes are usually progressive; in some patients, early arthritis in the hands, vertebral column and other areas.

The sparse scalp hair and poor self-image because of the shape of the nose, deformed fingers and in some patients short stature, may cause problems, especially in girls and women.

Differential diagnosis: Trichorhinophalangeal dysplasia type II (Langer–Giedion syndrome) (232).

Treatment: Orthopaedic and orthodontic care, plastic surgery (nose), and a wig may be indicated. Psychological support.

Genetic counselling.

Illustrations:

1–6 A 15-year-old, 167.5 cm tall school boy showing the typical syndrome, apparently inherited from his father. Scalp hair, lateral eyebrows and body hair sparse. Narrowly spaced teeth with relatively small lower jaw. Nails thin and extremely brittle; skin of the fingerpads also very tender and sensitive. Nails of the halluces ingrown, with inflammation. Painless enlargement and slight flexion of the proximal interphalangeal joints but good mobility. Thumbs and halluces especially short and broad.

References:

Spranger J W, Langer Jr L O, Wiedemann H-R: *Bone dysplasias. An atlas of constitutional disorders of skeletal development.* Stuttgart and Philadephia: G Fischer and W B Saunders; 1974.

Frias J L, Felman A H, Garnica A D *et al*: Variable expressivity in the trichorhinophalangeal syndrome type I. *Birth Defects Orig Art Ser* 1979, 15(5B):361.

Ranke M B, Heitkamp H-C: Tricho-rhino-phalangeales Syndrom. *Mschr Kinderheilk* 1980, **128**:208.

Goodman R M, Trilling R, Hertz M *et al*: New clinical observations in the trichorhinophalangeal syndrome. *J Craniofacial Genet Dev Biol* 1981, **1**:15.

Gaardsted C, Madsen E H, Friedrich U: A Danish kindred with tricho-rhino-phalangeal syndrome type I. *Eur J Pediatr* 1982, **139**:84–87.

Fryns J P, Van den Berghe H: 8q24.12 Interstitial deletion in trichorhinophalangeal syndrome type I. *Hum Genet* 1986, **74**:188–189.

Goldblatt J, Smart R D: Tricho-rhino-phalangeal syndrome without exostoses, with an interstitial deletion of 8q23. *Clin Genet* 1986, **29**:434–438.

Howell C J, Wynne-Davies R: The tricho-rhino-phalangeal syndrome... 14 cases in 7 kindreds. *J Bone Jt Surg* 1986, **68B**:311–314.

Schlesinger A E, Poznanski A K: Flattening of the distal femoral epiphyses in the trichorhinophalangeal syndrome. *Pediatr Radiol* 1986, **16**:498–500.

Bühler E M, Bühler U K *et al*: A final word on the tricho-rhino-phalangeal syndromes. *Clin Genet* 1987, **31**:273–275.

Yamamoto Y, Oguro N *et al*: Prometaphase chromosomes in the tricho-rhino-phalangeal syndrome type I. *Am J Med Genet* 1989, **32**:524–527.

Hamers A, Jongbloet *et al*: Severe mental retardation in a patient with tricho-rhino-phalangeal syndrome type I and 8q deletion. *Eur J Pediatr* 1990, 149:618–620.

Marchau F E *et al*: Tricho-rhino-phalangeal syndrome type I... *Am J Med Genet* 1993, **45**:450–455.

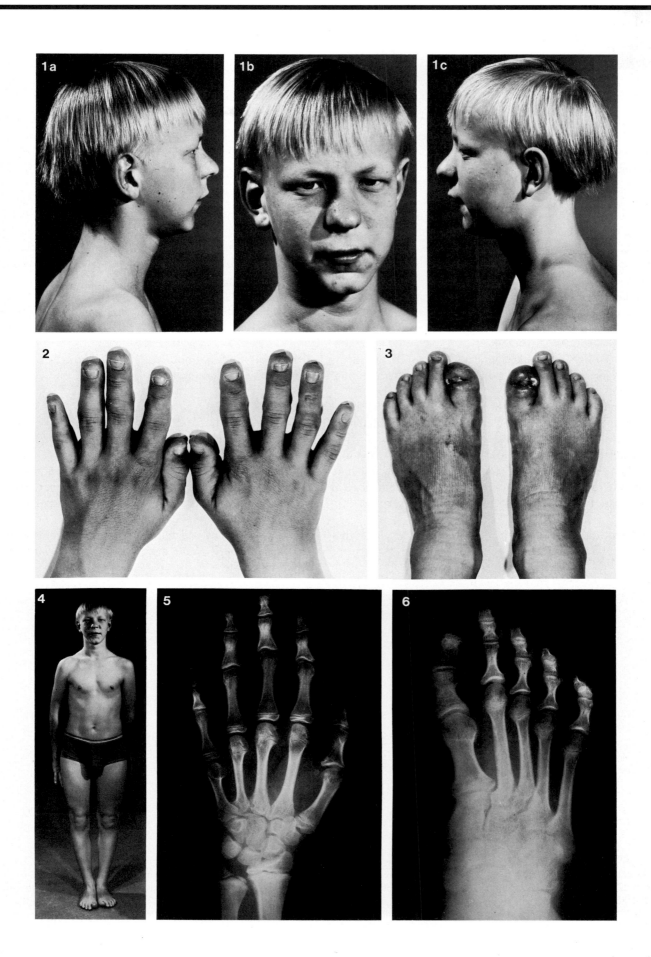

Oculodento-osseous Dysplasia

(Oculodentodigital Dysplasia, Meyer–Schwickerath Syndrome, Osteodentodigital Dysplasia)

J.K.

A characteristic syndrome with microcornea, hypoplastic alae nasi, enamel hypoplasia, bilateral syndactyly of the fourth and fifth fingers and hypoplasia or aplasia of the phalanges of the toes.

Main signs:

- Microcornea (in most patients with normal-sized eyeball), dysplasia of the iris.
- Long, thin nose with pronounced nasal columella, hypoplastic alae nasi and narrow nostrils.
- Enamel hypoplasia or dysplasia.
- Syndactyly of the fourth and fifth fingers bilaterally; dysplasia, hypoplasia or aplasia of one or more middle phalanges of the toes (seen on radiograph).

Supplementary findings: Narrow palpebral fissures, medial epicanthus, refraction anomalies, strabismus, glaucoma.

Clinodactyly, camptodactyly, cranial hyperostosis, thickened mandible, broad clavicles, thickened ribs, deficient tubulation of the long bones.

Generalized hair-growth anomaly, including eyebrows and eyelashes: hypotrichosis, trichorrhexis; lusterless, brittle hair.

Rarely, conductive hearing impairment and neurological signs in the form of hyperreflexia, ataxia, dysarthria.

Manifestation: At birth; other features, such as glaucoma, later.

Aetiology: Usually autosomal dominant disorder with variable expression but also sporadic cases (dominant new mutations, increased paternal age). Individual cases caused by autosomal recessive inheritance? Possible heterogeneity.

Frequency: Barely 100 patients reported up to 1991.

Course, prognosis: As a rule, normal psychomotor development; approximately 10% of patients show mild mental retardation. Impaired vision.

Differential diagnosis: Craniotubular hyperostoses, sclerosteosis, Pyle disease.

Treatment: Ophthalmological (glaucoma). Possible hand surgery. Genetic counselling.

Illustrations:

1a and b Female newborn; hypoplastic alae nasi, symmetrical syndactyly of the fourth and fifth fingers.

2a–f A 6-month-old boy: thin, sparse eyebrows and eyelashes. Microcornea, medial epicanthi, pronounced nasal columella with hypoplastic alae nasi; syndactyly of the fourth and fifth digits bilaterally; absent middle phalanges of the toes and hypoplastic distal phalanges.

3a and b A 3-day-old female newborn; depressed nasal bridge, hypoplastic alae nasi, syndactyly of third to fifth digits bilaterally.

References:

Beighton P, Hamersma H, Raad M: Oculo-dento-osseous dysplasia: heterogeneity or variable expression. *Clin Genet* 1979, **16**:169–177.

Judisch G F, Martin-Casals A, Hanson J W *et al*: Oculodentodigital dysplasia. Four new reports and a literature review. *Arch Ophthalmol* 1979, **97**:878–884.

Patton M A, Laurence K M: Three new cases of oculodentodigital (ODD) syndrome: development of the facial phenotype. *J Med Genet* 1985, **22**:386–389.

Traboulsi E I, Faris B M, Der Kaloustian V M: Persistent hyperplastic primary vitreous and recessive oculo-dento-osseous dysplasia. *Am J Med Genet* 1986, **24**:95–100.

Gutman D H, Zackai E H *et al*: Oculodentodigital dysplasia syndrome associated with abnormal white matter. *Am J Med Genet* 1991, **41**:18–20.

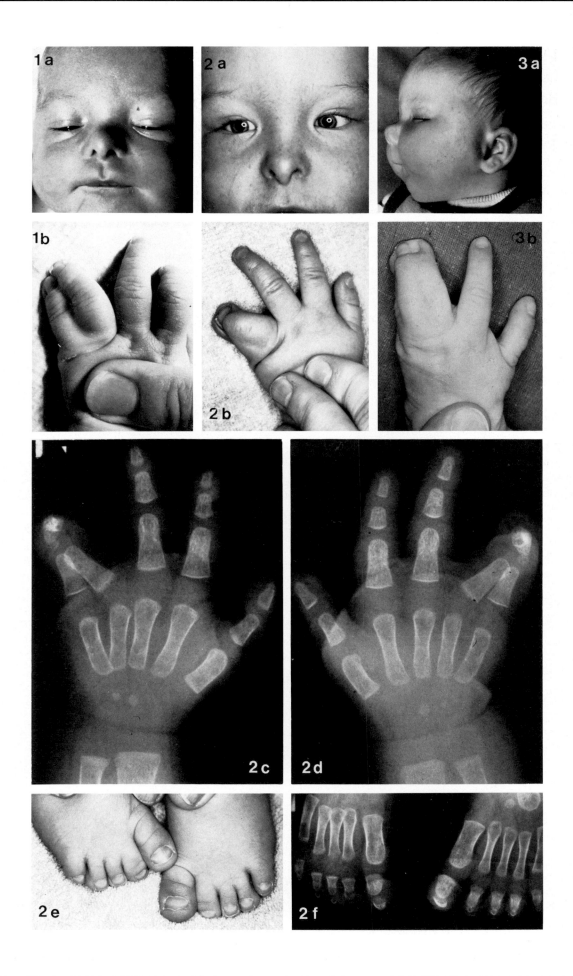

241 Symphalangism–Brachydactyly Syndrome with Conductive Hearing Impairment

(Facio-audiosymphalangism Syndrome, Syndrome of Multiple Synostoses with Conductive Hearing Impairment)

H.-R.W

A syndrome of malformations of the hands and feet, characteristic facies and defective hearing.

Main signs:
- Congenital limitation of movement at the proximal interphalangeal joints of the second to fifth fingers (radiologically, phalangeal fusion may not be seen until later) with absence of the normal articular creases; possible limited movement at the elbow joints and, later, at the wrist and ankle joints, in some patients with abnormal gait.
- Brachydactyly, possible absence of distal segments of fingers (or toes), cutaneous syndactylies (**1 and 2**).
- Unusual facies: long and rather narrow face with long, prominent nose, broad nasal bridge, asymmetrical mouth with thin upper lip (**1**).
- Conductive hearing impairment, possibly first apparent in adolescence (ankylosis of the auditory ossicles).

Supplementary findings: Normal height but possible abnormal proportions because of short arms.

On radiograph, abnormally short first metacarpals and metatarsals; gradual development of symphalangism of the proximal phalanges of the second to fourth fingers (**3 and 4**); later, ankylosis also of the carpals (**4**) and tarsals; various anomalies of the elbow region, even radio-humeral synostosis (**5**).

Manifestation: At birth and thereafter.

Aetiology: Hereditary disorder, autosomal dominant. Considerable intrafamilial variability.

Frequency: Very low (up to 1985, only 20 documented observations).

Course, prognosis: Symphalangism, ankylosis in the wrist and ankle region, and hearing impairment tend to progress.

Treatment: Corrective surgical measures for the extremities should only be carried out for exceptional patients and with utmost care. Early evaluation of hearing; treatment as indicated.

Genetic counselling.

Illustrations:
1–3, 5 A 2-year-old boy.
4 A raidiograph of his father's hand.

References:
Maroteaux P, Bouvet J P et al: La maladie des synostoses multiples. *Nouv Presse Méd* 1972, 1:3041–3047.
Herrmann J: Symphalangism and brachydactyly syndrome... *Birth Defects Orig Art Ser X* 1974, 5:23–53.
Königsmark B W, Gorlin R J: Dominant symphalangism and conduction deafness. In: *Genetic and metabolic deafness*. Philadelphia: W B Saunders 1976.
Poisson D, Zerbib M et al: Maladies des synostoses multiples. *Arch Fr Pédiatr* 1983, 40:35–37.
da-Silva E O, Filho S M et al: Multiple synostosis syndrome... *Am J Med Genet* 1984, 18:237–247.
Hurvitz S A, Goodman R M et al: The facio-audio-symphalangism syndrome... review of the literature. *Clin Genet* 1985, 28:61–68.

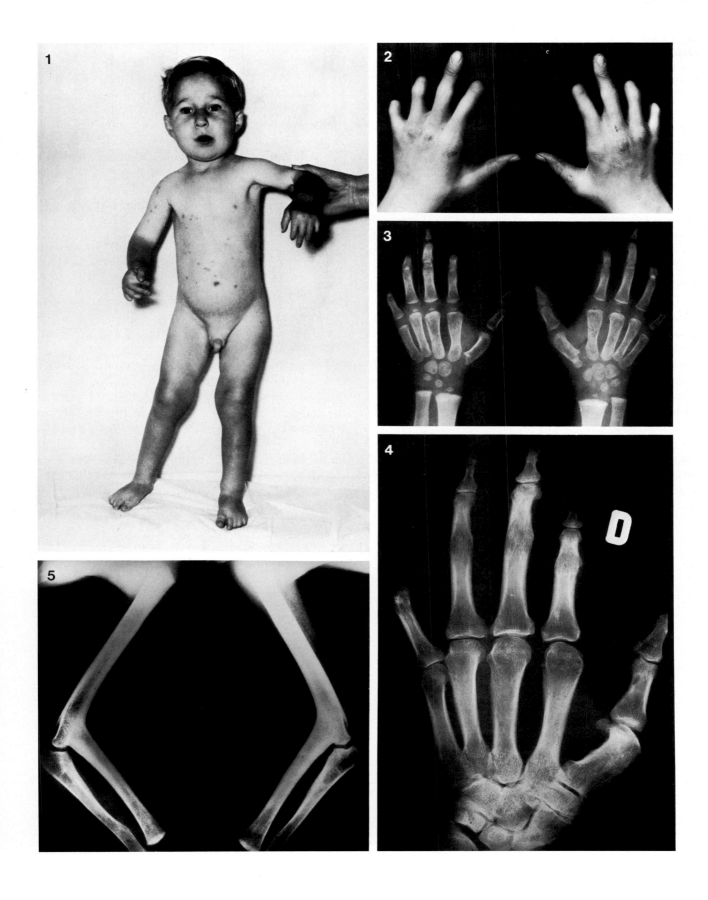

H.-R.W

A syndrome of psychomotor retardation with microcephaly, unusual facies and other diverse anomalies.

Main signs:
- Primary psychomotor retardation; (brachycephaly) microcephaly.
- Facies: slight antimongoloid slant of the palpebral fissures, left more than right; right epicanthus; relatively narrow palpebral fissures; thin alae nasi; large mouth. Low-set, prominent, simple ears (**1 and 2**). Microretrognathia. High-arched palate.
- Broad wrists, barely distinguishable from the forearms (**4**) and shapeless, pillar-like lower legs (**1, 3**). Progressive right-convex scoliosis of the thoracic spine (**3c**). Short hands with proximal cutaneous syndactyly between the second to fourth fingers bilaterally, clinodactyly of the left index finger and short tapering fingers with hypoplastic terminal phalanges (**4**). Limited movement at the ankles. Recurrent dislocation of the left patella. Short feet in club-foot position with dysdactyly; elongated halluces (**6 and 7**).

Supplementary findings: Short stature (below the 10th percentile). Suggestion of pterygium colli. Relatively sparse hair growth. Bilateral undescended testes (at 4 years) and left cryptorchidism (at 12 years and 9 months); small penis. Small atrial septal defect; possible small ventricular septal defect.

Radiologically: poorly modelled clavicles, high narrow pelvis, marked coxa valga. Clubbing of the proximal ends of the metacarpals, especially fifth, bilaterally. Slender fingers with strikingly short terminal phalanges (**5**). Dysdactyly of the feet (**7**).

Manifestation: At birth and later.

Aetiology: Not clear.

Treatment: Symptomatic.

Illustrations:
1–7 The patient at 12 years and 9 months and 15 years and 6 months, the third child of healthy, non-consanguineous parents (father 43 and mother 33 years old at the patient's birth). Unremarkable pregnancy; normal birth 3 weeks before term with weight 2500 g and length 49 cm.
Endocrinological and laboratory examinations negative; repeated chromosomal analyses unremarkable (including banded preparations).

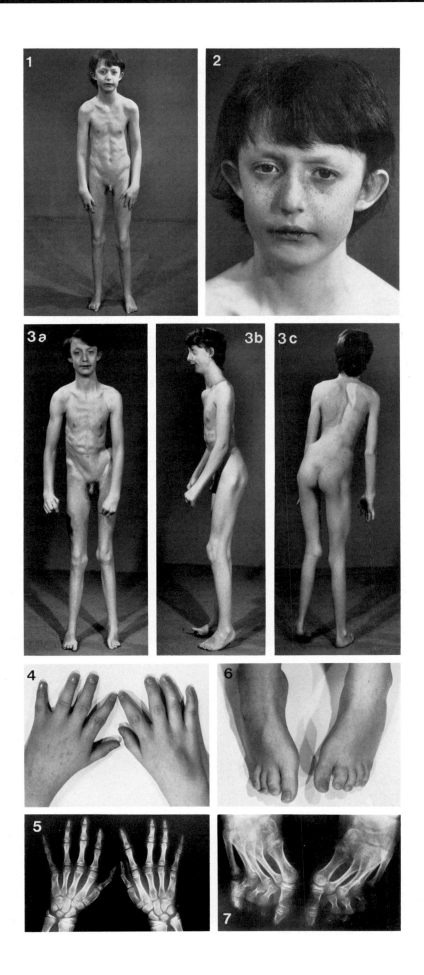

Hereditary Carpotarsal Osteolysis with Nephropathy
(Idiopathic Multicentric Osteolysis)

H.-R.W

A hereditary disorder with progressive carpotarsal osteolysis and chronic progressive nephropathy.

Main signs:
- Gradual shortening of wrists, ankles, metacarpus and metatarsus bilaterally and usually symmetrically as a result of progressive osteolysis starting in the carpals and tarsals (1, 3, 5–10). Possibly preceded or accompanied by soft-tissue swelling, tenderness, limited mobility, and warming of the affected region. Increasing deformity with ulnar deviation or volar subluxation of the shortened hands and eventual formation of claw hands or short pes cavus with overlapping toes (7).
- Progressive nephropathy (proteinuria, possible haematuria; development of arterial hypertension and so on).

Supplementary findings: Kyphoscoliosis not infrequent; development of muscular atrophy, especially in the distal extremities and of flexion contractures of the large joints.
  Unusual facies with mild exophthalmos, hypoplasia of the upper jaw and micrognathia has been noted; furthermore, mental retardation and short adult stature in isolated patients.

Manifestation: Osteolysis apparent in the first decade of life, generally in the toddler, rarely as early as the first year of life. Nephropathy towards the end of the first decade or during the second.

Aetiology: Autosomal dominant disorder with basic defect unknown. Autosomal recessive inheritance also reported. Possible genetic heterogeneity.

Frequency: Very low (30–40 observations have been reported).

Course, prognosis: Usually slow progression of the osteolysis, sometimes leading to complete dissolution of the carpal and tarsal bones and 'licked candy-stick' appearance of the shortened and narrowed ends of the adjacent long bones (9). Thus, gradual shortening of the forearms and sometimes of the lower legs; possible analogous involvement of the elbow regions and other joints, with corresponding limitation of movement. Skeletal changes may stabilize toward the end of the second decade of life. However, the nephropathy runs a protracted course, with possibly poor prognosis.

Differential diagnosis: Other osteolysis syndromes (*244, 245*). Rheumatoid arthritis may be considered at the onset of the illness but is easily excluded.

Treatment: Symptomatic. Career guidance. Genetic counselling. Kidney transplantation may be indicated.

Illustrations:
1, 2, 5, 7, 9 A 39-year-old woman.
3, 4, 6, 8, 10 Her 9-year-old, mildly mentally retarded son.
  Two older children healthy. Mother and son of normal height; both show a slightly receding chin; the mother finds her son's broad nasal bridge unusual ('unknown in the family'). In both, onset of symptoms in the left hand in early school years, subsequently less severe involvement of the right hand; feet more severely affected (left more than right). The mother's narrowed, shortened left hand, with markedly limited mobility, as in the son, shows a Dupuytren-like picture; similar development of connective tissue nodules and cords on the plantar fascia bilaterally. Proteinuria in both mother and son (in the former, fluctuating hypertension) varying from 1 g to 3 g/day.

References:
Erickson C M, Hirschberger M, Stickler G B: Carpal-tarsal osteolysis. *J Pediatr* 1978, **93**:779.
Fryns J P: Ostéolyse essentielle à début carpien et tarsien. *J Génét Hum 30 Suppl* 1982, 5:423–428.
Carnevale A, Canún S *et al*: Idiopathic multicentric osteolysis with facial anomalies and nephropathy. *Am J Med Genet* 1987, **26**:877–886.
Turner M C, Gonzalez O R *et al*: Multicentric osteolysis: report of the second successful renal transplant. *Pediatr Nephrol* 1987, 1:42–45.
Pai G S, Macpherson R I: Idiopathic multicentric osteolysis... review of the literature. *Am J Med Genet* 1988, **29**:929–936.
Barr R J, Hughes A E *et al*: Idiopathic multicentric osteolysis... *Am J Med Genet* 1989, **32**:556.
Shinohara O, Kubota C *et al*: Essential osteolysis associated with nephropathy... *Am J Med Genet* 1991, **41**:482–486.
Choi I H, Lee D Y *et al*: Carpal and tarsal osteolysis... *Pediatr Radiol* 1993, **23**:553–555.

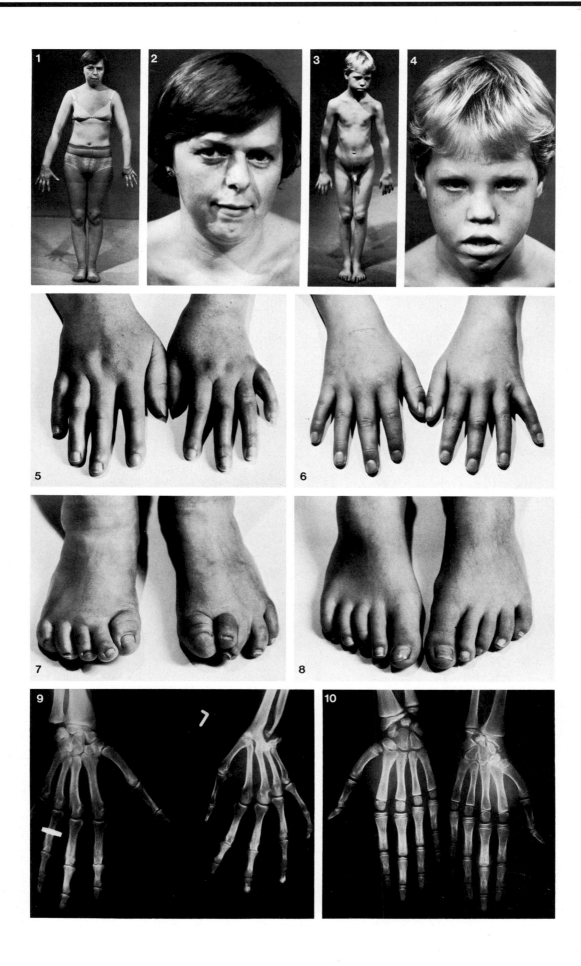

(Dystrophia Dermo-Chondro-Cornealis Familiaris)

H.-R.W

A hereditary syndrome of progressive carpotarsal osteolysis with skin and corneal changes.

Main signs:
- Gradual shortening of the wrist, ankle, metatarsus and metacarpus bilaterally (preceded by tenderness, warming and soft-tissue swelling) as a result of progressive osteolysis starting in the wrists and ankles (3–5). Increasing deformity (ulnar deviation of the shortened hands, eventual claw-hand [1 and 2]; short pes cavus).
- In some patients, impaired vision from school age on.
- Xanthomatous nodules, for example, on the hands, elbows, face.

Supplementary findings: Subepithelial and central corneal clouding, possibly only seen on slit-lamp examination.
  Idiopathic nephropathy with proteinuria in some patients.

Manifestation: Usually at a preschool or school age.

Aetiology: Monogenic disorder, autosomal recessive.

Frequency: Very low.

Course, prognosis: Slow progression of osteolysis with corresponding physical handicap. Life expectancy, without nephropathy, probably unaffected; with nephropathy, possibly unfavourable.

Differential diagnosis: Other osteolysis syndromes (243, 245). Rheumatoid arthritis may be considered early in the disease but is easily excluded.

Treatment: Symptomatic. Renal transplantation may be indicated. Genetic counselling.

Illustrations:
1–5 A 16-year-old girl; bone changes manifest in early childhood; xanthomatous nodules; corneal clouding noted at age 14 years with slit-lamp examination; nephropathy since early school age; death at 22 years from nephrosclerosis.

References:
Wiedemann H-R: Zur François'schen Krankheit. *Ärztl Wschr* 1958, 13:905.
Spranger J W, Langer Jr L O, Wiedemann H-R: *Bone dysplasias. An atlas of constitutional disorders of skeletal development*. Stuttgart and Philadephia: G Fischer and W B Saunders; 1974.
Maldonado R, Tamayo L, Velazquez E: Dystrophie dermo-chondro-cornéenne familiale (syndrome de François). *Ann Dermatol Venereol* 1977, 104:475–478.

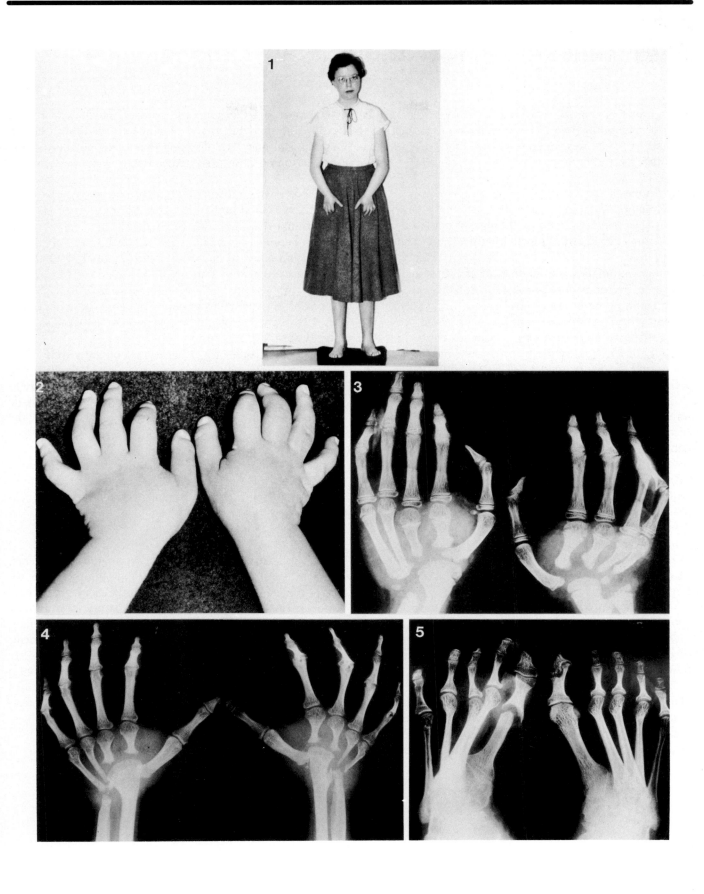

245 Hajdu–Cheney Syndrome
(Idiopathic Osteolysis, Hajdu–Cheney Type)

A syndrome of characteristic facies, persistence of cranial sutures and fontanelles, hyperextensible joints, increased tendency to fractures, premature loss of teeth and acro-osteolysis on radiograph.

Main signs:
- Characteristic facies: broad and strikingly heavy eyebrows; maxillary and mandibular hypoplasia; broad philtrum; broad, thin-lipped mouth (1). Coarse, thick scalp hair.
- Cranial anomalies: persistence of the fontanelles and sutures; eventual development of dolichocephaly with protruding occiput.
- Joint laxity; usually short stature with short neck; tendency to pathological fractures; carious teeth.
- Short, broad tips of the fingers and sometimes of the toes, which may be tender or painful and possibly associated with nail deformities (2).

Supplementary findings: Coarse skin in some patients, often with hypertrichosis. Hoarse voice common. Possible conductive hearing impairment; possible defective vision or other eye anomalies.

Radiologically: persistence of fontanelles and sutures with numerous wormian bones especially within the lambdoid suture (5, 6); later, in addition, dolichocephaly with protruding occiput, platybasia, elongation of the sella (6); small jaw, deficient pneumatization of the sinuses.

Osteolysis, in particular acro-osteolysis with formation of typical transverse clefts of the distal phalanges of the fingers (3 and 4).

Generalized osteoporosis in some patients, with corresponding changes in shape of the vertebral bodies and secondary kyphoscoliosis in some patients; multiple fractures; also abnormal modelling or deformity of the long bones.

Manifestation: The characteristic facies, abundant body hair and hoarse voice may come to attention in the newborn. Changes in the ends of the fingers with radiologically demonstrable osteolysis and generalized osteoporosis, sometimes with spontaneous fractures, may be apparent in early childhood but may not come to medical attention until much later. The diagnosis has often not been made until adolescence or even adulthood.

Aetiology: An autosomal dominant gene is apparently responsible. Predominantly sporadic occurrence (as new mutations).

Frequency: Low; to date, only approximately 30 patients are described in the literature.

Course, prognosis: Progressive increase in extent and severity of changes, including secondary changes, is usual.

Differential diagnosis: Other types of osteolysis (243, 244) as well as pyknodysostosis (108) and cleidocranial dysplasia (19) are usually easy to rule out. Normal mental development immediately excludes the Brachmann–de Lange syndrome (98), which may be suggested by the facies.

Treatment: Early audiological and ophthalmological assessment; adequate care as needed. Dental attention. Orthopaedic care and treatment of secondary complications. Genetic counselling.

Illustrations:
1–6 A girl, the third child of non-consanguineous parents, at ages 7 years (1, 2, 4) and 2 years and 3 months (3, 5, 6). At 7 years: short stature (third percentile), short neck, pectus excavatum and scoliosis; general laxity of the joints and muscular hypotonia. Coarse skin with abundant hair, bristly scalp hair; defective dentition; hearing impairment, hoarse voice; normal intellect. Radiographs show early dolichocephaly, widened sutures with wormian bones; generalized osteoporosis, platyspondyly; multiple fractures (since age 5 years); short terminal phalanges of the feet, acro-osteolysis of the terminal phalanges of the first, second and fifth fingers now more pronounced.

References:
Weleber R G, Beals R K: The Hajdu–Cheney syndrome. *J Pediatr* 1976, 88:243.
Wendel U, Kemperdick H: Idiopathische Osteolyse vom Typ Hajdu–Cheney, *Mschr Kinderheilk* 1979, 127:581.
Udell J, Schumacher H R *et al*: Idiopathic familial acroosteolysis:... review of the Hajdu–Cheney syndrome. *Arthritis Rheum* 1986, 29:1032–1038.
Diren H B *et al*: The Hajdu–Cheney syndrome... *Pediatr Radiol* 1990, 20:568–569.
Kaler S G *et al*: Hajdu–Cheney syndrome... *Dysmorphol Clin Genet* 1990, 4:43–47.
Laudi B *et al*: Hajdu–Cheney syndrome. *Dtsch Med Wschr* 1991, 116:1285–1289.

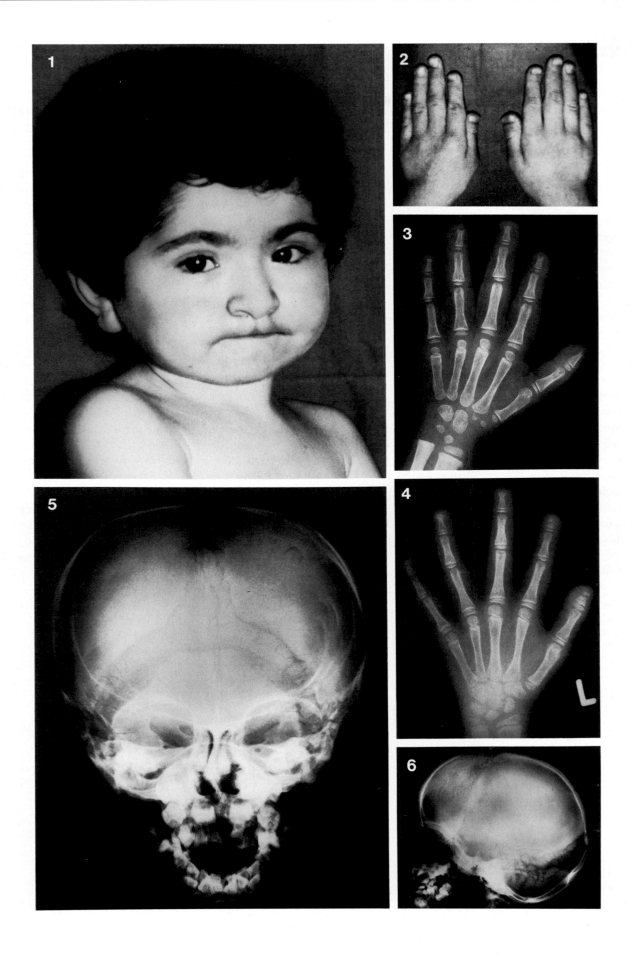

246 Syndrome of Triphalangism of the First Rays of the Hands, Thrombasthenia and Sensorineural Hearing Impairment

H.-R.W

A syndrome comprising triphalangeal digits instead of thumbs, a thrombasthenic bleeding diathesis and sensorineural hearing impairment.

Main signs:
- Well-developed or hypoplastic triphalangeal digits instead of thumbs (**4–6**), possibly with hypoplasia of the forearm (**1a and b**) or of the radius and with radiological anomalies of the wrist.
- Bleeding diathesis with episodes of skin and mucous membrane bleeding.
- Sensorineural hearing impairment.

Supplementary findings: Facial dysmorphism (hypertelorism, broad nasal bridge, prognathism).

Normal platelet count. Pathologically prolonged bleeding time and further findings of Glanzmann's thrombasthenia.

Manifestation: At birth and early in life.

Aetiology: Probable monogenic disorder, presumably autosomal recessive transmission in view of the thrombasthaenia.

Frequency: Probably very low.

Course, prognosis: As far as can be determined, relatively favourable.

Differential diagnosis: Fanconi anaemia (*249*), Aase syndrome (*247*), TAR syndrome (*209*), Holt–Oram syndrome (*248*), Blackfan–Diamond syndrome and IVIC syndrome.

Treatment: Symptomatic (transfusions of fresh blood or platelet concentrate for bleeding episodes; surgical correction of finger contractures).

Illustrations:
1–6 A girl, aged 13 years and 3 months, normal birth, robust development and normal height; recurrent, sometimes severe, skin and mucous membrane bleeding from 12 months of age. Repeated hospital admissions and transfusions required. No bleeding into the joints; heavy menstrual bleeding. Probably congenital sensorineural hearing impairment. Triphalangeal, strong, non-opposable digit in the thumb position on the right with broad, thenar-like bridge of soft tissue to the second ray; hypoplastic, triphalangeal digit contracted in flexion in the thumb position of the left hand (which as a whole is somewhat smaller than the right). Various asymmetrical anomalies of the wrist (**4–6**).

Relatively coarse facies with hypertelorism, broad nose and prognathism (**1a, 1c**). Large area of alopecia on the scalp (**2**). Pigmented naevus on the right side of the back (**1b, 3**). Multiple haematomas (e.g. on the inner surfaces of the left arm and left lower leg, **1a**). Pelvic kidney on the right. Normal platelet count, extremely prolonged bleeding time, detailed haematological findings as in Glanzmann's thrombasthaenia. Chromosomal analysis unremarkable.

References:

Arias S, Penchaszadeh V B *et al*: The IVIC syndrome: a new autosomal dominant complex pleiotropic syndrome with radial ray hypoplasia, hearing impairment, external ophthalmoplegia, and thrombocytopenia. *Am J Med Genet* 1980, **6**:25–59.
Schlegelberger B, Grote W, Wiedemann H-R: Probable autosomal recessive syndrome with triphalangia of thumbs, thrombasthenia Glanzmann and deafness of internal ear. *Klin Pädiatr* 1986, **198**:337–339.
Quazi Q, Kassner E G: Triphalangeal thumb. *J Med Genet* 1988, **25**:505–520.

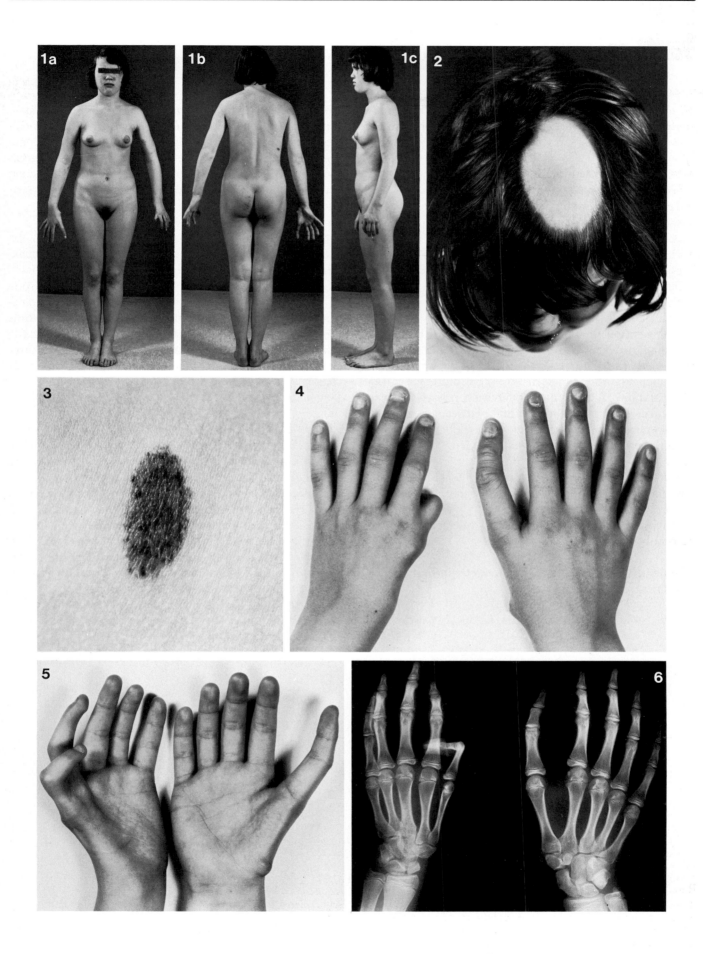

507

247 Syndrome of Hypoplastic Anaemia with Triphalangeal Thumbs

(Aase Syndrome, Aase–Smith Syndrome II)

H.-R.W

A characteristic syndrome with triphalangeal thumbs, early manifested hypoplastic anaemia and short stature.

Main signs:

- Intra-uterine growth retardation and decreased postnatal growth (with some degree of catch-up growth eventually).
- Triphalangeal thumb (with possible hypoplasia of the thenar eminence and radius); possible unilateral occurrence.
- Hypoplastic (and thus normochromic, normocytic) anaemia manifest from infancy (low reticulocyte count, decreased erythropoiesis in the marrow).
- Possible mild mental retardation.

Supplementary findings: The following have been noted in some patients: unusual facial appearance, antimongoloid slant of the palpebral fissures, cleft lip or palate, low nuchal hairline, unusual skin pigmentation, ventricular septal defect, anomalies of clavicles, ribs and pelvis.

Normal values for leukocytes and platelets and their precursors. Possibly increased foetal hemoglobin. No increase of chromosome breakage.

Manifestation: At birth (anaemia may also be present during the first year of life, usually in the first 6 months).

Aetiology: Presumed monogenic disorder with recessive transmission.

Frequency: Very low (up to 1990, only approximately 12 documented patients).

Course, prognosis: On the whole, favourable.

Differential diagnosis: Fanconi anaemia (249), in which, however, the blood disorder is usually manifest much later, initially with thrombocytopaenia, then pancytopaenia; hypoplasia or aplasia of the thumbs in the great majority; increased chromosome breakage. Blackfan–Diamond anaemia. Compare also with syndrome 246.

Treatment: Blood transfusion, corticosteroids may be indicated. (Iron medication contraindicated.) Surgical correction of the hands in some patients.

Genetic counselling.

Comment: Some authors consider that this syndrome falls within the spectrum of Diamond–Blackfan hypoplastic anaemia. However, in the latter the dysmorphic features are absent (especially triphalangeal thumbs) in the great majority of patients and this disorder does not appear to be genetically consistent.

Illustrations:

1–4 A boy, aged 12 years and 6 months. Hypoplastic anaemia since early infancy. On admission to the hospital, haemoglobin 8.3 g/dl; 2.5 million erythrocytes; 0.6% reticulocytes; leukopoiesis and thrombopoiesis normal. Shortly after increasing corticosteroids: haemoglobin 10.3 g/dl; 2.8 million erythrocytes; 7.8% reticulocytes. Short stature (height of a child aged 9 years and 6 months). Triphalangeal thumbs, low nuchal hairline, pigmented moles. IQ 77. Ocular fundi normal, no clefts, no organomegaly, testes normally descended. Haemoglobin electrophoresis unremarkable. Radiographs: no radial dysplasia; in the right wrist, absence of the navicular, fusion of the carpal bones (3).

References:

Aase J M, Smith D W: Congenital anemia and triphalangeal thumbs: a new syndrome. *J Pediatr* 1969, **74**:471.
Terheggen F G: Hypoplastische Anämie mit dreigliedrigem Daumen. *Z Kinderheilk* 1974, **118**:71.
Wood V E: Treatment of the triphalangeal thumb. *Clin Orthopaed* 1976, **120**:188.
Alter B P: Thumbs and anemia. *Pediatrics* 1978, **62**:613.
Pfeiffer R A, Ambs E: Das Aase-Syndrom… *Mschr Kinderheilk* 1983, **131**:235–237.
Patton M A, Sharma A *et al*: The Aase–Smith syndrome. *Clin Genet* 1985, **28**:521–525.
Muis N, Beemer F A *et al*: The Aase syndrome… review of the literature. *Eur J Pediatr* 1986, **145**:153–157.
Quazi Q, Kassner E G: Triphalangeal thumb. *J Med Genet* 1988, **25**:505–520.
Hurst J A, Baraitser M, Wonke B: Autosomal dominant transmission of congenital erythroid hypoplastic anemia with radial abnormalities. *Am J Med Genet* 1991, **40**:482–484.
Hing A V, Dowton S B: Aase syndrome: novel radiographic features. *Am J Med Genet* 1993, **45**:413–425.

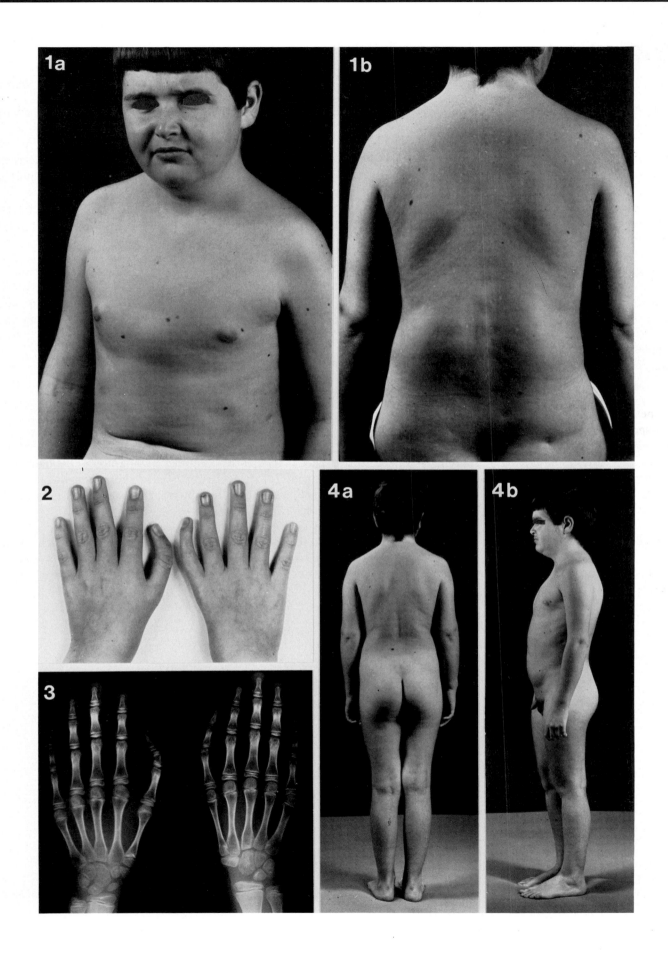

248 Holt–Oram Syndrome
(Heart–Hand Syndrome; Cardio-Digital Syndrome)

H.-R.W/ J.K.

A hereditary disorder with malformations of the heart and upper extremities.

Main signs:
- Malformations of the upper extremities, which may be symmetrical or asymmetrical. Triphalangism (**3a; 2c** left), hypoplasia (**1a and b**) or even aplasia of the thumbs; more extensive defects of the first ray in some patients (dysplasia or aplasia of the radius; dysplasia of the upper arm).
- Congenital heart defect (**2d, 3**) in the form of septal defects (frequent atrial septal defect, secundum type; possibly with dysrhythmia) or other cardiac malformations.

Supplementary findings: Possible dysplasia of the little fingers (note clinodactyly: **1a and b**), of the wrist (**3a** right), of the elbow joints and of the shoulder girdle (clavicles, scapulae and others **3**). On X-ray: spur formation on the lateral ends of the clavicles as a characteristic (but non-specific) finding; radial and humero-ulnar synostoses; hypoplasia of the humerus, clavicles and scapulae; pectus excavatum and carinatum, anomalies of the ribs, malformations of the vertebral bodies, scoliosis.

Manifestation: At birth (malformations of the upper extremities) and later, depending on the severity of the cardiac malformation.

Aetiology: Monogenic disorder, autosomal dominant with complete penetrance and variable expression: often more severe in females. Between 50% and 85% of the patients represent new mutations. Gene locus: 12q2.

Frequency: Relatively low, however, a series of affected sibships and several hundred patients have been reported.

Course, prognosis: Dependent for each patient on the severity of the cardiac defect and on the scope for surgical correction.

Differential diagnosis: TAR syndrome (*209*), Fanconi anaemia (*249*), thalidomide syndrome (*206*). Additionally: heart–hand syndrome II (Tabatznik syndrome), heart–hand syndrome III (Spanish type) and heart–hand syndrome IV (Rogers syndrome).

Treatment: Adequate care of the specific anomalies. Genetic counselling.

Illustrations:
1 and 2 Mother and daughter.
1a and b Hands of the mother.
2a–c Hands of the daughter. Radiograph of the daughter's hands (**2c**) shows triphalangeal thumb on the left with hypoplasia of the first metacarpal, of the wrist and of the radius.
2d Chest radiograph of the daughter.
3a Radiographs from another girl; note shoulder anomalies (os acromiale on the left, among others) and the almost symmetrical triphalangeal thumbs with asymmetry of the wrists.

References:
Holt M, Oram S: Familial heart disease with skeletal malformations. *Br Heart J* 1960, 22:236.
Kaufmann R L, Rimoin D L, McAlister W H, Hartmann A F: Variable expression of the Holt–Oram syndrome. *Am J Dis Child* 1974, **127**:21.
Capek-Schachner E, May L, Schwarzbach E: Holt–Oram-Syndrom. *Pädiatr Prax* 1979, **21**:607.
Smith A T, Sack G H, Taylor G J: Holt–Oram syndrome. *J Pediatr* 1979, 95:538.
Gladstone I Jr, Sybert V P: Holt–Oram syndrome: penetrance of the gene and lack of maternal effect. *Clin Genet* 1982, 21:98–103.
Regemorter N van, Haumont D *et al*: Holt–Oram syndrome mistaken for thalidomide embryopathy... *Eur J Pediatr* 1982, 138:77–80.
Najjar H, Mardini M *et al*: Variability of the Holt–Oram syndrome... *Am J Med Genet* 1988, 29:851–855.
Cox H, Viljoen D *et al*: Radial ray defects... *Clin Genet* 1989, 35:322–330.
Pfeiffer R A, Böwing B, Deeg K H: Varianten der radialen Hemimelie mit und ohne Vitium cordis (Holt–Oram-Syndrom) in zwei Familien. *Mschr Kinderheilk* 1989, **137**:275–279.
Hurst J A, Hall C M, Baraitser M: Syndrome of the month. The Holt–Oram syndrome. *J Med Genet* 1991, 28:406–410.
Kullmann F, Grimm T: Holt–Oram-Syndrom. *Dtsch Med Wschr* 1993, 118:1455–1462.
Basson C T, Cowley G S *et al*: The clinical and genetic spectrum of the Holt–Oram syndrome (heart–hand syndrome). *N Engl J Med* 1994, 330:885–891.

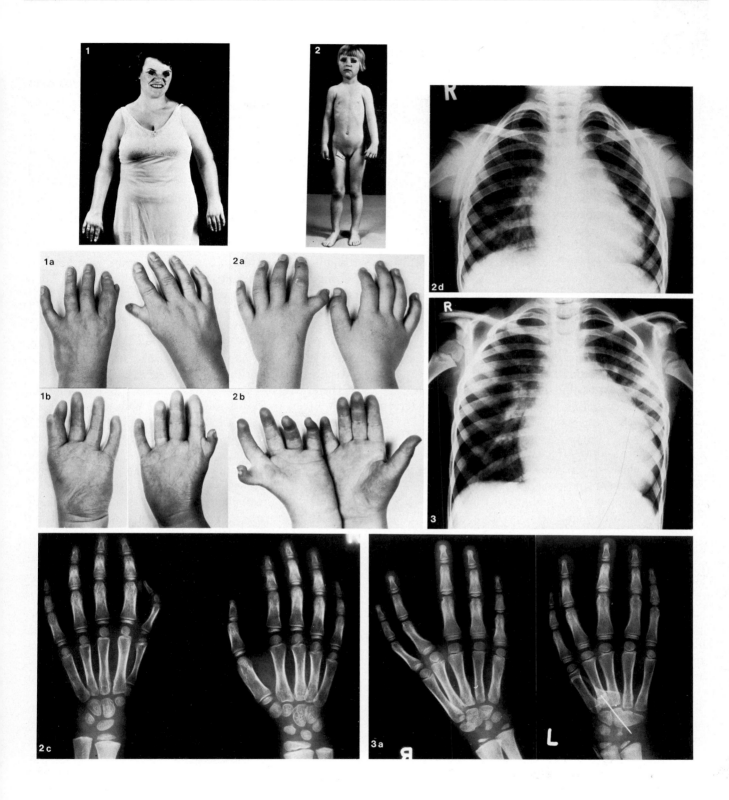

J.K./ H.-R.W

A characteristic syndrome of reduction malformations of the thumbs and radii, short stature, hyperpigmentation and signs of aplastic anaemia.

Main signs:
- Pronounced prenatal and postnatal growth deficiency; hypoplasia or aplasia of the thumbs (also, duplication or triphalangism), short or absent radii (**4, 5, 7, 8**). Extensive or patchy dirty brown skin pigmentation, especially truncal and in skin creases.
- Unusual facies (**3, 6**). Possible microphthalmos (20%), strabismus, nystagmus, coloboma.
- Microcephaly, even relative to body size; moderate mental retardation in approximately 20% of patients. Short stature (30%).

Supplementary findings: Hypoplastic male genitalia, undescended testes, hypospadias.

Ear deformities, possible deafness. Hyper-reflexia.

Renal malformations. Occasional cardiac defects. Increased infections.

Pancytopenia (also lymphocytopaenia); aplastic anaemia. Increased foetal haemoglobin.

Increased chromosome breakage with exchange figures in heterologous chromosome pairs.

Increased frequency of malignant tumours, especially leukaemia. Retarded bone age on radiograph (**5, 7**).

Comment: One-quarter of all patients are clinically normal.

Manifestation: Malformations and chromosome breakage present at birth. Increasing pigmentation from birth or later. Signs of pancytopaenia usually between 5 and 10 years of age; rarely, during infancy or not until the third decade. Initially, reduced numbers of platelets, then of leukocytes and erythrocytes. Chromosomal findings are of particular importance, as other signs may be only partially expressed.

Aetiology: Autosomal recessive disorder with exceptionally variable picture; heterogeneity. Increased chromosome breakage and sister chromatid exchange (frequency of heterozygotes = 1:300–600), increased incidence of short stature, thrombocytopaenia and other signs also possible in heterozygotes. DNA repair defect.

Frequency: Not particularly low (approximately 1:40000 newborns).

Course, prognosis: Chronic, progressive. Untreated patients survive approximately two years after onset of haematological signs; survival has increased significantly since the introduction of therapy. Death from bone marrow failure or malignancy, especially leukaemia (approximately 10%), hepatocellular carcinoma, squamous carcinoma. Additionally: recurrent infections, growth hormone deficiency, increased sensitivity to chemotherapeutics. Eighty per cent mortality by 12 years of age.

Treatment: Testosterone, in some patients with corticosteroids; bone marrow transplantation. Genetic counselling. Prenatal diagnosis possible.

Differential diagnosis:
- Holt–Oram syndrome (*248*): shows only similar thumb and arm malformations and cardiac anomalies, the latter rarely present in Fanconi anaemia.
- Thrombocytopaenia–radial aplasia (TAR) syndrome (*209*): always shows radial aplasia with thumbs present; thrombocytopaenia alone, beginning in the first year of life; good prognosis once thrombocytopaenic episodes have been overcome.
- Hypoplastic anaemia with triphalangeal thumbs syndrome (*247*): shows only the signs of the name.
- Syndrome of triphalangism of the first ray of the hands, thrombasthaenia, and sensorineural hearing deficit (*246*): normal platelet count.

Illustrations:

1–5 A patient, aged 3 years and 3 months; mother only 1.52 m tall. Birth measurements 2250 g, 45 cm. Present height 79 cm (=~16 months), 8.8 kg (=~8 months), head circumference 48 cm (normal for body size). Bone age 4–5 months. Mental age 2 years and 6 months. Isolated areas of hyperpigmentation. Bilateral microphthalmos with coloboma on the right. Hypoplastic genitalia. Haematologically, only mild thrombocytopaenia to date.

6–8 2-year-old patient. Birth measurements 2640 g, 48 cm. Present height 80 cm (=~17 months); 8.8 kg (=~8 months); head circumference 43 cm (5 months). Bone age 3 months. Psychomotor development about normal for age. Generalized hyperpigmentation. Persistent foramen ovale. Genital hypoplasia. Elevated foetal haemoglobin. Thrombocytopaenia and anaemia since the age of 13 months.

References:

Voss R, Kohn G, Shaham M *et al*: Prenatal diagnosis of Fanconi anemia. *Clin Genet* 1981, **20**:185.

Druckworth-Rysiecki G, Hultén M *et al*: Clinical and cytogenetic diversity in Fanconi's anaemia. *J Med Genet* 1984, **21**:197–203.

Schindler D, Kubbies M *et al*: Presymptomatic diagnosis of Fanconi's anaemia. *Lancet* 1985, I:937.

Rosendorff R, Bernstein R *et al*: Fanconi anemia... *Am J Med Genet* 1987, **27**:793–797.

Digweed M, Zakrezewski S *et al*: Fanconi's anaemia... *Hum Genet* 1988, **78**:51–54.

Giampietro P F, Adler-Brecher B *et al*: The need for more accurate and timely diagnosis in Fanconi anaemia: a report from the international Fanconi anemia registry. *Pediatrics* 1993, **91**:1116–1120.

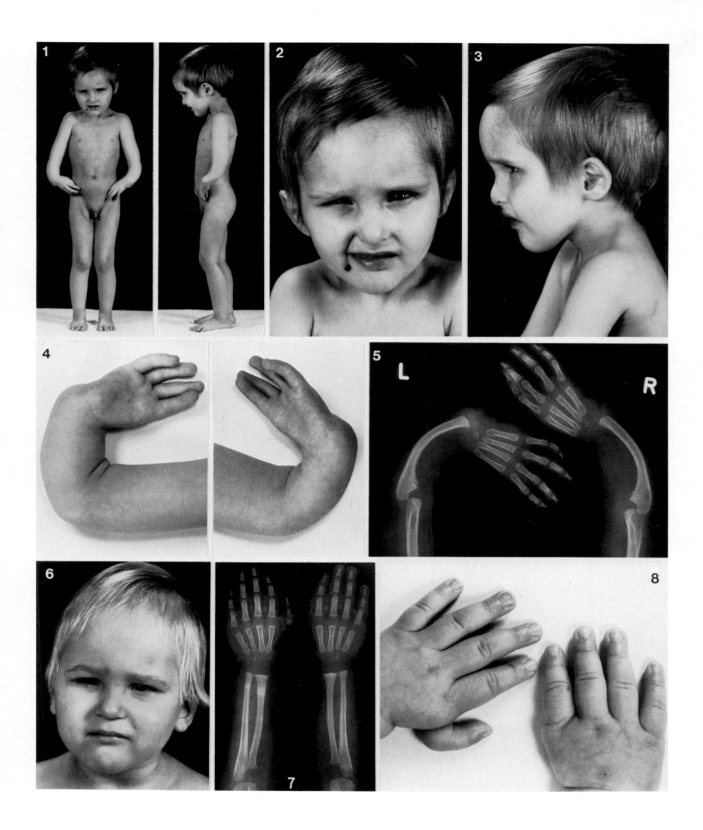

250 Alpha Thalassaemia with Mental Retardation, X-Linked Recessive

(ATR-X Syndrome)

J.K.

A sex-linked hereditary syndrome with severe mental retardation, microcephaly, facial dysmorphism, seizures and evidence of haemoglobin-H inclusions.

Main signs:
- Severe muscular hypotonia, drinking difficulties, gastro-oesophageal reflux.
- Cryptorchidism, hypoplastic scrotum, labioscrotal fusion, shawl scrotum, labia minora and uterine structures absent, male pseudohermaphroditism.
- Facial deformities: hypertelorism, horizontal nystagmus, epicanthus medialis, depressed nasal bridge, small triangular nose, anteverted nostrils, large tongue with protrusion, low-set rotated ears, nuchal skin folds, flat face, widely spaced teeth, everted lower lip.
- Microcephaly.
- Pes planus, club foot, malpositioning of the toes, scoliosis, kyphosis, hemivertebrae, short stature.
- Central nervous system seizures. No speech development. No control over the bladder and intestine. Delayed unassisted walking (not until 3 or even 5 years of age).
- Detection of haemoglobin H cells (alpha thalassaemia). Stain blood smears with 1% brilliant cresyl blue. Additionally, perform haemoglobin electrophoresis.

Supplementary findings: Inguinal hernias, umbilical hernias, coxa valga, cardiac defect. Unilateral renal agenesis.

Manifestation: Soon after birth.

Aetiology: X-linked recessive inheritance. A few haemoglobin H cells detected in one-half of the female carriers.

Pathogenesis: Unknown.

Frequency: Approximately 25 patients have been reported to date.

Course, prognosis: Epilepsy, delay in unassisted walking. Poor communication with absence of speech development. No control over the bladder and intestine.

Differential diagnosis: Angelman syndrome (53), Smith–Lemli–Opitz syndrome (281), Coffin–Lowry syndrome (15), FG syndrome.

Treatment: Seizure control. Around-the-clock nursing.

Illustrations:

1a and b Aged 3 years and 2 months, craniofacial dysplasia: dolichocephaly, high forehead, prominent cheeks, eyebrows absent medially, mouth open and arched, malocclusion, dysplastic ears.

2 Three cells with characteristic haemoglobin H inclusions.

References:

Weatherall D J, Diggs D R et al: Hemoglobin H disease and mental retardation: a new syndrome or a remarkable coincidence? N Engl J Med 1981, 305:607–612.

Wilkie A O, Zeitlin H C et al: Clinical features and molecular analysis of the alpha-Thalassaemia/mental retardation syndromes. Am J Med Genet 1990, 46:1127–1140.

Wilkie A O M, Pembrey M E: The non-deletion type of alpha-thalassaemia/mental retardation: a recognizable dysmorphic syndrome with X-linked inheritance. J Med Genet 1991, 28:724.

Gibbons R J, Wilkie A O M et al: A newly defined X-linked mental retardation syndrome associated with alpha thalassaemia. J Med Genet 1991, 28:729–733.

Cole T R P, May A, Hughes H E: Alpha thalassaemia/mental retardation syndrome (non-deletional type): report of a family supporting X linked inheritance. J Med Genet 1991, 28:734–737.

Wilkie A O M, Gibbons R J et al: X linked alpha thalassaemia/mental retardation: spectrum of clinical features in three related males. J Med Genet 1991, 28:738–741.

Donnai D, Clayton-Smith J et al: The non-deletion alpha-thalassaemia/mental retardation syndrome further support for X-linkage. J Med Genet 1991, 28:742–745.

Gibbons R J, Suthers K G et al: X-linked alpha-thalassaemia/mental retardation (ATR-X) syndrome: localization to Xq12-q21-31 by X-inactivation and linkage analysis. Am J Hum Genet 1992, 51:1136–1149.

Cohen M, Stengel-Rutkowski S, Kohne E, Enders H: Alpha-Thalassämie und mentale Retardierung, X-gebunden (ATR-X-Syndrom). Medizinische Genetik 1993, 4:364–366.

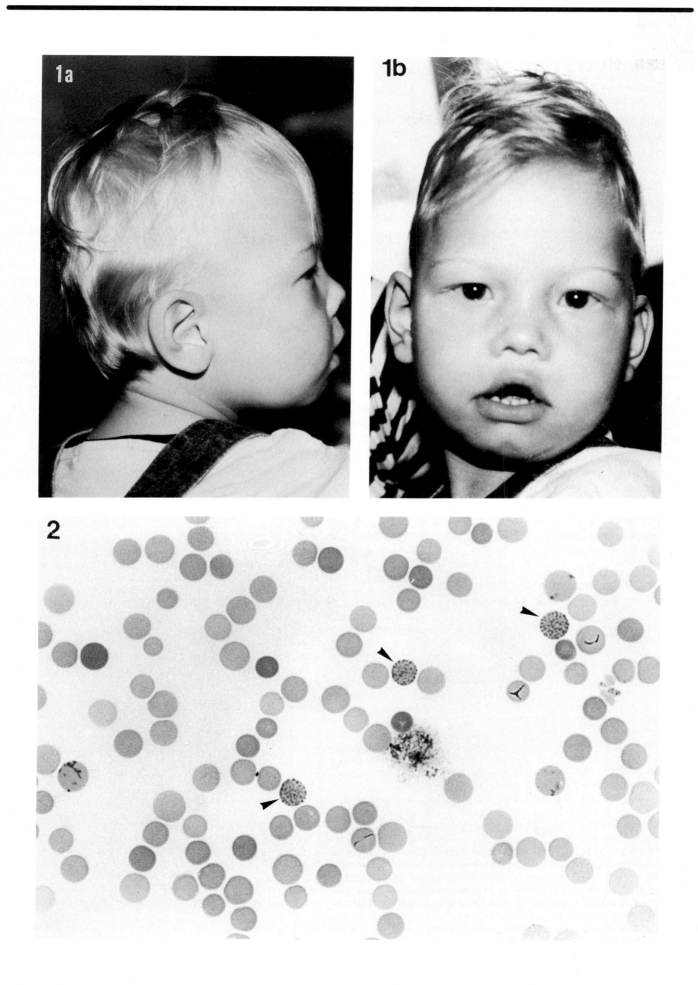

(Acrorenal Syndrome)

J.K.

A combination of acral and renal malformations of widely varying aetiologies.

Main signs:
- Morphological anomalies in the radial rays: pre-axial polydactyly, triphalangeal thumbs, mild to severe hypoplasia of the thumbs, syndactyly, acromicria, amelia, terminal transverse defects, phocomelia, central axis defects, tetra-ectrodactyly (split hand or foot).
- Malrotation of the kidneys, ectopia renis, ureteral anomalies, vesico-ureteral reflux, vesical diverticulum, unilateral renal agenesis, bilateral renal hypoplasia, hydronephrosis.

Supplementary findings: As a result of the varying aetiologies, there may also be: ocular anomalies, auricular dysplasia, congenital deafness, weakness of the facial nerve, cardiac defects, musculoskeletal anomalies, omphalocoele, body wall defects, internal genital anomalies, diaphragmatic defects, anal atresia, central nervous system malformations such as an encephalocoele, hydrocephalus, spina bifida, exstrophy of the bladder, scoliosis, malformed abdomen, oligomeganephronia, oesophageal atresia, tracheal fistula, cleft lip and palate, defects of the vertebral column.

Manifestation: At birth. Impaired renal function may in some patients occur later.

Aetiology: A complex of developmental field disorders. Sporadic occurrence, not infrequently autosomal dominant. A complex of at least 25 aetiologically distinct congenital anomalies, for example, Fanconi anaemia, Sorsby syndrome, acrorenomandibular syndrome, acrorenoocular syndrome and so on (compare with Temtamy–McKusick).

Frequency: The complex has only been diagnosed on a significant scale in recent years. 1:20 000 newborns and 16% of children with malformed extremities have disorders of the urogenital system.

Course, prognosis: Dependent on malformations of specific organs, for example, the kidney.

Treatment: Symptomatic and surgery where indicated.

Differential diagnosis: Acrorenomandibular syndrome, acroreno-ocular syndrome, Fanconi anaemia (*249*), Sorsby syndrome, VATER association (*311*), VATERL plus hydrocephalus (*312*), Poland anomaly (*220*), trisomy 18 (*48*).

Illustrations:
1 An infant with hypospadias and bilateral vesico-ureteral reflux, grade IV.
1a Hypoplastic thumbs bilaterally, absent nail.
1b In addition, hypoplastic hallures bilaterally.
2a and b The child's father, with small, delicate thumbs (compared with his large hands and fingers and tall stature. The father has been aware of his small thumbs since childhood.).
2b His short hallures with hypoplastic nails bilaterally.

References:
Halal F, Homsy M, Perreault G: Acro-renal-ocular symdrome: autosomal dominant thumb hypoplasia, renal ectopia, and eye defect. *Am J Med Genet* 1984, **17**:753–762.
Temtamy S, McKusick V: The genetics of hand malformations. *Birth Defects Orig Art Ser* 1984, **XIV**(3):171–172.
Johnson V P, Munson D P: A new syndrome of aphalangy, hemivertebrae, and urogenital-intestinal dysgenesis. *Clin Genet* 1990, **38**:346–352.
Hedge H R, Leung A K C, Robson W L M: Acro-renal polytopic defect. *Am J Med Genet* 1991, **39**:239.
Houlston R, MacDermot K: Acrorenal syndrome: further observations. *Clin Dysmorphol* 1992, **1**:23–28.
Miltenyi M, Czeizel A E, Balogh L, Detre Z: Autosomal recessive acrorenal syndrome. *Am J Med Genet* 1992, **43**:789–790.
Evans J A, Vitez M, Czeizel A: Patterns of acrorenal malformation associations. *Am J Med Genet* 1992, **44**:413–419.
Akl K: Acrorenal syndrome in a child with renal failure. *Am J Med Genet* 1994, **49**:447.

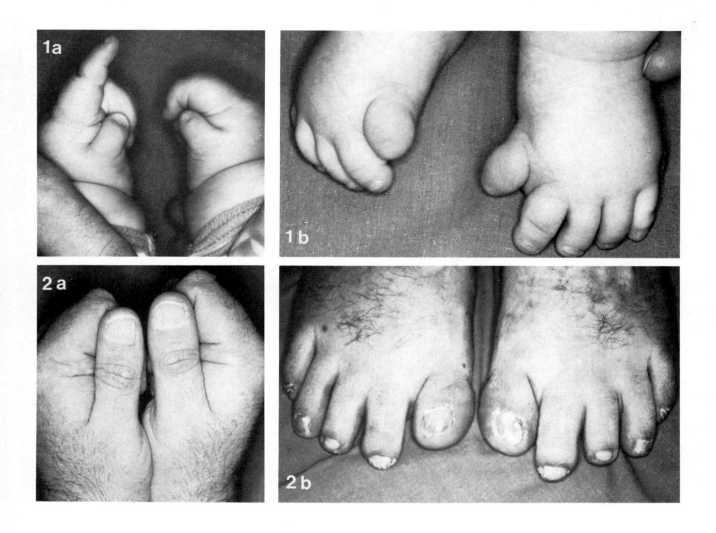

H.-R.W/ J.K.

A syndrome of congenital microdactyly of the halluces, also often of the thumbs and (usually not until later) dysplastic connective-tissue swellings with subsequent ossification intramuscularly and extramuscularly.

Main signs:

- Congenital shortening and valgus position of the halluces (**8, 11, 12**) caused by dysplasia of the first metatarsal; less often, analogous shortening of the thumbs (**5, 6, 9, 10**) and inward curving of the little finger (clinodactyly, **5, 6, 9**) or reduction defects of all fingers.
- Soft-tissue swellings (occasionally with pain and fever), which may be noted perinatally but usually appear during the first 2 years of life and on into the first decade; preferentially located in the occipitonuchal region, neck and shoulder girdle ('torticollis', **1 and 2**). Risk of subsequent ossification. Intermittent progressive course with new episodes of ossification affecting further body and muscle regions in a craniocaudal direction and causing increasing limitation of movement (**3 and 4**), in some patients on to almost complete mechanical 'freezing'.

Supplementary findings: Hearing impairment or deafness not infrequent. Possible mental retardation, loss of scalp hair, dental anomalies (frequent) and disorders of sexual maturation.

Aetiology: Monogenic disorder, autosomal dominant with complete penetrance but variable expression. Most patients represent new mutations, often associated with above-average paternal age. Gene locus 20p12. Basic defect unknown.

Frequency: Not particularly low. Up to 1958, over 300 patients reported in the literature; the great majority of subsequent observations have not come to publication.

Prognosis: In patients with the typical dysplastic connective-tissue swellings: subsequent progressive ectopic ossifications from infancy and early childhood are unfavourable for life expectancy; not infrequently, death before the end of the second decade of life from pulmonary disease or heart failure after the thorax has become immobile. After completion of the growth period, slowing or cessation of the ossification process.

Diagnosis, differential diagnosis: Soft-tissue swellings appearing in an individual with anomalies of the extremities should suggest the diagnosis and thus avoidance of active procedures. Minor trauma can provoke new swelling and ossification. Thus, absolute avoidance of incisions (for suspected inflammation) or biopsy (for suspected tumour); also avoid electromyography.

Treatment: Although 'diphosphonate' (EHDP), which was administered recently during exacerbations, seemed to limit further calcification and ossification in a few patients, this therapeutic trial has also proved disappointing. Psychological support. Genetic counselling.

Illustrations:

1 and 2 A 2-year-old boy with an acute attack of occipito-nuchal-dorsal soft-tissue swelling with torticollis and marked limitation of movement, still without calcifications.
3 and 4 A boy, aged 6 years and 6 months, with typical stiff posture, numerous sites of ossification in the musculature of the back, bizarre, clasp-like new-bone formation on radiograph.
5, 7 Radiographs of the hands and feet of the child in **2**.
6, 9, 8, 11 Hands and feet of the boy in **4**.
10, 12 Hands and feet of a 13-year-old girl with Münchmeyer syndrome.

References:

Becker P E, v Knorre G: Myositis ossificans progressiva. *Ergeb Inn Med Kinderheilk* N F 1968, **27**:1.
v Schnakenburg K, Groß-Selbeck G, Wiedemann, H-R: Zur Behandlung der Fibrodysplasia ossificans progressiva mit 'Diphosphonat' (EHDP). *Dtsch Med Wschr* 1972, **97**:1873.
Azmy A, Bensted J P M, Eckstein H B: Myostitis ossificans progressiva. *Z Kinderchir* 1979, **26**:252.
Holmsen H, Ljunghall S, Hierton T: Myositis ossificans progressiva. *Acta Orthopaed Scand* 1979, **50**:33.
Connor J M, Evans D A: Fibrodysplasia ossificans progressiva... 34 patients. *J Bone Jt Surg* 1982, **64B**:76–83. By the same authors: Genetic aspects of fibrodysplasia ossificans progressiva. *J Med Genet* 1982, **19**:35–39.
Schulze-Solce N, Lanser K: Fibrodysplasia ossificans progressiva. *Medwelt* 1984, 407–410.
Lindhout D, Golding R P et al: Fibrodysplasia ossificans progressiva... *Pediatr Radiol* 1985, **15**:211–213.
Carter S R, Davies A M, Evans N et al: Value of bone scanning... in fibrodysplasia ossificans progressiva. *Br J Radiol* 1989, **62**(735):269.
Daltroff G et al: Fibromatose et fibrodysplasie ossifiante progressive. *Arch Fr Pédiatr* 1992, **49**:441–444.
Kalifa G et al: Fibrodysplasia ossificans progressiva and synovial chondromatosis. *Pediatr Radiol* 1993, **23**:91–93.

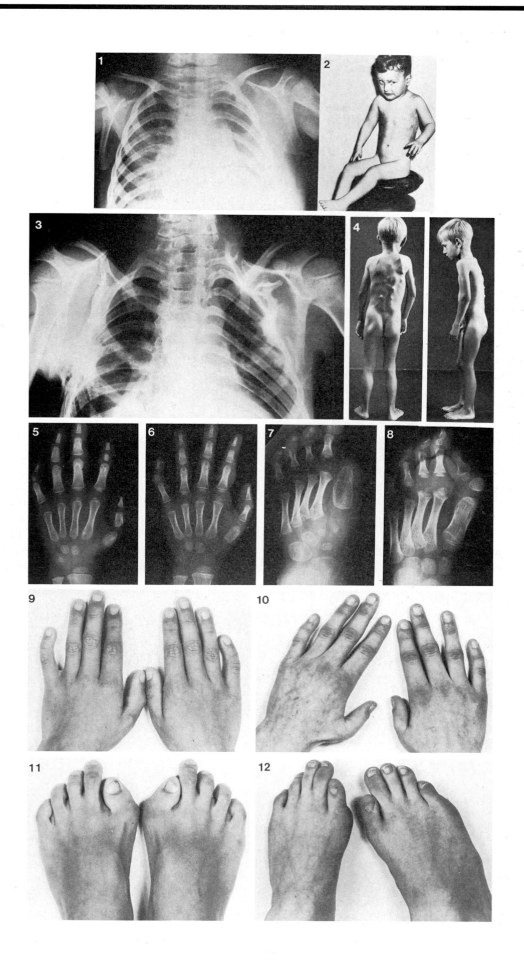

253 Rigid Spine Syndrome

J.K.

A characteristic, slowly progressive syndrome with impaired flexion, stiffness and hyperextension of the entire spinal column ('reverse Bechterew'); decrease in subcutaneous fatty tissue; reduced muscle mass; joint contractures.

Main signs:
- Markedly limited flexion of the entire vertebral column with hyperextension of the cervical, thoracic and lumbar regions ('reverse Bechterew'), contracture of the extensor muscles.
- Generalized muscular hypotonia and weakness, permanently elevated shoulders, decrease of muscle mass.
- Decrease of adipose tissue.

Supplementary findings: Not consistent. Depending on the aetiology: absent or normal tendon reflexes; decreased nerve conduction velocity and normal biochemistry in some patients but pathologic electromyogram and elevated creatine kinase in others; possible cardiomyopathy with sudden death but normal cardiac findings also possible; different muscle biopsy findings with normal structure, or muscle fibre type 1 or 2 atrophy with or without connective-tissue changes.

Manifestation: From birth on into adulthood, peak between the second and 12th years of life.

Aetiology: Genetic heterogeneity: X-linked recessive (the most frequent), autosomal recessive and autosomal dominant inheritance have all been observed but also sporadic cases.

Frequency: Low; approximately 50 patients have been described.

Prognosis, course: Depending on aetiology, minimal, slow or rapid progression with sudden cardiac death in all age groups.

Differential diagnosis:
- X-linked recessive, benign Emery–Dreifuss muscular dystrophy (also called Cestan–LeJonne disease).
- Scapuloperoneal atrophies and myopathies.
- Mitochondrial myopathies.
- Congenital muscular dystrophies; Fukuyama muscular dystrophy.
- Autosomal dominant fibrodysplasia ossificans progressiva.
- Hypertrophic cardiomyopathy in children of diabetic mothers, Pompe glycogen storage disease, Friedreich ataxia.

Treatment: Symptomatic. Surgical intervention for joint contractures; physiotherapy. Cardiac pacemaker, for example, for Emery–Dreifuss muscular dystrophy.

Illustrations:
1a–c, 2a–c Young men with shoulders permanently elevated in the typical manner, hyperextension in the cervical, thoracic and lumbar regions ('reverse Bechterew').

References:
Colver A F, Steer C R, Godman M J et al: Rigid spine syndrome and fatal cardiomyopathy. *Arch Dis Child* 1981, 56:148–151.
Echenne B, Astruc J, Brunel D et al: Congenital muscular dystrophy and rigid spine syndrome. *Neuropediatrics* 1983, 14:97–101.
Pavonne L, Gullotta F, La Rosa M et al: Rigid spine syndrome. Some evidence of varying pathological patterns. *Helv Paediatr Acta* 1983, 38:367–372.
Rowland L P, Layzer R B: Emery–Dreifuss muscular dystrophy. In: *Handbook for clinical neurology.* P J Vinken, G W Bruyn (Eds.). Vol 40: Disease of Muscle. Part I. Amsterdam, New York, Oxford: North-Holland Publ. 1979, 389–392.
Hanefeld F, von Maltzan V, Stoltenburg G: Mitochondriale Myopathie bei Rigid Spine Syndrom. *Monatsschr Kinderheilkd* 1982, 130:648.
Poewe W, Willeit H, Sluga E, Mayr U: The rigid spine syndrome — a myopathy of uncertain nosological position. *J Neurol Neurosurg Psychiatry* 1985, 48:887–893.
Goto I, Ishimoto S, Yamady T, Hara H, Kuroiwa Y: The rigid spine syndrome and Emery–Dreifuss muscular dystrophy. *Clin Neurol.Neurosurg* 1986, 88:293–298.
Emery A E H: Emery-Dreifuss syndrome. *J Med Genet* 1989, 26:637–641.

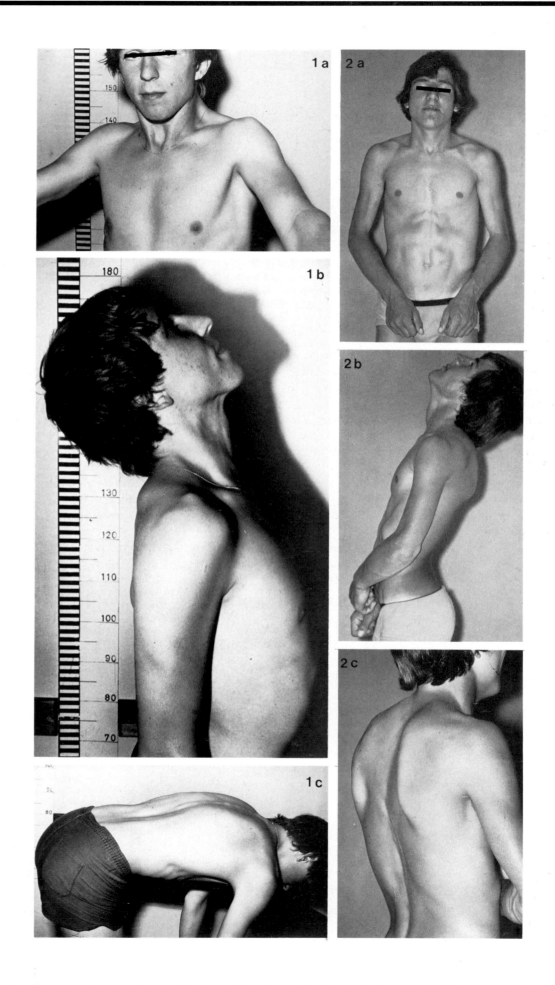

Nail–Patella Syndrome

(Nail–Patella–Elbow Syndrome with Iliac Horns; Osteo-Onycho Dysplasia; [Österreicher-] Turner–Kieser Syndrome)

H.-R.W/ J.K.

A characteristic syndrome particularly of skeletal anomalies, dysplasia of nails and frequently renal disease.

Main signs:

- Hypoplasia and dysplasia of the nails (softness, discoloration, longitudinal ridging, abnormal splitting), preferentially involving the thumb and index fingers (**1 and 2**).
- Hypoplasia of the patellae (**5**) with frequent lateral dislocation; occasionally aplasia.
- Hypoplasia of the radial head with frequent dorsal dislocation and impaired mobility (**6**).
- Iliac horns (symmetrically located pyramidal outgrowths of the dorsal surfaces of the iliac wings [**4**], usually readily palpable or seen on radiograph or computerized tomography scan).

Supplementary findings: Hypoplasia of the scapulae; radiologically, hypoplasia of the lateral femoral condyle, coxa valga and other findings.

Poorly defined, darkly pigmented pupillary margin of the iris.

Proteinuria and nephropathy in some patients, not infrequently beginning in childhood.

Possible development of cords or webbing over the elbow joints (**3**); also muscle aplasias.

Manifestation: Although diagnosis is possible in the newborn, the child usually first comes to attention because of difficulties in walking, related to the patellar abnormality.

Aetiology: Monogenic disorder, autosomal dominant with very variable expressivity. Gene localized to the distal long arm of chromosome 9 (9q34), linked to the ABO blood group locus.

Frequency: Not particularly low. Well over 500 patients described in the literature; estimate (1965) of 22 carriers of the trait out of 1 million of the general population.

Prognosis: Dependent on the development and course of renal disease, which occurs in over 50% of patients (unusual slowly progressive nephropathy, with unfavourable outcome in at least 10%).

For a patient with nail–patella syndrome and nephropathy, the risk for nephropathy in a child is approximately 1:4.

Treatment: Orthopaedic care; renal follow-up. Genetic counselling.

Illustrations:

1–6 A 14-year-old affected boy with nephropathy.

1 and 2 Dysplasia of the nails (fingers much more than toes).

3 Firm 'web' formation at both elbow joints.

4 Iliac horns.

5 Patellar hypoplasia; angular appearance of the flexed knees.

6 Elbow joint with distinct dorsal dislocation of the radial head.

References:

Caliebe M-R, Rohwedder H-J, Wiedemann H-R: Über das Mißbildungs-Erbsyndrom Osteo-Onycho-Dysplasie mit Nierenbeteiligung. *Arch Kinderheilk* 1963, **169**:149.

Spranger J W, Langer Jr L O, Wiedemann H-R: *Bone dysplasias. An atlas of constitutional disorders of skeletal development.* Stuttgart and Philadephia: G Fischer and W B Saunders; 1974.

Sabnis S G, Antonovych T T *et al*: Nail-patella syndrome. *Clin Nephrol* 1980, **14**:148–153.

Reed D, Nichols D M: Computed tomography of 'iliac horns' in hereditary osteo-onychodysplasia... *Pediatr Radiol* 1987, **17**:168–169.

Looij B J, Teslaa B L *et al*: Genetic counseling in... nail-patella syndrome with nephropathy. *J Med Genet* 1988, **25**:682–686.

Drut R M *et al*: Nail-patella syndrome... study of the kidneys. *Am J Med Genet* 1992, **43**:693–696; and: Gubler M-C. *et al*: (Letter) *Am J Med Genet* 1993, **47**:122–123.

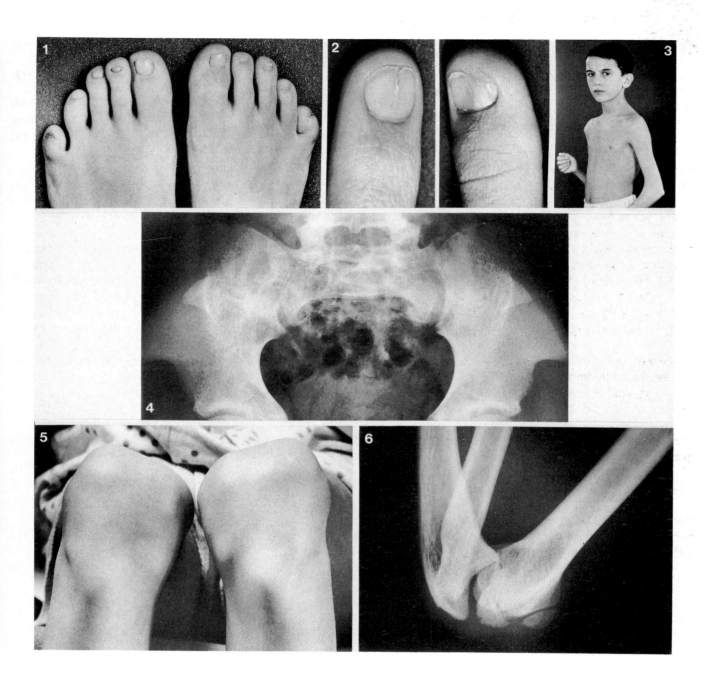

523

A syndrome of mostly minor malformations regarded as being caused by anti-epileptic medication with hydantoin, phenobarbital or carbamazepine.

Main signs:

- Hypoplasia of the distal phalanges of the fingers; shortening of the distal phalanges and hypoplasia or aplasia of the nails (**5 and 6**). Possible simian creases.
- Facial dysmorphism, mainly involving the mid-face: short, broad nose with anteverted nostrils; broad, low nasal bridge; hypertelorism; possible epicanthic folds; low-set, poorly modelled ears (**1–4**).

Supplementary findings:

- Not infrequently, prental and postnatal growth retardation but with compensation possible. Microcephaly (phenobarbital).
- Major malformations also possible, for example, cardiac defects, myelomeningocoeles, cleft lip and palate.
- Possible psychomotor retardation.

Comment: Even independent of anticonvulsant medication, children of epileptic mothers have a higher risk of major malformations, primarily cleft lip or palate and cardiac anomaly (approximately 13%).

Manifestation: At birth.

Aetiology: Anti-epileptics *in utero*. Direct teratogenic effect.

Pathogenesis: Epoxide formation, folic acid deficiency.

Frequency: Minor anomalies and malformations present in around 50% of all newborns of mothers treated with anticonvulsives during pregnancy; lower with monotherapy (48%), increased with polytherapy (56%). Prevalence of myelomeningocoeles after carbamazepine therapy: 1%.

Illustrations:

1–6 A series of typically affected children of various ages.

References:

Dieterich E: Antiepileptika-Embryopathien. Ergeb. *Inn Med Kinderheilk N F* 1979, **43**:93.

Dieterich E, Lukas A, Steveling A *et al*: Art und Ausmaß von Fehlbildungen bzw. Fehlbildungsmustern bei Kindern antiepileptisch behandelter Väter und Mütter. In: *Epilepsie 1979.* H Doose *et al.* (eds). Stuttgart, New York: Thieme, 1980, 47.

Van Dyke D C, Hodge S *et al*: Family studies in fetal phenytoin exposure. *J Pediatr* 1988, **113**:301–306.

Karpathios T, Zervoudakis A, Venieris F *et al*: Genetics and fetal hydantoin syndrome. *Acta Paediatr Scand* 1989, **78**:125–126.

Jones K L, Lacro R V, Johnson K A, Adams J: Pattern of malformations in the children of women treated with carbamazepine during pregnancy. *N Engl J Med* 1989, **320**:1661–1666.

Buehler B A, Delimont D, van Waes M, Finnell R: Prenatal prediction of the fetal hydantoin syndrome. *N Engl J Med* 1990, **322**:1567–1572.

D'Souza S W, Robertson I G, Donnai D, Mawer G: Fetal phenytoin exposure, hypoplastic nails, and jitteriness. *Arch Dis Child* 1990, **65**:320–324.

Rosa F W: Spina bifida in infants of women treated with carbamazepine during pregnancy. *N Engl J Med* 1991, **324**:674–677.

Koch S, Lösche G, Jäger-Roman E *et al*: Major and minor birth malformations and antiepileptic drugs. *Neurol* 1992, **42**(S):83–88.

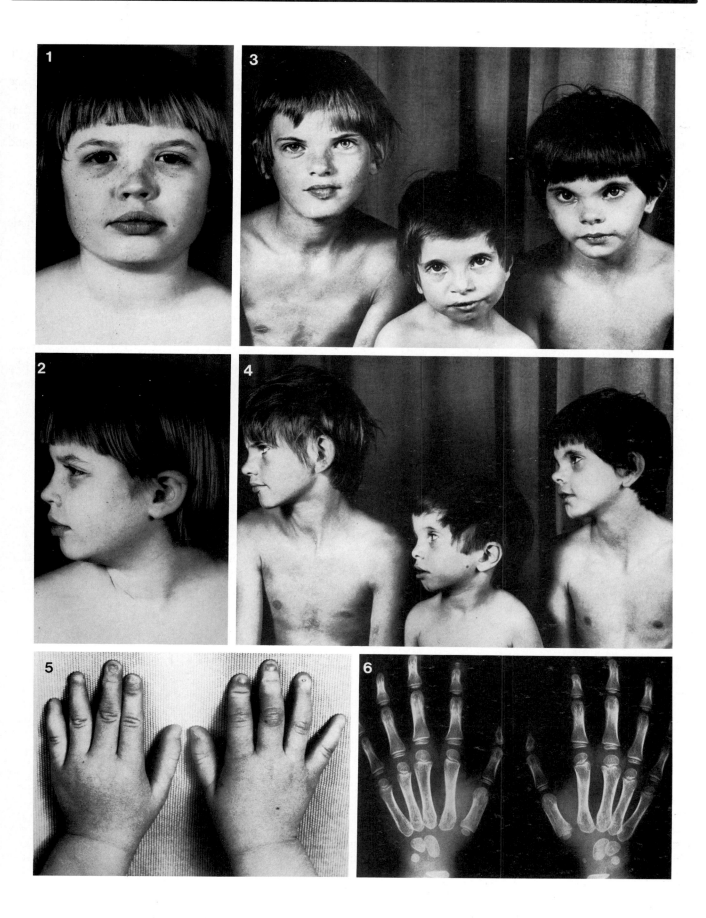

Embryofoetal Valproic Acid Syndrome

(Foetal Valproate Syndrome, Valproic Acid Embryopathy)

J.K./ H.-R.W

A syndrome of fairly characteristic craniofacial abnormalities, frequent developmental delay and, in some patients, serious malformations after valproate treatment of the mother in the first trimester of pregnancy.

Main signs:
- Facial phenotype: metopic ridge, prominent glabella, or trigonocephaly because of early closure of the metopic suture. Unusually narrow forehead, poorly developed outer orbital ridges. Hypoplasia of the mid-face. Epicanthic folds. Short pug nose with broad or flat bridge. Long and flat philtrum and long, narrow upper lip. Small mouth. Retrognathia. Slight deformity of the external ears in some patients.
- Developmental retardation, usually mild to moderate, or neurological abnormalities in (as far as can be judged at present) over 50% of the children.
- Possible lumbrosacral neural tube defects (myelomeningocoele or meningocoele) (in 2%); club feet. Long fingers and toes. Cleft lip and palate; tracheomalacia. Cardiac defect.

Pre-axial malformations had been reported in nine newborns up to 1993: pre-axial polydactyly, triphalangeal thumbs, radial aplasia, proximal phocomelia, club hand, syndactyly of the fingers, aplasia of the thumbs; tibial and pre-axial defect of the lower extremities.

Supplementary findings:
- Frequent hyperexcitability in the early postnatal period as part of a withdrawal syndrome (especially pronounced when the mother required additional anticonvulsants). Possible hypotonia, delayed motor and, not infrequently, speech development.
- Possible cardiac or urogenital anomalies (e.g. hypospadias, cryptorchidism), hernias.
- Combinations of valproic acid with other anticonvulsant treatment in expectant mothers may lead to further defects: microcephaly, postnatal growth delay and others.

Manifestation: At birth and later.

Aetiology: Valproate treatment of the expectant mother, especially in the first trimester.

Frequency: Approximately 75% of newborns of mothers exposed to valproic acid in the first trimester of pregnancy show minor anomalies and malformations. Major malformations are also increased.

Course, prognosis: Dependent on the extent of expression of the syndrome (e.g. myelocoele).

Diagnosis, differential diagnosis: Despite many similar features, the syndrome differs from hydantoin–barbiturate embryofoetopathy (255). Diagnostic differentiation from monogenic syndromes with pre-axial disorders, the VATER association (311), and the Cornelia–de-Lange syndrome (98).

Treatment: As indicated: symptomatic. Prenatal diagnosis using amniocentesis and ultrasound, especially of the lower vertebral column.

Illustrations:

1 and 2 The fairly characteristic facies of an infant with embryofoetal valproic acid syndrome: narrow, prominent forehead, slight mongoloid slant of the palpebral fissures, epicanthic folds, short pug nose with low bridge, flat dorsum, long flat philtrum, thin upper lip and retrognathia.
3 Patient 2: female, 3 days old, with facial dysmorphism.
4 Patient 3: male, 3 days old, with pre-axial hexadactyly.
5 Patient 4: male, severe myelomeningocoele.
6a–d Patient 5: male newborn, radial aplasia right, radial hypoplasia left.

References:
Di Liberti J H, Farndon P A, Dennis N R *et al*: The fetal valproate syndrome. *Am J Med Genet* 1984, **19**:473–481.
Jäger-Roman E, Deichl A, Jakob S *et al*: Fetal growth, major malformations, and minor anomalies in infants born to mothers receiving valproic acid. *J Pediatr* 1986, **108**:997–1004.
Winter R M, Donnai D, Burn J *et al*: Fetal valproate syndrome: is there a recognisable phenotype? *J Med Genet* 1987, **24**:692–695.
Ardinger H A, Atkin J F, Blackston R D *et al*: Verification of the fetal valproate syndrome phenotype. *Am J Med Genet* 1988, **29**:171–185.
Chitayat S, Farrell K *et al*: Congenital abnormalities in two sibs exposed to valproic acid in utero. *Am J Med Genet* 1988, **31**:369–373.
Verloes A, Frikiche A, Gremillet C *et al*: Proximal phocomelia and radial aplasia in fetal valproic syndrome. *Eur J Pediatr* 1990, **149**:266–267.
Martinez-Frias M L: Colinical manifestation of prenatal exposure to valproic acid using case reports and epidemiologic information. *Am J Med Genet* 1990, **37**:277–282.
Buntinx I M: Preaxial polydactyly in the fetal valproat syndrome. *Eur J Pediatr* 1992, **151**:919–920.
Omtzigt J G C, Los F J *et al*: Prenatal diagnosis of spina bifida aperta after first-trimester valproate exposure. *Prenat Diagn* 1992, **12**:893–897 .
Sharony R, Garber A *et al*: Preaxial ray reduction defects as part of valproic acid embryofetopathy. *Prenat Diagn* 1993, **13**:909–918.

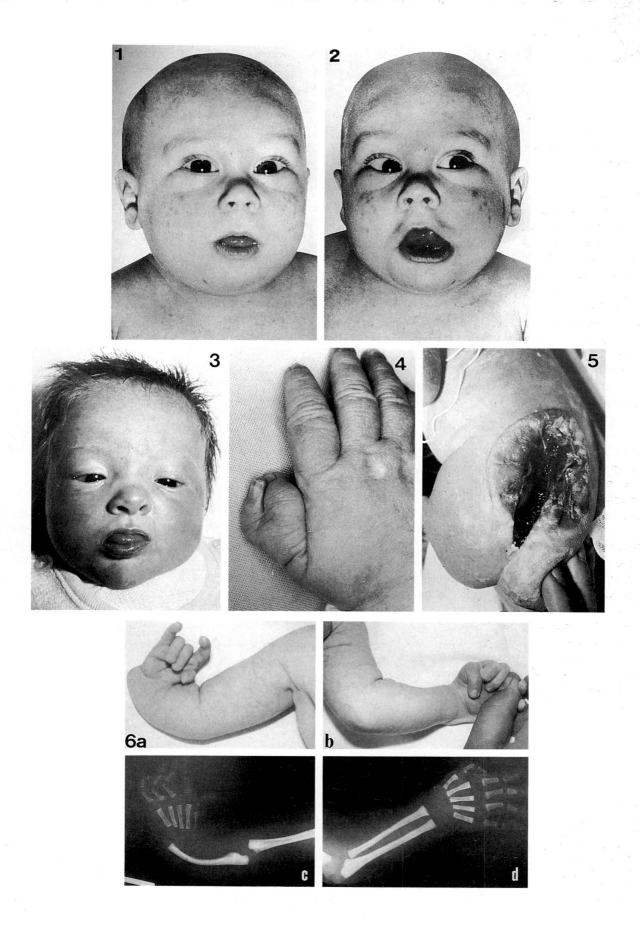

H.-R.W/ J.K.

A hereditary disorder of poikiloderma, nail dystrophy, leukoplakia and possibly pancytopaenia.

Main signs:

- Skin: Formation of subepidermal blisters (clinically usually not very prominent), reticular hyperpigmentation and depigmentation, atrophy and telangiectasia, which result in a 'mottled skin' appearance (poikiloderma) (**1**). Palmar and plantar erythemas, hyperkeratoses, hyperhidrosis.
- Mucous membranes (especially those bordering on the external integument): blisters, ulcers, scars, stenoses, and strictures and also hyperkeratoses and leukoplakia or leukokeratoses (**3**).
- Nails: Severely dystrophic (longitudinal ridges, splitting, shortness, atrophy) (**2, 4–6**).
- Eyes: Blepharitis, lacrimal conjunctivitis with obliteration of the lacrimal puncta and disturbance of the flow of tears; possible ectropion and loss of eyelashes.

Supplementary findings: Development of pancytopaenia (panmyelophthisis) in approximately 50% of patients.

'Connective-tissue weakness' with hyperextensible joints (**2**), tendency to hernias and so on. Sparse, thin hair growth or alopecia. Various anomalies have been observed around the eyes, teeth, skeletal system and the respiratory, oesophageal and urogenital tracts.

Manifestation: Usually between the third and 10th years of life (pancytopaenia tends to develop during the second or third decade).

Aetiology: Hereditary disorder; definite preponderance of males. Hence the prevailing view favours X-linked inheritance (maybe Xq28). Basic defect unknown.
An autosomal recessive form may also exist.

Frequency: Low. Nevertheless, over 100 patients had been described up to 1988.

Course, prognosis: Shortened life expectancy for patients with pancytopaenia, especially from possible malignant transformation of precancerous hyperkeratoses of the mucous membranes.

Diagnosis: Apart from the facial poikiloderma, lacrimal conjunctivitis and nail changes are the most important signs. Differentiate from Fanconi anaemia (*249*).

Treatment: Symptomatic. Close haematological and oncological follow-up; excision of leukoplakia patches. Genetic counselling.

Illustrations:

1, 3, 5, 6 A 10-year-old boy. Hyperpigmentation of the lower eyelids, reticular hyperpigmentation paranasally; lacrimal conjunctivitis, blepharitis, obliteration of the lacrimal puncta. Pancytopaenia.
2, 4 A 13-year-old boy.

References:
Reich H: Zinsser–Cole–Engman-Syndrom. *Med Klin* 1973, **68**:283.
Trowbridge A A, Sirinavin C H, Linman J W: Dyskeratosis congenita: hematologic evaluation of a sibship and review of the literature. *Am J Hematol* 1977, **3**:143.
Rodermund O E, Hausmann G, Hausmann D: Zinsser–Cole–Engman-Syndrom. *Z Hautkr* 1979, **54**:273.
De Boeck K, Degreef H, Verwilghen R *et al*: Thrombocytopenia: first symptom in a patient with dyskeratosis congenita. *Pediatrics* 1981, **67**:898.
Kelly T E, Stelling C B: Dyskeratosis congenita: radiologic features. *Pediatr Radiol* 1982, **12**:31.
Womer R, Clark J E *et al*: Dyskeratosis congenita: two examples of this multisystem disorder. *Pediatrics* 1983, **71**:603–607.
Davidson H R, Connor J M: Dyskeratosis congenita. *J Med Genet* 1988, **25**:843–846.
Shashidhar Pai G, Morgan S, Whetsell C: Etiologic heterogeneity in dyskeratosis congenita. *Am J Med Genet* 1989, **32**:63–66.
De Bauche D M *et al*: Enhanced G 2 chromatid radiosensitivity in dyskeratosis congenita fibroblasts. *Am J Hum Genet* 1990, **46**:350–357.

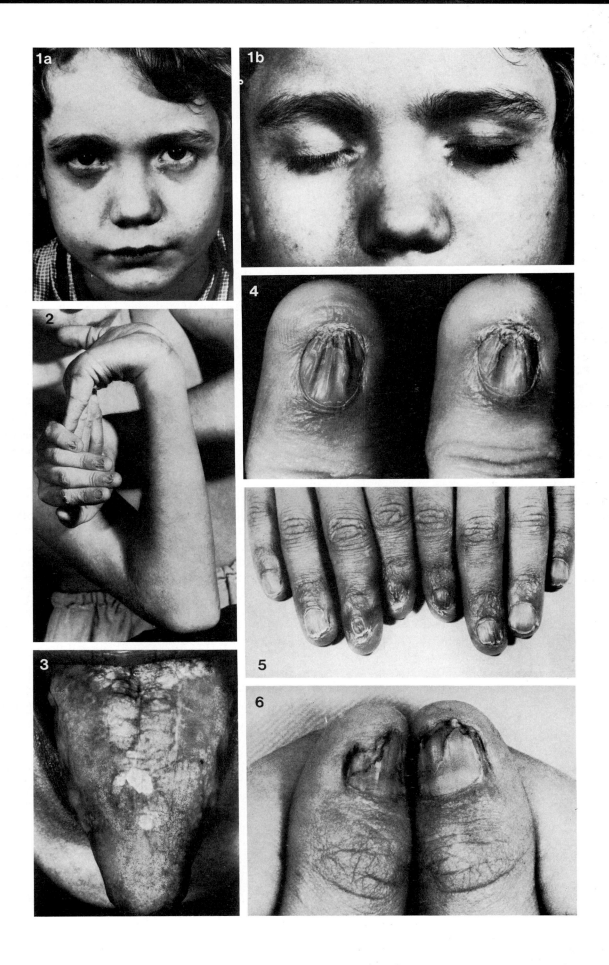

Hypohidrotic Ectodermal Dysplasia
(Christ–Siemens–Touraine Syndrome)

H.-R.W/ J.K.

A highly characteristic hereditary disorder of 'anhidrosis' with the danger of recurrent hyperthermia, hypotrichosis, hypodontia or anodontia and typical facies.

Main signs:
- Characteristic facies with bulging forehead, prominent supra-orbital ridges, hypertelorism, low nasal bridge and short nose with hypoplastic alae nasi, maxillary hypoplasia, full pouting lips, prognathism and possible prominent ears pointed at the top ('satyr ears') (**1, 2, 6**).
- Sparse, light scalp hair; short, fine and dry. Eyebrows and eyelashes absent or extremely sparse. Fine wrinkling of the peri-ocular and sometimes peri-oral skin, often heavily pigmented (**1–4**).
  Premature baldness.
- Alveolar ridges almost absent, with anodontia or hypodontia (**5**).
- Skin is hypoplastic, translucent, soft and very dry, virtually no sweat formation. Possible papular changes on the face and axillae; frequent depigmentation of the nuchal and genital regions. Possible hyperkeratosis of the palms and soles. No lanugo hair in the neonate. Later, little or no body hair.
- Rise in body temperature even with minimal physical exertion (especially in early childhood and infancy) or increased environmental temperature; heat intolerance; failure to thrive.

Supplementary findings: Dry, sensitive mucous membranes with tendency to atrophy. Possible deficiency of tears, conjunctivitis. Frequent photophobia. Tendency to chronic atrophic rhinitis. Possible hyposmia; hoarseness.
  Not infrequently, eczema.
  Possible mild dystrophy of the nails.
  Possible hypoplasia or aplasia of the mamillary glands and nipples.
  Mental retardation in some patients, presumably as the result of cerebral damage from repeated severe hyperthermia.
  Possible sensorineural hearing impairment.
  On biopsy, hypoplasia or aplasia of the exocrine sweat glands and sebaceous glands of the skin and hypoplasia or absence of mucous glands in the mucous membranes.

Manifestation: At birth.

Aetiology: Recessive, sex-linked hereditary disorder affecting males; in females only minor features; identification of female carriers important. Gene locus: Xq12.2-13.1.

Frequency: Approximately 1:100 000 newborns; hundreds of patients described in the literature.

Course, prognosis: Initially, survival or cerebral function endangered by episodes of hyperthermia. Mortality in childhood approximately 30%. In adults, life expectancy and functioning usually no longer appreciably affected.

Diagnosis: Ectodermal dysplasia should be ruled out in all cases of unexplained fever in small infants, even when other signs are minimal. Caution with sweat tests in suspected patients.
  Female carriers of the X-linked recessive form often show dental dysplasia, decreased ability to sweat (regional aplasia of sweat glands; linear distribution of hypohidrotic areas along the V-shaped lines of Blaschko over the back), minimal breast development.

Differential diagnosis: Other ectodermal dysplasia syndromes (*260*). Kohlschütter syndrome (*259*).

Treatment: Immediate cooling for hyperthermia; beware convulsions and brain damage. Protection against overheating and sunstroke; possible move to cooler climate.
  Eyedrops may be required. Otological care. Dentures, possibly from early childhood. A wig may be indicated. Skin care. Genetic counselling.

Illustrations:
1 Infant with hypotrichosis, 'satyr ears', prominent forehead, fine creases in eyelids, full lips. Deficient tears; rhinitis sicca; dysphonia and hoarseness. Aplasia of the dental germs. Dry scaly skin. History of life-threatening episodes of hyperthermia.
2–6 A 2-year-old cousin of the patient in **1**, also with the full clinical picture. Hypoplastic nipples. Skin biopsy showed aplasia of sweat and sebaceous glands.

References:
Zonana J, Clarke A *et al*: X-linked hypohidrotic ectodermal dysplasia: localization within the region Xq11-21.1 by linkage analysis and implications for carrier detection and prenatal diagnosis. *Am J Hum Genet* 1988, 43:75–85.
Clarke A *et al*: Sweat testing to identify female carriers... *J Med Genet* 1991, 28:330–333.
Happle R: Association of pigmentary anomalies with... mosaicism... (Letter). *Am J Hum Genet* 1991, 48:1013–1014.
Zonana J *et al*: Detection of de novo mutations... in... hyphidrotic ectodermal dysplasia. *J Med Genet* 1994, **31**:287–292.

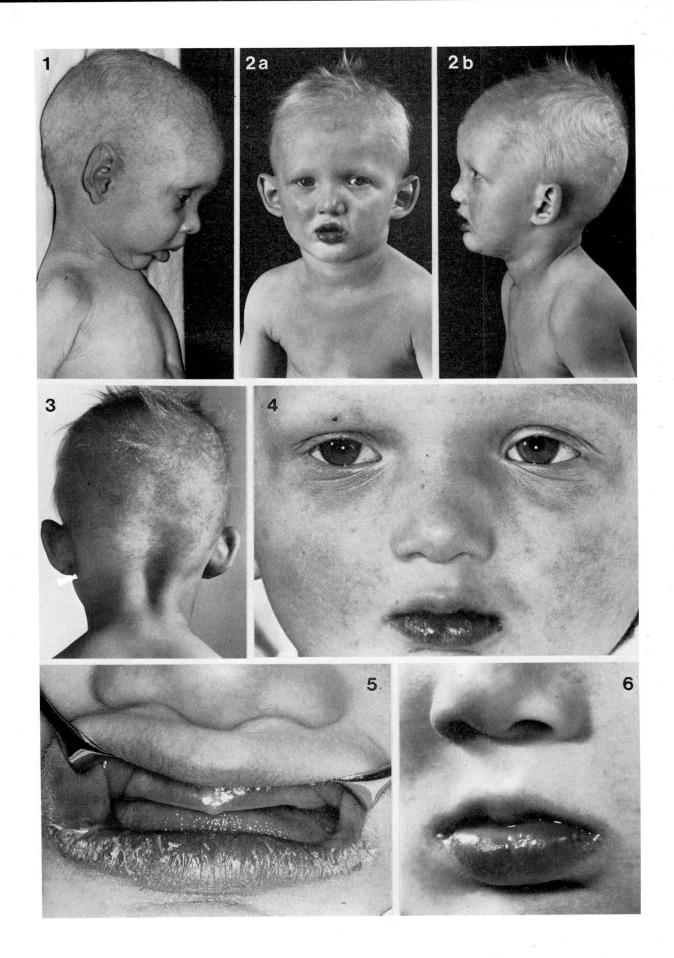

J.K.

A syndrome comprising the triad of amelogenesis imperfecta, cerebral seizures and hypohidrosis.

Main signs:
- Thin, hypoplastic tooth enamel with light amber colouring (amelogenesis imperfecta) of both the primary and secondary dentition.
- Severe epileptic seizures between the 11th month and the fourth year of life.
- Hypohidrosis.

Supplementary findings: Spastic, progressive mental retardation. Nerve conduction velocity and the histology of peripheral nerves are normal. Microcephalic development. Reduced number of sweat glands, increased potassium levels in the sweat.

Manifestation: Amelogenesis recognizable during primary dentition. Neurological anomalies from the end of the first year of life.

Aetiology: Autosomal recessive disorder. We observed two siblings of different sexes.

Pathogenesis: Unknown. Neuro-ectodermal clinical picture.

Course, prognosis: Most patients die in the first decade of life.

Differential diagnosis: Amelo-onychohypohidrotic syndrome, hypohidrotic ectodermal dysplasia, Christ–Siemens–Touraine type (*258*).

Treatment: Seizure control. Dental treatment.

Illustrations:

1 and 2 Brother and sister, aged 5 and 3 years, with amelogenesis imperfecta (light amber teeth colouring); brittle teeth, therapy-resistant epilepsy and retardation.

1 and 2 from:
M. Petermöller, J. Kunze, G. Groß-Selbeck: Kohlschütter syndrome: syndrome of epilepsy, dementia, amelogenesis imperfecta. *Neuropediatrics* 1993, 24:337–338.

References:
Kohlschütter A, Chappuis D, Meter C, Tönz O, Vasella F, Herschkowitz N: Familial epilepsy and yellow teeth — a disease of the central nervous system associated with enamel hypoplasia. *Helv Paediatr Acta* 1974, 29:283–294.
Christodoulou J, Hall R, Menahem S, Hopkins I, Rogers J: A syndrome of epilepsy, dementia, and amelogenesis imperfecta: genetic and clinical features. *J Med Genet* 1988, 25:827–830.
Zlotogora J, Fuks A, Borochowitz Z, Tal, A: Kohlschütter-Tönz syndrome: epilepsy, dementia and amelogenesis imperfecta. *Am J Med Genet* 1993, 46:453–454.
Petermöller M, Kunze J, Groß-Selbeck G: Kohlschütter syndrome: syndrome of epilepsy-dementia-amelogenesis imperfecta. *Neuropediatrics* 1993, 24:337–338.

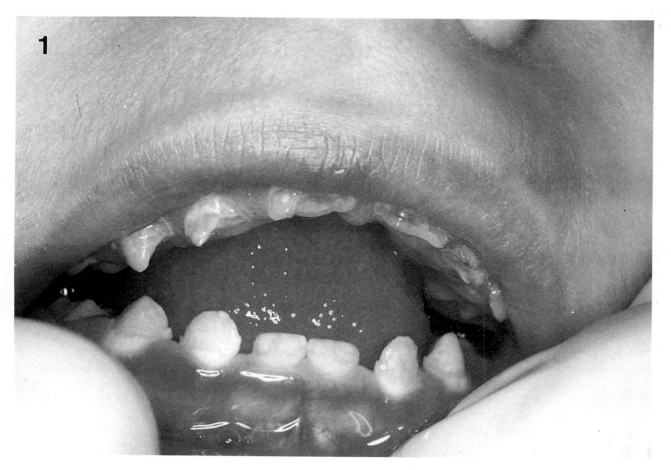

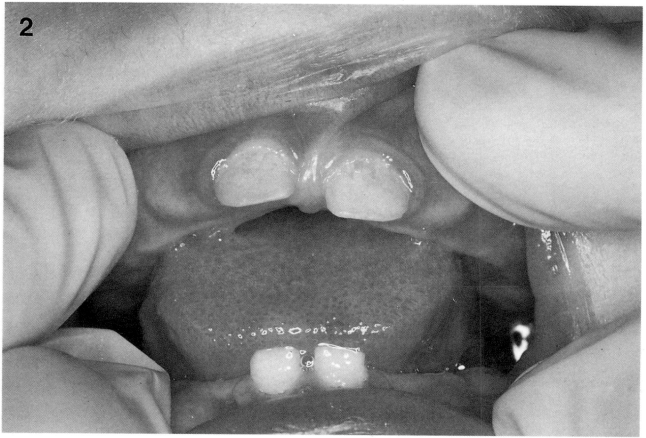

H.-R.W

A syndrome of hypotrichosis with pili torti, dental hypoplasia, ichthyosiform skin changes and cutaneous syndactyly of the hands and feet.

Main signs:
- Hypotrichosis of the scalp, eyebrows and eyelashes (**1, 4–9**). Helical twisting of the hair (pili torti).
- Generalized dryness of the skin, with hyperkeratosis especially on the lower trunk, lower extremities, palms, and soles, with sparing of the axillae and elbows (**10c, 10d**)
- Cutaneous syndactyly of various grades on the hands (III and IV greater than II and III, **10a–d, 12**) and feet (II and III greater than III and IV; **11a–c**).
- Marked hypoplasia of the crowns of the teeth with normal number of teeth and dental germs. (Slight delay in loss of deciduous teeth and eruption of permanent dentition and atypical order of eruption.) Hyperlordosis.

Supplementary findings: No hyperthermia. A dermatological sweat test (using 1,4-dehydroxy anthrachinon powder and an electric cradle) is positive (axillae, elbows, soles of the feet, anterior sweat grooves, anogenital area, thighs, popliteal areas). Thickening and yellow discoloration of some of the toenails.
Bilateral simian creases.
  Absence of hypertelorism, of low nasal bridge and short nose, of full lips, of peri-ocular or peri-oral wrinkling of the skin and of 'satyr' (pointed) ears.
  High palate, normal alveolar processes. Unremarkable mucous membranes.
  Very fine lens opacities on ophthalmoscopic examination. No photophobia. Slight hyperopia.
  Normal mental development. Normal audiometric results.
Normal height and skeletal maturity. Normally formed nipples.
  Unusual familial resemblance of the affected persons.

Manifestations: At birth.

Aetiology: Hereditary disorder; probably autosomal recessive transmission as a result of close parental consanguinity.

Frequency: Unknown; presumably low.

Course, prognosis: Favourable.

Differential diagnosis: Other ectodermal dysplasias (a great variety of types described in the literature).

Treatment: Dental care. A wig may be indicated for both cosmetic and psychological reasons. Genetic counselling.

Illustrations:
1–12 Three siblings aged 12, 6, and 3 years (two other siblings healthy). Pili torti; other parts of hair smooth or wavy; hair mostly white–blond, fine and soft, other parts darker, stronger and firm; very variable length because of easy breakage.
Eyebrows merely suggested; very scanty eyelashes.
Bilateral simian creases in all three children.
  Patient 1 (**1, 2, 4, 7, 10a, 11c**) shows additionally a blind fistula below the tragus of each ear. On ophthalmological examination, very tiny peripheral punctate lens opacities.
  Patient 2 (**3, 5, 8, 10b, 10c, 11b**) has had surgical correction of syndactyly of the left hand. Ophthalmologically, small subcapsular opacities of the right lens at the dorsal pole.
  Patient 3 (**3, 6, 9, 10d, 11a, 12**) was allegedly 'hairless' at birth. Both hands surgically corrected for syndactyly.

Note: *P. Meinecke* (Hamburg) has observed further patients with this syndrome (paper given by *P. Meinecke and H-R. Wiedemann* during the 1st Frankfurt Dysmorphology Workshop from 19-20.11.1993; joint publication in preparation).

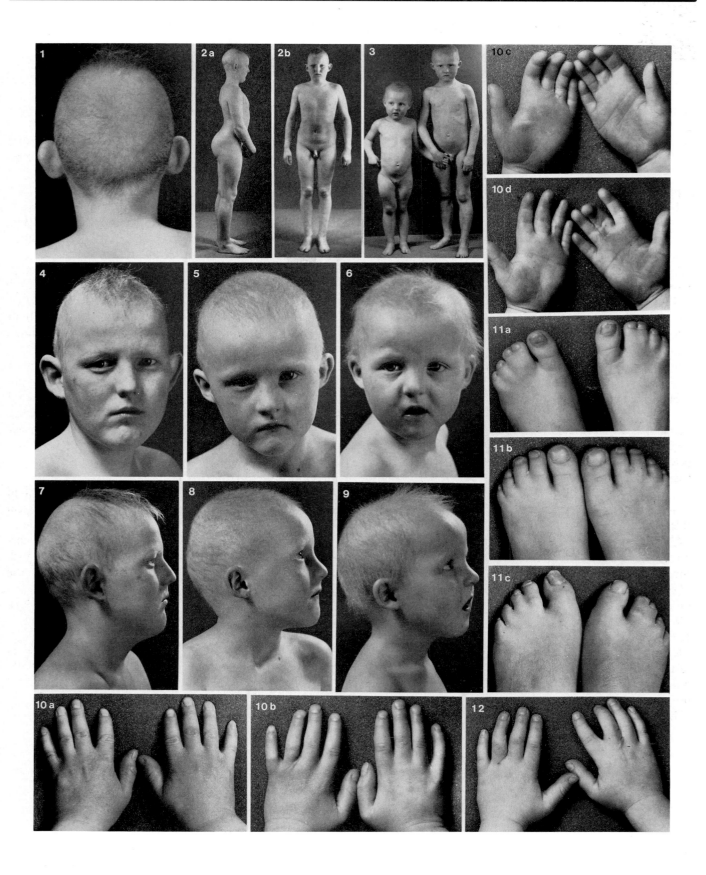

Nonne–Milroy Syndrome
Hereditary Lymphoedema Type I.

J.K.

Main signs:
Lymphoedema of the lower extremities below the inguinal ligament, painless, soft, without signs of inflammation, no ulceration.

Supplementary findings: Sometimes confined to one foot or individual toes.

Manifestation: At birth.

Aetiology: Autosomal dominant disorder with variable expression.

Frequency: 1:6000.

Pathogenesis: Congenital developmental defect of the lymphatic drainage system.

Course, prognosis: Mild pitting, fluctuation of the oedema over the course of the day. Poor local healing after traumatic injury. In adulthood, development of lymphangiosarcomas, squamous epidermoid carcinomas with 50% mortality within 24 months of diagnosis. Without tumours, normal life expectancy.

Differential diagnosis: Lymphoedema type II (Meige), hemihypertrophy (*309*), Ullrich–Turner syndrome (*103*), microcephaly-lymphoedema syndrome with normal intelligence, lymphoedema-distichiasis syndrome (*263*). Hereditary early-onset lymphoedema (*262*).

Treatment: Symptomatic: diuretics, bed rest. Excision of subcutaneous tissue followed by skin graft?

Illustrations:
1–4 Male newborn with lymphoedema of the lower extremities.

References:
Esterly J R: Congenital hereditary lymphedema. *J Med Genet* 1965, **2**:93–98.
Leung A K: Dominantly inherited syndrome of microcephaly and congenital lymphedema. *Clin Genet* 1985, **27**:611–612.
Watts G T: Lymphedema (non-pitting) and simple (pitting) edema are different. *Lancet* 1985, **II**:1414–1415.
Crowe C A, Dickerman L H: A genetic association between microcephaly and lymphedema. *Am J Med Genet* 1986, **24**:131–135.
Opitz J M: On congenital edema (Editorial). *Am J Med Genet* 1986, **24**:127–129.

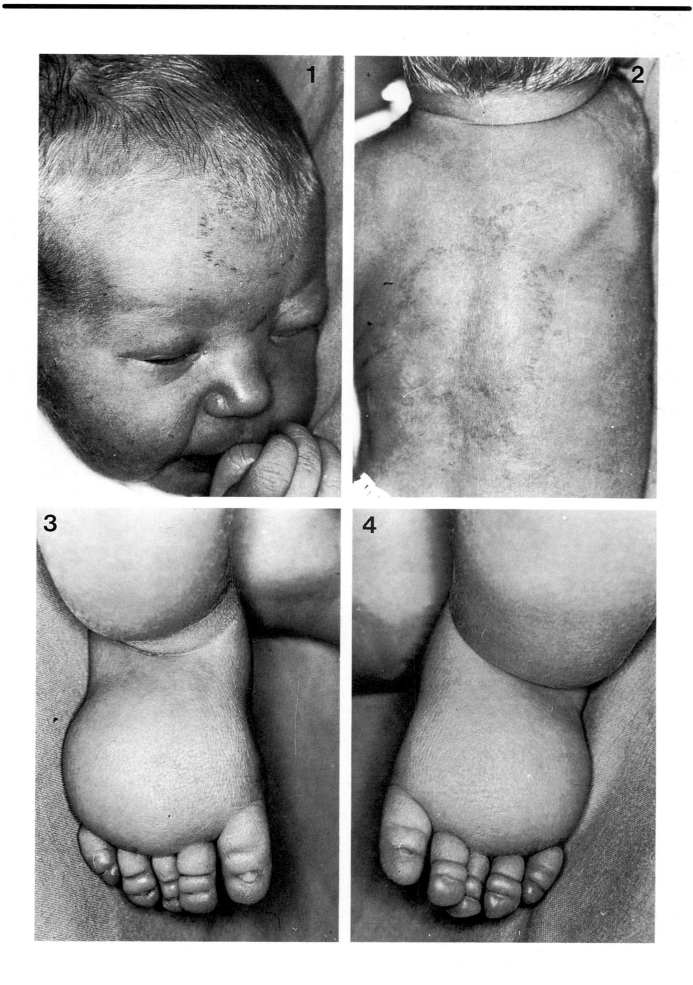

J.K.

A generalized lymphoedema, beginning *in utero*, with facial anomalies, secondary genital anomalies, chemosis and hypo-albuminaemia.

Main signs:
- Severe, generalized lymphoedema with prenatal onset, pronounced in the lower extremities, less marked in the hands and eyelids.
- Intestinal lymphoedema with deep Kerckring's folds (plicae circulares).
- Hypertrophic prepuce.
- Facial anomalies: antimongoloid slant of the palpebral fissures, euryblepharon (lateral dislocation of the lower outer edge of the lid), full cheeks, long upper lip, retrognathia, conjunctival chemosis.

Supplementary findings: Coarctation of the aorta, patent ductus arteriosus. Hypoplasia of the pelvic veins, hypo-albuminaemia, dysproteinaemia.

Manifestation: Prenatal and postnatal.

Aetiology: Autosomal recessive disorder (possibly X-linked recessive).

Pathogenesis: Aplasia or hypoplasia of the lymphatic vessels with dilated extralymphatic spaces.

Frequency: To date only reported in three sibships (twice in brothers and sisters, once in two brothers).

Course, prognosis: Still inconsistent; growth normal or near the third percentile. Increasing chemosis of the sclera. Lymphoedemas unchanged. One patient (11 years and 6 months old) has learning difficulties.

Differential diagnosis: Ullrich–Turner syndrome (*103*), Noonan syndrome (*105*), lymphoedema-distichiasis syndrome (*263*), Nonne–Milroy–Meige syndrome (*261*), intestinal lymphangiectasia.

Treatment: Protein supplementation, triglycerides, elevation of the legs.

Illustrations:
1 Two brothers aged 28 months and 11 years and 5 months.
2 Age 11 years and 5 months, antimongoloid slant of the palpebral fissures, euryblepharon (lateral dislocation of the lower outer edge of the lid), long upper lip, micrognathia.
3 Age 28 months, identical to his brother.
4 Hypertrophic prepuce at 4 months and lymphoedema of the dorsum pedis and lower leg (patient from **2**).
5 Patient from **2** at age 5 years: prepuce still hypertrophic with lymphatic drainage disorder.
6 Chemosis and conjunctival injection.

1-6 from:
J. Mücke et al. Early onset lymphoedema, recessive form. *Eur J Pediatr* 1986, **145**:195–198.

References:
Kajii T, Tsukahar M: Congenital lymphedema in two siblings. *Jpn J Hum Genet* 1985, **30**:31–34.
Kajii T, Tsukahara M: Autosomal recessive lymphedema? (Letter) *Jpn J Hum Genet* 1986, **31**:57.
Mücke J, Hoepffner W, Scheerschmidt G, Gornig H, Beyreiss K: Early onset lymphedema, recessive form — a new form of genetic lymphedema syndrome. *Eur J Pediatr* 1986, **145**:195–198.

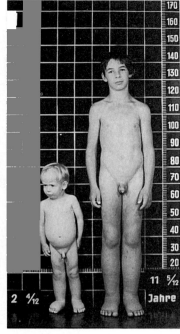
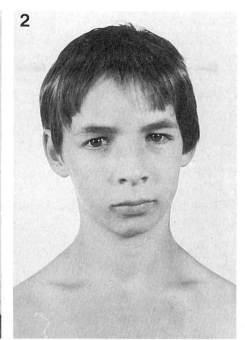
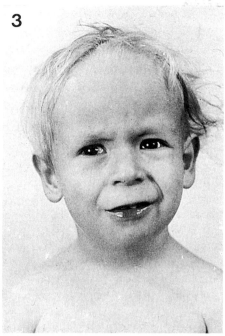

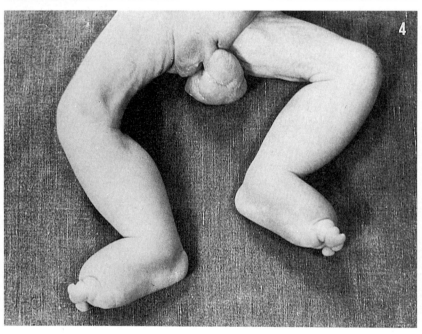
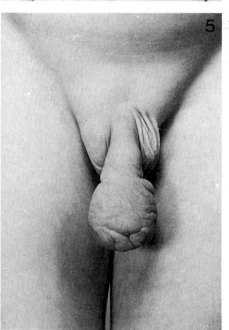

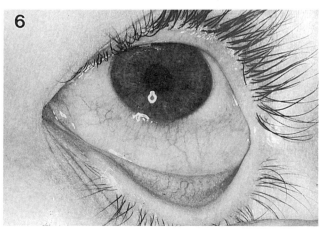

H.-R.W

A hereditary disorder of late-onset lymphoedema of the lower extremities combined with double rows of lashes on the eyelids (distichiasis) and other anomalies.

Main signs:
- Lymphoedema of the legs (2), especially from the knees downward, in males also possibly with considerable scrotal swelling.
- Double rows of eyelashes on the upper and lower lids (3).

Supplementary findings: Ectropion of the lower lids; unilateral or bilateral ptosis; webbed neck (1); dilatation of the spinal canal; formation of arachnoidal and extradural spinal cysts, in some patients with neurological signs; diverse anomalies of the vertebral column have been repeatedly observed. Likewise, congenital cardiac defects, dysrhythmia and development of a dilated cardiomyopathy.

Manifestation: Lymphoedema usually presents from the second half of the first decade of life but possibly not until the second decade or later. One side may be affected many years before the other.

Aetiology: Autosomal dominant disorder with incomplete penetrance and variable expression.

Frequency: Low; approximately 85 patients reported up to 1980.

Course, prognosis: For the most part dependent on the extent and severity of oedema and on development of spinal column complications.

Differential diagnosis: Other forms of late-onset Meige-type lymphoedema.

Treatment: Symptomatic (compression, elevation; diuretics). Removal of annoying lid hair (irritating the conjunctiva or even the cornea). Surgical treatment of oedematous regions not very successful. Genetic counselling.

Illustrations:
1 and 2 A 31-year-old woman, 1.60 m tall, with extensive oedema of the lower legs: on the right leg, since the age of 13 years; on the left leg, increasing since her third pregnancy. Double rows of eyelashes on all four eyelids; ptosis of the right upper eyelid. A dysplastic left auricle and neck webbing have been surgically corrected. Aneurysm of the ascending aorta, tilted kidneys.
Two sons of the proband, aged 11 years and 9 years and 6 months, also show distichiasis; no oedema to date. Further members of the family affected.
3 The lower lid of one of the sons: double row of lashes, some having been removed.

References:
Holmes L G, Fields J P, Zabriskie J B: Hereditary late-onset lymphedema. *Pediatrics* 1978, **61**:575.
Fuhrmann-Rieger A: Familiäres Distichiasis-Lymphödem-Syndrom. In: Klinische *Genetik in der Pädiatrie. I. Symposion in Kiel.* M Tolksdorf, J Spranger (eds). Stuttgart: Thieme 1979.
Schwartz J F, O'Brien M S, Hoffmann J C Jr: Hereditary spinal arachnoid cysts. distichiasis, and lymphedema. *Ann Neurol* 1980, **7**:340.
Pap Z, Biró T et al: Syndrome of lymphoedema and distichiasis. *Hum Genet* 1980, **53**:309–310.
Dale R F: Primary lymphoedema when found with distichiasis is of the type defined as bilateral hyperplasia by lymphography. *J Med Genet* 1987, **24**:170–171.
Hilliard R I, McKendry J B J et al: Congenital abnormalities of the lymphatic system: a new clinical classification. *Pediatrics* 1990, **86**:988–994.
Kolin T, Johns K J et al: Hereditary lymphedema and Distichiasis. *Arch Ophthalmol* 1991, **109**:980–981.
Temple I K, Collin J R O: Distichiasis-lymphoedema syndrome: a famimly report. *Clin Dysmorphol* 1994, **3**:139–142.

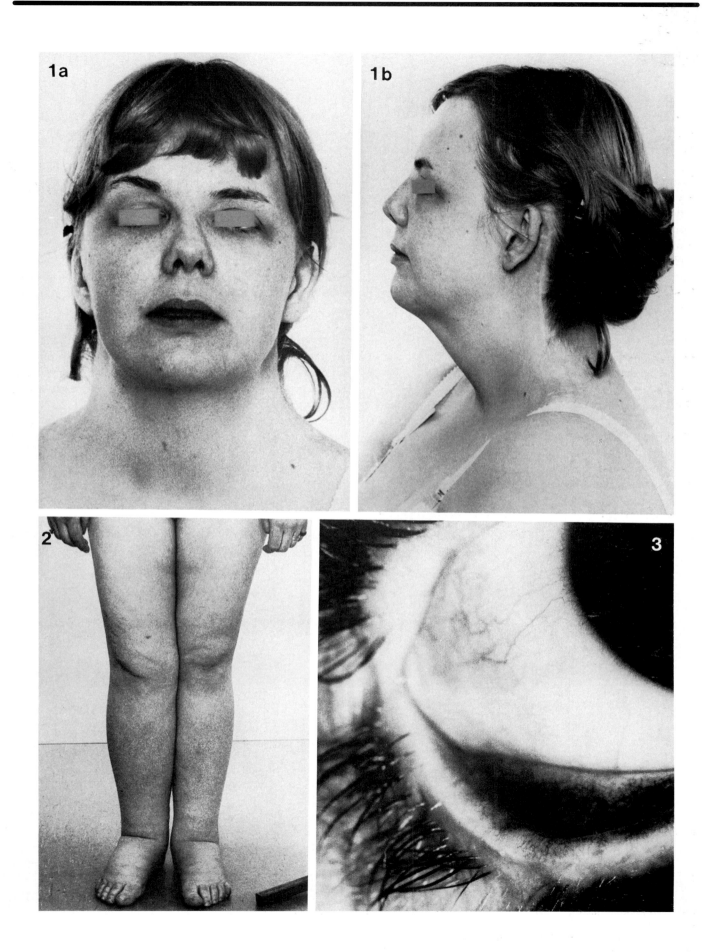

H.-R.W

A hereditary disorder, frequently with an intermittent course, of peri-orificial and acral skin changes, alopecia, and diarrhoea caused by a disorder of zinc metabolism.

Main signs:
- A distinctive skin disorder usually with initial vesico-bullous eruptions, which later become dry-crusted and scaly-lamellar (or psoriatic), at first distributed in symmetrical groups around the body orifices (especially the anogenital region) and eyes (**1**), then the back of the head and neck, elbows, knees, hands and feet. Nails and spaces between the fingers and toes are often significantly involved (**3 and 4**). Frequent secondary bacterial or parasitic infections.
- Alopecia (possibly even total loss of scalp hair, eyebrows and eyelashes) (**1**).
- Possible diarrhoea (various grades of severity).

Supplementary findings: In addition to failure to thrive, poor growth and severe psychological problems: frequent secondary glossitis (**2**) and stomatitis, conjunctivitis, blepharitis and photophobia (**1**) as well as severe nail dystrophies (**3b**) and even loss of nails.
Increased susceptibility to infections.
Low serum and urinary zinc levels (plus low serum alkaline phosphatase and reduced metallo-enzymes).

Manifestation: Usually presents during the first year of life; often after weaning from breast milk; occasionally not until later.

Aetiology: Autosomal recessive disorder (disorder of zinc metabolism with zinc malabsorption and its sequelae).

Frequency: Low.

Course, prognosis: Without therapy, intermittent but relentlessly progressive course usually leading to early death. With adequate treatment, usually normal life expectancy.

Treatment: Oral zinc substitution (usually with zinc sulphate) brings about dramatic improvement and healing of all lesions within a few weeks. Follow up and specific treatment, if necessary, of accompanying secondary infections. Lifelong zinc substitution required.
Genetic counselling.

Illustrations:
An 8-year-old boy (**1, 3a**) and a 3-year-old girl (**2, 3b, 4**), both with the fully developed clinical picture.

References:
Lombeck I, Schnippering H G, Kasperek K *et al*: Akrodermatitis enteropathica - eine Zinkstoffwechselstörung mit Zinkmalabsorption. *Z Kinderheilk* 1975, **120**:181.
Chandra R K: Acrodermatitis enteropathica: zinc levels and cell-mediated immunity. *Pediatrics* 1980, **66**:789.
Brenton D P, Jackson M J *et al*: Two pregnancies in a patient with acrodermatitis enteropathica treated with zinc sulphate. *Lancet* 1981, **II**:500–502.
Gordon E F, Gordon R C *et al*: Zinc metabolism: basic, clinical and behavioral aspects. *J Pediatr* 1981, **99**:341–349.
Ohlsson A: Acrodermatitis enteropathica: reversibility of cerebral atrophy with zinc therapy. *Acta Paediat Scand* 1981, **70**:269–273.

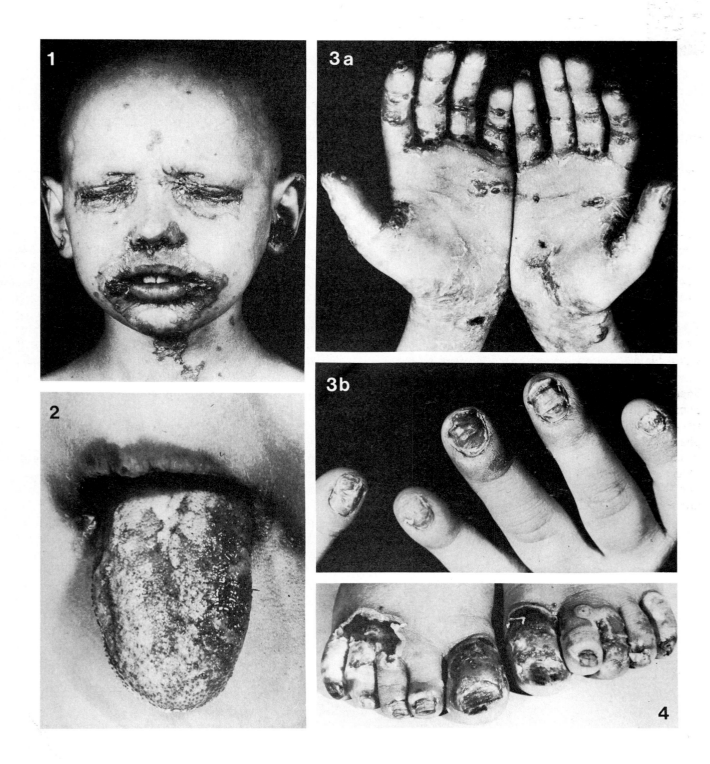

Ichthyosis congenita is a heterogeneous group of diseases with at least seven different genotypes.

Main signs: A group of genetically and clinically heterogeneous clinical pictures, symptomatic from birth, involving the large flexion creases and possibly the palms and soles; no association with other clinical signs. Three groups of disorders are delineated: the lamellar ichthyoses, the bullous ichthyoses and a group with two specific variants.

Lamellar ichthyoses: Non-bullous, non-epidermolytic (except for the harlequin foetus), congenital ichthyoses: often initially coming to clinical attention as collodion baby, self-healing. Subclassified as autosomal dominant lamellar ichthyoses, erythrodermal ichthyoses and non-erythrodermal lamellar ichthyoses.

Autosomal dominant lamellar ichthyoses: present at birth, not a collodion baby; the entire body (including the palms and soles) is covered with large dark grey scales; flexion surfaces less severely affected; lichenification of the dorsum pedis. Severe caries from early infancy.

Erythrodermal lamellar ichthyoses: ichthyosiform erythroderma at birth; usually collodion baby; scaling of the flexion surfaces, hyperkeratosis of the hands and feet. Ectropion.

Non-erythrodermal lamellar ichthyoses: no erythroderma at birth but the large, disc-shaped, dark grey scales are interspersed with red lines, which are less marked on the surfaces of the hands and feet than in erythrodermal lamellar ichthyoses.

Bullous ichthyoses: Brocq-type bullous, ichthyosiform erythroderma and Siemens-type ichthyosis bullosa. Histologically, epidermolytic hyperkeratoses (acanthokeratolysis) are grouped together.

Brocq-type bullous, ichthyosiform erythroderma: Immediately *post partum*, ichthyosiform erythroderma and severe blistering (*enfants brûlés*); towards the end of the first year the erythroderma fades, giving way to a spine-like hyperkeratosis, sometimes protruding as much as 1 cm (hystrix-like), especially in the large flexion areas. On the trunk, lichenification, blistering after skin lesions, sparing the palms and soles.

Siemens-type ichthyosis bullosa: blistering at birth, dark grey hyperkeratoses also in the flexion areas, with lichenification on the extensor surfaces of the major joints. Localized areas of the axilla spared centrally and localized hyperkeratoses on the trunk. Blistering after minor traumas. In most patients, superficial desquamation ('moulting') on the hands and feet. Palms and soles clear.

Special variants: ichthyosis hystrix (as reported by *Curth* and *Macklin*) and the harlequin foetus.

Curth–Macklin ichthyosis hystrix: Spine-like, keratotic masses cover the body, including the flexion areas and the palms and soles. Variable picture.

'Harlequin' foetus (266).

Manifestation: Prenatal and at birth.

Aetiology: The lamellar ichthyoses are inherited as autosomal recessive traits, with the exception of one autosomal dominant type. Prenatal diagnosis is not possible before the 22nd week of pregnancy because of the later keratinization of the skin (except for two subtypes with earlier keratinization). The bullous ichthyoses and Curth–Macklin ichthyosis hystrix are inherited as autosomal dominant traits. Prenatal diagnosis is possible in the 20th week of pregnancy by foetal skin biopsy (ultrastructural examination).

Pathogenesis: Disturbed keratinization of the epidermis, basement membrane and the stratum granulosum and changes within the stratum corneum.

Frequency: Gene frequencies of 1:20 000 are given.

Course, prognosis: Dependent on the type of disorder. Complications are: pruritis, skin infections (impetigo), hyperhidrosis, alopecia ichthyotica, cosmetic problems, body odour.

Differential diagnosis: Associated congenital ichthyoses: KID syndrome (keratitis–ichthyosis–deafness), X-linked dominant ichthyosis, Comel–Netherton syndrome, neutral fat storage disease, Sjögren–Larsson syndrome (267), HID syndrome (hystrix-like ichthyosis and deafness), IFAP syndrome (ichthyosis follicularis, atrichia and photophobia).

Treatment: Keratolysis, humidity: uric acid, propylene glycol, acetylsalicylic acid, sodium chloride, lactic acid. A maritime climate is favourable, likewise a hot climate. Treat body odour with daily potassium permanganate baths.

Illustrations:

1a–c A 4-day-old boy. 'Collodion baby' with a taut, shiny 'skin armour'; desquamation in progress.

2 A 5-day-old girl, sister of the patient in 1; identical picture.

3 A further 'collodion child'. 3a, at 10 days; 3b, at 3 weeks with sheet-like desquamation.

4a and b A brother of the child in 3, at age 2 days: O-shaped mouth; fingers and toes firmly enclosed by a shiny layer of skin; deep cracks in the sheets of skin on the trunk.

5a and b A further patient. Fingers and toes enveloped in an armour-like covering.

References:

Anton-Lamprecht I: Hereditäre Ichthyosen. In: *Pädiatrische Dermatologie*. J J Herzberg, G W Korting (eds). Stuttgart, New York: Schattauer, 1978, 161–182.

Anton-Lamprecht I: Prenatal diagnosis of genetic disorders of the skin by means of electron microscopy. *Hum Genet* 1981, 59:392–405.

Traupe H: *The ichthyoses. A guide to clinical diagnosis, genetic counselling, and therapy.* Berlin: Springer, 1989.

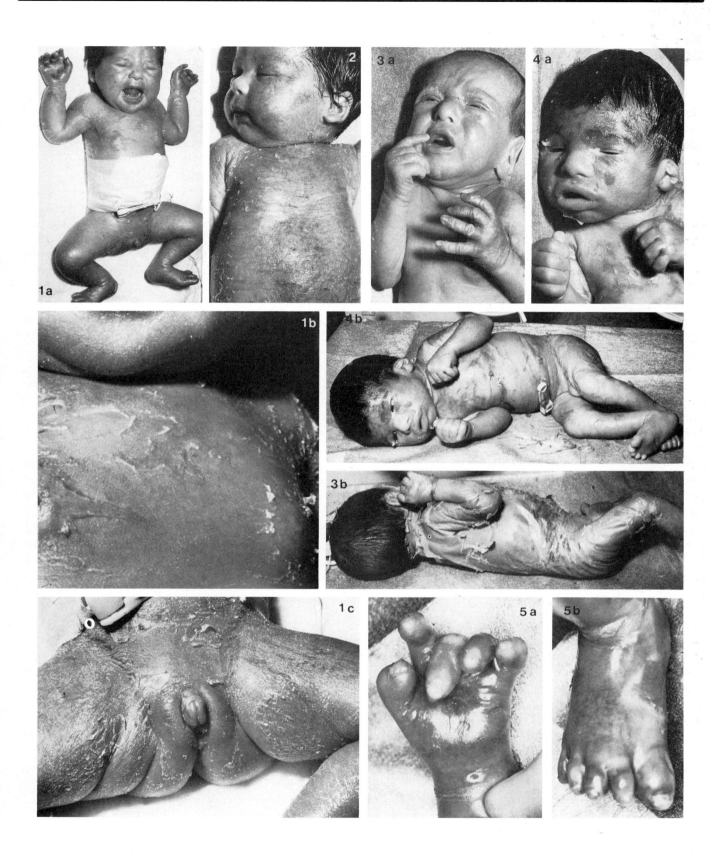

J.K.

An extreme, lethal form of ichthyosis congenita with a severe disorder of skin keratinization. As the horny skin masses split or tear in a rhomboidal pattern *post partum*, such children have also been called 'harlequin' foetuses.

Main signs:

- Postnatally, the infant appears to be constricted in a thick, yellow–white 'skin armour'. Shortly after birth, cracks up to a centimetre deep appear in the skin: the hyperkeratotic epidermis takes on polygonal, rhomboidal forms (resembling a harlequin costume). Dark red cutis is visible at the base of the clefts (1–3).
- The face is altered past recognition with ectropion of the mouth and eyes (2). The ears appear packed in armour (1, 3).
- Hands and feet are also firmly constricted and the fingers and toes immobilized. Clawlike position (1, 3).

Supplementary findings: Histologically, a markedly thickened lamellar horny layer with absence of the stratum granulosum in some areas.

Manifestation: Prenatally (from the sixth month of pregnancy) and *post partum*.

Aetiology: Autosomal recessive inheritance. Several affected siblings observed.

In one child, the horny mass showed beta-keratins instead of alpha-keratin and an abnormal amino acid composition.

Frequency: 1:300 000 newborns.

Course, prognosis: Death in the newborn period as a result of infection, sepsis, respiratory disorders. Since 1985, there have been reports of patients surviving for several years after administration of oral retinoids. Clinical progression to erythrodermal lamellar ichthyosis. Normal intelligence.

Differential diagnosis: Neu Laxova syndrome, restrictive dermopathy (*271*), Sjögren–Larsson syndrome (*267*), Rud syndrome (*268*), Tay syndrome (*270*).

Treatment: Attempt to peel off the horny plates in a humid incubator environment and use of oral retinoids, oil.

Prenatal diagnosis possible from the 20th week of pregnancy (foetal skin biopsy, ultrastructural examination).

Illustrations:

1–3 A characteristically affected newborn; immediate death *post partum*.

References:

Anton-Lamprecht I: Hereditäre Ichthyosen. In: *Pädiatrische Dermatologie*. J. J. Herzberg, G. W. Korting (eds). Stuttgart, New York: Schattauer, 1978, 161–183.

Brenndorff A I v: Ichthyosis congenita. *Pädiatr Prax* 1983, 28:499–506 (1983).

Blanchet-Bardon C, Dumez Y, Luzner M-A *et al*: Prenatal diagnosis of harlequin fetus. *Lancet* 1983, I:132.

Lawlor F, Peiris S: Harlequin fetus successfully treated with etretinate. *Br J Dermatol* 1985, 112:585–590.

Arnold M L, Andon-Lamprecht I: Prenatal diagnosis of epidermal disorders. *Curr Probl Dermatol* 1987, 16:120–128.

Unamuno P, Pierola J M *et al*: Harlequin foetus in four siblings. *Br J Dermatol* 1987, 116:569–572.

Lawlor F: Progress of a Harlequin fetus to nonbullous ichthyosiform erythroderma. *Pediatrics* 1988, 82:870–873.

Herterich R, Hofweber K, Hammerschmid K, Steijlen P M, Happle R: Harlequin-Ichthyosis. Erfolgreiche Therapie mit oralen Retinoiden. *Pädiatr Prax* 1993/94, 46:93–99.

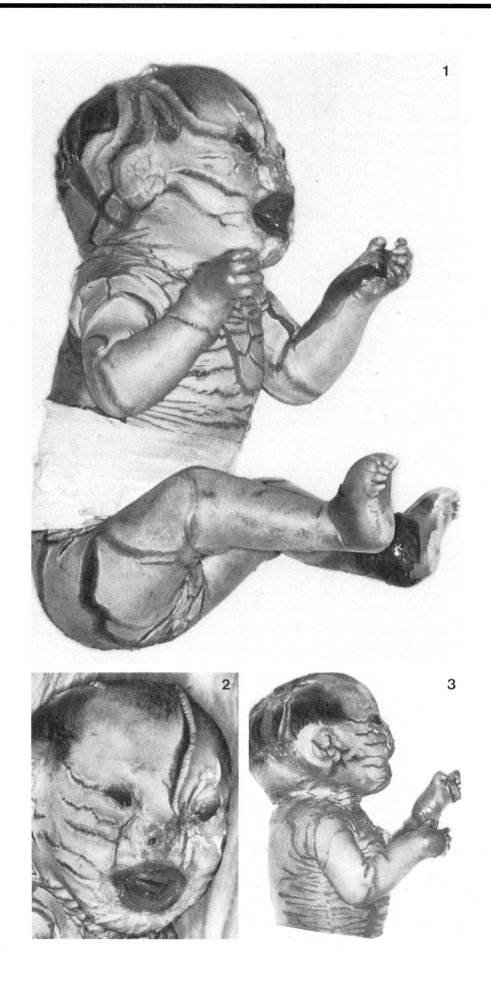

J.K./ H.-R.W

A familial disorder with congenital ichthyosis, spastic paraparesis, mental retardation and short stature.

Main signs:

- Congenital ichthyosis, especially of the nuchal, axillary, and other flexion areas; the face may remain clear. Possible hyperkeratoses of the hands and feet. In the neonatal period, marked ichthyosis on the lower trunk, transient erythema. Ichthyosis fully expressed at age 12 months. The erythema fades.
- Spastic paraplegia (to tetraplegia) plegia, developing between the fourth and 30th month of life. Joint contractures. Restricted movement of the vertebral column.
- Considerable mental retardation (IQ generally between 30 and 60); usually a speech disorder of variable severity. Borderline intelligence (IQ 70–79) has also been observed.
- Short stature (often below the 10th percentile).

Supplementary findings: Seizures in approximately one-third of patients. Blepharitis, conjunctivitis, punctate corneal erosions. Pigmentary degeneration of the retina, reflective spots seen foveally and parafoveally in approximately 25–30% of patients.

Decreased ability to sweat. Hypoplasia of teeth and enamel. Scalp hair may be sparse.

Manifestation: Ichthyosis, scaling and hyperkeratosis from birth. The central nervous system manifestations become apparent in the first 3 years of life. Small size may be apparent at birth.

Aetiology: Autosomal recessive disorder. In fibroblasts the fatty alcohol-(nicotinamide-adenine-dinucleotide) oxireductase levels are reduced. Even in heterozygotes, fatty alcohol oxireductase or fatty aldehyde dehydrogenase levels are reduced. Differentiate from other ichthyoses using enzyme-histochemical evidence of hexanol-dehydrogenase activity from skin biopsies.

Frequency: Varies regionally, increased in certain areas where inbreeding is common; otherwise rare. In Sweden 1:1 million. Over 200 patients documented in the literature.

Course, prognosis: Very dependent on the severity of mental retardation, diplegia and possible visual impairment. Three quarters of all patients are confined to a wheelchair.

Differential diagnosis: Rud syndrome (*268*), ichthyosis congenita (*265*), Tay syndrome (*270*).

Treatment: Symptomatic. Genetic counselling. Prenatal diagnosis: measurement of fatty alcohol oxireductase activity in amniotic or chorionic cells. Foetal skin biopsy in the 23rd week of pregnancy (ultrastructural examination).

Illustrations:

1 and 2 A mentally retarded boy with spastic diplegia and congenital ichthyosis with hyperkeratosis.

3 A girl at age 4 years and 8 months: spastic diplegia, cerebral shunt with hydrocephalus.

4 Generalized ichthyosis congenita.

References:

Theile U: Sjögren–Larsson syndrome. Oligophrenia-ichthyosis-di/tetraplegia. *Humangenetik* 1974, 22:91.
Jagell S, Lidén S: Ichthyosis in the Sjögren–Larsson syndrome. *Clin Genet* 1982, 21:243.
Jagell S, Heijbel J: Sjögren–Larsson syndrome: physical and neurological findings. *Helv Paediatr Acta* 1982, 37:519–530.
Kousseff B G, Matsuoka L Y *et al*: Prenatal diagnosis of Sjögren–Larsson syndrome. *J Pediatr* 1982, 101:998–1001.
Gedde-Dahl T Jr, Rajka, G et al: Autosomal recessive ichthyosis in Norway: II. Sjögren–Larsson like ichthyosis without CNS or eye involvement. *Clin Genet* 1984, 26:242–244.
Chaves-Carballo E: Sjögren–Larsson syndrome. In: *Neurocutaneous diseases*. M R Gomez (ed). Boston: Butterworth, 1987, 219–224).
Iselius L, Jagell S: Sjögren–Larsson syndrome in Sweden: distribution of the gene. *Clin Genet* 1989, 35:272–275.
Rizzo W B, Dammann A L *et al*: Sjögren–Larsson syndrome: Inherited defect in the fatty alcohol cycle. *J Pediatr* 1989, 115:228–234.
Lake B D, Smith V V *et al*: Hexanol dehydrogenase activity shown by enzyme histochemistry on skin biopsies allows differentiation of Sjögren–Larsson syndrome from other ichthyoses. *J Inher Metab Dis* 1991, 14:338–340.
Levisohn D, Dintiman B, Rizzo W B: Sjögren–Larsson syndrome: Case reports. *Pediatr Dermatol* 1991, 8:217–220.
Kelson T L, Craft D A, Rizzo W B: Carrier detection for Sjögren–Larsson syndrome. *J Inher Metab Dis* 1992, 15:105–111.
Rizzo W B, Craft D A *et al*: Prenatal diagnosis of Sjögren–Larsson syndrome using enzymatic methods. Prenat Diagn 1994 14:577–578

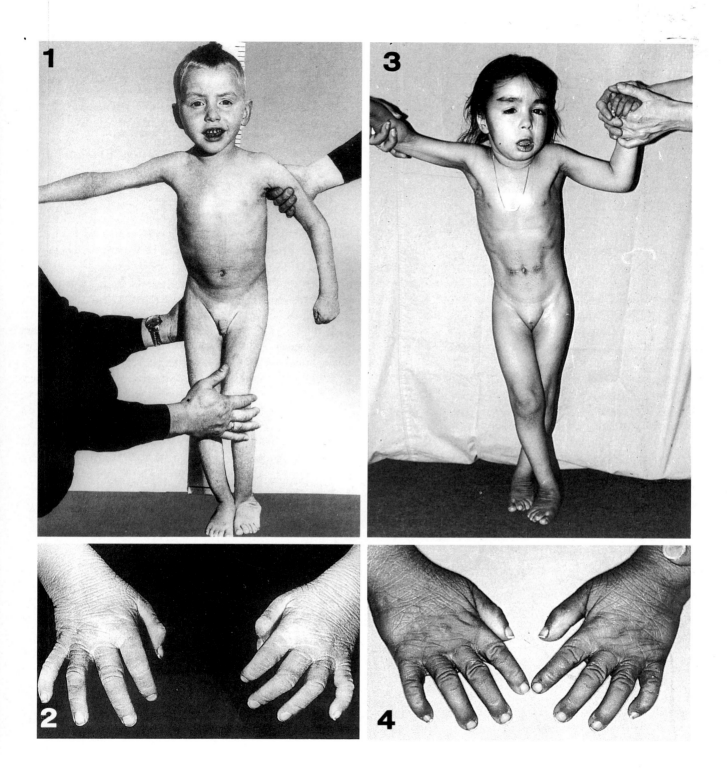

Rud Syndrome

(Ichthyosis–Hypogonadism–Mental Retardation–Epilepsy Syndrome)

H.-R.W

A hereditary disorder comprising ichthyosis, mental retardation, epilepsy and (almost invariably) hypogonadism.

Main signs:
- Ichthyosis, usually from early infancy.
- Psychomotor retardation of variable severity (IQ between 30 and 80).
- Seizure disorder (time of onset variable).

Supplementary findings: Hypogonadism with eunuchoid habitus and in some patients fairly distinct sexual infantilism.

Short stature, possible hypoplastic teeth and nails, possible eye or hearing disorders.

Manifestation: At birth or later.

Aetiology: Uniformity of this syndrome questionable. No doubt of a genetic basis. Sporadic occurrence in most patients. Autosomal recessive transmission has been presumed. An X-linked recessive type may also occur.

Frequency: Low.

Course, prognosis: Very dependent on the degree of mental retardation and severity of epilepsy.

Differential diagnosis: Sjögren–Larsson syndrome (267), ichthyosis congenita (265), Tay syndrome (270).

Treatment: Symptomatic. Genetic counselling.

Illustrations:
1–9 Three brothers, the children of healthy parents; one brother of the mother has ichthyosis congenita.
5, 8 The oldest boy at 16 years and 3 months: moderate ichthyosis since birth. Developmental retardation, low intelligence; no seizures (to date), genitalia in **8**.
1–4, 7 The 'middle' brother at 10 years (**4**) and 13 years and 6 months (**1–3**): ichthyosis since birth, mental retardation, seizure disorder, hypogenitalism (**7**).
6, 9 The youngest brother at 10 years. Moderately severe ichthyosis since birth, low-normal mental development, no seizures (to date), genitalia in **9** (undescended testis on the right).

Chromosomal analyses of the three brothers unremarkable (with banding). A sister, aged 14 years and 6 months, healthy and normally developed for her age.

References:

Maldonaldo R R *et al*: Neuroichthyosis with hypogonadism (Rud's syndrome). *Int J Dermatol* 1975, **14**:347.
Larbisseau A, Carpenter St: Rud syndrome... *Neuropediatrics* 1982, **13**:95.
Münke M, Kruse K *et al*: Genetic heterogeneity of the ichthyosis, hypogonadism, mental retardation, and epilepsy syndrome... *Eur J Pediatr* 1983, **141**:8–13.
Traupe H, Müller-Migl C R *et al*: Ichthyosis vulgaris with hypogenitalism and hypogonadism: evidence for different genotypes... *Clin Genet* 1984, **25**:42–51.
Scribanis R, Buoncompagni A *et al*: La sindrome di Rud. *Min Pediatr* 1985, **37**:823–826.
Marxmiller J, Trenkle I *et al*: Rud syndrome revisited... *Dev Med Child Neurol* 1985, **27**:335–343.
Wisniewski K, Levis A *et al*: X-linked inheritance of the Rud syndrome (Abstract). *Am J Hum Genet* 1985, **37A**:83.

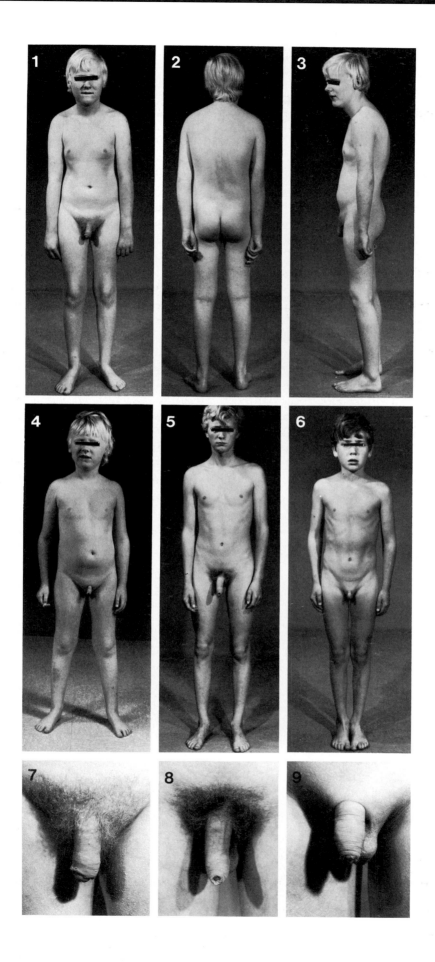

269 Hyperkeratosis Palmoplantaris with Periodontoclasia
(Papillon–Lefèvre Syndrome)

J.K./ H.-R.W

A syndrome of plantopalmar hyperkeratoses, periodontopathy and loss of teeth.

Main signs:
- Hyperkeratosis of the soles of the feet and the palms of the hands, the latter usually being less severely affected (**2 and 3**).
- Severe periodontal destruction of the deciduous and subsequent teeth with loosening and loss of all teeth (**1**).

Supplementary findings: Severe secondary periodontitis and gingivostomatitis.

Possible mental retardation, intracranial calcification, nail dysplasia and increased susceptibility to infections. Increased brittleness of the nails, alopecia, cysts on the eyelids.

Manifestation: Reddening and hyperkeratosis of the palms and soles may be apparent from birth and, when an older sibling is typically affected, allows for early diagnosis. Otherwise the diagnosis cannot be made until eruption of the primary dentition and the immediate onset of dental problems.

Aetiology: Autosomal recessive disorder.

Frequency: Low. Estimated one out of 1 million of the general population; 126 patients known in the literature up to 1979.

Course, prognosis: Severe periodontosis (and secondary periodontitis) affects the primary and later the secondary dentition with loss of all teeth. The deciduous teeth are lost at age 5–6 years, and the permanent teeth at 13–14 years.

No occupational difficulties from the palmar skin disorder.

Treatment: Symptomatic. Special oral hygiene. Dental care. Dental prostheses (upper and lower) at the appropriate time. Treatment with oral retinoids. Genetic counselling.

Illustrations:

1–4 A Turkish boy, aged 3 years and 9 months, family history not available. Dyskeratotic–hyperkeratotic changes of the palms and soles with garland-like, sharply delineated border to the healthy skin at the level of the malleoli and the heels. Reddening of the volar and plantar skin. Bilateral hyperkeratoses of the patellar regions. Early loss of deciduous teeth in both jaws; a few remaining, loose teeth with the necks extensively exposed; periodontosis.

References:

Giasanti J S *et al*: Palmar-plantar hyperkeratosis and concomitant periodontal destruction (Papillon–Lefèvre syndrome). *Oral Surg* 1973, **36**:40.
Hacham-Zadeh S, Schaap T *et al*: A genetic analysis of the Papillon–Lefèvre syndrome... *Am J Med Genet* 1978, 2:153–157.
Haneke E: The Papillon–Lefèvre syndrome... report of a case and review... *Hum Genet* 1979, 51:1–35.
Geormaneanu M, Ciofu C *et al*: Maladie de Papillon–Lefèvre... *Ann Génét* 1982, 25:189–192.
Nazzaro V, Blanchet-Bardoon C, Mimoz C, Revuz J, Puissant A: Papillon–Lefèvre syndrome: ultrastructural study and successful treatment with acitretin. *Arch Dermatol* 1988, **124**:533–539.

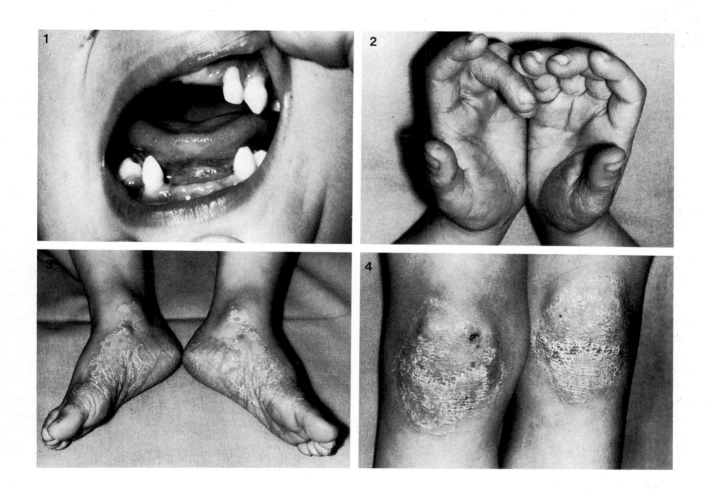

270 Tay Syndrome

(Amish, Brittle Hair Syndrome; PIBIDS Syndrome [Photosensitivity, Ichthyosis, Brittle Hair, Impaired Intelligence, Decreased Fertility, Short Stature])

J.K.

A syndrome characterized by trichothiodystrophy (brittle hair), congenital ichthyosis and microcephaly.

Main signs:
- Prenatal dystrophy.
- Congenital ichthyosis or ichthyosiform erythroderma, sometimes 'collodion baby', flexion surfaces of the extremities remain clear. Appearance of progeria.
- Disturbed hair growth: sparse, short, thin, brittle (trichothiodystrophy). Dysplasia of the nails.
- Microcephaly; non-progressive, mild mental deterioration.
- Short stature.

Supplementary findings: Examination under a polarizing or electron microscope reveals pili torti, trichoschisis, trichorrhexis nodosa, a zigzag, banded pattern, alternately light and dark (polarizing microscopy: 'tiger-tail' appearance). Cysteine deficiency (50% of normal levels). Over one half of all patients suffer from photophobia. Mottled lesions on exposure of the skin to sunlight.
Facial deformities: prominent nose because of reduced subcutaneous tissue, micrognathia, large protruding ears.
Neurology: defective co-ordination when performing precise movements, unsteady gait, ataxia, intention tremor, rigidity, spasticity, mild sensorineural deafness, intracerebral calcification, electroencephalogram changes. Mild mental retardation (microcephaly). Punctate cataract.
Dysphonia: hoarse, croaking, high voice.
Partial anodontia, severe caries, yellowing of the teeth.
Severe susceptibility to infection.

Delayed postpubertal development with cryptorchidism, genital hypoplasia, disturbance of secondary sexual characteristics.

Manifestation: In the first weeks and months after birth.

Aetiology: Autosomal recessive disorder. Approximately 75 patients reported to date.

Pathogenesis: Hypothetically, the ectodermal changes have been attributed to a cysteine deficiency and the mental retardation to an absence of sulphurous amino acids in the brain.

Course, prognosis: Reduced life expectancy, reduced fertility.

Differential diagnosis: Xeroderma pigmentosum (*181*).

Treatment: Symptomatic treatment of infections with antibiotics. Treatment of the hair and skin with topical ointments. Avoidance of sunlight.

Illustrations:
1–4 An 11-month-old female infant: large ears, microcephalic. Brittle hair since birth (breaks where the head rests against the support).
5 Hair has an alternately light and dark zigzag pattern under a polarizing microscope.
6 Congenital ichthyosis.

References:
Happle R, Traupe H, Gröbe H, Bonsmann G: The Tay syndrome (congenital ichthyosis with trichothiodystrophy). *Eur J Pediatr* 1984, **141**:147–152.
Blomquist H H, Back O, Fagerlund M, Holmgren G, Stecksen-Blicks C: Tay or IBIDS syndrome: a case with growth and mental retardation, congenital ichthyosis and brittle hair. *Acta Paediatr Scand* 1991, 80:1241–1245.
Price V H: Trichothiodystrophy: update. *Pediatr Dermatol* 1992, 9:369–370.

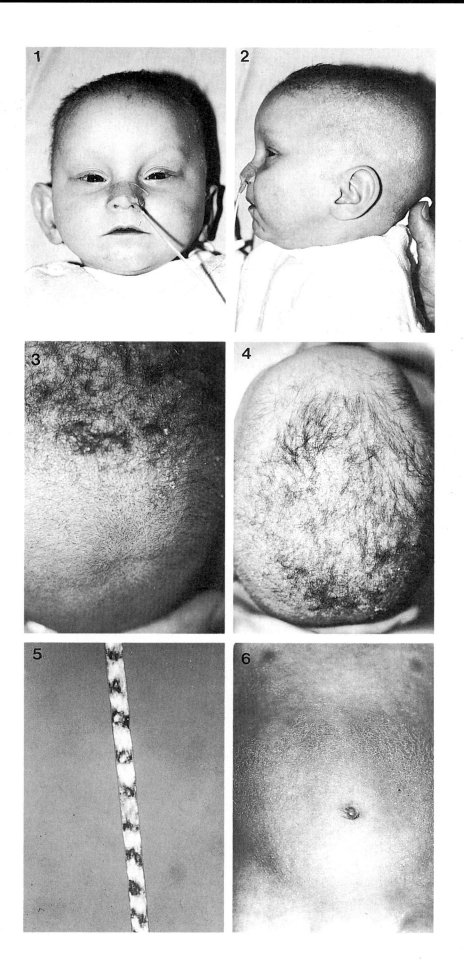

J.K.

A lethal genodermatosis with congenital contractures, hyperkeratosis and characteristic facial dysmorphism.

Main signs:

- Premature births between the 31st and 33rd week of pregnancy, birth weight below the third to 25th percentile, head circumference between the fifth and 50th percentile. Hydramnios, large placenta, short umbilical cord.
- Variable skin signs from birth: in some patients, a hard, shell-like structure, sometimes thin, translucent skin with prominent vessels and diffuse erythema.
- Generalized contractures of the knee, elbow, wrist and ankle joints in the flexed position. 'Rocker-bottom feet'.
- Facial dysmorphism: hypertelorism, ectropion, absent eyelashes, small nose, deep-set dysplastic ears, micrognathia, microstomia, open mouth. Anterior fontanelle wide open.
- Organic involvement: hypoplasia of the lungs, pseudohypertrophy of the breasts, hepatosplenomegaly.

Supplementary findings: Teeth present at birth, premature dentition. Microcephaly, choanal atresia, submucous cleft palate, hypospadias. Ureteral duplication, kyphoscoliosis, patent ductus arteriosus, ventricular septal defect, absent adrenal cortex. Hypoplastic clavicles, scapulae and long bones.

  Histology: thickening of the epidermis, hyperkeratosis of the stratum corneum. Hypoplasia of the sebaceous and sweat glands. Thin skin, hypoplasia of the elastic fibres. Abnormal subcutaneous fat.

Manifestation: Prenatally and at birth.

Aetiology: Autosomal recessive disorder. Several reports in siblings of both sexes.

Pathogenesis: Unknown.

Frequency: Reported in 28 newborns from 22 families. First reports in 1929 and 1938.

Course, prognosis: Death within few days or weeks of birth; the longest surviving patient lived for 120 days.

Differential diagnosis: Stiff skin syndrome, foetal akinesia, aplasia cutis congenita, Neu-Laxova syndrome, ichthyosis congenita gravis (266).

Treatment: Unknown. Retinoids? Possible prenatal diagnosis by electron-microscopic examination of foetal skin biopsy.

Illustrations:

1 Premature male infant (29th week of pregnancy, 1180 g), who died within 2 h of asphyxia. One has the impression that the child is enclosed in 'skin armour' that is too small. Arms and legs are fixed in a flexed position.
2 Typical facies with hypoplasia of the nose and chin, open mouth, downward slanting palpebral fissures, erosion of the skin, through which the vessels on the forehead and trunk are visible.
3 Diffuse hyperkeratosis with lamellar desquamation (left foot).

1–3 from:
R. Happle *et al*. Restrictive dermopathy in two brothers. *Arch Dermatol* 1992, **128**:232–235.

References:
Toriello H V: Restrictive dermopathy and report of another case. (Invited editorial comment). *Am J Med Genet* 1986, **24**:625–629.
Witt D R, Hayden M R *et al*: Restrictive dermopathy: a newly recognized autosomal recessive skin dysplasia. *Am J Med Genet* 1986, **24**:631–648.
Gillerot Y, Loulischer L: Restrictive dermopathy. (Letter to the editor). *Am J Med Genet* 1987, **27**:239–240.
Mok Q, Curley R *et al*: Restrictive dermopathy: a report of three cases. *J Med Genet* 1990, **27**:315–319.
van Hoestenberghe M-R, Legius E *et al*: Restrictive dermopathy with distinct morphological abnormalities. *Am J Med Genet* 1990, **36**:297–300.
Happle R, Schuurmanns Stekhoven H *et al*: Restrictive dermopathy in two brothers. *Arch Dermatol* 1992, **128**:232–235.
Verloes A, Mullies N *et al*: Restrictive dermopathy, a lethal form of arthrogryposis multiplex with skin and bone dysplasias: three new cases and review of the literature. *Am J Med Genet* 1992, **43**:539–547.
Hamel B C J, Happle R *et al*: False-negative prenatal diagnosis of restrictive dermopathy. *Am J Med Genet* 1992 **44**:824–826.
Dean J C S, Gray E S *et al*: Restrictive dermopathy: a disorder of skin differentiation with abnormal integrin expression. *Clin Genet* 1993, **44**:287–291.
Reed M H, Chudley A E *et al*: Restrictive dermopathy: a lethal congenital skin disorder. *Eur J Pediatr* 1993, **152**:95–98.
Lenz W, Meschede D: Historical note on restrictive dermopathy and report of two new cases. *Am J Med Genet* 1993, **47**:1235–1237.

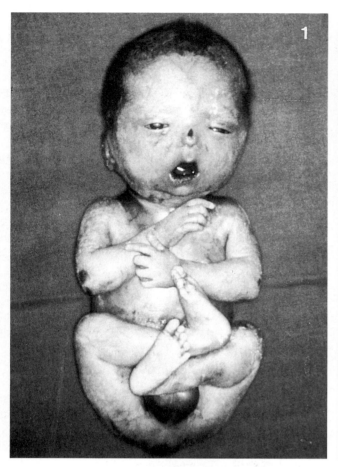

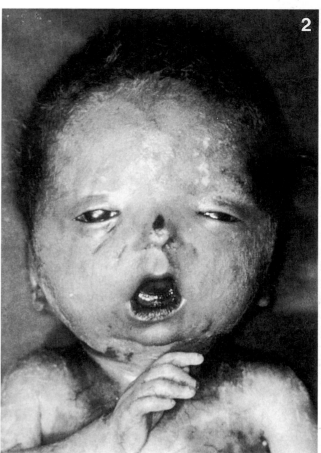

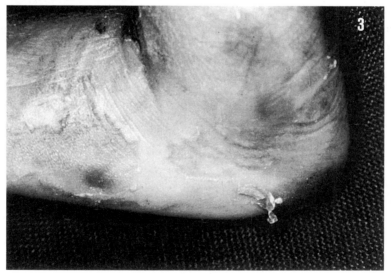

J.K./ H.-R.W

A collective term for a group of genodermatoses in which very mild trauma or mechanical or other factors lead to blistering of the skin.

Main signs:

Divided into three large groups: epidermolysis bullosa simplex (EBS), epidermolysis bullosa atrophicans (EBA) and epidermolysis bullosa dystrophica (EBD).

- EBS: intra-epidermal blistering from birth, generalized or local after mild trauma. Heals without scars or atrophy. Involvement of the mucous membranes. Nine subtypes in all.
- EBA: junctional blistering *in utero*, generalized. Nails and teeth also involved with severe caries. Six subtypes.
- EBD: dermolytic blistering at birth, traumatic or spontaneous with tendency to heal slowly, dystrophic scars, atrophies and milia. Nail dystrophy. Twelve subtypes.

Manifestation: EBS and EBD at birth or in the first weeks of life, EBA *in utero*.

Aetiology: More than 27 subtypes in total.

Seven subtypes are inherited as autosomal dominant traits, EBS Mendes da Costa is X-linked recessive and the lethal type is autosomal recessive.

All types of EBA are autosomal recessive.

With EBD, the Cockayne–Touraine and Pasini types, the pretibial type and the Bart type are autosomal dominant, the remaining eight subtypes being autosomal recessive.

Pathogenesis:

EBS: a keratin disorder has recently been postulated (point mutations that control the formation of K14 and K5 keratins).

EBD: collagen VII defect.

Frequency: More than 50 000 Americans have epidermolysis bullosa.

Course, prognosis:

EBS: impetiginization of the blisters. Microcephaly with the Mendes da Costa type. Normal life expectancy with the exception of the lethal autosomal recessive type.

EBA: early death with two forms because of sepsis, dehydration and respiratory disorders. Otherwise, mild caries. Local skin infections. Oesophageal strictures.

EBD: oesophageal strictures with the Hallopeau–Siemens type. Corneal ulcers. Urethral strictures. Squamous Cockayne–Touraine-type carcinomas. Severe caries.

Differential diagnosis: Ritter's exfoliative dermatitis, pemphigoid. Lyell's syndrome, scalding, acrodermatitis enteropathica (*264*), congenital porphyria, dermatitis herpetiformis, pemphigus, incontinentia pigmenti Bloch–Sulzberger (*187*).

Treatment:

EBS: symptomatic, local; vitamins, cortisone, antibacterials. Recognition after prenatal skin biopsy and ultrastructural examinations.

EBA: local therapy, as for EBS; no cortisones. Prenatal diagnosis after foetal skin biopsy.

EBD: local therapy, as for EBS; systemically with vitamin E. Treatment of Hallopeau–Siemens type with diphenyl hydantoin, which reduces the collagenase, is of limited value. Likewise limited success with retinoids.

Illustrations:

1a and b A 2-day-old newborn.

2a–d A 3-year-old girl with alopecia, lesions of the lips and teeth, nail dystrophy. Both **1** and **2** show autosomal recessive forms of the disorder.

3a and b The lower leg of a newborn and the hand of his father with an autosomal dominant form of the disease.

References:

Voigtländer V, Schnyder U W, Anton-Lamprecht I: Hereditäre Epidermolysen. In: Korting G W. (eds): *Dermatologie in Praxis und Klinik, Vol III.* Stuttgart: Thieme, 1979.

Rodeck C H, Eady R A J, Gosden C M: Prenatal diagnosis of epidermolysis bullosa letalis. *Lancet* 1980, I:979.

Anton-Lamprecht I: Prenatal diagnosis of genetic disorders of the skin by means of electron microscopy. *Hum Genet* 1981, 59:392–405.

Anton-Lamprecht I, Rauskolb R *et al*: Prenatal diagnosis of epidermolysis bullosa dystrophica... *Lancet* 1980, II:1077.

Gedde-Dahl T Jr, Anton-Lamprecht I: Epidermolysis bullosa. In: *Principles and practice of medical genetics.* A E H Emery, D L Rimoin (eds). Edinburgh: Churchill Livingstone 1983, 672–687.

Beighton P *et al*: International nosology of heritable disorders of connective tissue. Berlin 1986. *Am J Med Genet* 1988, **29**:581–594.

Editorial: Epidermolysis bullosa simplex: a disorder of Keratin. *Lancet* 1992, 339:29–30.

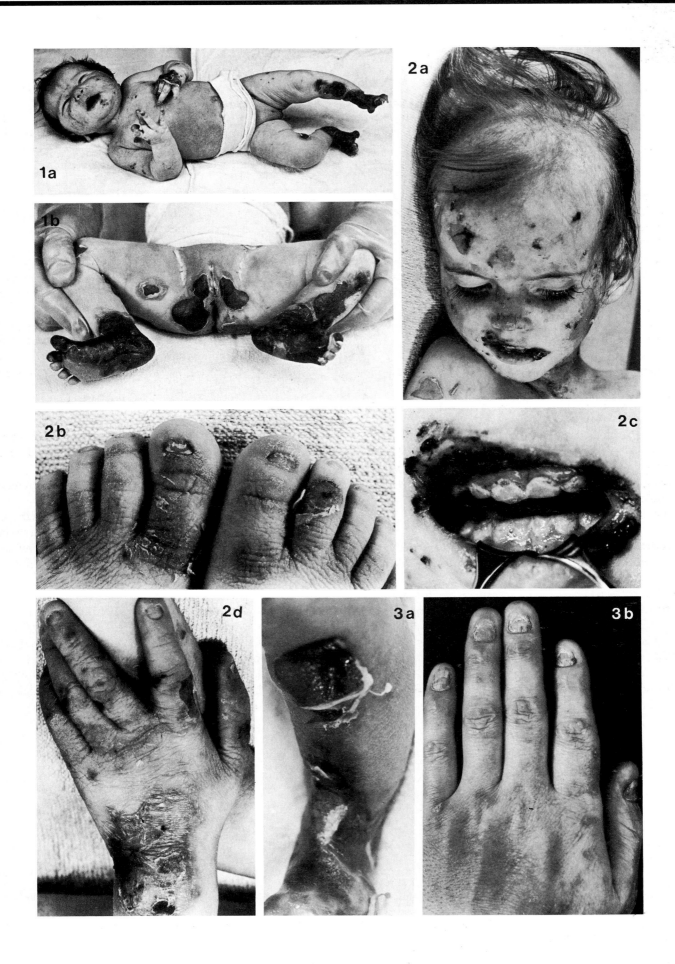

J.K.

An X-linked recessive disorder with the following triad of signs: eczema, thrombocytopenia with bleeding tendency and recurrent infections.

Main signs:
- Clinical onset frequently with eczema (T cell defect) in the first 6 months of life, indistinguishable from atopic dermatitis. Recurrent staphylococcal skin infections.
- Thrombocytopaenia, bleeding tendency: haematemesis, melena, chronic diarrhoea, purpura, petechiae.
- Recurrent pneumococcal infections. Otitis media, pneumonia, meningitis, sepsis. Later pneumocystis carinii, herpesvirus infections.

Supplementary findings:
- Disorder of humoral immunity with dysgammaglobulinemia, selective disorders of B and T lymphocytes, qualitative changes of the thrombocytes and their accoelerated removal by the reticulo-endothelial system, deficient formation of blood-group iso-antibodies and cutaneous anergy.
- Markedly elevated IgE; IgA is also elevated, IgM is depressed or absent; IgG levels are normal or variable.
- Severe auto-immune disorders: Coombs-positive haemolytic anaemia, juvenile rheumatoid arthritis, auto-immune thrombocytopaenia.

Manifestation: Eczema and irreversible thrombocytopaenia frequently in the first weeks and months of life.

Aetiology: X-linked recessive disease. Two different, parallel strategies are pursued for diagnosing female carriers: A segregation analysis is carried out in the family using DNA probes from the proximal X_p (indirect genotype analysis). Additionally, the pattern of X-inactivation is determined in the peripheral blood cells of high-risk females. It is known that female carriers of WAS show a unilaterally displaced inactivation pattern: in the overwhelming majority of peripheral blood cells, the same X-chromosome (with the WAS mutation) is always inactivated. The WAS has been localized to the proximal short arm of the X-chromosome (Xp11.22) and shows a close link with the loci DXS14, DXS255, TIMP, and OATL1; recent data also suggest that it is flanked by TIMP and DXS255.

Frequency: Four new patients in 1 million live-born boys.

Course, prognosis: Median survival for those born before 1935 was 8 months. For those born after 1964, median survival increased to 6.5 years. Currently, 25% of the 301 patients reported have lived for 10 years (with a total life span of up to 36 years in isolated cases). Development of lymphoreticular tumours and leukaemias in 12% of patients (risk of tumours 100 times greater than in the general population). The most frequent cause of death are infections (e.g. pneumonia, sepsis; in 59%), followed by generalized bleeding (e.g. central nervous system, intestinal; in 27%), malignancies (in 5%) and various other problems (e.g. asphyxia, shock, aplastic anaemia, vascular occlusion, pulmonary oedema with cardiac failure, altogether 9%).

Differential diagnosis: Can be differentiated easily from congenital and acquired thrombocytopaenias.

Treatment: Allogenic bone marrow transplantation. Administration of transfer factor. Possible splenectomy. Genetic counselling. Possible prenatal diagnosis.

Illustrations:

1 A male patient, aged 9 months, generalized eczematous skin changes with sharply delineated round or oval erythematous foci, which coalesce into larger honeycombed and multicentric areas.
2 A boy, aged 23 months, with generalized thrombocytopaenic bleeding of the skin, particularly around the mouth.

References:

Perry G S, Spector B D, Schuman L M et al: The Wiskott–Aldrich Syndrome in the United States and Canada (1892-1979). J Pediatr 1980, 97:72–78.
Erttmann R, Thöne I, Landbeck G: Wiskott–Aldrich-Syndrom. Monatsschr Kinderheilkd 1983, 131:524–527.
Holmberg L, Gustavii B, Jönsson A: A prenatal study of platelet count and size with application to the fetus at risk for Wiskott-Aldrich syndrome. J Pediatr 1983, 102:773–776.
Mallory S B, Krafchik B R: What syndrome is this? Pediatr Dermatol 1991, 8:250–252.
Brochstein J A, Gillio A P et al: Marrow transplantation from human leucocyte-antigen-identical or haploidentical donors for correction of Wiskott–Aldrich syndrome. J Pediatr 1991, 119:907–912.
Notarangelo L D, Parolini O et al: Analysis of X-chromosome inactivation and presumptive expression of the Wiskott–Aldrich syndrome (WAS) gene in hematopoietic cell lines of a thrombocytopenic carrier female of WAS. Hum Genet 1991, 8:237–241.
Greer W L, Peacocke M, Siminovitch K A: The Wiskott–Aldrich syndrome: refinement of the localization on Xp and identification of another closely linked marker locus. OATL1. Hum Genet 1992, 88:453–456.
Basile G. de Saint, Notarangelo L D et al: Wiskott-Aldrich syndrome carrier detection with the hypervariable marker M27β. Hum Genet 1992, 89:223–228.
Orth U, Rosenkranz W, Schwinger E, Holzgreve W, Gal A: Molekulargenetische Diagnostik beim Wiskott-Aldrich-Syndrome. Monatsschr Kinderheilkd 1993, 141:728–731.

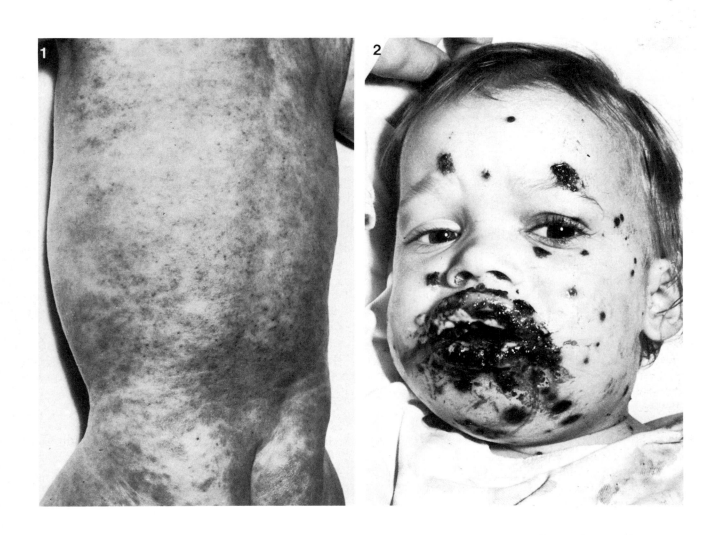

274 Abt–Letterer–Siwe Disease
(Acute Disseminated Histiocytosis X)

J.K.

A generalized malignant form of histiocytosis X in infants and children with seborrheic, macular or petechial skin rash; generalized lymphadenopathy; hepatosplenomegaly and pulmonary involvement.

Main signs:
- Seborrheic dermatitis, maculopapular yellow–brown skin rash with petechial bleeding.
- Hepatosplenomegaly.
- Generalized lymphadenopathy.
- Pulmonary infiltration with respiratory distress and coughing.
- Haematological disorders: anaemia, leukopaenia, thrombocytopenia.

Supplementary findings: Sepsis-like clinical picture with recurrent fever. Histologically, demonstration of atypical histiocytes in the upper dermis. Electron-microscopic demonstration of 'Langerhans cell granules'. Diabetes insipidus.

On radiograph, osteolytic bone lesions, especially in the cranial region.

Manifestation: Infancy and childhood.

Aetiology: Many pairs of affected siblings known. Autosomal recessive inheritance presumed.

Frequency: Approximately 1:100 000 for the first year of life; 0.2:100 000 for children under 15 years.

Course, prognosis: Lethal in up to 30% of patients. Untreated, outcome always fatal. Dramatic clinical picture in infants and toddlers.

Differential diagnosis: Initially, diaper rash, fungal infections and scabies. Later, Hand–Schüller–Christian disease and eosinophilic granuloma.

Treatment: Chemotherapy using vinca alkaloids, antimetabolites, alkylating agents and glucocorticoids. Possible splenectomy.

Illustrations:

1 and 2 Maculopapular, petechial skin rash mainly affecting the trunk; enlarged lymph nodes.

References:

Any paediatric textbook.

Frisell E, Björksten B, Holmgren G *et al*: Familial occurrence of histiocytosis. *Clin Genet* 1977, **11**:163–170.

Wolff H H, Janka G E: Morbus Abt-Letterer-Siwe. Zur Diagnostik und Therapie. *Monatsschr Kinderheilk* 1978, **126**:425–430.

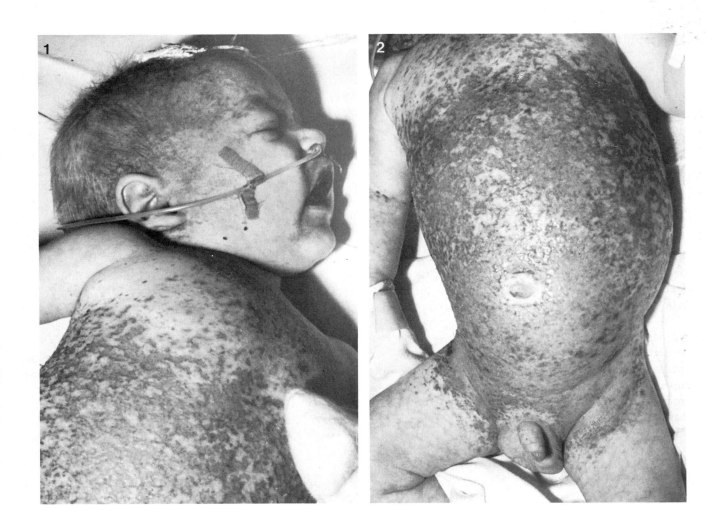

A teratogenic disorder of mental and motor development, typical facies with microcephaly and growth deficiency, multiple further gross and subtle anomalies and behavioural signs in children of chronic alcoholic mothers.

Main signs:

- Marked prenatal and postnatal growth retardation, disproportionate small stature and microcephaly.
- Craniofacial dysmorphism: short palpebral fissures (blepharophimosis); epicanthus, ptosis; short, flat nasal bridge; hypoplastic philtrum; thin upper lip with narrow prolabium; flat mid-face (maxillary hypoplasia); frequent minor ear anomalies.
- Delayed motor development with muscular hypotonia; marked postnatal irritability; transition to marked hyperactivity possible.
- Central nervous system disorder: mild to severe mental retardation, psychological disorders, unusual behaviour, impaired concentration and learning. Severe eating disorders, recurrent infections, otitis in the first and second years of life, impaired hearing and vision.

Supplementary findings: Gross anomalies: cardiac defect in 30%, renal malformation in 10%, cleft palate, minor anomalies of the genitalia (hypoplasia of the labia majora, glandular hypospadias, cryptorchidism). Lesser anomalies: abnormal hand creases, clinodactyly, camptodactyly, limited supination, hypoplasia of the distal phalanges and nails, dislocation of the hips, coccygeal pits, hernias, haemangiomas, pectus excavatum, myopia.

Classification into three grades of severity as recommended by the Research Society on Alcoholism:
I. Foetal Alcohol Syndrome (FAS):
Alongside established maternal alcohol abuse
I. Prenatal and postnatal growth retardation
II. Central nervous system dysfunction (any neurological abnormality, developmental delay or intellectual retardation)
III. Two of the following characteristic signs of craniofacial dysmorphism:
  a) microcephaly (below third percentile)
  b) microphthalmos, blepharophimosis
  c) flat philtrum or narrow prolabium
  d) flat mid-face or maxillary hypoplasia.
II. Foetal Alcohol Effects (FAE):
Two of the three symptom complexes given under FAS.

Manifestation: At birth.

Aetiology: The teratogenicity of alcohol *in utero* is still unknown. This embryopathy has only been observed in children of chronic alcoholic women. Whether ethyl alcohol or acetaldehyde plus additional secondary deficiencies of the mother are pathogenetically responsible remains unclear. A third of all children of chronic alcoholic mothers show diagnosable AE. Approximately 60–70% show partial teratogenic effects. Individual genetic factors are probably responsible for the differences in vulnerability.

Frequency: Next to Down syndrome and myelocele, AE is the most frequent congenital cause of mental retardation. The frequency varies markedly and is dependent on the drinking habits of women in different cultural groups (e.g. one out of 100 in some Indian reservations in America). The frequency is 1:750 in the USA, 1:600 in Sweden, and in France, where milder patients are also registered, 1:212. In Germany, probably 1000–1500 children with AE are born per year, with a large, unknown number of mild or aborted patients.

Illustrations:
1–3 A 3-month-old child. Mother a chronic alcoholic. Birth weight 1590 g after unknown gestation period. Measurements at 9 months: length 68.5 cm; weight 5700 g; head circumference 42 cm. Typical facies. Premature synostosis of the frontal suture, cardiac defect, psychomotor retardation.
4 and 5 Two more typically affected young children.

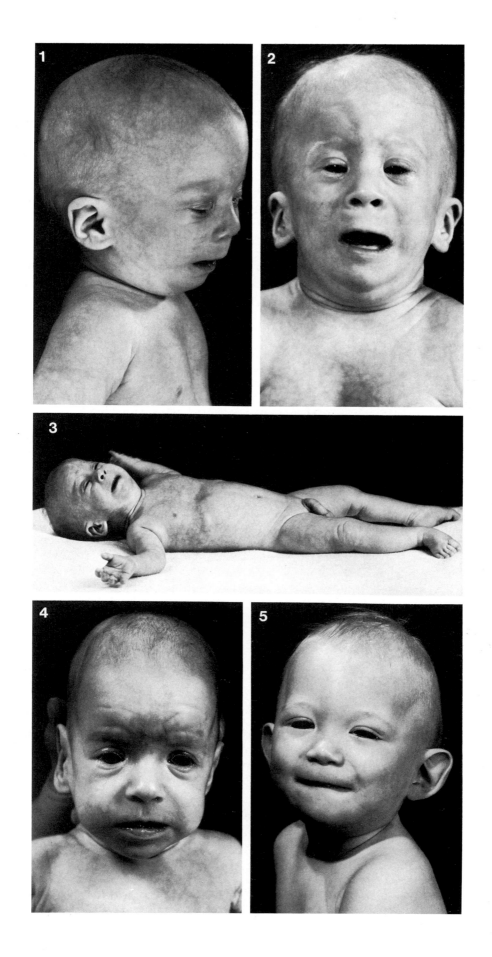

Course, prognosis: Perinatal mortality is not increased. Frequent infections in the first 2 years of life, failure to thrive and need for surgery are responsible for numerous hospital admissions. The extent of permanent mental retardation is of decisive importance for the patient's life. Even when all mild patients are included, only 20% can attend a normal school. For approximately 50% of the children, special schools for learning disability or for the mentally retarded must be considered. Approximately one-third of patients are severely retarded. The frequency of alcohol embryopathy is growing with increasing maternal alcoholism.

Recent long-term studies confirm persistent physical and especially mental retardation.

Differential diagnosis: Trisomy 18 (*48*), which shows extremely severe mental impairment, death almost always within the first year of life, characteristic chromosome findings. Dubowitz syndrome (*95*) and Noonan syndrome (*105*) should also not be difficult to rule out (especially considering the absence of the corresponding social history).

Treatment: Symptomatic; prolonged hospital admissions frequently necessary at first, operative correction of cleft palate, cardiac defects, hernias, correction of impaired vision and hearing. All appropriate measures to help the handicapped. Only one-third of the children live with one of their biological parents. Residential care or referral to special therapy centres is often necessary. Most importantly: AE is a preventable form of mental retardation, so measures to prevent chronic maternal alcoholism are imperative.

Illustrations:
Infants and young children with alcohol embryopathy. Horizontally, first row: children in the first 3 months of life; second row: children from 4 to 11 months; third row: 1–2-year-old children; fourth row: children of 2 years and 3 months, 2 years and 6 months and 5 years and 3 months.

References:
Lemoine P, Harousseau H, Boteyru J P *et al*: Les enfants de parents alcooliques: anomalies observées. Apropos de 127 cas. *Quest Med* 1968, **25**:477.
Jones K L, Smith D W, Ulleland C *et al*: Pattern of malformation in offspring of chronic alcoholic mothers. *Lancet* 1973, I:1267.
Hanson J W, Jones K L, Smith D W: Fetal alcohol syndrome. Experience with 41 patients. *JAMA* 1976, **235**:1458.
Majewski F, Bierich J R, Löser H *et al*: Zur Klinik und Pathogenese der Alkoholembryopathie (Bericht über 68 Patienten) *Münch Med Wschr* 1976, **118**:1635.
Clarren S K, Smith D W: The fetal alcohol syndrome. Experience with 65 patients and a review of the world literature. *N Engl J Med* 1978, **298**:1063.
Hanson J W, Steissguth A P, Smith D W: The effects of moderate alcohol consumption during pregnancy on fetal growth and morphogenesis. *J Pediatr* 1978, **92**:457.
Streissguth A P, Herman S, Smith D W: Intelligence, behavior and dysmorphogenesis in the fetal alcohol syndrome: a report on 20 patients. *J Pediatr* 1978, **92**:363.
Nestler V M, Spohr H L, Steinhausen H C: *Die Alkoholembryopathie.* Stuttgart: Enke 1981.
Spohr H L, Steinhausen H C: Follow-up studies of children with fetal alcohol syndrome. *Neuropediatrics* 1987, **18**:13–17.
Sokolowski F, Sokolowski A, Majewski F: Risiken für die Nachkommen alkoholkranker Frauen. *Pädiatr Prax* 1989, **38**:373–387.
Sokohl R J, Clarren S K: Guidelines for use of terminology describing the impact of prenatal alcohol on the offspring. *Alcoholism* 1989, **13**:597–598.
Streissguth A P, Aase J M, Clarren S K, Randels S P, La Due R A, Smith D F: Fetal alcohol syndrome in adolescents and adults. *JAMA* 1991, **265**:1991–1967.
Spohr H L, Steinhausen H C, Willms J. Prenatal alcohol exposure and long-term developmental consequences. *Lancet* 1993, **341**:907–910.
Spohr H L, Willms J, Steinhausen H C: The fetal alcohol syndrome in adolescence. *Acta Paediatr* 1994, 404:19–26.

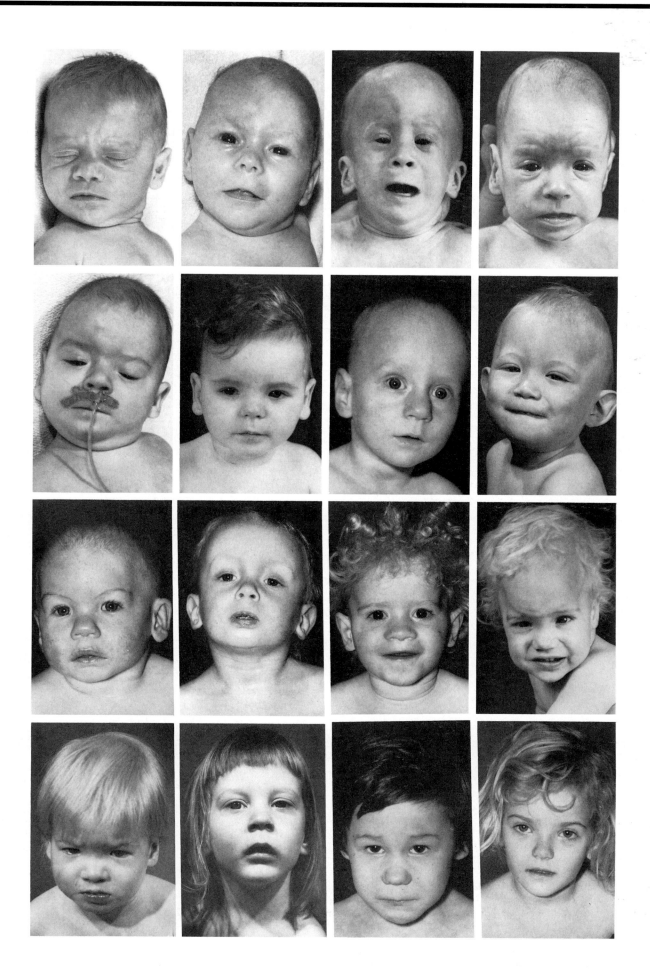

H.-R.W

R. Pankau

A malformation–retardation syndrome with typical facial dysmorphism, short stature, mental retardation, vascular stenosis, renal anomalies and (infrequently) hypercalcaemia.

Main signs:
- Facies essentially characterized by a broad forehead, suprapalpebral fullness, short palpebral fissures, hypertelorism or hypotelorism, epicanthus, low nasal bridge, hypoplasia of the mid-face, slightly anteverted nostrils, long philtrum, full cheeks, large mouth and occasionally drooping lips (1, 2, 6–8).
- Internal strabismus (6).
- Hypoplastic teeth (5), occasionally hypodontia. Hypoplasia of the enamel and malpositioned teeth.
- Short stature, microcephaly.
- Mild to moderate mental retardation (IQ 35–70) but normal intellectual development is also possible. Friendly, lively disposition; hoarse voice. Good memory for faces and places.

Supplementary findings: Vascular stenosis, especially supravalvular aortic stenosis, peripheral pulmonary stenoses, stenosis of the aortic root, extensive hypoplasia of the aorta, stenosis of the renal vessels.

Ventricular and atrial septal defects. Frequent mitral insufficiency in adulthood.

Renal anomalies (20%), radio-ulnar synostoses (9%). Frequently inguinal hernias.

Hypercalcaemia infrequent, usually limited to early infancy and, if present, associated with the related clinical signs (anorexia, constipation, failure to thrive and so on) metastatic calcification, especially of the kidneys.

Osteosclerosis (especially of the skull, metaphyses 3 and 4). Possible craniosynostosis, kyphoscoliosis.

Short, hypoplastic nails; hallux valgus; radial deviation of the fifth finger.

Whitish inclusions of the iris, resembling wheel spokes.

Manifestation: From birth; the typical facies cannot usually be recognized until the second year of life.

Aetiology: Usually sporadic occurrence. An autosomal dominant gene with variable expression; there appear to be deletions involving the elastin gene on 7q11.23. Contiguous gene syndrome.

Frequency: Not low (approximately one out of 10 000 newborns); hundreds of patients in the literature.

Prognosis: Infrequently, early death (infarctions?). Course otherwise dependent on the significance of the stenosed vessels, the severity of the stenosis and its operability. Arterial hypertension frequent in infancy but also gastro-intestinal and urogenital problems as the condition progresses.

Treatment: Operative relief of vascular stenoses. Treatment of hypercalcaemia where indicated. All necessary support from an early age.

Illustrations:
1–5 Patient 1 at 2 years and 9 months (1, 3); and at 4 years and 9 months (2, 4, 5). Severe primary psychomotor retardation. On initial examination at 2 years and 9 months, height 79 cm (50th percentile for a 14-month-old girl); under-weight by 1 kg in relation to height; head circumference 46 cm (normal for height); persistent hypercalcaemia, up to 15 mg% (3.75 mmol/l). At 4 years and 9 months, calcium still as high as 3.3 mmol/l. Death from uraemia at 5 years and 3 months. On autopsy: nephrocalcinosis; calcium deposits in the heart muscle, thyroid gland and bronchial cartilages; left ventricular hypertrophy; stenosis of the aortic root.
6–8 Patient 2 at 15 months (6 and 7) and at 24 years (8). Since the second 6 months of life: anorexia, insufficient weight gain. On initial examination at 15 months, height within normal limits, underweight by 1.5 kg for height. Head circumference normal. Calcium values as high as 4.35 mmol/l; supravalvular aortic stenosis with hypoplastic aorta; hypoplastic pulmonary vascular tree, two superior venae cavae. Mental impairment first recognized at 9 years. Height at that time (124 cm) in the low normal range.

References:
Beuren A J: Supravalvular aortic stenosis: a complex syndrome with and without mental retardation. *Birth Defects Orig Art Ser VIII* 1972, 5:45
Jones K L, Smith D W: The Williams elfin facies syndrome. *J Pediatr* 1975, 86:718.
Editorial: Williams syndrome — the enigma continues. *Lancet* 1988, II:490.
Morris C A, Demsey S A et al: Natural history of Williams syndrome... *J Pediatr* 1988, 113:318–326.
Udwin O: A survey of adults with Williams syndrome... *Dev Med Child Neurol* 1990, 32:129–147.
Kruse K et al: Calcium metabolism in Williams Beuren syndrome. *J Pediatr* 1992, 121:902–907.
Pober B R et al: Renal findings in 40 individuals with Williams syndrome. *Am J Med Genet* 1993, 46:271–274.
Morris C A et al: Williams syndrome: autosomal dominant inheritance. *Am J Med Genet* 1993, 47:478–481.
Plissart L, Borghgraef M et al: Adults with Williams–Beuren syndrome... *Clin Genet* 1994, 46:161–167.
Wessel A, Pankau R et al: Three decades follow-up of aortic and pulmonary vascular lesions in the Williams–Beuren syndrome. *Am J Med Genet* 1994, 52:297–301.

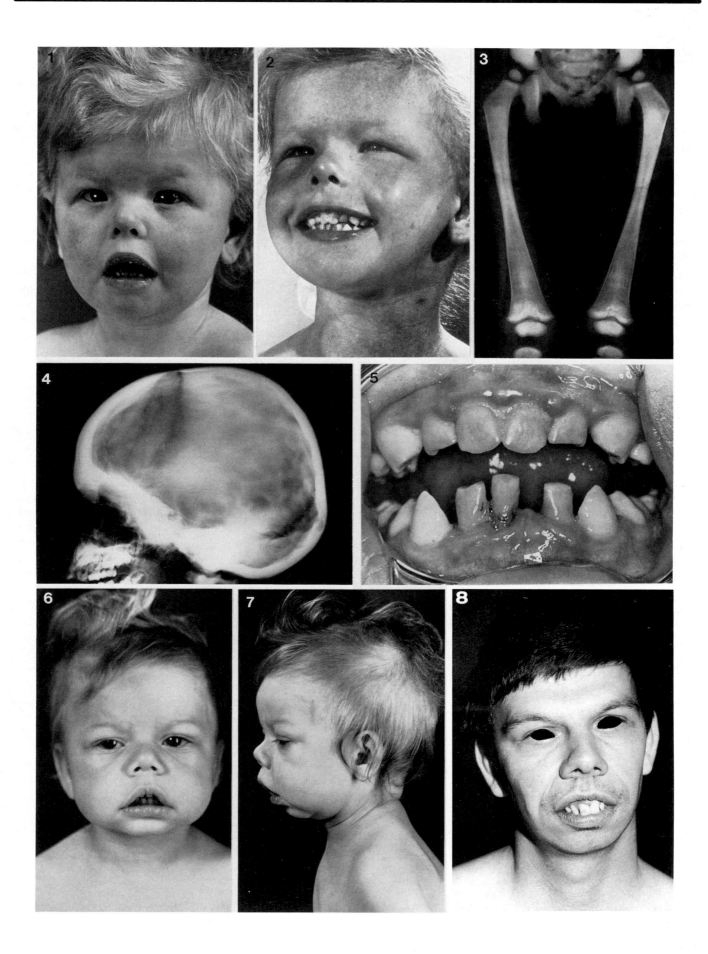

H.-R.W

A syndrome of somewhat unusual appearance, goitre (familial), peculiarities of the hands and body proportions and cardiovascular anomalies.

Main signs:
- Facies: pronounced supra-orbital ridges; almond-shaped eyes; small nose with narrow bridge; hypoplasia of the zygomatic arches; large, prominent, simply modelled ears; microstomia, prognathism (**1 and 2**).
- Whorl of hair at the back of the neck.
- Goitre (familial).
- Short, unusual hands with approximately equal lengths of second and fourth digits bilaterally; clinodactyly of second and fifth digits bilaterally (**3**). Short toes (**5**).
- Lanky appearance (height approximately 75th percentile) with excessively long extremities and an almost feminine-appearing pelvic region. Winging of the scapulae with elevation of the left shoulder (**7–9**).
- Cardiologically: partial transposition of the pulmonary veins with drainage into the left brachiocephalic vein; small atrial septal defect.

Supplementary findings: Radiologically, brachymesophalangism of the little fingers and of the second to fifth toes bilaterally (**4, 6**).

Manifestation: At birth and later.

Aetiology: Not known.

Treatment: Symptomatic.

Illustrations:

1–9 An 11-year-old boy with normal mental development, the second child of non-consanguineous parents; father 46 years, mother 36 years at the patient's birth. (Patient has had diffuse euthyrotic goitre since age 6 years. Mother of the boy and five of her siblings are similarly affected, as is the older sister of the proband.)

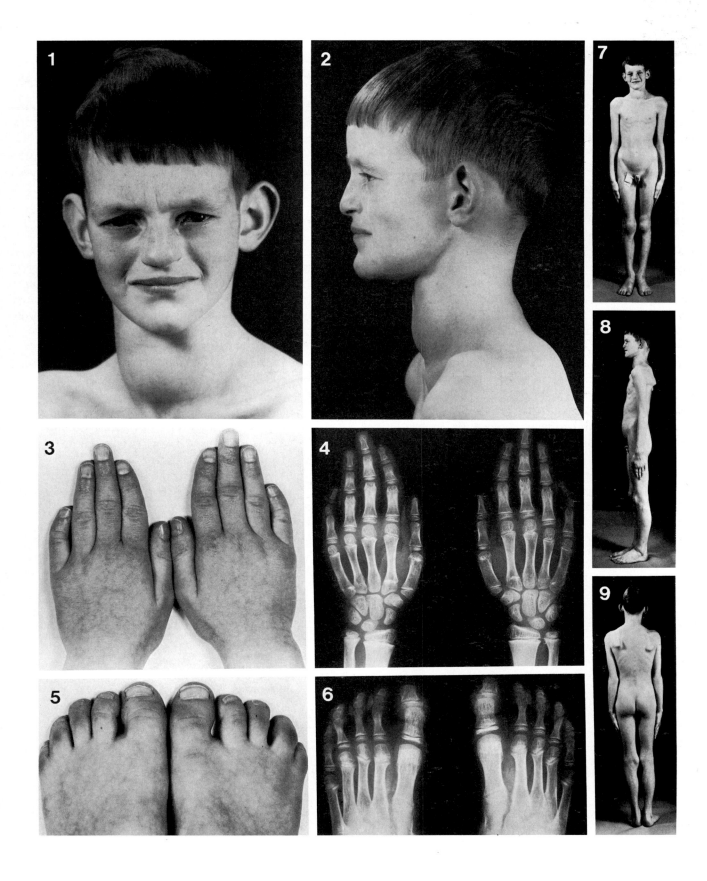

H.-R.W

A malformation–retardation syndrome of characteristic facies, usually moderate mental retardation, cleft palate and cardiovascular anomalies.

Main signs:
- Typical appearance: long, narrow face with micrognathia (and malocclusion), prominent nose with broad bridge and hypoplastic alae nasi, slightly deformed ears. Frequently, abundant scalp hair (**1–6**).
- Mild to moderate mental retardation with learning disability. Behavioural anomalies and (in more than 10%) psychiatric disorders in adulthood.
- Cleft palate (open or submucous); hypernasal speech.
- Cardiovascular anomalies such as ventricular septal defect, tetralogy of Fallot or others.

Supplementary findings: Not infrequently, structural (and possibly metabolic) cerebral anomalies, also microcephaly; eye anomalies. Growth deficiency; narrow hands and fingers; possible scoliosis. Hernias. Secondary hearing and possible speech problems. Frequently, increased susceptibility to infections.

Manifestation: At birth and later.

Aetiology: An autosomal dominant disorder with very variable expression; microdeletion on chromosome 22q11.

Note: The syndrome shows phenotypic overlap with the DiGeorge sequence, which is likewise associated with monosomy of a region of chromosome 22q11.

Frequency: Not low.

Course, prognosis: Essentially dependent on the type and severity of cardiac defect, on the severity of mental retardation or on the development of a psychiatric disorder.

Diagnosis, differential diagnosis: Early recognition important, not least to prevent secondary handicaps.

Treatment: Surgery for cardiac defects; in some patients hearing, speech and other aids.

Illustrations:
1–4 Four boys (aged 7 years, 5 years, 7 months and 6 years) with Shprintzen syndrome, from different families.
5 An affected 25 year old with her 8-month-old daughter.
6 On the right, the girl shown as an infant in **5**, now 9 years old; on the left, her similarly affected sister, aged 7 years and 9 months.

References:
Shprintzen R J, Goldberg R B, Lewin H L *et al*: A new syndrome involving cleft palate, cardiac anomalies, typical facies, and learning disabilities: velo-cardio-facial syndrome. *Cleft Palate J* 1978, **15**:56–62.
Meinecke P, Beemer F A, Schinzel A *et al*: The velo-cardio-facial (Shprintzen) syndrome. *Eur J Pediatr* 1986, **145**:539–544.
Letters to the editor by Pagon R A, Shprintzen R J, Beemer F A *et al* re CHARGE versus velo-cardio-facial syndrome: *Am J Med Genet* 1987, **28**, 751–758.
Lipson A H *et al*: Velocardiofacial (Shprintzen) syndrome... *J Med Genet* 1991, **28**:596–604.
Scambler P J *et al*: Velo-cardio-facial syndrome associated with chromosome 22 deletions... *Lancet* 1992, **339**(I):1138.
Shprintzen R J *et al*: Late-onset psychosis in the velo-cardio-facial syndrome (Letter). *Am J Med Genet* 1992, **42**:141–142.
Goldberg R *et al*: Velo-cardio-facial syndrome: a review of 120 patients. *Am J Med Genet* 1993, **45**:313–319.
Motzkin B *et al*: Variable phenotypes in velocardiofacial syndrome with chromosomal deletion. *J Pediatr* 1993, **123**:406–410.
Scott D *et al*: Velo-cardio-facial syndrome. Intrafamililal variability of the phenotype. *AJDC* 1993, **147**:1212–1216.
Kelly D *et al*: Confirmation that the velo-cardio-facial syndrome is associated with haplo-insufficiency of genes at chromosome 22q11. *Am J Med Genet* 1993, **45**:308–312.
Mitnick R J *et al*: Brain anomalies in velo-cardio-facial syndrome. *Am J Med Genet (Neuropsych Genet)* 1994, **54**:100–106.
Chow E W C *et al*: Velo-cardio-facial syndrome and psychotic disorders... *Am J Med Genet Neuropsych Genet* 1994, **54**:107–112.
Nickel R E, Pillers De-Ann M *et al*: Velo-cardio-facial syndrome synd DiGeorge sequence... *Am J Med Genet* 1994, **52**:445–449.
Shprintzen R J: Velocardiofacial syndrome and DiGeorge sequence (Letter). *J Med Genet* 1994, **31**:423–424.

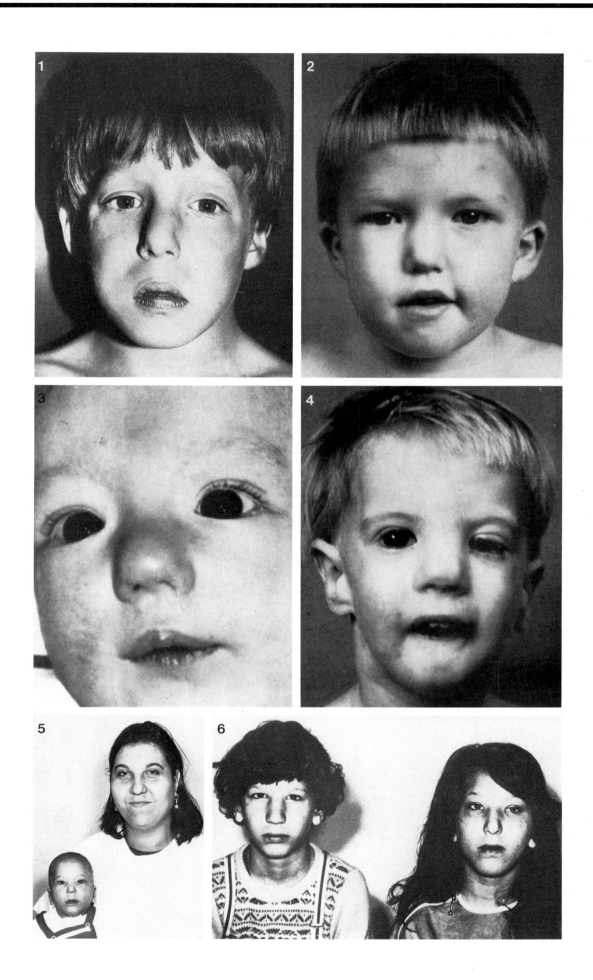

Rabenhorst Syndrome

F.R. Grosse
H.-R.W

A syndrome of typical facial dysmorphism, cardiac defect and multiple lesser anomalies.

Main signs:
- Narrow face with high narrow nose, slight mongoloid slant of the palpebral fissures, microstomia, prognathism, adherent ear lobes. High palate. Dolichocephaly (**1 and 2**).
- Markedly asthenic physique (**3**).
- Limited mobility of the distal interphalangeal joints with hypoplasia of the corresponding articular creases. Simian crease. Syndactyly of the second and third toes.

Supplementary findings: Ventricular septal defect with pulmonary stenosis.

Manifestation: At birth.

Aetiology: Probable autosomal dominant disorder.

Frequency: Two patients reported to date.

Prognosis: As far as can be determined from the small number of patients, relatively good.

Treatment: Correction of the cardiac defect.

Illustrations:
1–4 A father and his 4-year-old daughter (**2–4**). Both had ventricular septal defect with pulmonary stenosis. In the meantime the girl has undergone successful surgery.

References:
Grosse F-R: Rabenhorst syndrome. A cardio-acro-facial syndrome. *Z Kinderheilk* 1974, **117**:109.

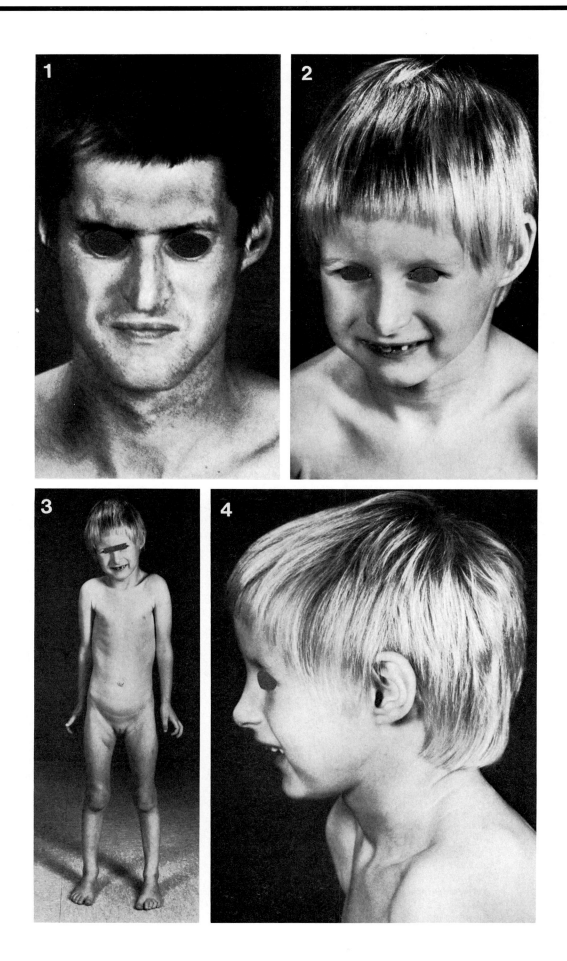

H.-R.W/ J.K.

A clinical picture comprising congenital, generally bilateral, cranial nerve (usually facial-abducent) paralysis with malformation of the extremities.

Main signs:
- Expressionless face; disorders of drinking, swallowing and speech; strabismus and ptosis of the lids (1–3) due to congenital defect of the following cranial nerves: most frequently, the facial (not infrequently with preservation of the oral branch) and abducent nerves; less frequently, the oculomotor (usually a partial defect with no internal paralysis) and hypoglossal nerves; very seldom, the motor portion of the trigeminal and trochlear nerves, the hypoglossal, glossopharyngeal and vagus nerves.
- Unilateral and bilateral club feet in one-third of patients (1).

Supplementary findings: Various hand anomalies, usually symbrachydactyly, also with ipsilateral aplasia of the pectoralis muscle (Poland anomaly), terminal transverse defects, stiff index finger, arthrogryposis multiplex congenita.

Ear anomalies: ears of different sizes and protruding, cartilage anomalies, occasionally deafness.

Aplasia of the lacrimal puncta.

Occasionally, mental retardation (approximately 10% of cases), mild in most cases.

Additionally: Microstomia, micrognathia, short palpebral fissures, bilateral epicanthus medialis, hypertelorism, bifid uvula, cleft palate, rib defects, Klippel–Feil anomaly, anomalies of the brachialis muscle, association with anosmia, hypogonadotropic hypogonadism (Kallmann syndrome, 307).

Manifestation: At birth.

Aetiology: Hereditary occurrence has been described with autosomal dominant and autosomal recessive transmission. Heterogeneity, pleiotropism; interfamilial and intrafamilial variability.

Most cases are sporadic and of unknown aetiology; risk of recurrence then around 2%. In recent years, vascular disruptions in the early embryonic stage have been postulated (subclavian artery supply disruption sequence = SASDS): atrophy of the brain stem, calcifications in the pons and medulla region, capillary telangiectasis in the mesencephalon and pons.

Misoprostol (synthetic prostaglandin analog) possibly as an abortifacient.

Frequency: Low (between 1888 and 1980 approximately 180 observations were reported in the literature).

Course, prognosis: Feeding problems in the neonatal period and early infancy, danger of aspiration.

Tendency for the paralysis to improve in some patients.

Normal life expectancy in 90% of cases.

Differential diagnosis: Oral-acral 'syndrome' (212), of which Möbius sequence can be considered a partial manifestation; Poland anomaly (220). Facio-scapulo-humeral muscular dystrophy, infantile myotonic dystrophy (286), Charcot-Marie-Tooth.

Treatment: Nurse the young infant prone and tube-feed. Begin speech therapy at the appropriate time. Multidisciplinary care and support. Genetic counselling.

Illustrations:

1–3 A 10-year-old girl with paralysis of the facial and abducent nerves; surgically corrected club feet.

References:

Henderson, J L: The congenital facial diplegia syndrome: clinical features, pathology and aaetiology. A review of 61 cases. Brain 1939, 62:381.

Szabo L: Möbius-Syndrom und Polandsche Anomalie. Z Orthop u Grenzgeb 1976, 114:211.

Herrmann J, Pallister P D, Gilbert E F et al: Nosologic studies in the Hanhart and the Möbius syndrome. Eur J Pediat 1976, 122:19.

Meyerson M D, Foushee D R: Speech, language and hearing in Moebius syndrome: a study of 22 patients. Dev Med Child Neurol 1978, 20:357.

Legum C, Godel V, Nemet P et al: Heterogeneity and pleiotropism in the Moebius syndrome. Clin Genet 1981, 20:254–259; also ibid 1982, 21:290.

Benney H, Kinzinger W: Kinder mit Moebius-Syndrom… Pädiat Prax 1978, 26:237.

Collins D L, Schimke R N: Moebius syndrome in a child and extremity defect in her father. Clin Genet 1982, 22:312–314.

Stabile M, Cavaliere M L et al: Abnormal B.A.E.P. in a family with Moebius syndrome… Clin Genet 1984, 25:459–463.

Bavnick J N B, Weaver D D: Subclavian artery supply disruption sequence: hypothesis of a vascular etiology for Poland, Klippel-Feil and Moebius anomalies. Am J Med Genet 1986, 23:903–918.

Kumar D: Moebius syndrome. J Med Genet 1990, 27:122–126.

Fujita I, Koyanagi T et al: Moebius syndrome with central hypoventilation and brainstem calcification: a case report. Eur J Pediatr 1991, 150:582–583.

Gonzales C H, Vargas F et al: Limb deficiency with or without Möbius sequence in seven Brazilian children associated with Misoprostol use in the first trimester of pregnancy. Am J Med Genet 1993, 47:59–64.

Charles S S, DiMario F J Jr, Grunnet M L: Möbius sequence: Further in vivo support for the subclavian artery supply disruption sequence. Am J Med Genet 1993, 47:289–293.

D'Cruz O F, Swisher C N et al: Möbius syndrome: evidence for a vascular aetiology. J Child Neurol 1993, 8:260–265.

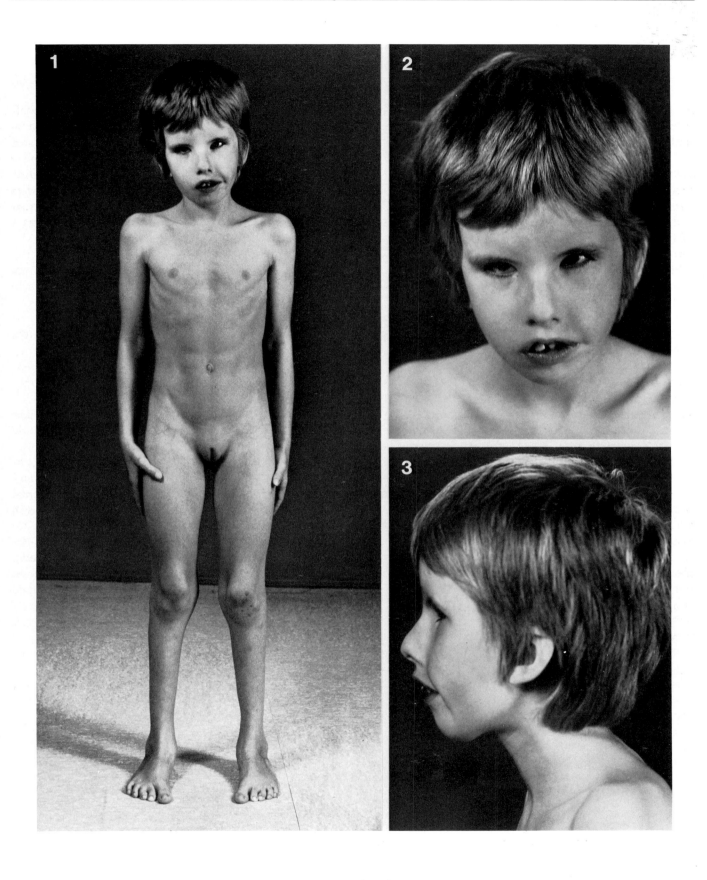

281 Smith–Lemli–Opitz Syndrome
(SLO Syndrome; RSH Syndrome)

A very variable hereditary disorder of primordial growth deficiency, mental retardation with microcephaly, unusual facies, genital anomalies in males and other abnormalities.

Main signs:
- Primordial growth deficiency (with failure to thrive and frequent vomiting in infancy).
- Microcephaly (with metopic ridge in some patients), high forehead.
- Facies: blepharophimosis, ptosis, epicanthi, possible strabismus; posteriorly rotated or low-set ears; pug nose with broad tip; small tongue; broad alveolar ridge; micrognathia (**3 and 4**).
- Hypospadias (**9**), small penis, possible cryptorchidism or even a clinical appearance of pseudohermaphroditism in males.
- Syndactyly of the second and third toes (**8**); abnormal palmar creases (**6**) and dermatoglyphics. Possible postaxial polydactyly.
- Psychomotor retardation with various grades of severity (often considerable) with abnormal muscle tone (**2**).

Supplementary findings: Possible cataracts; prominent lateral palatine ridges (**5**) or cleft palate (**5**); abnormally positioned fingers (**7**) and toes; hip dysplasia; cutis laxa; hernias; cerebral, cardiac and urogenital anomalies and other severe internal malformations. Hyperexcitability. Low resistance to infections.

Manifestation: At birth (predominantly breech presentation).

Aetiology: Autosomal recessive disorder; very variable interfamilial (not intrafamilial) expression of the gene. Gene locus probably on the long arm of chromosome 7 (7q32.1?).
  Chromosomal analysis always indicated.
  Defective cholesterol biosynthesis in addition to other biochemical anomalies: significant lowering of cholesterol and elevation of 7-dehydrocholesterol in blood or tissue.

Frequency: Not low; 1:20 000 has been estimated, possibly higher.

Comment: The spectrum of the syndrome is very broad. It appears that patients with polydactyly, male hermaphroditism, cleft palate and cataract also show severe internal malformations: diverse cardiac anomalies, incomplete lobar development of the lungs, gastro-intestinal defects such as malrotation, agangliosis of the colon, hypoplasia of the kidneys and cerebral or other anomalies. Whether such a 'genitopalatocardiac' SLO syndrome represents a separate 'type II' entity is highly questionable.

Course, prognosis: Unfavourable, especially in view of the severity of mental retardation. In severe cases, death in the neonatal period or the first years of life.

Treatment: Symptomatic (high-cholesterol diet in the experimental stage).
  Genetic counselling of the parents. Prenatal diagnosis by ultrasound or biochemical methods.

Differential diagnosis: In severe cases, Meckel–Gruber syndrome (*45*) or hydrolethalus syndrome (*323*) should be considered.

Illustrations:
1–9 A 2-year-old child of young, healthy parents; pregnancy unremarkable with birth at term, breech presentation (birth measurements unknown). Present measurements: length 76 cm; weight 6.4 kg; head circumference 43.5 cm (all well below the second percentile). Typical facies. Cleft palate. Asymmetry of the nipples. Short first metacarpals; clinodactyly of the second and third fingers with ulnar deviation; cutaneous syndactyly of the second and third toes to the middle phalanges bilaterally, dysplasia of the third toes. Very severe psychomotor impairment, considerable muscular hypotonia and hyperirritability with attacks of dystonia (**2**). Severe failure to thrive; frequent vomiting. Abnormal electroencephalogram. Chromosomal analysis (including banded preparations) normal.

References:
Lowry R B: Variability in the Smith-Lemli-Opitz syndrome... *Am J Med Genet* 1983, **14**:429–433.
Bialer M G *et al*: Female external genitalia... in a 46.XY infant... *Am J Med Genet* 1987, **28**:723–731.
Irons M *et al*: Defective cholesterol biosynthesis in Smith-Lemli-Opitz syndrome. *Lancet* 1993, **341**:1414.
Irons M *et al*: Abnormal cholesterol metabolism in the Smith-Lemli-Opitz syndrome... *Am J Med Genet* 1994, **50**:347–352.
Opitz J M *et al*: Cholesterol metabolism in the... Smith-Lemli-Opitz syndrome (Conference summary). *Am J Med Genet* 1994, **50**:326–338.
Opitz J M: RSH/SLO... syndrome... *Am J Med Genet* 1994, **50**:344–346.
Tint G S *et al*: Defective cholesterol biosynthesis... *N Engl J Med* 1994, **330**:107–113, 1685–1687.
Wallace M *et al*: Smith-Lemli-Opitz syndrome... 7q32... *Am J Med Genet* 1994, **50**:368–374.

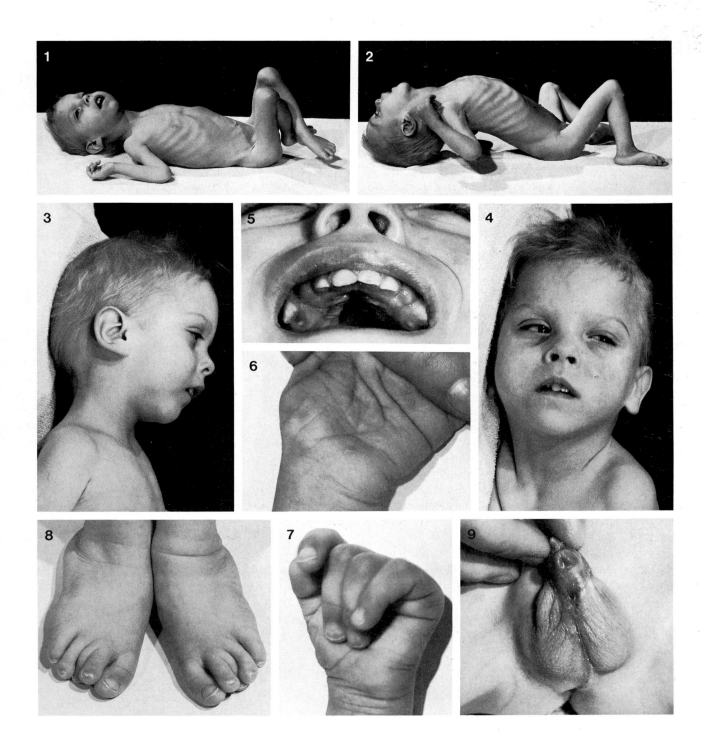

J.K.

A characteristic syndrome of ophthalmoplegia, ptosis, expressionless face, decrease in muscle mass, moderate to severe muscular hypotonia, severe respiratory disorder and disorders of swallowing.

Main signs:
- Autosomal recessive form: onset in the neonatal period with respiratory disorders, ptosis, strabismus, expressionless, 'sleepy' face (myopathic facies), weak cry, difficulties with drinking, atrophy of the sternocleidomastoid muscle and of the muscles of the extremities, usually most marked proximally. Nasal speech. Tendon reflexes reduced or absent. Long face, high palate, club feet.
- X-linked recessive form: similar to the autosomal recessive form but more severe. Breathing difficulties caused by atrophy of the respiratory musculature. 'Floppy infant', weak cry, no active sucking, swallowing disorders. Bilateral ptosis, facial diplegia, reduced eye movements, cardiomyopathy. Maternal polyhydramnios. Increased miscarriages, perinatal death of male infants.
- Autosomal dominant form: onset between the first and third decades of life. Muscular hypotonia of the pelvic girdle, slow progression. Involvement of the facial musculature. Gait disturbance, wheelchair required later in life.

Supplementary findings: Proptosis, strabismus, mild cataracts. Joint contractures; slender, fragile bones; 'excess skin', cryptorchidism.

On biopsy, abnormal type 1 muscle fibres with atrophy, central nucleus, formation of rows of nuclei and perinuclear myofibril-free haloes. Clusters of mitochondria, lipopigments, glycogen, rough endoplasmic reticulum, and Golgi apparatus in the perinuclear zone.

Hypertrophy of type 2 muscle fibres, frequently accompanied by abnormal electromyogram.

Manifestation: Onset of the autosomal recessive and X-linked recessive forms soon after birth; with the autosomal dominant type, after the first decade of life.

Aetiology: Three genetically distinct forms: autosomal recessive, X-linked recessive and autosomal dominant. Gene locus for the X-linked form: Xq28. Diagnosis of heterozygotes after muscle biopsy?

Frequency: No accurate figures available for any of the forms.

Course, prognosis: Dependent on the hereditary type. In autosomal recessive patients, it may be difficult to differentiate adults with an autosomal dominant course, who show scoliosis, lordosis, protruding scapulae. Wheelchairs are required later. Seizures in 18% of patients. X-linked recessive disease is usually manifest at birth with severe asphyxia and an early fatal outcome. Additional complications: aspiration pneumonia, myogenic heart failure.

Differential diagnosis: Myotonic dystrophy (286), mitochondrial myopathy (283).

Treatment: Physiotherapy. Anticonvulsive therapy.

Illustrations:

1 A 12-year-old boy. Ptosis, myopathic facies, external ophthalmoplegia, muscular hypotonia.

References:

Mortier W E, Michaelis E, Becker J et al: Centronucleäre Myopathie mit autosomal-dominantem Erbgang. *Humangenetik* 1975, 27:199–215.

Pavone L, Mollica F, Grasso A et al: Familial centronuclear myopathy. *Acta Neurol Scand* 1980, 62:33–40.

Sarnat H B, Roth S J, Yimenez J F: Neonatal myotubular myopathy: neuropathy and failure of postnatal maturation of fetal muscle. *Can J Neurol Sci* 1981, 8:313–320.

Heckmatt J Z, Sewry C A, Hodes D et al: Congenital centronuclear (myotubular) myopathy. a clinical, pathological, and genetic study in eight children. *Brain* 1985, 108:941–964.

Breningstall G, Marks H: Maternal muscle biopsy in severe neonatal centronuclear (myotubular) myopathy. *Am J Med Genet* 1986, 25:722–723.

Bucher H U, Boltshauser E, Briner J et al: Severe neonatal centronuclear (myotubular) myopathy: an X-linked recessive disorder. *Helv Paediatr Acta* 1986, 41:291–300.

Keppen L D, Husain M M, Woody R C: X-linked myotubular myopathy: intrafamilial variability and normal muscle biopsy in a heterozygous female. *Clin Genet* 1987, 32:95–99.

Braga S E, Gerber A, Meier C, Weiersmuller A, Zimmermann A et al: Severe neonatal asphyxia due to X-linked centronuclear myopathy. *Eur J Pediatr* 1990, 150:132–135.

Thomas N S T, Williams H, Cole G et al: X-linked neonatal centronuclear/myotubular myopathy: evidence for linkage to Xq28 DNA marker loci. *J Med Genet* 1990, 27:284–287.

Breningstall G N, Grover W D, Marks H G: Maternal muscle biopsy in X-linked recessive centronuclear (myotubular) myopathy. *Am J Med Genet* 1991, 39:13–18.

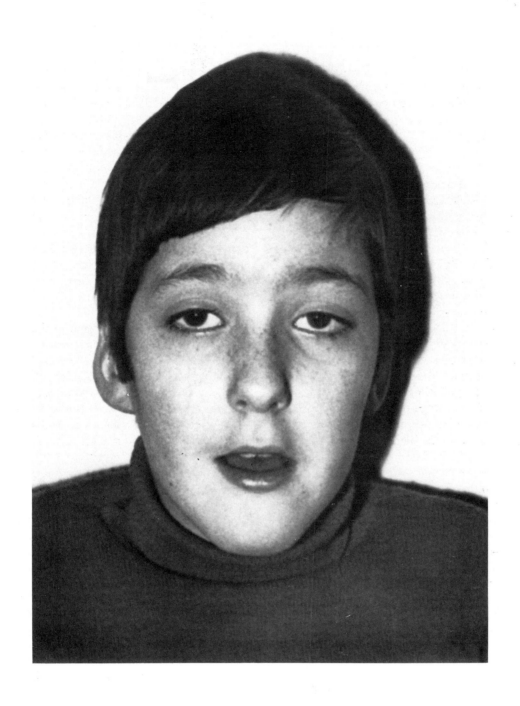

J.K

A group of diseases with the characteristics of a primary dysfunction of the central nervous system, the musculature or both as a result of a disorder of oxidative metabolism in the mitochondria.

Main signs:
- Disorder of central nervous system function: spinocerebellar degeneration, cortical blindness. Sensorineural hearing loss. Seizures. Psychomotor retardation. Ataxia, choreo-athetosis. Hemiparesis. Respiratory disorder, somnolence, apathy. Confusion.
- External ophthalmoplegia. Pigmented retinopathy, hemianopia, optic atrophy. Peripheral sensory neuropathy.
- Muscle weakness, muscular hypotonia, fatigability with slow proximal to distal progression. Cardiomyopathy. Macroglossia.
- Short stature. Microcephaly. Vomiting, headaches.

Supplementary findings: On electroencephalogram, generalized slowing with foci of hypersynchronic activity. Electromyogram with myopathic and neurogenic lesions but often normal findings. Computerized axial tomography of the skull shows cerebral atrophy, cerebellar atrophy, decreased density of the silent area, dysmyelinization, multiple infarcts, calcification of the basal ganglia.

Muscle biopsy: accumulation of mitochondria at the periphery of the muscle fibres (ragged-red fibres), abnormal mitochondria (abnormal size, unusual structure, paracrystalline inclusions).

Oral glucose tolerance test shows an abnormal increase in serum lactate and pyruvate. Similar findings after a 24-h fasting test.

Manifestation: Onset in childhood of progressive muscular hypotonia and initially obscure central nervous disorders.

Aetiology: Biochemical defect of abnormal mitochondria. Usually sporadic cases. Familial cases may be autosomal dominant, autosomal recessive or X-linked recessive. As mitochondrial DNA can only be maternally transmitted, a non-hereditary pattern of transmission must be expected. In 30 examined families, maternal transmission occurred 27 times. In 71 patients, paternal transmission never occurred, the increased risk for siblings was 3% and there was a 5.5% risk of further transmission by the index patient. Empirical recurrence risks depend on the basic biochemical defect.

Frequency: The number of diagnosed patients is increasing.

Course, prognosis: Progressive course; depending on the enzyme defect, lethal outcome possible during the neonatal period. However, the first manifestations may not occur until adulthood.

Differential diagnosis: Chronic progressive external ophthalmoplegia, Kearns–Sayre syndrome (*284*), familial myoclonus epilepsy syndrome with 'ragged-red fibres', mitochondrial myopathy (*283*), encephalopathy, lactic acidosis and stroke-like episodes, Alpers' progressive poliodystrophy, Canavan's spongy degeneration of the white matter, Leigh's subacute necrotizing encephalomyopathy, Menkes' kinky hair syndrome (*59*), Zellweger's cerebro-hepato-renal syndrome (*291*) and myotubular myopathy (*282*).

Treatment: No effective treatment known. With enzyme defects in the pyruvate dehydrogenase complex, a controlled ketogenic diet in isolated patients. Symptomatic therapy for seizures, hemiparesis and hearing impairment.

Illustrations:

1a–c A 15-year-old boy, progressive external ophthalmoplegia, bilateral abducent weakness, ptosis (tapetoretinal degeneration).

2a and b A boy, aged 14 years and 6 months, progressive external ophthalmoplegia, ptosis (pigmented retinopathy).

References:

Egger J, Wilson, J: Mitochondral inheritance in a mitochondrially mediated disease. *N Engl J Med* 1983, 309:142–146.

Sengers R C A, Stadhouders A M, Trijbels J M F: Mitochondrial myopathies. Clinical, morphological and biochemical aspects. *Eur J Pediatr* 1984, 141:192–207.

Siemes H: Mitochondriale Myopathien und Encephalomyopathien. Neuromuskuläre und zentralnervöse Erkrankungen infolge von Defekten des mitochondrialen oxydativen Stoffwechsels. *Monatsschr Kinderheilkd* 1985, 133:798–805.

Reichmann H, Rohkamm R, Rikker K *et al*: Mitochondriale Myopathien. *Dtsch Med Wschr* 1988, 113:106–113.

Smeitink J A M, Senger R C A *et al*: Fatal neonatal cardiomyopathy associated with cataract and mitochondrial myopathy. *Eur J Pediatr* 1989, 148:656–659.

Zeviani M, Gellera C *et al*: Tissue distribution and transmission of mitochondrial DNA deletions in mitochondrial myopathies. *Ann Neurol* 1990, 28:94–97.

Tulinius M H, Holme E *et al*: Mitochondrial encephalomyopathies in childhood. I. Biochemical and morphologic investigations. *J Pediatr* 1991, 119:251–259.

Tulinius M H, Holme E *et al*: Mitochondrial encephalomyopathies in childhood. II. Clinical manifestations and syndromes. *J Pediatr* 1991, 119:251–259.

van Hellenberg Hubar J L M, Gabreels F J M *et al*: MELAS syndrome. Report of two patients, and comparison with data of 24 patients derived from the literature. *Neuropediatrics* 1991, 22:10–14.

Ciafaloni E, Ricci E *et al*: MELAS: clinical features, biochemistry, and molecular genetics. *Ann Neurol* 1992, 31:391–398.

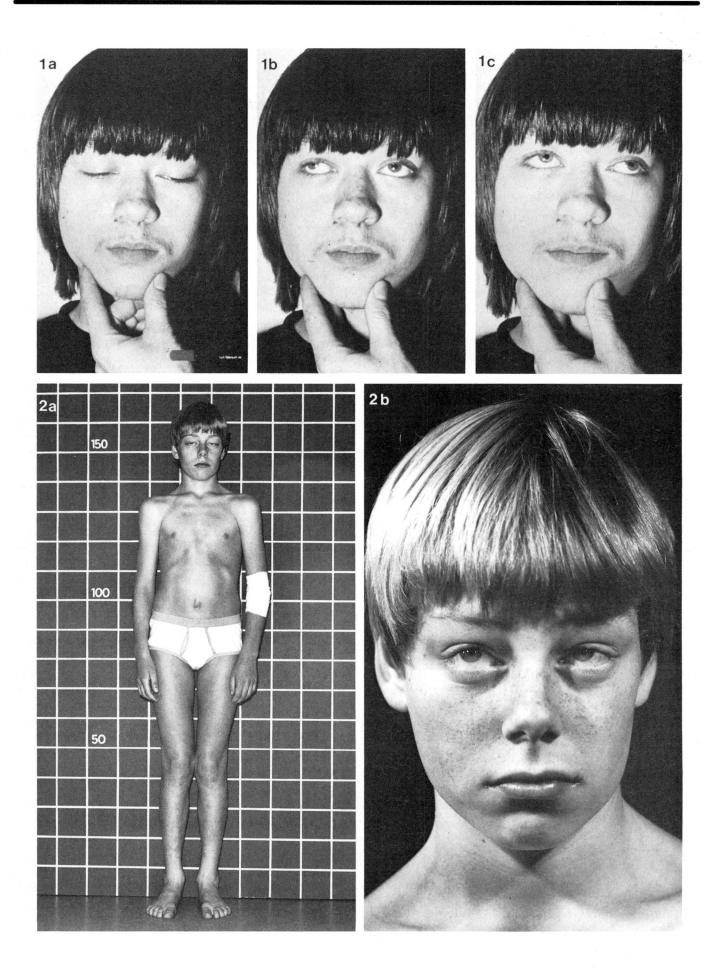

H.-R.W

A mitochondrial encephalomyopathy with chronic, progressive external ophthalmoplegia and further neuromuscular defects, intracardiac conduction defect, tapetoretinal degeneration and characteristic appearance.

Main signs:
- Chronic, progressive external ophthalmoplegia (**1 and 2**).
- Disorders of intracardiac conduction or bundle branch block.
- Pigmentary degeneration of the retina.
- Characteristic appearance, especially typical facies (**1 and 2**).

Supplementary findings: Many different defects of the central and peripheral nervous systems: optic atrophy, hearing impairment and vestibular defect, cerebellar ataxia, pareses and pyramidal signs; myopathy of the proximal skeletal musculature; increased protein and sometimes cell count in the spinal fluid; electroencephalogram changes. In some patients, signs of spongy degeneration of the brain on computerized axial tomography.

Not infrequently, poor intellectual development or mental deterioration.

Possible hypogonadism, hypoparathyroidism, diabetes mellitus, renal dysfunction.

Electromyographic evidence of a generalized myopathy; on muscle biopsy, characteristic (but nonspecific) 'ragged-red fibres' (special mitochondrial changes with paracrystalline inclusions, which may also be demonstrable in other organs).

Often considerable short stature. This and the lax posture, poor musculature, frequent secondary kyphoscoliosis, hyperlordosis, frequent wasting and typical facies all contribute to the characteristic general appearance (**1 and 2**). Biochemistry: Increased lactate in plasma, urine, cerebrospihal fluid.

Manifestation: Possibly as early as the first year of life (ptosis), but onset is more frequently toward the end of the first decade of life or later. Progressive external ophthalmoplegia, in some patients facial paresis, high-tone deafness, dysphonia, dysphagia, ataxia, spasticity, mental decline, congestive cardiomyopathy and other signs.

Aetiology: Mitochondrial inheritance has been postulated; findings of heteroplasmy for a partial mitochondrial DNA deletion. Predominantly sporadic cases have been described, familial occurrence (autosomal dominant and recessive) less frequently; heterogeneity.

Frequency:
Not so very low; since the first description, well over 150 'complete' (and probably a corresponding number of 'incomplete') patients have been described.

Course, prognosis:
Apparently, the earlier the onset, the more unfavourable the prognosis. Sudden deterioration and (cardiac or brainstem) death can occur even with the best possible cardiac care.

Comment: The group of mitochondrial encephalomyopathies is not small; see also mitochondrial myopathy (**283**). Pearson syndrome may be a precursor of Kearns–Sayre syndrome.

Treatment: Symptomatic. Careful cardiac follow-up with early, possibly preventative implantation of a pacemaker. Surgical treatment of severe ptosis may be indicated. Hearing assessments. Physiotherapy and orthopaedic measures. Hormone replacement (if indicated). Replacement of coenzyme Q10 and carnitine appears to improve eye mobility, ptosis and, to some extent, ataxia and electrocardiogram changes.

Genetic counselling.

Illustrations:

1 and 2 A girl aged 15 years and 9 months, the fourth child of healthy parents after three healthy siblings. Primary delay of motor development; bilateral ptosis at 4 years (multiple operations). Total ophthalmoplegia, retinitis pigmentosa, hypo-acusis, dysphagia, complete left bundle branch block (preventative implantation of a pacemaker), myopathy especially of the proximal limb musculature, ataxia, short stature (below the third percentile), poor intellectual development, emaciation.

References:

Kearns T R, Sayre, G P: Retinitis pigmentosa, external ophthalmoplegia and complete heart block. *Arch Ophthalmol* 1958, **60**:280.
Egger J, Wilson J: Mitochondrial inheritance in a mitochondrially mediated disease. *N Engl J Med* 1983, **309**:142–146.
Machraoui A, Breviere G M *et al*: Syndrome de Kearns familial. *Ann Pédiatr* 1985, **32**:701–711.
Siemes, H: Mitochondriale Myopathien und Encephalomyopathien... *Mschr Kinderheilk* 1985, **133**:798–805.
Ogasahara S, Nishikawa Y *et al*: Treatment of Kearns-Sayre syndrome with coenzyme Q10. *Neurology* 1986, **36**:45–53.
Zeviani M, Moraes C T *et al*: Deletions of mitochondrial DNA in Kearns-Sayre syndrome. *Neurology* 1988 **38**:1339–1346.
Nelson I *et al*: Kearns-Sayre syndrome with sideroblastic anemia... *Neuropediatrics* 1992, **23**:119–205.
Nørby S *et al*: Juvenile Kearns-Sayre syndrome... *J Med Genet* 1994, **31**:45–50.

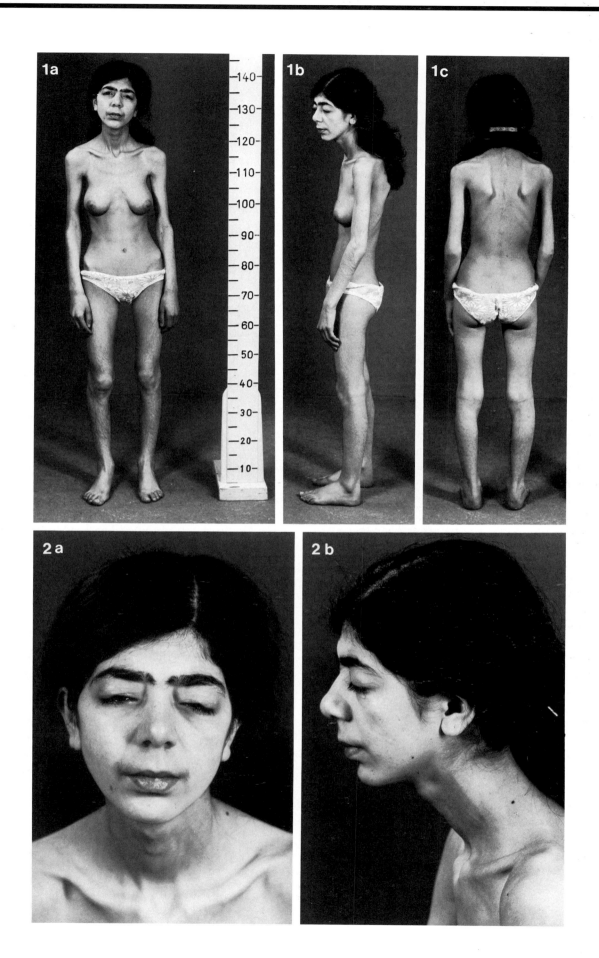

J.K.

Myasthenia is characterized by signs of abnormal muscular fatigue after physical exercise with recovery taking several minutes to hours.

Main signs:
- Transient neonatal form (10% of patients seen in childhood forms) in 15% of newborns of myasthenic mothers between the first and third days of life: generalized muscular hypotonia, decreased movements, weak sucking, difficulties swallowing, ptosis.
- Persistent neonatal form (20% of childhood patients), the same signs as above but persisting.
- Juvenile myasthenia (the most frequent form in childhood), usually occurs after the 10th year of life. Girls:boys = 6:1. First signs frequently postinfectious with unilateral or bilateral ptosis. Occasionally it is also generalized with ophthalmoplegia and weakness of facial and limb musculature. Persistence of features until the fourth to sixth decade of life.

Supplementary findings: Myasthenic crises can be life threatening with infections, stress or surgery.

Manifestation:
Transient neonatal form: at birth.
Persistent neonatal form: before the second year of life.
Juvenile myasthenia: after age 10 years.

Aetiology: The result of autoimmune reactions against muscle acetylcholine receptors. Other immunological disorders may also be present. Hyperplasia of the thymus, thymomas, lupus erythematosus. The demonstration of an association between HLA-B8 and myasthenia gravis indicates genetic factors. In familial cases, siblings frequently are affected. The rare infantile familial forms show severe respiratory distress and recurrent apnoeic episodes and are probably transmitted by autosomal dominant inheritance.

Frequency: 1:15 000–200 000, worldwide. Familial cases rare; usually sporadic occurrence.

Course, prognosis: The transient neonatal form (in children of myasthenic mothers) may lead to death within hours or days *post partum* if untreated. The persisting myasthenia of newborns (with healthy mothers) has a good prognosis for life once diagnosed. With the juvenile form, intervening crises must be anticipated.

Differential diagnosis: Myasthenic syndrome with disorders of thyroid function and lupus erythematosus. Additionally: familial infantile myasthenia: slow channel type of myasthenia.

Treatment:
- Thymectomy in patients who do not respond well to cholinesterase inhibitors.
- Cholinergics: pyridostigmine bromide, neostigmine.
- Immunosuppressive therapy with prednisone. (Avoid: tranquilizers, barbiturates, narcotics, local anaesthetics, anti-arrhythmic agents and certain antibiotics, including tetracycline, neomycin, colistin, lincomycin.)

Illustrations:
1a and 2a A patient aged 9 years and 6 months, with recent onset of ocular myasthenia (ptosis of the upper lids, double vision).
1b and 2b The same girl immediately after intravenous administration of 10 mg edrophonium chloride (Tensilon®).

References:
Gordon N: Congenital myasthenia. *Dev Med Child Neurol* 1986, 28:803–813.
Haas J: Myasthenia gravis. Aktuelle Therapie unter pathophysiologischen Aspekten. *Dt Ärztebl* 1988, 85:C–114–C–118.
Any textbook on paediatrics and internal medicine.

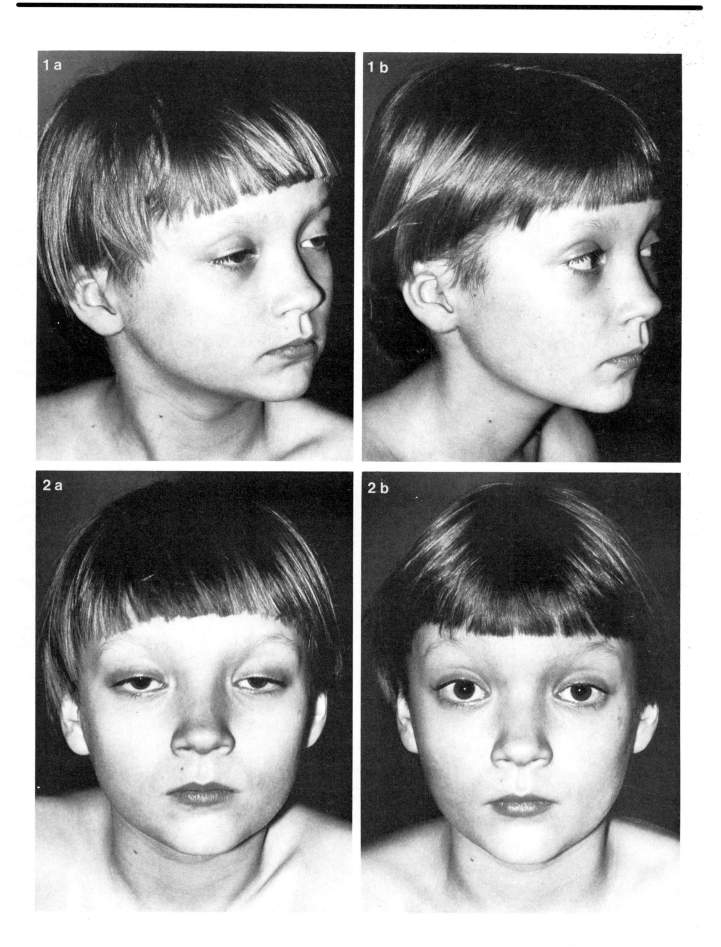

J.K./ H.-R.W

An autosomal dominant disorder with severe myotonic signs in newborns, transmitted by mildly affected mothers.

Main signs:
- Neonatal form: severe generalized muscular hypotonia with symmetric weakness of the facial muscles, triangular open ('tent-shaped') mouth and ptosis (facial diplegia). Initially, good deep-tendon reflexes. Frequently disorders of sucking, swallowing and respiration (often life threatening) during the first days to weeks. Global development delay common.
- Adult form: myotonic facies, localized muscular atrophy, cataract, frontal baldness. Characteristic inability to 'bury the eyelashes' by tightly closing the lids.

Supplementary findings:
- Neonatal form: mother with myotonic dystrophy (usually only mild signs).
Frequent pes equinovarus; high palate and other minor signs. Possible oedema, tendency to bleed into the skin, liver, brain. Enlarged cerebral ventricles.
- Adult form: Hollow temples, myotonic reaction on thenar percussion, rapid fatigue with repeated clenching of the fist (recuperation pauses required when typewriting). Mild endocrinopathies. In 65% of patients, cardiac involvement. Decreased fertility in both males and females (small testes with progressive involution of the seminiferous tubules; menstrual disorders). High-risk patients for anaesthesia.

Manifestation: At birth for the neonatal form, frequently after weak foetal movements during pregnancy and often with hydramnios.

Aetiology: Autosomal dominant disorder. Mildly affected mothers have to expect a high risk with their children: 12% stillbirths or neonatal deaths; 9% severely affected (survival); 29% affected later. Affected fathers rarely have children with the severe neonatal form. Intrafamilial variability. New mutations very rare. Always search for affected parents (mothers), especially with severely affected newborns.
Gene localized to chromosome 19: 19q13.3. Molecular genetic techniques succeeded in showing an amplification of a triplet of base pairs, CTG, in affected individuals to between 50 and 2000 (compared with a maximum of 37 in healthy individuals). The expansion of the maternal nucleotide sequence into the next generation explains the anticipation effect: increasing severity of the disease from generation to generation.

Frequency: Differs with geographic location. Estimated at between 1:20 000 and 1:40 000. In Switzerland, 50 affected individuals out of 1 million of the general population. Estimated mutation rate 1.3×10^{-5}.

Course, prognosis: Up to 50% neonatal mortality from severe respiratory insufficiency. After survival through this dangerous initial phase, however, there is little (if any) progression of muscle weakness in early childhood and little or no sign of myotonia. Motor development delayed, but patients usually learn to walk. In later years, increasing muscle weakness and atrophy, especially in the face (flaccid, expressionless, myotonic facies with open mouth), the neck (sternocleidomastoids), the distal extremities (e.g. extensors of the hands and fingers, levators of the feet) and other areas. Impaired articulation in most patients. Deep reflexes often reduced, moderate myotonic signs present. The endocrine features and cataracts of the adult form are not present in the first decade of life.
Summary: Poor long-term prognosis with little hope of an independent existence (mental retardation, increasing muscular atrophy). In adulthood, progressive cataracts; early death from pulmonary infections or cardiac arrhythmia.

Diagnosis: In the neonate, a clinical diagnosis is possible. On close examination of the parents: inability to 'bury' the eyelashes is an unfailing sign even in individuals not previously recognized as affected (at least 15%). Slit-lamp examination of the lenses (cataract) and muscle biopsy frequently confirm the diagnosis in adults. Frequent myopathic electromyogram. Creatine kinase often normal (a slight elevation requires especially critical evaluation). Reliable diagnosis now possible by demonstration of CTG amplification in excess of 50.

Differential diagnosis: In the neonatal period, the various causes of 'floppy infants', cerebral anoxia, trauma, medication, neonatal myasthenia (285), Prader–Willi syndrome (158), Werdnig–Hoffmann (293) and many more.

Treatment: Difficult ethical problem in severely ill neonates with respiratory insufficiency. Genetic counselling. Molecular genetic diagnosis and prenatal diagnosis possible in informative families.

Illustrations: 1–3 Female first-born with congenital form; in **1**, as a neonate; in **2 and 3**, at 4 weeks. The mother, her brother and father: myotonic dystrophy. **4** A woman (previously not known to be affected) and her typically affected newborn. The mother was unable, on request, to 'bury' her eyelashes. **5** Father and son; neither able to close their eyes tightly.

References:
Glanz A, Fraser F C: Risk... myotonic dystrophy. *J Med Genet* 1984, **21**:186.
Rutherford M A *et al*: Congenital myotonic dystrophy. *Arch Dis Child* 1989, **64**:191.
Sutherland G R: Myotonic dystrophy: from linkage with secretor status to mutation detection. *Clin Genet* 1993, **43**:273–275.

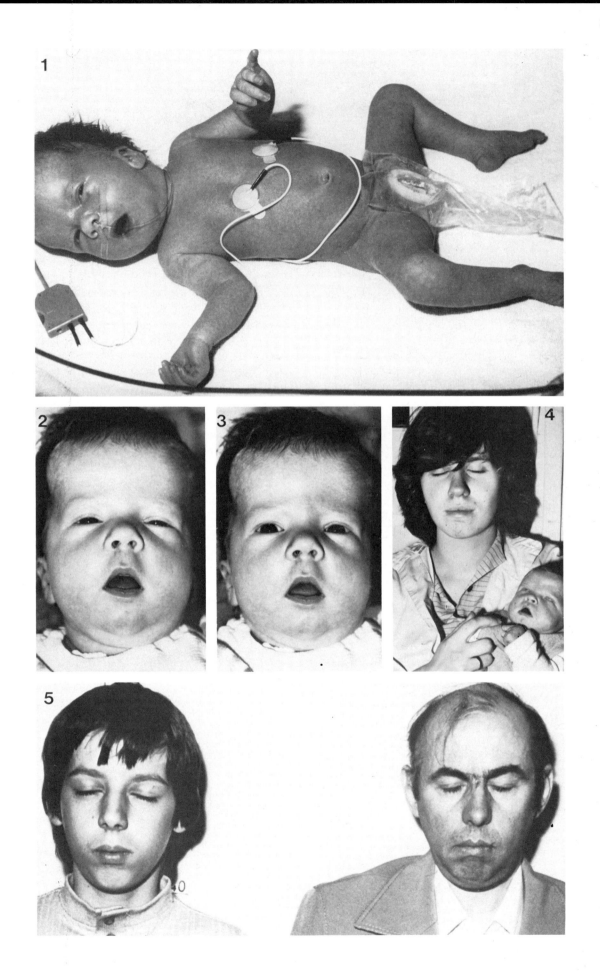

287 Myotonia Congenita, Becker Type

H.-R.W

An autosomal recessive myotonia causing increasing clinical handicap and associated with distinct muscular hypertrophy.

Main signs:
- Strong or sudden stimuli elicit a state of tonic contraction of the innervated striated muscles (especially in the extremities but also the external eye muscles and so on), the rigidity resolving only after a few seconds, becoming less marked and finally no longer occurring when the movement is carried out repeatedly.
- Onset of symptoms in the legs, then the hands and arms, later the throat and masticatory muscles and so on becoming generalized by adulthood.
- Distinct hypertrophy of the musculature (1–3) with no increase in general strength.
- Limited dorsiflexion of the hands and feet.

Supplementary findings: Reflexes and sensation normal. Diagnostically, the patient cannot open his or her fist immediately after (on request) clenching it suddenly and forcefully; tapping the thenar eminence, tongue or biceps briefly with a reflex hammer elicits a persisting contraction depression as a myotonic reaction; characteristic myotonic pattern on electromyogram.

Manifestation: Usually between the fourth and 12th years of life; in males, possibly later. Onset usually in the legs.

Aetiology: Autosomal recessive disorder.

Frequency: Approximately 1:500 000. Thomsen type = 4.4:1 000 000.

Course, prognosis: A generalized progressive disorder leading to increasing weakness and atrophy of the musculature.

Differential diagnosis: In Thomsen-type autosomal dominant myotonia congenita, pronounced muscle hypertrophy is an exception; the disorder runs a milder course and usually does not cause the individual to seek medical help.

Treatment: Protection from cold; avoidance of a high-potassium diet.
In patients with particular complaints because of the myotonic reaction, treatment may be initiated with quinidine sulphate or procainamide and diphenyl hydantoin. Genetic counselling.

Illustrations:
1–3 A boy aged 12 years and 5 months, mentally normal, from a healthy family. Myotonia, manifest since the age of 8 years, was initially limited to his lower extremities (at first, disturbance of gait; difficulties with starts in sports) and is now generalized, including involvement of m. levator palpebrae and m. orbicularis oculi. Pronounced muscle hypertrophy and slightly reduced general strength. A myotonic reaction can be elicited mechanically on the tongue and thenar eminences; characteristic electromyogram findings.

References:
Any specialist textbook on paediatrics, internal medicine or neurology.
Zellweger H, Pavone L, Biondi A *et al*: Autosomal recessive generalized myotonia. *Muscle Nerve* 1980 3:176.
Sun S F, Streib E W: Autosomal recessive generalized myotonia. *Muscle Nerve* 1983, 6:143–148.
Treatment of myotonia (Editorial). *Lancet* 1987; 1242–1244.

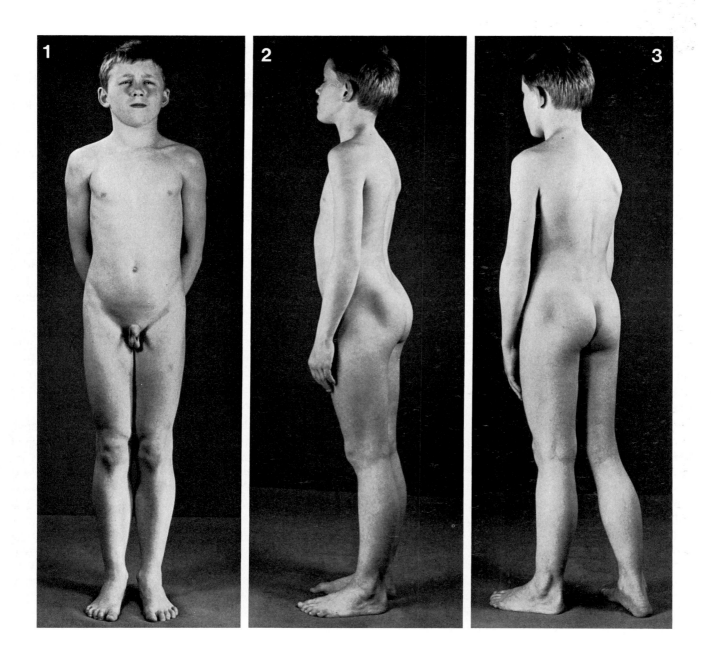

288

Schwartz–Jampel Syndrome

(Catel–Schwartz–Jampel Syndrome; Chondrodystrophic Myotonia)

H.-R.W

A characteristic hereditary disorder with postnatal development of myotonic signs, typical facies, growth retardation and osteo-articular changes.

Main signs:
- Flat, full-cheeked face, which appears small in relation to the normal-sized cranium, small-appearing mouth, small chin and fixed expression. Eyes appear deep set; narrow, palpebral fissures (possibly with slight antimongoloid slant) as a result of blepharospasm of variable severity. Tightly closed, puckered mouth which is difficult to open. The facial expression may be described as 'a frozen smile' but also 'sad' or 'as when crying' and rarely relaxes (2 and 4).
- Increasing growth retardation of intra-uterine onset; linear growth often below the third percentile. 'Truncal dwarfism', that is, a short trunk with disproportionately long extremities (3 and 4).
- Poor motor function, rapid fatigability caused by 'stiffness' of the palpably firm, sometimes hypertrophic, musculature of the trunk and extremities. (Myotonic reaction usually readily elicited on the thenar eminences.) Early flexion contractures of most large joints; corresponding gait and posture. Hyporeflexia.
- Early onset of pain, especially in the legs. On radiograph, dysplasia especially of the femoral head (6); all in all, a picture of moderately severe spondylo-epimetaphyseal dysplasia. Osteoporosis.

Supplementary findings: Horizontal wrinkling of the brow and raised eyebrows because of the contracted facial musculature. Large, low-set ears (2). Possible distichiasis; ptosis in some patients; frequent, possibly severe myopia. Alae nasi sometimes hypoplastic; high palate; possible dimpled chin. High, nasal voice (occasionally stridor).

Short neck; elevated shoulders (3); pectus carinatum; increased dorsal kyphosis and lumbar lordosis; also scoliosis. Possibly retarded bone age.

Electromyogram: non-specific findings resembling myotonia. No biochemical abnormalities.

Mental development normal in 80% of patients.

Manifestation: Slowing of growth and motor development, facial changes and motor impairment usually become distinct in the second year of life or later; onset of pain and rapid fatigability at about the same time. Manifestation at birth or in infancy is unusual.

Aetiology: Autosomal recessive disorder with very variable expression. Basic defect unknown.

Frequency: Low; 60 patients described up to 1987.

Course, prognosis: Life expectancy apparently not affected in most patients. The myotonic manifestations may remain stationary soon after appearing in early childhood; motor function may improve. However, further (generally slow) progression over a number of years is also possible.

Diagnosis, differential diagnosis: Growth retardation and conspicuous osteo-articular signs with 'peculiar facies' may so dominate the clinical picture that the myotonia and thus the diagnosis are overlooked. Myotonia must be confirmed electromyographically.

The Freeman–Sheldon syndrome (27) shows considerable overlap with this syndrome. However the former, present at birth, does not show multiple bony dysplasias or a myotonic electromyogram and as a rule is transmitted by autosomal dominant inheritance.

Easily differentiated from myotonia congenita (287), paramyotonia and myotonic dystrophy (286).

Treatment: Carbamazepine can be beneficial. Remedial orthopaedic measures; ophthalmological attention; psychological support. Beware: increased risk with anaesthesia. Genetic counselling. Prenatal diagnosis.

Illustrations:

1–5 A boy as a toddler, before the characteristic facies were distinctly manifest (1) and at 6 years and 6 months, with the full clinical picture (2–5; on his back, a pigmented naevus).

6 Typical hip findings in this boy (the first child of healthy parents). Disorder manifest at age 2 years ('eyes closed slowly'). Smooth, shiny facial skin with taut musculature. Blepharophimosis right greater than left; marked difficulty in opening his contracted, snout-like mouth. High, narrow palate. Stiffness, impaired mobility and contractures; leg pain. Typical electromyogram findings. Short stature. Normal intellect. Some improvement of function later.

References:

Seay A R *et al*: Malignant hyperpyrexia in... Schwartz-Jampel syndrome. *J Pediatr* 1983, 93:83.
Farrell S A *et al*: Neonatal Schwartz-Jampel syndrome. *Am J Med Genet* 1987 27:799.
Hunziker U A *et al*: Prenatal diagnosis... *Prenat Diagn* 1989, 9:127.
Topaloglu H *et al*: Improvement of myotonia with carbamazepine in... Schwartz-Jampel syndrome. *Neuropediatrics* 1993, 24:232.
Al Gazali L I: The Schwartz-Jampel syndrome. *Clin Dysmorphol* 1993, 2:47–54.

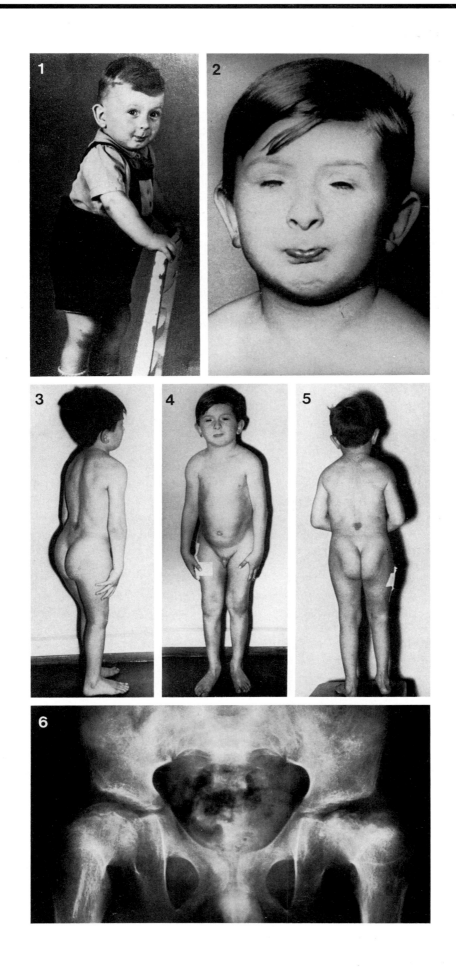

289

Syndrome of Blepharophimosis, Pterygium Colli, Flexion Contractures of the Fingers and Toes and Osteodysplasia

H.-R.W

A syndrome of unusual facies, short neck with mild pterygium, development of flexion contractures of fingers and toes and of spondylo-epiphyseal dysplasia.

Main signs:
- Facies: round with blepharophimosis, broad nasal bridge, epicanthus and small mouth with very narrow prolabium (**1**). 'A congenital strabismus syndrome of convergent microstrabismus with bilateral dissociated vertical squint and rotary nystagmus'. Left-sided amblyopia.
- Short neck; nuchal hairline somewhat low; slight pterygium colli (**1 and 2**).
- Flexion contractures of the (very long) second to fifth fingers bilaterally, especially of the proximal interphalangeal joints, and of all toes (**3 and 4**) with subluxation of the distal joints of the second to fifth bilaterally.
- Somewhat short stature (approximately 10th percentile) with the extremities being disproportionately long. Dysgenesis of vertebral bodies and epiphyses (**5**).

Supplementary findings: Freely mobile large joints. Winging of the scapulae. Mild pectus carinatum; S-form scoliosis. Genu valgum. Flat feet.

On radiograph, slight flattening of the vertebral bodies dorsally, causing slightly ovoid configuration.

Flattening of both femoral heads with irregularly honeycombed and markedly sclerotic changes, left greater than right (**5**), both resembling the changes seen in Perthes disease. Coxa vara.

Slight flattening of the epiphyses of the knee joints; somewhat plaque-like structure of the patellae.

Varus deformity of the toes bilaterally (**6**).

Normal intellectual development. No evidence of a neurological or muscular disorder.

Normal biochemical findings.

Normal female karyotype.

Manifestation: Partly at birth (facies), partly later in infancy and early childhood (flexion contractures of fingers and toes; osteodysplasia).

Aetiology: Not clear. Genetic basis assumed. (The unusual appearance with narrow palpebral fissures and lips is also present in the child's mother and maternal grandfather; on the other hand, the deceased paternal grandmother and her mother are said to have suffered from severely twisted toes. The child's father is unremarkable.)

Comment: The clinical picture presented here shows certain similarities to disorders as diverse as Stickler dysplasia (arthro-ophthalmopathy, *302*), chondrodystrophic myotonia (Schwartz–Jampel syndrome, *288*), and Ullrich–Turner syndrome (*103*), none of which is present here.

Illustrations:
1–6 The proband at 9 years. The second child of young, healthy, nonconsanguineous parents; older brother unremarkable. Birth and early development normal. Later in early childhood, manifestation of finger and toe contractures, which have not progressed since then and do not handicap the patient. At approximately the same time, clinical manifestation of hip dysplasia (especially on the left) with pain in the left leg, which tired easily and which she favoured. Subsequent surgery of the hip joint by bilateral intertrochanteric osteotomy with re-alignment. Patient now free of pain.

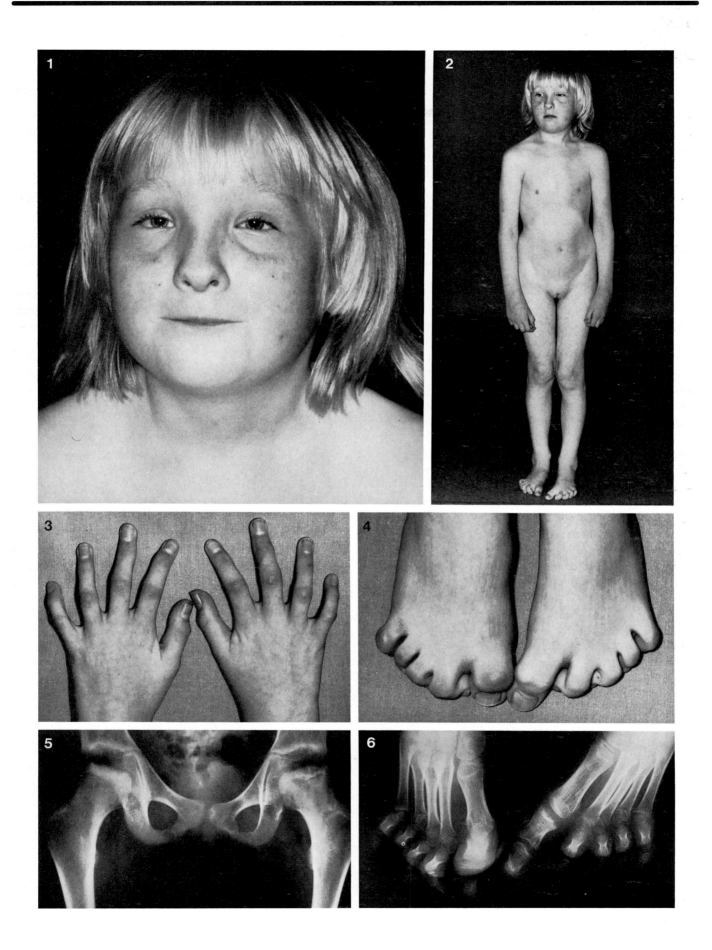

290

Lowe Syndrome
(Oculo-Cerebro-Renal Syndrome)

J.K.

An X-linked recessive syndrome with congenital cataract, muscular hypotonia, areflexia, severe psychomotor retardation, tubular proteinuria, and amino-aciduria.

Main signs:
- Male patients. Bilateral central cataracts, occasionally with glaucoma, buphthalmos, corneal clouding, enophthalmos.
- Severe progressive psychomotor retardation; disturbance of growth; high shrill cry. Growth retardation after the first year of life.
- Muscular hypotonia, areflexia; myopathic electromyogram.
- Tubular proteinuria, amino-aciduria.

Supplementary findings: Prominent forehead, thin hair, pale skin. Adiposity in the first year of life, later wasting. Cryptorchidism. Hyperphosphaturia with hypophosphataemic rickets; metabolic acidosis, intermittent glycosuria. Often constant low-grade fever. Elevated creatine kinase values. Peripheral neuropathy, central demyelination.

Manifestation: Eye signs and muscular hypotonia at birth. Later, distinct motor and intellectual deterioration.

Aetiology: X-linked recessive disorder. Female carriers may show cataracts or corneal clouding on slit-lamp examination. Gene locus: Xq25-q26.1. Prenatal diagnosis by restriction fragment length polymorphism.

Frequency: More than 100 patients have been described.

Course, prognosis: Most patients die in childhood, in the first decade of life. Few attain adulthood, severely handicapped. Mean IQ is 40–54, with 25% over 70.

Treatment: Correction of eye anomalies, acidosis, hypophosphataemia and rickets. Alkalinizing therapy. Substitution therapy with potassium, phosphate, calcium or carnitine.

Differential diagnosis: Zellweger cerebrohepatorenal syndrome (291).

Illustrations:
1 A 6-year-old boy; enophthalmos on the left, corneal clouding on the right.
2 A 17-year-old; bilateral corneal clouding.

References:

Abassi V, Lowe C U, Calcagno P L: Oculo-cerebro-renal syndrome. A review. *Am J Dis Child* 1968, 115:145.

Pallisgaard G, Goldschmidt E: The oculo-cerebro-renal sydrome of Lowe in four generations of one family. *Acta Paediatr Scand* 1971, 60:146–148.

Gardner R J M, Brown N: Lowe's syndrome: identification of carriers by lens examination. *J Med Genet* 1976, 13:449–454.

Hanefeld F, Stephani U, Lennert T et al: Congenitale Myopathie bei Kindern mit Lowe-Syndrom. In: *Fortschritte der Myologie* 1981, VI:63–66. Deutsche Gesellschaft für 'Bekämpfung der Muskelkrankheiten e.V', Freiburg, Germany.

Tripathi R C, Cibis G W, Harris D J et al: Lowe's syndrome. Birth Defects, *Orig Art Ser* 1982, 18(6):629–644.

Kownatzki R: Das okulo-zerebro-renale Syndrom (Lowe-Syndrom). *Pädiat Prax* 1985/68, 32:511–519.

Hodgson S V, Heckmatt J Z, Hughes E et al: A balanced de novo X/autosome translocation in a girl with manifestations of Lowe syndrome. *Am J Med Genet* 1986, 23:837–847.

Charnas L, Bernar J et al: MRI findings and peripheral neuropathy in Lowe's syndrome. *Neuropediatrics* 1988, 19:7–9.

Gazit E., Brand N et al: Prenatal diagnosis of Lowe's syndrome: a case report with evidence of de novo mutation. *Prenat Diagn* 1990, 10:257–260.

Mueller O T, Hartsfield J K Jr et al: Lowe oculocerebrorenal syndrome in a female with a balanced X,20 translocation: mapping of the X chromosome breakpoint. *Am J Hum Genet* 1991, 49:804–810.

Charnas L R, Bernardini I et al: Clinical and laboratory findings in the oculocerebrorenal syndrome of Lowe, with special reference to growth and renal function. *N Engl J Med* 1991, 324:1318–1325.

Kenworthy L, Park T, Charnas L R: Cognitive and behavioral profile of the oculocerebrorenal syndrome of Lowe. *Am J Med Genet* 1993, 46:297–303.

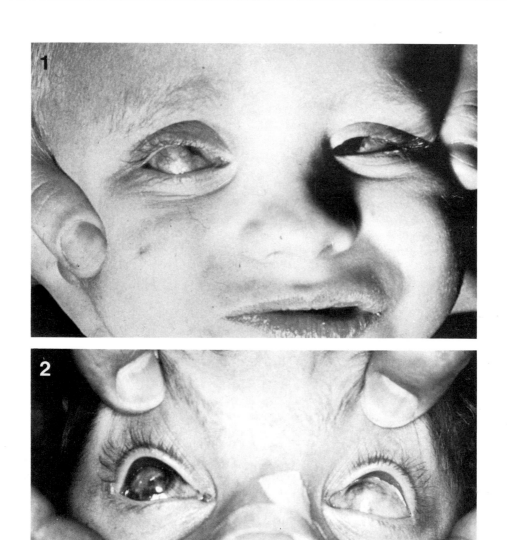

An autosomal recessive, peroxisomal metabolic-dysplasia syndrome with characteristic facies, extreme muscular hypotonia, hepatomegaly, practically absent psychomotor development and usually early death.

Main signs:

- Characteristic facies with high forehead, increased interocular distance, flat nasal bridge, possible slight mongoloid slant of the palpebral fissures and epicanthi, anteverted nares, dysplastic ears, 'full' cheeks and micrognathia. Wide-open fontanelles and cranial sutures, persistent frontal suture; high palate (**1, 3**).
- Extreme muscular hypotonia (**4**) with absence of deep-tendon reflexes and weak sucking and swallowing reflexes. Central nervous system seizures.
- Minimal psychomotor development. Deafness.
- Hepatomegaly (fibrosis, cirrhosis), occasionally also splenomegaly, liver function disorders, gastro-intestinal bleeding.
- Retarded growth.
- Absent or severely reduced peroxisomes.

Supplementary findings: Corneal clouding, glaucoma, cataract, nystagmus, pallor of the optic discs, retinal changes.

Cubitus valgus, contractures of the finger joints, simian crease; club feet, clitoral hypertrophy or cryptorchidism, hypospadias.

Renal cortical cysts, albuminuria, amino-aciduria.

Cardiovascular anomalies.

Punctate calcifications of the skeleton (**2**), similar to those in chondrodysplasia punctata (*123–125*).

Anomalies of the central nervous system. Neuronal migration defects, malformations of the cerebral cortex.

Frequently, elevated serum iron and copper levels, siderosis of the reticulo-endothelial system. Elevated serum levels of long-chain fatty acids and of pipecolic and other acids and further abnormal biochemical characteristics (depressed plasmalogen, signs of adrenal insufficiency).

Manifestation: At birth (hepatomegaly usually later).

Aetiology: Autosomal recessive disorder; peroxisomal enzyme defect ('peroxisomopathy'). Prenatal diagnosis by detection of long-chain fatty acids.

Frequency: Not so very low: over 200 patients since the first patient was described in 1964. Estimated at 1:50000 newborns.

Course, prognosis: Death usually within the first 6 months of life. (Apparently, elevated serum iron levels and siderosis of the reticulo-endothelial system are more likely to show in younger patients, whereas fibrosis and cirrhosis of the liver are found primarily in somewhat older patients.) Occurrence also of a milder variant.

Treatment: Treatment by diet still in the experimental stage but initial success has been recorded.

Transplantation of bone marrow, kidneys, liver.

Genetic counselling; prenatal diagnosis possible.

Illustrations:

1–4 A female patient, death at age 6 months. Serum iron levels markedly elevated on several occasions in the first months of life; on follow-up at age 6 months, normal. The initially markedly elevated transaminases also showed a tendency to decrease with increasing age. Hypoprothrombinaemia, no icterus. Central nervous system seizures. No psychomotor development.

At autopsy: arrhinencephaly, moderate hydrocephaly; liver fibrosis; renal cortical cysts.

References:

Bleeker-Wagemaker E M, Oorthuys J W E *et al*: Long term survival of a patient with the cerebro-hepato-renal... syndrome. *Clin Genet* 1986, 29:160–164.

Wilson G N, Holmes R G *et al*: Zellweger syndrome: diagnostic assays, syndrome delineation, and potential therapy. *Am J Med Genet* 1986, 24:69–82.

Zellweger H: The cerebro-hepato-renal... syndrome... *Dev Med Child Neurol* 1987, 29:821–829.

Stephenson J B P: Inherited peroxisomal disorders involving the nervous system. *Arch Dis Child* 1988, 63:767–770.

Wilson G N, Holmes R D *et al*: Peroxisomal disorders... *Am J Med Genet* 1988, 30:771–792.

Wanders R J A, Schutgens R B H *et al*: Prenatal diagnosis of inborn errors in peroxisomal β-oxidation. *Prenat Diagn* 1991, 11:25–261.

Theil A C, Schutgens R B H *et al*: Clinical recognition of patients affected by a peroxisomal disorder: a retrospective study in 40 patients. *Eur J Pediatr* 1992, 151:117–120.

Brown F R, Voigt R, Singh A K, Singh I: Peroxisomal disorders. Neurodevelopmental and biochemical aspects. *AJDC* 1993, 147:617–626.

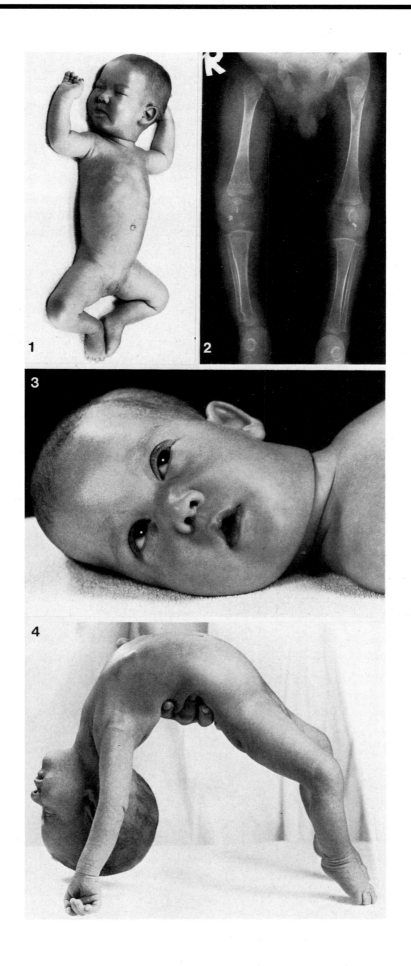

Glycanosis Carbohydrate-Deficient Glycoprotein

(Carbohydrate-Deficient Glycoprotein Syndrome, CDG Syndrome; Disialotransferrin-Developmental Deficiency Syndrome, DDD Syndrome)

J.K.

A metabolic dysmorphic syndrome resulting from defective glycoprotein metabolism with encephalopathy, hepatopathy, enteropathy, endocrinopathy, cardiopathy, nephropathy and metabolic disorders.

Main signs:
• Age-dependent signs, progressive, can be divided into four stages:

I. Infantile multi-system stage: Failure to thrive from birth, muscular hypotonia, growth retardation, severely delayed development and the following alarming, episodically occurring multi-organ system signs: liver insufficiency, pericardial effusions, cardiac tamponades and stupors or epileptoid attacks.

Phenotypically unusual fat-pads formed above and to the side of the gluteal region: many patients have a thick, pasty skin (like 'tallow, orange peel'), especially on the legs. Some develop lipotrophic striation of the skin. Noticeable facial characteristics are a high nasal bridge, prominent jaw, large ears, restricted movement of the joints of the lower extremities. Inversion of the nipples in nearly 100%. Mild hepatomegaly with elevated transaminase.

Onset of dystrophy from the sixth month of life, simultaneous reduction in length and weight (from the second to third year of life, below the third percentile). Secondary microcephaly in some cases. Parallel onset of delayed development from the fourth to fifth month. Tendon reflexes no longer detectable from the 2nd/3rd year. In isolated cases, pericardial effusions, neonatal cerebral haemorrhage, subcutaneous bleeding.

Increased mortality in infancy and early childhood in 15–20%.

II. Stage of ataxia and mental retardation (3–10 years): IQ around 50–60, no further regression. Abnormal gait; few patients learn to walk but the performance of precise movements improves: ataxia, impaired sense of balance, dyskinesia. Loss of tendon reflexes, peripheral neuropathy, strabismus with abduction disorder. Retinitis pigmentosa (progressive). Signs of seizure during and after acute infections from the fourth to fifth year of life, associated with comatose or stuporous conditions; in some patients, hemiplegia. Recovery can take several hours or several days. Temporary blindness has also been reported.

III. Teenage stage: atrophy of the legs: Extrovert behaviour, happiness. Now distinct short stature, additional kyphosis, scoliosis, pectus carinatum. Renewed development of fat-pads and lipotrophic striae. Generalized muscular hypotonia, progressive atrophy of the lower motor neurons with involvement of the legs, cerebellar ataxia and impaired co-ordination.

IV. Adult stage: hypogonadism: Premature ageing, neurologically stable, constricted thorax with disproportionately long arms and legs. Eventual height 130–140 cm. Testicular atrophy, hypergonadotropic hypogonadism in females. In some patients, normal puberty and sexual characteristics.

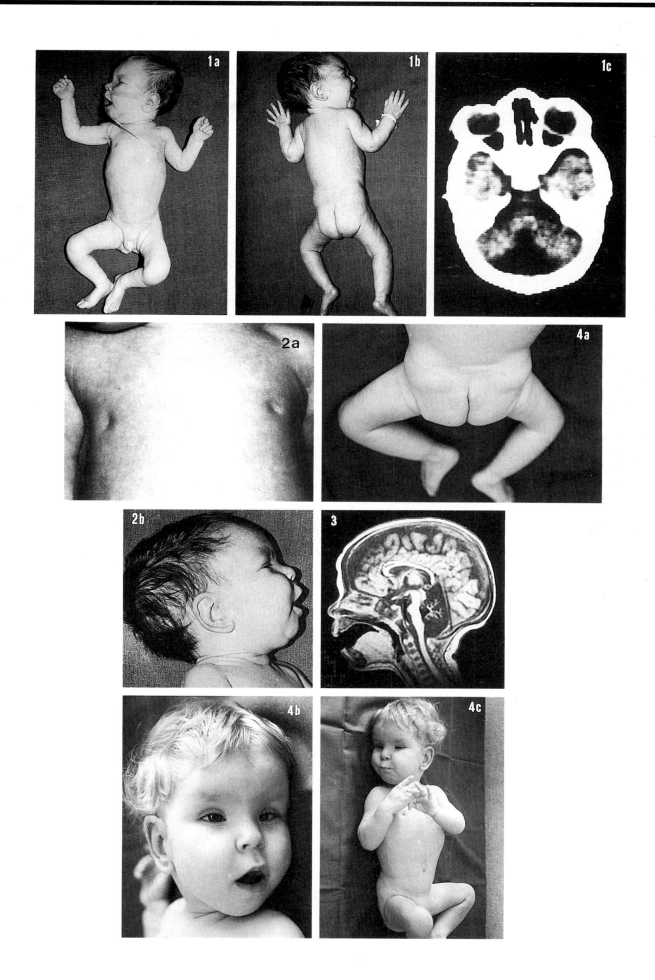

J.K.

Supplementary findings: Detection of a secretory glyco-protein that is partially deficient in carbohydrate and particularly deficient in serum transferrin. Tubular protein-uria, slightly elevated transaminases, significantly depressed total cholesterol, normalization in infancy.

Hypobetalipoproteinaemia. Depressed serum albumin.

Fatty liver and granular/lamellar lysosomal inclusion bodies.

Cerebrospinal fluid protein slightly elevated. Delayed nerve conduction velocity after the first year of life. Cerebellar atrophy as in olivopontocerebellar atrophy.

Elevated excretion of prolactin, growth hormone, insulin and follicle stimulating hormone; luteotropic hormone normal. Thyroxin-binding globulin depressed in 75% of patients.

Manifestation: Between the third and fifth months of life.

Aetiology: Autosomal recessive inheritance.

Pathogenesis: Multisystemic clinical picture resulting from systemic disturbance of the glycosylation of macromolecules. Only the carbohydrate (glycan) components of various soluble glycoproteins are affected. The disturbance relates to a step in the synthesis of the branched (N) glycans of the complex type.

Frequency: Nearly 50 patients known. Approximately 1:40 000–60 000.

Course, prognosis: Death in late infancy and early childhood 15–20%. The oldest surviving patient is 48 years old. For later course see stages I–IV. Milder forms and monosymptomatic variants probably exist.

Treatment: Symptomatic. Prenatal diagnosis by determination of the ratio of total transferrin/carbohydrate-deficient isotransferrin.

Illustrations:
Previous page:
1a and b Age 3 months, supragluteal fat-pad.
1c Computerized tomography with cerebellar hypoplasia.
2a and b Patient 2 at age 3 months: Magnetic resonance imaging shows cerebellar hypoplasia.
4a–c Patient 2 at age 2 years: marked supragluteal pads, strabismus.
Opposite page:
5a–d Patient 3 at age 12 years and 1 month: strabismus, unable to stand without support, right nipple inverted, supra-umbilical (**5b and d**) median striate fatty atrophy.

References:
Jacken J, Stibler H, Hagberg B (eds): The carbohydrate-deficient glycoprotein syndrome. *Acta Paediatr Scand Suppl* 1991, **375**:5–71.
Heyne K, Weidinger S: Diagnostik und Nosologie der Glykanose CDG (Carbohydrate-deficient glycoprotein syndrome). *Monatsschr Kinderheilkd* 1992, **140**:822–827.
Heyne K, Weidinger S: Drei neue biochemische Marker bei Glykanose CDG (Carbohydrate-deficient glycoprotein syndrome). *Monatsschr Kinderheilkd* 1994, **142**:199–204.
Eyskens F, Centerick C *et al*: CDG-syndrome with previously unreported features. *Acta Paediatr* 1994, **83**:892–896.

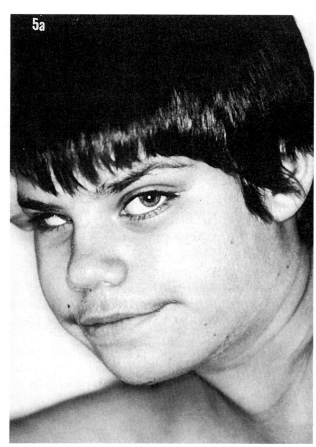

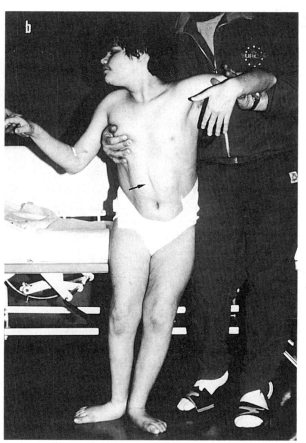

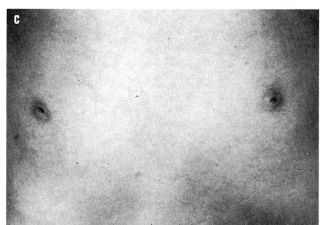

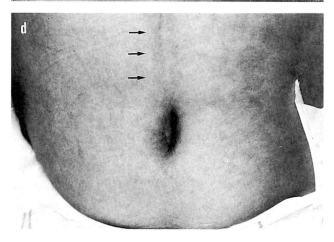

A characteristic picture with onset of progressive muscular atrophy in infancy, loss of deep-tendon reflexes and appearance of further signs of denervation with intelligence, sensorium, sensation and sphincter function remaining unaffected.

Main signs:
- Weakness and decreased movements, at first of the pelvic, then the leg muscles and finally also of the arm muscles. Lower extremities externally rotated, flaccid; upper extremities abducted, flaccid, 'handle' appearance. The diaphragm is not affected: paradoxical respiration (diaphragmatic breathing). Long, narrow, bell-shaped thorax. Little facial expression.
- Disappearance of tendon reflexes. Sensorium intact; absence of pain. Sensation, sphincter function and intelligence unaffected.
- Muscle fasciculation, predominantly of the tongue.

Supplementary findings: Contractures of the large joints, kyphoscoliosis, deformity of the thorax. Neurogenic atrophy pattern on electromyogram and muscle biopsy.

Manifestation: In some cases, the mother may note a lack or gradual decrease of foetal movements and the diagnosis can be established immediately after birth.

Aetiology: Autosomal recessive inheritance. Comprises 74% of all forms of infantile spinal muscular atrophy. Gene locus: chromosome 5p11.2-13.3.
Prenatal diagnosis with restriction fragment length polymorphism markers and highly polymorphic microsatellite markers (reliability of over 96%). Hypothesis: the three different forms are probably allelic mutations of the same gene.

Pathogenesis: Degeneration of the α-motor neurons in the anterior horn of the spinal cord, in part also of the bulbar cranial nerve nuclei.

Frequency: 1:10 000. Heterozygote frequency: 1:50.
Course, prognosis: Acute, progressive course, death by age 18 months. Absence of control over the head, inability to sit up or walk without assistance. Severe respiratory complications with hypostatic and aspiration pneumonia. Frequent bulbar signs. Cardiomyopathy, cardiac arrhythmia. Occasionally arthrogryposis.

Differential diagnosis: SMA type II = intermediate chronic form (like I but onset between the third and 24th month of life, bulbar signs less frequent, positive control over the head, life expectancy 15 years); and type III SMA (Kugelberg–Welander) slowly progressive, chronic form (like I, but onset between 2 and 20 years of age, fasciculation of the tongue less frequent, fasciculation of other muscles, bulbar signs infrequent, ability to sit up and walk unassisted, life expectancy into the sixth decade).

Treatment: Symptomatic: care by a physiotherapist; prevention of contractures. High-protein diet; prevention of obesity. Antibiotic protection in the event of respiratory infections. Intellectual stimulation. Psychological support.

Illustrations:
1–3 Patient 1, almost 4 months old: at 4 weeks, rapidly progressive muscle weakness and paralysis noted. Exclusively diaphragmatic respiration; thorax deformity. Contractures of the knee and hip joints. Generalized areflexia. Complete reaction of degeneration. Little facial expression. Mental development normal. Soon thereafter, death from respiratory paralysis. Diagnosis confirmed histopathologically. A similarly affected sibling died at age 2 months.
4 and 5 Patient 2 at 8 years and almost 11 years. Diagnosed clinically and by muscle biopsy in infancy. With optimal care, survival of multiple episodes of pneumonia. Extreme muscle atrophy, pectus excavatum, kyphoscoliosis, joint contractures; absolutely no head control; little facial expression; intellectual responses normal for age. Signs of denervation. Puffy deformity of the tongue with marked fasciculations.

References:
Zerres K, Rudnik-Schöneborn S, Röhrig D, Wirth B: Spinale Muskelatrophien des Kindesalters, *Monatsschr Kinderheilkd* 1993, **141**:848–854.
Heber U, Müller C R: Indirekte molekulargenetische Familienuntersuchung und Pränataldiagnostik bei kindlichen spinalen Muskelatrophien (SMA). *Klin Pädiatr* 1994, **206**:30–35.

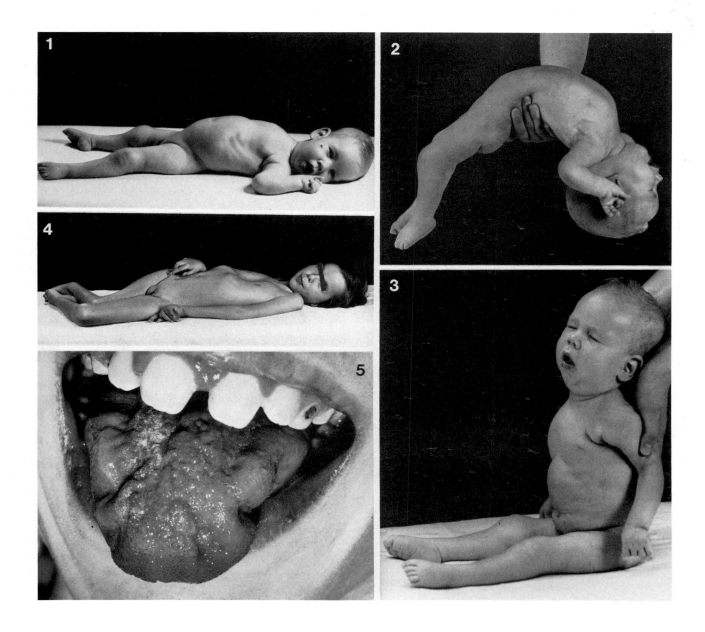

J.K./ H.-R.W

A characteristic hereditary syndrome in males, with onset in childhood of 'ascending' muscle atrophy beginning in the pelvis and thigh regions, at first obscured by fatty infiltration and associated with a corresponding progressive decrease in performance (with simultaneous slowing of mental development in approximately one-third of patients).

Main signs:
- After learning to walk, often poorly and with delay (with frequent falling), development of a rocking, weaving or waddling gait. Rapid fatigue when climbing stairs (possibly accomplished 'on all fours'); difficulty getting up from the floor, eventually 'climbing up himself' (Gower's sign; **1**).
- Hyperlordosis with protruding abdomen (**1c, 3**). Broad-based stance (**1–3**). Prominent, 'loose' shoulders (**2 and 3a**).
- Pseudohypertrophy (fatty infiltration) especially of the calves, also of the thigh and buttock musculature (**1–3**), less frequently of other muscle regions.
- Ascending degeneration of the musculature starting at the pelvic girdle and thighs, clinically involving the rest of the trunk, then the shoulder girdle, upper arm and other regions. Tendency for contractures to develop, especially in the legs: relatively early tendency to develop talipes equinus and toe-walking.
- Mental retardation in approximately 30% of the children (IQ = 70–85). Dyslexia especially noticeable. No progression.

Supplementary findings: Absence of pain, disordered sensation or denervation phenomena. Gradual weakening and eventual loss of tendon reflexes. Myocardial involvement frequently demonstrable on electrocardiogram.

Short stature. Frequent development of scoliosis; coxa valga. Secondary obesity not unusual.

Markedly increased serum creatine kinase activity (also of some other enzyme activities to a lesser degree), especially in the initial stages of the process. Absence of dystrophin can be shown immunohistologically.

Manifestation: Between 3 and 5 years of age.

Aetiology: X-linked recessive disorder; 65% of patients with Duchenne- and Becker-type muscular dystrophy show deletion mutations; 5–10% show duplications or insertions in the dystrophin gene. Duchenne and Becker are allelic. The gene product, dystrophin is deficient; in Duchenne patients, it is almost completely absent, in Becker patients it is synthesized in reduced quantities or in a modified form. Direct genetic diagnosis. New mutations in approximately one-third of patients. Genetic defect in the short arm of the X chromosome (Xp21.2).

Frequency: Not so very low (at least 1 in 4000 male newborns).

Course, prognosis: Relentless progression. Dependence (wheelchair) usually around the end of the first decade of life, and death in the course of the second (pneumonias).

Differential diagnosis: Becker-type progressive muscular dystrophy, which has its onset in late infancy with primary involvement of the pelvic musculature, slow progression; life expectancy 30–55 years.

Treatment: Maximum possible improvement and conservation of physical mobility. Physiotherapy, swimming, prevention of contractures, avoidance of any unnecessary bed confinement or inactivity; use of a breathing mask at home (vital capacity less than 1000), surgery to stabilize the vertebral column. Gene therapy may be possible. Intellectual stimulation and promotion of social contact. Psychological support.

Identification of female carriers is possible by enzyme level determination (60% show elevated creative kinase levels) and more recently also by direct or indirect demonstration of the deletion. Prenatal diagnosis for such a 'carrier' during pregnancy. New mutations (mother not a carrier) have an estimated recurrence risk of 10%, based on the germ-cell mosaic.

Illustrations:

1–3 Three typically affected patients, aged 6 years, 7 years and 6 months and 8 years, showing pseudohypertrophy, Gower's sign (**1**), hyperlordosis, winging of the scapulae, waddling gait, inability to climb stairs. Mental retardation in two of the boys.

References:

Hejtmancik J F, Harris S G et al: Carrier diagnosis of Duchenne muscular dystrophy using restriction fragment length polymorphisms. *Neurology* 1986, **36**:1553–1562.
Darras B T, Harper J F et al: Prenatal diagnosis and detection of carriers with DNA probes in Duchenne's muscular dystrophy. *N Engl J Med* 1987, **316**:985–992.
Hyser C L, Doherty R A et al: Carrier assessment for mothers and sisters of isolated Duchenne dystrophy cases: the importance of serum enzyme determinations. *Neurology* 1987, **37**:1476–1480.
Gutman D H, Fischbeck K H: Molecular biology of Duchenne and Becker's muscular dystrophy: clinical applications. *Ann Neurol* 1989, **26**:189–194.
Nudel V et al: Duchenne muscular dystrophy gene product is not identical in muscle and brain. *Nature* 1989, **337**:76–78.
Darras B T: Molecular genetics of Duchenne and Becker muscular dystrophy. *J Pediatr* 1990, **117**:1–15.
Janka M, Grimm T: Bedeutung des Keimzellmosaiks für die genetische Beratung von Familien mit Muskeldystrophie Duchenne und Becker. *Klin Pädiatr* 1991, **203**:354–358.
Engel A G: Gene therapy for Duchenne dystrophy (Editorial). *Ann Neurol* 1993, **34**:3–4.

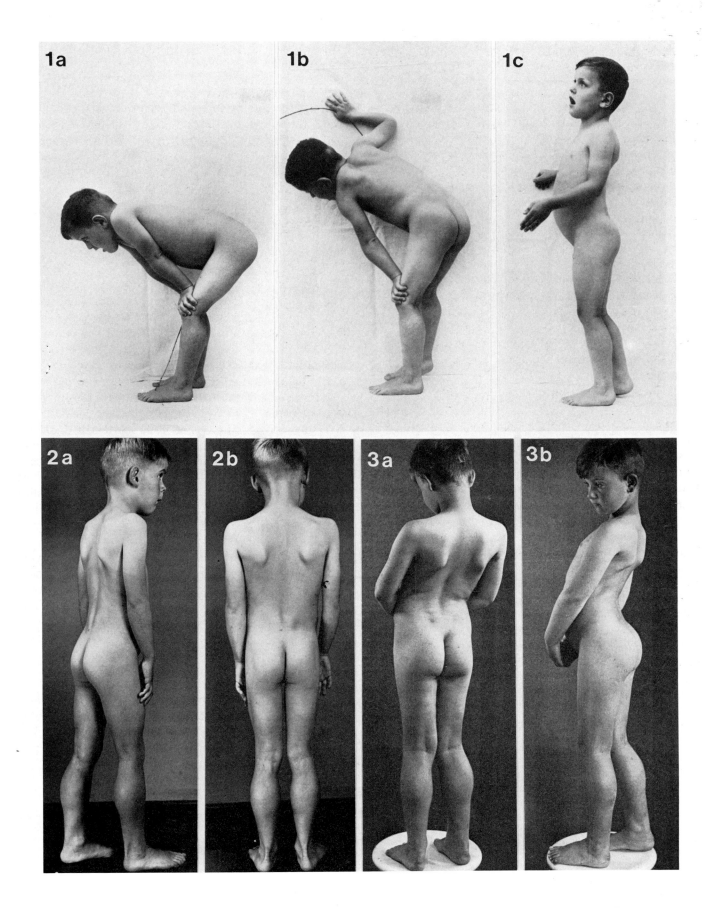

295 Progressive Diaphyseal Dysplasia
(Camurati–Engelmann Syndrome)

H.-R.W

Hereditary systemic hyperostosis and sclerosis of the diaphyses of the long tubular bones and of the cranium, associated with myopathy of the skeletal musculature.

Main signs:
- Waddling or dragging gait and rapid fatigability especially of the lower extremities; also complaints of limb pain after exertion.
- Unusual proportions with relatively short trunk and over-long, very slender extremities (thin muscles, little subcutaneous fat) (1).
- Radiologically, widening and densification of the diaphyses of the long bones (4–8) caused by endosteal and periosteal proliferation; also sclerosis of the skull (2 and 3), base greater than calvaria.

Supplementary findings: Neurologically unremarkable as a rule.

Slight (usually transitory) short stature in childhood; occipital and frontal bossing (1) and mild exophthalmos possible. Genu varum or valgum in some patients.

Delayed sexual maturity not unusual.

On biopsy and electron microscopy, atrophy of the muscle fibres and other signs; laboratory analysis may reveal increases in serum alkaline phosphatase and excretion of hydroxyproline in the urine, together with anaemia and reduced levels of muscle carnitine.

Manifestation: Very often in early childhood but variable. Not infrequently, delay in learning to walk without support; then abnormal gait and general failure to thrive. Later, variable decrease in general vitality, with possible spontaneous remission in this respect during or after adolescence.

Mild cases of this syndrome may be recognized only from an incidental finding on radiograph.

Aetiology: Autosomal dominant disorder; often distinct intrafamilial differences in expression. High proportion of new mutations.

Frequency: Low: approximately 150 patients described in the literature.

Prognosis: Life expectancy not affected. Late complications caused by cranial nerve compression (impaired sight or hearing, facial paralysis) relatively infrequent.

Treatment: Adequate orthopaedic follow-up and treatment as indicated. Definite improvement has been repeatedly observed with long-term, low-dose corticosteroid treatment.

Genetic counselling.

Illustrations:
1 An 11-year-old boy.
2, 4–7 His radiographs.
3 Skull radiograph of the same patient at age 32 years; later optic nerve damage in the optic canal.
8 and 9 Progression of the changes at 15 and 21 years.

References:

Wiedemann H R: Systematisierte sklerotische Hyperostose des Kindesalters mit Myopathie. *Z Kinderheilk* 1948, **65**:346.

Hansen H G: Progressive diaphysäre Dysplasie. *Handbuch der Kinderheilkunde* 1967, 6:356.

Spranger J W, Langer L O Jr, Wiedemann H R: Bone dysplasias. *An atlas of constitutional disorders of skeletal development*. Stuttgart and Philadelphia: G Fischer and W B Saunders 1974.

Kuhlencordt F, Kruse H P, Hellner K A *et al*: Diaphysäre Dysplasie (Camurati-Engelmann-Syndrom) mit fortschreitendem Visusverlust. *Dtsch Med Wschr* 1981, **106**:617.

Sheldon J, Reeve J, Clayton B: Engelmann's disease (progressive diaphysial dysplasia). A review and presentation of two cases with abnormal phosphate retention. *Metab Bone Dis Rel Res* 1981, 2:307.

Naveh Y, Kaftori J K *et al*: Progressive diaphyseal dysplasia... *Pediatrics* 1984, 74:399–405.

Naveh Y, Alon U *et al*: Progressive diaphyseal dysplasia: evaluation of corticosteroid therapy. *Pediatrics* 1985, 75:321–323.

Naveh Y, Ludatshcer *et al*: Muscle involvement in progressive diaphyseal dysplasia. *Pediatrics* 1985, **76**:944–949.

Bosselmann E, Dietzmann K Braun, H S: Myopathische Veränderungen bei der diaphysären Dysplasie Camurati-Engelmann. *Beitr Orthop Traumatol* 1987, **34**:316–321.

Bye A M E, Hodson E, Kewley G, Kozlowski K: Progressive diaphyseal dysplasia and a low muscle carnitine. *Pediatr Radiol* 1988, **18**:340.

Ghosal S P, Mukherjee A K *et al*: Diaphyseal dysplasia associated with anemia. *J Pediatr* 1988, **113**:49–57.

Gorlin R J: Craniotubular bone disorders. *Pediatr Radiol* 1994, 24:392–406.

Voit T: Personal communications. 1994.

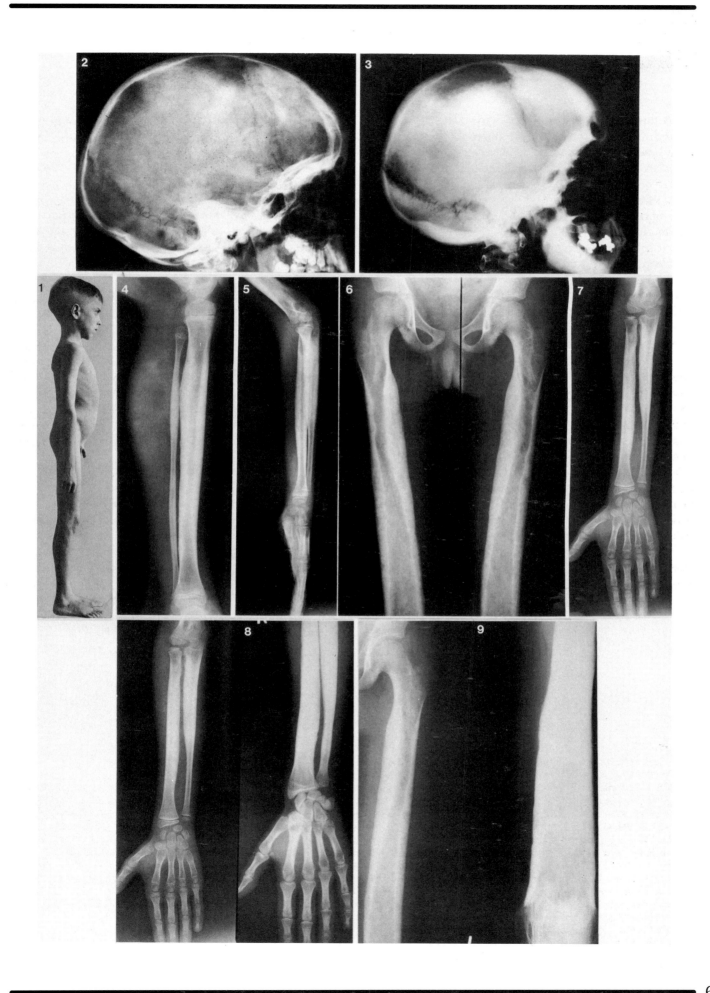

H.-R.W

An X-linked recessive disorder in males who show a cerebral disorder with dystonia, choreo-athetosis, mental retardation and a marked tendency to self-mutilation, associated with hyperuricaemia (and its typical sequelae).

Main signs:
- Cerebral disorder manifest as spastic paralysis, choreoathetoid hyperkinesia with severe dysarthria (if not anarthria) and severe mental defect (1).
- Pathognomonic bizarre, aggressive behaviour with frenzied biting and scratching especially in the form of self-mutilation (biting through or picking apart the lips [2 and 3], fingers and toes, scratching the eyelids, and so on until severely damaged).
- Development of signs of gout (with hyperuricaemia, haematuria, crystalluria, urolithiasis, progressive nephropathy and, usually not until much later, tophi and recurrent attacks of acute arthritis).

Supplementary findings: Short stature.
Macrocytic anaemia, usually of moderate severity, is a common finding.

Manifestation: First year of life onwards. (Initial generalized hypotonia developing into generalized spasticity. Mental retardation. Failure to thrive. Choreo-athetosis from the second year of life and from the third year, aggressive tendencies with frenzied biting, scratching and self-mutilation.)

Aetiology: X-linked recessive disorder with variable expression. Thus, exclusively males affected (absence of the enzyme hypoxanthine-guanine phosphoribosyltransferase, with corresponding effects on purine synthesis and purine base catabolism). Gene localized on the long arm of the X chromosome (Xq26-27.2).

Frequency: Approximately 1:100 000.

Course, prognosis: Patients at risk of renal involvement and nutritional problems as a result of choreo-athetoid dysphagia and frequent vomiting. Before the introduction of allopurinol therapy, patients rarely survived beyond the fifth year of life.

Diagnosis: In exceptional patients, mental deficiency and aggressive tendencies may be absent.

Treatment: Allopurinol on a long-term basis is very effective in the treatment of hyperuricaemia and all of its direct (gouty) consequences. However, it can neither prevent nor mitigate the cerebral disorder. Protection from automutilation as far as possible. Genetic counselling. Identification of heterozygotes possible. Prenatal diagnosis.

Illustrations:
1–3 A boy aged 2 years and 3 months, his parents' first child, with the typical clinical picture. Diagnosis, (heterozygosity in his mother), confirmed by determination of the rate of 14C-hypoxanthine incorporation. In the second pregnancy, prenatal recognition of a male foetus as affected; confirmation of the diagnosis after interruption of the pregnancy. The third pregnancy, again with a male foetus, resulted in the birth of a healthy child after prenatal exclusion of the disorder.

References:
Leiber B, Olbrich G: Lesch-Nyhan-Syndrom. *Mschr Kinderheilk* 1973, **121**:42.
Letts R M, Hobson D A: Special devices as aids in the management of child selfmutilation in the Lesch-Nyhan syndrome. *Pediatrics* 1975, **55**:852 .
Francke U, Felsenstein J, Gartler S M *et al*: The occurrence of new mutants in the... Lesch-Nyhan disease. *Am J Hum Genet* 1976, **28**:123.
Schneider W, Morgenstern E, Schindera I: Lesch-Nyhan-Syndrom ohne Selbstverstümmelungstendenz. *Dtsch Med Wschr* 1976, **101**:167.
Manzke H: Variable Expressivität der Genwirkung beim Lesch-Nyhan-Syndrom. *Dtsch Med Wschr* 1976, **101**:428.
Christie R, Bay C, Kaufman I A *et al*: Lesch-Nyhan disease: clinical experience with nineteen patients. *Dev Med Child Neurol* 1982, **24**:293.
Dempsey J L, Morley A A *et al*: Detection of the carrier state for... the Lesch-Nyhan syndrome... *Hum Genet* 1083, **64**:288–290.
Wilson J M, Young A B *et al*: Hypoxanthine-Guanine phosphoribosyltransferase deficiency. *N Engl J Med* 1983, **309**:900–910.
Gibbs D A, Crawfurd M *et al*: First-trimester diagnosis of Lesch-Nyhan syndrome. *Lancet* 1984, **II**:1180–1184.
Goldstein M, Anderson L T *et al*: Self-mutilation in Lesch-Nyhan disease is caused by dopaminergic denervation. *Lancet* 1985, **I**:338–339.
Mizuno T: Long-term follow-up of ten patients with Lesch-Nyhan syndrome. *Neuropediatrics* 1986, **17**:158–161.
Davidson B *et al*: Genetic basis... Lesch-Nyhan syndrome. *Hum Genet* 1988, **63**:331–336.
Davidson B. *et al*: Identification of 17 independent mutations responsible for... HPRT deficiency. *Am J Hum Genet* 1991, **48**:951–958.
Lightfoot T *et al*: The point mutation of... HRPT... *Hum Genet* 1992, **88**:695–696.
Tohyama J *et al*: Hypoxanthine-guanine phosphoribosyltransferase (HRPT) deficiency... *Hum Genet* 1994, **93**:175–181.

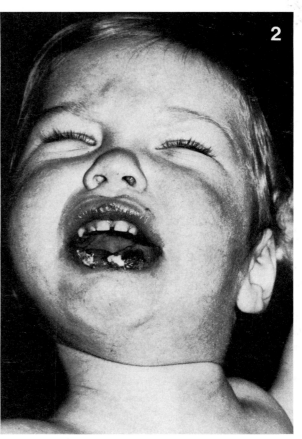

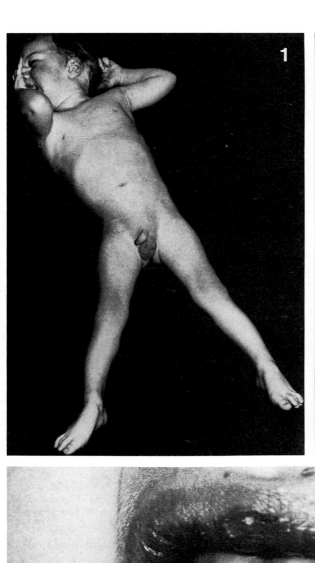

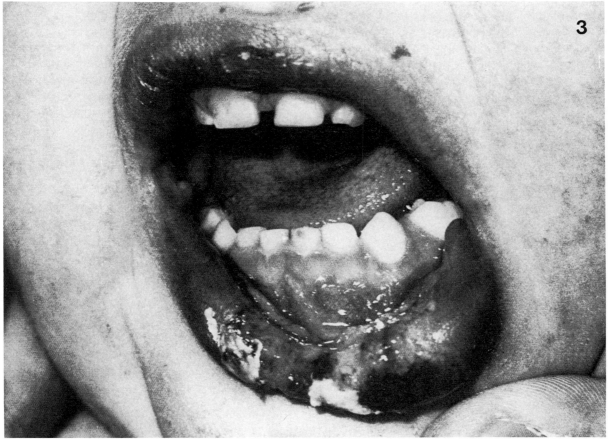

J.K./ H.-R.W

A characteristic hereditary syndrome with neurological, cutaneous and immunopathological signs.

Main signs:

- Progressive cerebellar ataxia, both at rest and with movement (beginning in early childhood) (1). Subsequent choreo-athetosis; later, dyssynergia and intention tremor. Deterioration of speech, disturbance of eye movements; flaccid, apathetic to mask-like facial expression (2) with slow development of a smile. Drooling. Stooped posture. Occasionally myoclonus.
Mental involvement beginning the end of the first decade in a proportion of patients, gradually increasing with age.
- Telangiectasia (from approximately the age of 3 years), at first mainly in areas of the bulbar conjunctiva that are exposed to light (3), later possibly on the lids, in a butterfly distribution on and alongside the nose, on the ears (4 and 5), palate, back of the neck, chest, elbows, knees and backs of the hands and feet. The vessels, which are initially delicate and attenuated, giving the impression in the eyes of mere conjunctival hyperaemia, become increasingly dilated and tortuous. Preferred areas are those most exposed to sunlight. Gradually, the ears become inelastic, the facial skin stretched and taut with loss of adipose tissue. Affected skin areas develop pigmentation disorders (areas of hyper- and depigmentation side by side) and become atrophic; patients show signs of seborrhoeic dermatitis. Also frequently café au lait spots. Progeroid changes: strands of grey hair, neurofibrillar structural anomalies and lipofuscin deposits in the brain. Premature onset of malignant changes such as basal cell carcinomas, uterine tumours.
- Immune deficiency (dysplasia of the thymolymphatic system), causing frequent or 'constant' signs of respiratory tract infections (sinobronchitis, frequently progressive bronchiectasis, pneumonias).

Supplementary findings: Short stature regularly present (usually first noted in the preschool child). Wasting. Later, disorders of sexual maturation and other endocrinological anomalies.
Possible lymphocytopenia. Serologically, deficiency primarily of IgA and IgE, also particularly of IgG_2 and IgG_4. Increased levels of α foetoprotein.
Chromosomal analysis shows an increased tendency to chromosome breakage; structural aberration of the long arm of chromosome 14 in 3–5% of cells.
Patients definitely have an increased risk of developing lymphoreticular malignancies (one-third of all affected individuals, the lymphoreticular system being involved in 80% of patients). Normal puberty. Severe fibrosis after exposure to radiation. Sterility caused by ovarian or testicular insufficiency.

Manifestation: Onset of ataxia from the beginning of the second year of life or later, appearance of telangiectases usually between the ages of 3 and 5 years; mental impairment, when present, often first apparent at an advanced stage of the disease.

Aetiology: Autosomal recessive disorder; heterogeneity. The pathogenetic relationships between the neurological disorder (primary cerebellar degeneration), the skin and mucous membrane changes and the immunological defect are still largely unexplained. Structural chromosome changes, in particular: 7p14, 7q35, 14q11, 14q32, 2p11, 22q11. Gene locus: 11p22-23.

Frequency: Between 1:30 000 and 1:100 000.

Course, prognosis: Progressive. Patients often confined to a wheelchair by the middle of the second decade of life and usually succumb to the sequelae of chronic pulmonary infections or of the neurological disorder itself or else to a malignancy before the end of the third decade. Heterozygotes are five times more likely to develop malignancies (breast, pancreas, liver); the risk of breast cancer is 6.8%. Nine per cent of all carcinomas of the breast in the USA are found in ataxia-telangiectasia patients, compared with a gene frequency of 1.4% (0.5–5%) for Louis–Bar.

Diagnosis: Unmistakable when telangiectases are present.

Treatment: Symptomatic. Particular benefit from conservative physiotherapy; timely antibiotic therapy for acute bacterial infections. Genetic counselling. Possibility of prenatal diagnosis.

Illustrations:
1–5 A 10-year-old girl, no longer able to stand alone. Completely unremarkable development until age 18 months then, onset of progressive ataxia. Telangiectases of the conjunctiva, eyelids, ears and upper arms. Mask-like, fixed, facial expression; frequent episodes of extrapyramidal dyskinesia, usually with torsion of the head to the right. Short stature, wasting, lymphocytopenia.

References:
Jaspers N G J, Bootsma D: Genetic heterogeneity in ataxia-teleangiectasia... *Proc Nat Acad Sci* 1982, 79:2641–2644.
Shaham M, Voss R, Becker Y *et al*: Prenatal diagnosis of ataxia teleangiectasia. *J Pediatr* 1982, 100:135.
Rosin M P, Ochs H D: In vivo chromosomal instability in ataxia-telangiectasia homozygotes and heterozygotes. *Hum Genet* 1986, 74:335–340.
Shiloh Y, Parshad R *et al*: Carrier detection in ataxia-teleangiectasia. *Lancet* 1986, I:689.
Leuzzi V, Antonelli A *et al*: Neurological and cytogenetic study in early onset ataxia-telangiectasia patients. *Eur J Pediatr* 1993, 152:609–612.

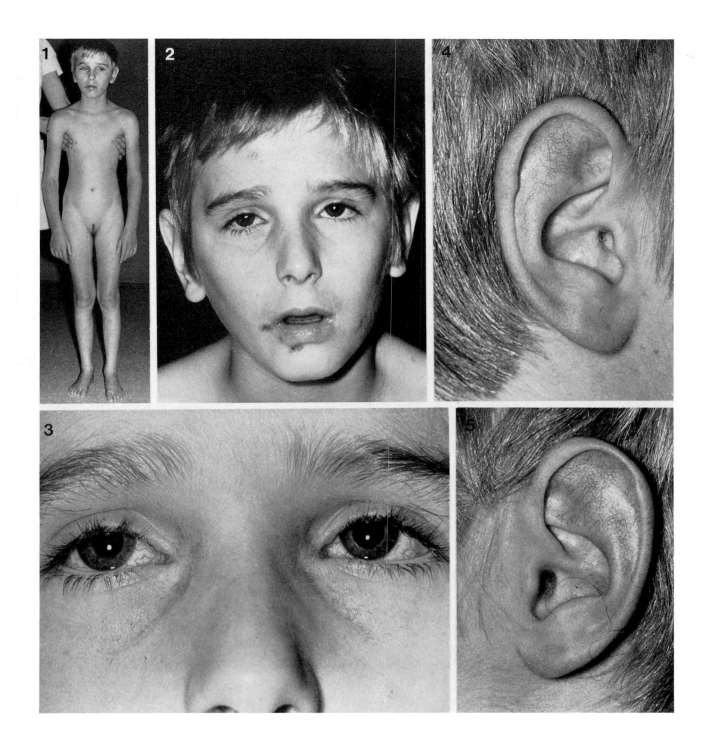

298 Marinesco–Sjögren Syndrome
(Cerebellolenticular Dystrophy with Mental Retardation)

H.-R.W

A syndrome of early manifest cataracts, mental retardation, ataxia myopathy and short stature.

Main signs:
- Spinocerebellar ataxia with a variable degree of motor impairment such as severe delay in and difficulty with walking.
- Primary mental retardation of variable grades of severity.
- 'Congenital' cataract.
- Myopathy (with elevated serum creatine kinase), muscular hypotonia and atrophy.
- Moderate growth deficiency.

Supplementary findings: Dysarthria, hypersalivation, strabismus, nystagmus; paralysis of the vertical conjugate gaze, ptosis.

Hypergonadotropic hypogonadism.

Possible development of scoliosis, pectus carinatum, pes planovalgus.

Computerized tomography: atrophy of the vermis and hemispheres of the cerebellum.

Manifestation: The first years of life.

Aetiology: Autosomal recessive disorder. Lysosomal storage disease?

Frequency: Low; approximately 80 patients described up to 1985.

Course, prognosis: Very dependent on the degree and progression of ataxia and on the severity of mental impairment.

Differential diagnosis: Other ataxia syndromes should be easy to differentiate, especially in view of the cataracts.

Treatment: Symptomatic. The ophthalmological care is especially important.

Genetic counselling.

Illustrations:

1–3 A 15-year-old girl, the second child of healthy parents with no known consanguinity. Cataract surgery in the first year of life. Primary mental retardation. Early manifest ataxia. Height 1.56 m. Strabismus, little change of facial expression. Micrognathia; genu valgum.

4–6 The 21-year-old sister of the proband, 1.60 m tall; similar development but not yet needing crutches. Both girls tend to be tearful.

References:

Andersen B: Marinesco-Sjögren syndrome: Spinocerebellar ataxia, congenital cataract, somatic and mental retardation. *Dev Med Child Neurol* 1965, 7:249.

Alter M, Kennedy W: The Marinesco-Sjögren syndrome. *Minn Med* 1968, 51:901.

Superneau D, Wertelecki W *et al*: The Marinesco-Sjögren syndrome described a quarter of a century before Marinesco. *Am J Med Genet* 1985, 22:647–648.

Walker P D, Blitzer M G *et al*: Marinesco-Sjögren syndrome: evidence for a lysosomal storage disorder. *Neurology* 1985, 35:415–419.

Superneau D W, Wertelecki W, Zellweger H, Bastian F: Myopathy in Marinesco-Sjögren syndrome. *Eur Neurol* 1987, 26:8–16.

Komiyama A, Nonaka I, Hirayama K: Muscle pathology in Marinesco-Sjögren syndrome. *J Neurol Sci* 1989, 89:103–113.

Tachi N, Nagata N, Wakai S, Chiba S: Congenital muscular dystrophy in Marinesco-Sjögren syndrome. *Pediatr Neurol* 1991, 7:296–298.

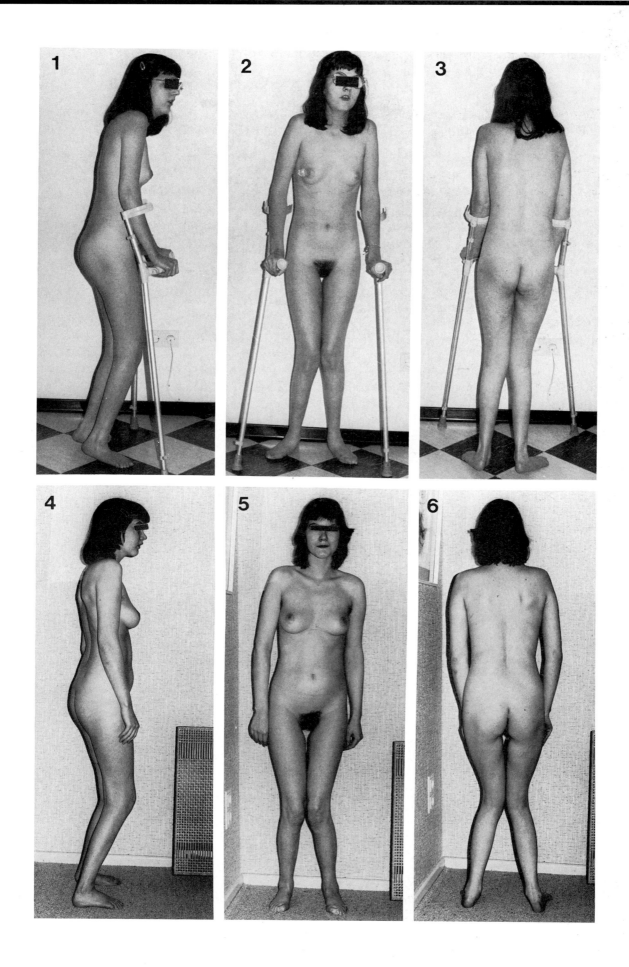

J.K.

Cardiac, intestinal, urogenital, central malformations of the foetus after inadequately controlled diabetes mellitus in the mother during foetal organogenesis.

Main signs:
There are no pathognomonic malformations. The spectrum of malformations is large and variable and includes:
- Congenital cardiac defects: transposition of the great vessels, ventricular septal defect, coarctation of the aorta, atrial septal defect, hypoplastic right heart, presence of only one umbilical artery.
- Hydronephrosis, renal agenesis, local anomalies, unilateral agenesis, bifid ureters, mega-ureter, megalovesica, multicystic kidneys.
- Duodenal atresias, anorectal atresias, small left colon syndrome.
- Caudal dysplasia (no regression) with absence of the sacrum, coccyx and several lumbar or thoracic vertebral bodies; anomalies of the ribs, club hands, femoral hypoplasia, possible unusual facies syndrome.
- Open neural tube defect, hydrocephalus (ten-fold increase in incidence compared with the normal population), anencephaly, holoprosencephaly (1%), mid-line cleft face syndrome.

Supplementary findings: Aplasia of the ears, atresia of the auditory canal, hairy ears. Cataract, coloboma of the iris, hypoplasia of the optic nerve. Cleft lip and palate. Occipital encephalocoele, gastro-intestinal malrotation, omphalocoele, gastroschisis, polysyndactyly, syndactyly, situs inversus. Frequent spontaneous abortions, still-births, premature births.

Manifestation: Prenatal and at birth.

Aetiology: Early teratogen exposure of a genetically predisposed foetus. In 0.3% of all pregnancies, the mother is diabetic. Malformations are up to seven times more frequent with uncontrolled diabetes mellitus in the first 10 weeks of pregnancy.

Pathogenesis: Maternal hyperglycemia as a key triggering factor. Vascular disruption is also possible. Insulin is not teratogenic because maternal insulin does not cross the placenta and the foetus produces insulin only after the eighth to 12th week of pregnancy. Gestational diabetes does not lead to embryopathy.

Course, prognosis: Up to 50% of children with embryopathy die. The deaths occur as a result of the malformations.

Diagnosis, differential diagnosis: Chromosomal disorders, holoprosencephalies (*24*). Femoral hypoplasia, unusual facies syndrome (*217*). Caudal dysplasia 'syndrome' (*168*), Currarino triad (*310*).

Treatment: Prevention of hyperglycemia and ketonemia in pregnant women, starting before conception. HbA1c levels around 7% or lower, blood sugar levels around 84 mg/dl. Weekly or fortnightly checks.

Illustrations:
1–4 Premature birth, 31st week of pregnancy, 1370g, club hands with radial aplasia, caudal dysplasia from L2. Arthrogryposis of the lower extremities. Anal atresia. Partial agenesis of the corpus callosum. Bilateral choanal atresia. Dystopia of the kidney(s). Microtia on the left side. Rectovestibular fistula.
5 Newborn child of a diabetic mother with hairy ear helix.

References:
Abnormal infants of diabetic mothers (Editorial). *Lancet* 1980, I:633–634.
Grix A Jr: Invited editorial comment: malformations in infants of diabetic mothers. *Am J Med Genet* 1982, **13**:131–137.
Fuhrmann K, Reiher H, Semmler K, Fischer F, Fischer M, Glöckner E: Prevention of congenital malformation in infants of insulin-dependent diabetic mothers. *Diabetes Care* 1983, **6**:219–223.
Dominick H C, Burkart W: Kinder diabetischer Mütter. *Monatsschr Kinderheilkd* 1984, **132**:886–892.
Diabetes in pregnancy (Editorial). *Lancet* 1965, I:961–962.
Sadler T W, Hunter E S, Balkan W, Horton W E Jr: Effects of maternal diabetes on embryogenesis. *Am J Perinat* 1988, **5**:319–326.
Mills J L, Knopp R H, Simpson J L *et al*: Lack of relation of increased malformation rates in infants of insulin-dependent diabetic mothers to glycemic control during organogenesis. *N Engl J Med* 1988, **318**:671–676.
Congenital abnormalities in infants of diabetic mothers. *Lancet* 1988, I:1313–1315.
Mills J L *et al*: Incidence of spontaneous abortion among normal women and insulin-dependent diabetic women whose pregnancies were identified within 21 days of conception. *N Engl J Med* 1988, **319**:1617–1623.
Pregnancy in diabetic women (Editorial). *N Engl J Med* 1988, **319**:1663–1665.
Becerra J E, Khoury M J, Cordero J F, Erickson J D: Diabetes mellitus during pregnancy and the risks for specific birth defects: a population-based case-control study. *Pediatrics* 1990 **85**:1–9.
Kalter H: Case reports of malformations associated with maternal diabetes: history and critique. *Clin Genet* 1993, **43**:174–179.
Martinez-Frias M L: Epidemiological analysis of outcomes of pregnancy in diabetic mothers: identification of the most characteristic and most congenital abnormalities. *Am J Med Genet* 1994, **51**:108–113.

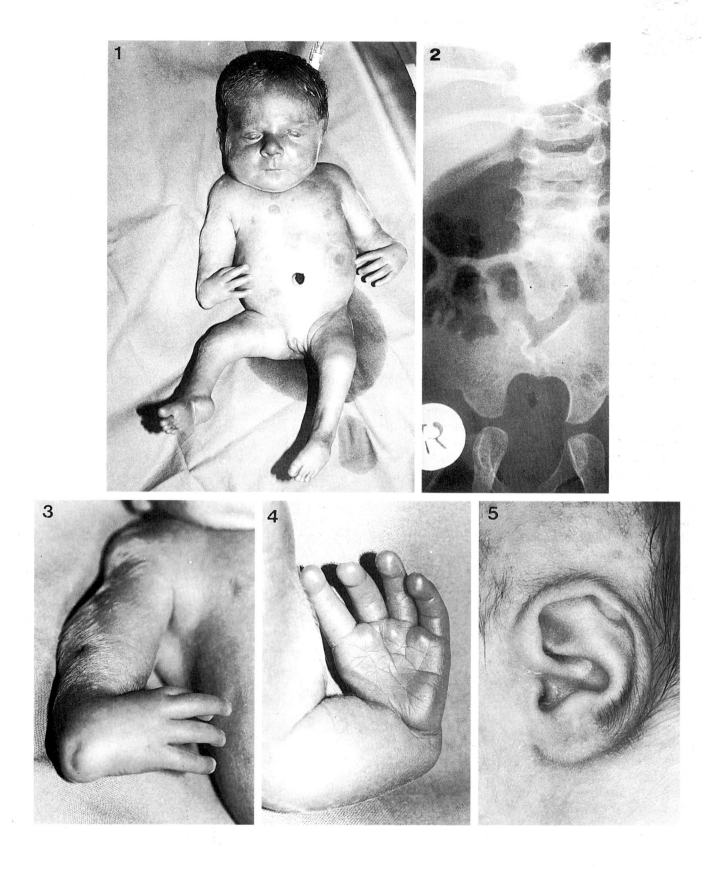

300 Rubella Embryofoetopathy

(Extended Gregg Syndrome)

J.K./ H.-R.W

A characteristic picture varying in extent, of embryonal or foetal damage caused by the rubella virus.

Mains signs:
- Syndrome of defects in older children (previously called Gregg syndrome) (1–3, 5–7, 9): Cataract, unilateral or bilateral, frequently with microphthalmos (and retinitis pigmentosa). Sensorineural hearing defect or deafness, unilateral or bilateral, frequently with signs of defective vestibular function.
- Microsomia, microcephaly (usually mild) in relation to linear growth and psychomotor retardation (mild to severe, with or without neurological signs).
- Cardiovascular anomalies: most frequently patent ductus arteriosus and pulmonary stenosis.
- Spectrum of disease and damage in newborns and infants (4, 8): Usually, small size at birth, failure to thrive and problems with early care.
- Cataract at birth or possibly manifest in the first weeks of life. Secondary glaucoma with corneal clouding may be present at birth or develop in subsequent weeks.
- Possible additional signs noted in 8: thrombocytopaenic purpura, hepatosplenomegaly, hepatitis, myocarditis, meningo-encephaloretinitis and so on.

Supplementary findings: Possible hypoplastic anaemia.
Radiograph evidence of metaphyseal lesions of the long bones during the first months of life.
Demonstration of rubella-specific IgM in the child's serum.
It is possible to show rubella virus in tissues, body fluid (especially cerebrospinal fluid) and excreta for months after birth.

Manifestation: At birth and in early infancy.

Aetiology: Infection of the embryo or foetus with rubella virus.

Frequency: Variable, depending on the virulence of the organism or on the extent to which young women have been immunized. In Germany, up to 200 patients per year can be anticipated.
Maternal rubella in the first trimester results in defects in all children (principally of the heart and auditory organ); maternal rubella in the ensuing period until the 16th week of pregnancy leads to defects in up to one-third of children (primarily hearing impairments).

Course, prognosis: Dependent on the type and extent of damage as well as on the intensity and quality of rehabilitation. Fatal outcome in the first months not infrequent.

Differential diagnosis: Microphthalmos, microcephaly, central nervous signs and deafness may also occur with embryofoetal cytomegalic virus infection or foetal toxoplasmosis; generally the signs of foetal rubella may resemble those of congenital infection from other, diverse pathogens. A hereditary syndrome of congenital cataract and cardiomyopathy should also be considered.

Treatment: Urgent treatment of glaucoma. Removal of cataracts generally after the sixth month of life. Operative correction of a cardiac defect as appropriate. Early application of hearing aids if hearing impairment present. Other appropriate handicap aids.
Prednisone recommended for thrombocytopaenic purpura and hypoplastic anaemia.
Prophylaxis: girls should be immunized against rubella at least twice during childhood.

Illustrations:
1, 7, 9 A 4-year-old patient; maternal rubella in the first and second months of pregnancy. Low birth weight, problems with early care; congenital cataracts and microphthalmos bilaterally; deafness; slight microcephaly, mental retardation, amblyopia and athetosis; short stature.
2 A 9-year-old patient; cataract, microphthalmos, mental retardation, patent ductus arteriosis, club foot, dysodontiasis.
3, 6 A 4-year-old patient; microphthalmos and cataract on the right, retinopathy on the left; sensorineural hearing defect (left greater than right); mild microcephaly, mental retardation, patent ductus arteriosis.
4 A 6-week-old patient; cataract, microphthalmos and corneal clouding bilaterally; patent ductus arteriosis and atrial septal defect; hepatosplenomegaly, icterus, anaemia, thrombocytopaenia; muscular hypotonia; prenatal dystrophy, maternal rubella in third to fourth months of pregnancy.
5 A 9-month-old patient; microcephaly, cataract, microphthalmos, amblyopia, cardiac defect, short stature.

References:
Miller E, Craddock-Watson J E et al: Consequences of confirmed maternal rubella at successive stages of pregnancy. Lancet 1982, II:781–784.
Daffos F, Forester F. et al: Prenatal diagnosis of congenital rubella. Lancet 1984, II:1–3.
Craddock-Watson J E, Anderson M J et al: Rubella reinfection and the fetus. Lancet 1985, I:1039.
Cruysberg J R M: Presumed congenital rubella syndrome: virus embryopathy or hereditary disease? Lancet 1988, I:529.
McIntosh E D et al: A fifty-year follow-up of congenital rubella. Lancet 1992, 340:414–415.

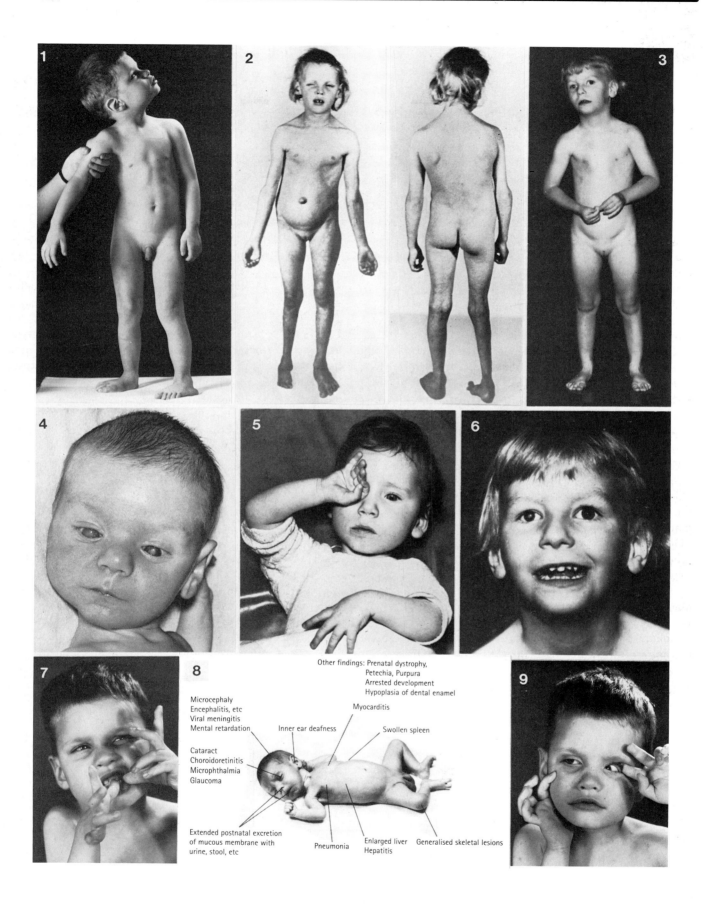

Other findings: Prenatal dystrophy,
Petechia, Purpura
Arrested development
Hypoplasia of dental enamel

Microcephaly
Encephalitis, etc
Viral meningitis
Mental retardation

Inner ear deafness

Myocarditis

Swollen spleen

Cataract
Choroidoretinitis
Microphthalmia
Glaucoma

Extended postnatal excretion
of mucous membrane with
urine, stool, etc

Pneumonia

Enlarged liver
Hepatitis

Generalised skeletal lesions

H.-R.W

A highly characteristic syndrome of dyscrania with hypotrichosis, anomalies of the face and especially of the eyes and short stature.

Main signs:
- Abnormalities of the skull (frontal or occipitoparietal bossing, delayed closure of fontanelles and sutures; relatively small face with flat orbits, hypoplasia of the jaw and micrognathia) (1–7).
- Microphthalmos; cataracts (congenital or manifest in the early postnatal period).
- Small, narrow nose, becoming increasingly 'beak-like' (3–5, 7).
- Congenital teeth and other dental anomalies; high, narrow palate.
- Atrophy of the skin, especially over the nose and cranial sutures; hypotrichosis, especially of the scalp, eyebrows, eyelashes (3–5, 7).
- Proportionate short stature.

Supplementary findings: Mental development is normal as a rule but exceptions are not uncommon.

Frequent amblyopic nystagmus, strabismus. Blue sclerae may occur.

On radiograph, hypoplasia of the ascending ramus of the mandible and anterior displacement of the temporo-mandibular joints.

Occurrence of pectus excavatum, winged scapulae and other skeletal anomalies. Also, right heart anomalies and hypogenitalism.

Manifestation: At birth.

Aetiology: Genetic basis certain but the causes remain unknown. Almost always sporadic occurrence perhaps as new mutations of an autosomal dominant gene. However, evidence also of possible autosomal recessive transmission. Possible heterogeneity.

Frequency: Low; over 150 patients described in the literature up to 1982.

Course, prognosis: In early infancy, glossoptosis or related anomalies may cause feeding and dangerous respiratory problems. Later, eye defects present the greatest problem (however, spontaneous resorption of the cataracts has been reported); vision often markedly decreased.

Adult height in females usually over 150 cm and in males over 155 cm.

Differential diagnosis: Progeria (149) and progeroid syndromes (150–154) are not difficult to rule out; mandibulofacial dysostosis (28), cleidocranial dysostosis (19) and pyknodysostosis (108) are even less difficult.

Treatment: Early ophthalmological and dental care are very important. There may be indications for growth hormone.

Genetic counselling.

Illustrations:

1–5 An 18-month-old boy with the complete picture of the syndrome. Congenital cataracts, congenital teeth. Mental development normal for age. Height below the third percentile. Cataract operation at age 5 months; vision well corrected with spectacles or contact lenses.

6 and 7 The same patient aged 10 years and 6 months. Height and weight below the third percentile. Bone-age retarded by approximately 3 years. Distinct partial HGH deficiency; growth hormone treatment was instituted. Mental development normal. He has one healthy sister, 3 years younger.

References:

Steele R W, Bass J W: Hallermann-Streiff syndrome. *Am J Dis Child* 1970, 20:462.

Suzuki Y, Fuji T, Fukuyama Y: Hallermann-Streiff syndrome. *Dev Med Child Neurol* 1970, **12**:496.

Dinwiddie R, Gewitz M, Taylor J F N: Cardiac defects in the Hallermann-Streiff syndrome. *J Pediatr* 1978, **92**:77.

Ronen S, Rozenmann Y, Isaacson M *et al*: The early management of a baby with Hallermann Streiff François syndrome. *J Pediatr Ophthalmol Stab* 1979, **16**/2:119.

François J: François' dyscephalic syndrome. *Birth Defects Orig Art Ser* 1982, **16**:6:595-619.

Huber J: Dento-alveolar abnormalities in oculomandibulodyscephaly (Hallermann-Streiff syndrome). *J Oral Path* 1984, **13**:147–154.

Symposion on the Hallermann-Streiff syndrome. *Am J Med Genet* 1991, **41**:487–523.

Al Khani A M, Al Herbish A S: Hallermann-Streiff syndrome in one of dizygotic twins (Letter). *Am J Med Genet* 1994, **49**:251–252.

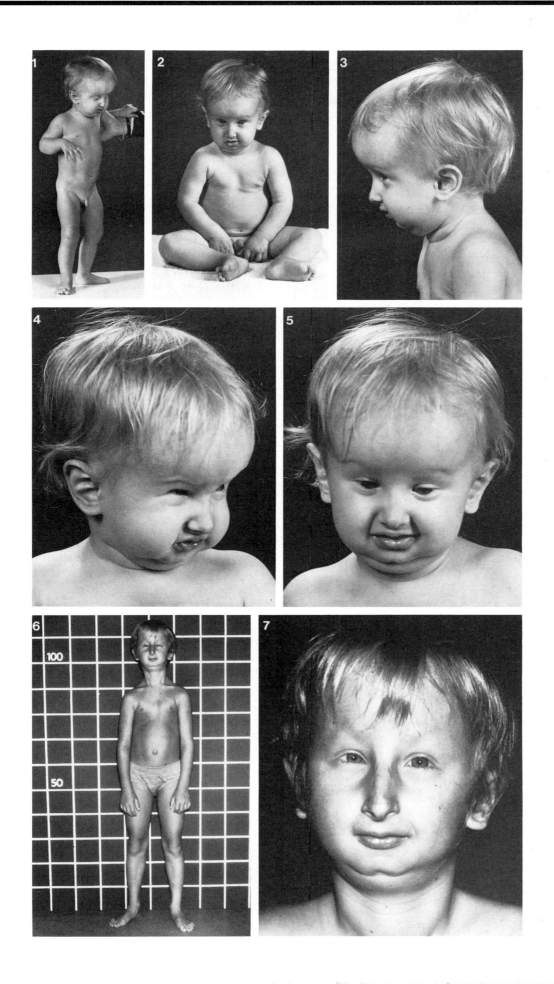

302 Arthro-ophthalmopathy

(Stickler Dysplasia, Stickler Syndrome, Stickler Phenotype)

H.-R.W

A relatively frequent and important autosomal dominant disorder of orofacial signs with abnormalities of the eyes, skeleton and joints.

Main signs:

- Flat, often asymmetrical face with variably depressed nasal bridge and nose (**1, 4**); epicanthic folds; hypoplasia of the mid-face (**1, 4**) or mandibles (**3**); cleft palate (hard or soft palate, sometimes with bifid uvula); frequently with fully expressed Robin triad (**39**).
- Early myopia of marked to extreme severity with changes of the fundi, possible glaucoma, cataract, retinal detachment and retinoschisis leading to blindness.
- Not infrequently, marfanoid habitus (**1, 2, 4**). Moderately developed, hypotonic musculature and hyperextensibility of large (and possibly also of small) joints; in some patients mild, rheumatoid arthropathies, even in childhood, severe arthropathies are also seen occasionally. Hip and knee joints most severely affected. The arthropathies are not constant and the least important sign.

Supplementary findings: Hearing impairment not so infrequent (conductive or sensorineural defect). Dental anomalies. Possible development of kyphosis or scoliosis; thoracic deformities; genu valgum (**1**) and so on.

Prolapse of the mitral valve frequent.

Radiologically, the picture of a mild spondylo-epiphyseal dysplasia with flattening of the vertebral bodies reminiscent of the picture in Scheuermann disease, narrow diaphyses and broad metaphyses of the long bones and changes of the knee and other joints (e.g. subluxation of the hip joints).

Manifestation: At birth (orofacial signs and possible conspicuous, bony prominence of the large joints, especially of the ankle, knee and wrist joints). Myopia usually manifest during early childhood; retinal detachment usually not until the second decade or later.

Aetiology: Autosomal dominant disorder (generalized stromal dysplasia) with very varied expression of individual signs, even intrafamilially and with incomplete penetrance. Heterogeneity. One gene locus: 12q13.11-q13.2. Collagen II structural defect. A further locus on chromosome 6.

Frequency: Not low (approximately 1:20 000). Stickler syndrome should be considered in every case of isolated cleft palate, Robin anomaly or dominantly occurring myopia and myopia should be ruled out in the former two conditions.

Course, prognosis: Usually normal life expectancy, intellectual development and height. Handicap caused by visual or joint disorders may occur, usually starting in the second decade (or even earlier).

Differential diagnosis: Marfan syndrome (76) and homocystinuria (79), spondylo-epiphyseal dysplasias (136, 137), osteodysplasia type Kniest (138) and possibly the Ehlers–Danlos syndrome (203) are usually easy to distinguish.

A few Stickler syndrome-like combinations of signs go by other names (Marshall syndrome, Weissenbacher–Zweymüller syndrome); their classification as separate entities does not yet seem to be unequivocally settled.

Treatment: Paediatric care of a Robin anomaly. From infancy, regular check-ups by a qualified ophthalmologist; glaucoma therapy may be indicated, operation for cataracts or specific treatment for retinal detachment. Closure of cleft palate and speech therapy as required. Audiometric assessment. Avoidance of physical strain. Cardiac assessment and treatment as needed.

Genetic counselling.

Illustrations:

1–4 A child and adolescents from a large sibship with Stickler syndrome.

1, 4 Mid-face hypoplasia.

3 Micrognathia.

References:

Meinecke P: Das Stickler-Syndrom, *Pädiat Prax* 1980/81, **24**:705.

Weingeist T A, Hermsen V *et al*: Ocular and systemic manifestations of Stickler's syndrome. *Birth Defects Orig Art Ser* 1982, 18(6):539–560.

Aymé S, Preus M: The Marshall and Stickler syndromes: objective rejection of lumping. *J Med Genet* 1984, **21**:34–38.

Liberfarb R M: Prevalence of mitral-valve prolapse in the Stickler syndrome. *Am J Med Genet* 1986, **24**:387–392.

Temple I K: Stickler's syndrome. *J Med Genet* 1989, **26**:119–126.

Ahmad N N *et al*: Stop codon in the procollagen II gene (COL2A1) in a family with the Stickler syndrome. *Proc Nat Acad Sci* 1991, **88**:6624–6627.

Vintimer G M *et al*: Genetic and clinical heterogeneity of Stickler syndrome. *Am J Med Genet* 1991, **41**:44–48.

Zlotgora J *et al*: Variability of Stickler syndrome. *Am J Med Genet* 1992, **42**:377–379.

Spranger J *et al*: The type II collagenopathies... *Eur J Pediatr* 1994, **153**:56–65.

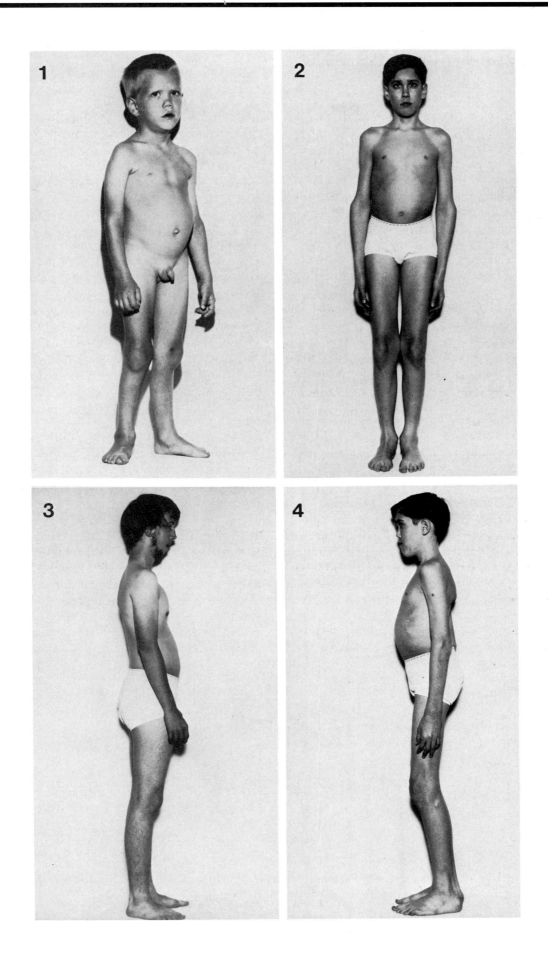

A Rare Malformation–Retardation Syndrome with Haemorrhagic Diathesis

H.-R.W

A syndrome of eye and skeletal anomalies, haemorrhagic diathesis and mental retardation.

Main signs:

- Ptosis, more severe on the right than the left (1) with deep-set eyes and myopia on the right. Loss of roundness of the iris on the right, typical coloboma of the iris on the left. Large coloboma of the choroid below the optic disc bilaterally. Large ears of simple configuration (1 and 2).
- Scoliosis, lumbar hyperlordosis (2); clinodactyly of the little and index fingers bilaterally (3); bilateral pes cavus.
- Haemorrhagic diathesis beginning at 6 years of age, with palm-size haematomas.
- Psychomotor retardation (IQ 66 at 11 years), uncertain whether primary or as a result of unilateral akinetic cerebral focal seizures that occurred from early infancy until about 4–5 years of age.

Supplementary findings: On radiograph, somewhat coarse, poorly modelled first rays of the hands and feet (4 and 5). Very coarse epiphyses of the terminal phalanges of the halluces and malformations of the ungual processes; atypical middle and terminal phalanges of the other toes (5). Mild clinodactyly of the fifth fingers, very pronounced pseudo-epiphyses of the second metacarpals (4). Haematologically: occasionally borderline platelet counts; prolonged periods of leukopaenia; normal erythrocytosis. Somewhat cell-poor bone marrow, without definite pathological findings. Good global thrombocyte function. No evidence of defective clotting factors. (Haemoglobin analysis negative. No erythrocyte enzyme defects demonstrable.)

Manifestation: At birth and later.

Aetiology: Unknown.

Course, prognosis: Apart from the mental deficiency, apparently favourable. At 14 years and 6 months, no further bleeding, platelet count normal; still slight 'constitutional' leukopaenia.

Comment: The patient has no cardiac defect (see Ho), no basis for Fanconi anaemia syndrome (249), nor for cat-eye syndrome (38) and so on.

Treatment: Symptomatic.

Illustrations:

1–5 The same boy at 7 years (4) and at 9 years (1–3, 5), the third child of healthy, young, nonconsanguineous parents after two healthy brothers. Pregnancy and delivery normal (3600 g; 51 cm). No hyperpigmentation. Normal linear growth (at 14 years and 6 months, 11 cm above average height). Normal head circumference. Normal genitalia and normal sexual maturation for age. Heart normal; renal pyelogram normal. Normal male karyotype and no increased chromosome breakage.

References:

Ho C K, Kaufman R L, Podos S M: Ocular colobomata, cardiac defect, and other anomlies: a study of seven cases including two sibs. *J Med Genet* 1975, 12:289.

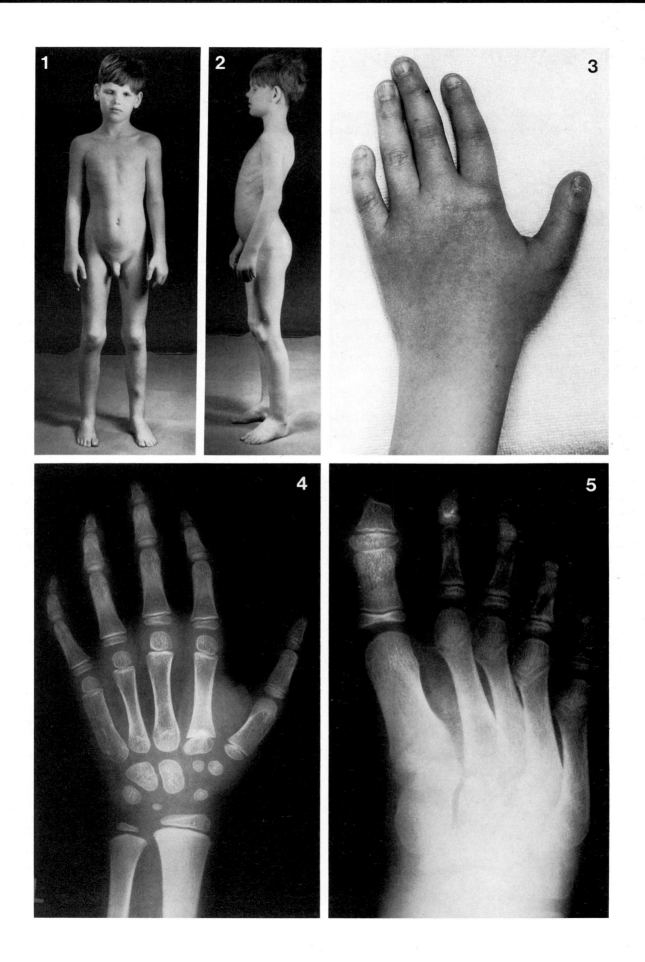

J.K.

A disorder of adrenal steroid biosynthesis (21-hydroxylase defect) with increased production of adrenal androgens causing virilization (or intersex in females), salt loss, and hyperkalaemia.

Main signs:
- Intersex of XX individuals: female pseudohermaphroditism with clitoral hypertrophy or complete masculinization (Prader stages I–V). Patients with stages I and II still have separate urethral and vaginal openings; with stages III–V, only one urogenital opening, which, however, may separate distally into urethra and vagina. XY patients show precocious pseudopuberty with enlargement of the penis and pigmented scrotum.
- Failure to thrive from the second week of life, with marked vomiting, fever, weight loss. Cortico-adrenal hyperplasia. Without treatment, death in the first weeks of life.

Supplementary findings: Increase of 17-ketosteroids and pregnanetriol in the urine and demonstration of pregnanetriolone, which is not normally present.

Manifestation: In females, at birth; in males (in the absence of salt-losing syndrome), diagnosis in later years. At least 40% of children with precocious puberty appear to be heterozygotes for the defective 21-hydroxylase gene.

Aetiology: Autosomal recessive 21-hydroxylase defect of adrenal steroid biosynthesis in the zona fasciculata and glomerulosa. The defective gene is linked with the HLA locus on chromosome 6 (6p21.3).

Frequency: The most frequent congenital disorder of steroid biosynthesis (approximately 90% of all patients). Worldwide regional differences, for example, 1:500 in the Eskimos of south-western Alaska; in the white population, incidence of 1:11 900 has been calculated following a screening. Salt-losing AGS is three times more frequent than without salt loss. General heterozygote frequency 1:55; for Alaska, 1:11.

Course, prognosis: Rapid growth, accelerated skeletal maturity, appearance of pubic hair at age 2–3 years and pronounced muscle contours. In girls, increased clitoral hypertrophy; in boys, signs of puberty with small testes (androgen production in the adrenals, no increase of gonadotropins). With continued absence of therapy, premature closure of the epiphyses (eighth year of life). Adult height approximately 145 cm. Men with AGS and appropriate therapy have no fertility problems. Complications with febrile illnesses, surgical procedures and trauma caused by increased demand for (unavailable) cortisol, resulting in: hypoglycemia, tachycardia, respiratory difficulties, seizures, somnolence, profuse sweating.

Prenatal diagnosis: This is important, because prenatal therapy appears possible. Either: diagnosis by determining 17-OH progesterone levels in amniotic fluid in the 16th week of pregnancy (beware the mother who is homozygous for the 21-hydroxylase defect); or HLA typing after a first child with AGS (HLA Bw47). More recently, it has been possible after an index patient to perform an indirect molecular genetic diagnosis (restriction fragment length polymorphism analysis) on chorionic villi.

Treatment: With the onset of acute vomiting, electrolyte replacement, aldosterone and prednisone parenterally. Long-term replacement therapy with hydrocortisone during childhood. After cessation of growth, prednisone. 9α-fludrocortisone as mineralocorticoid. Individual adjustment of dosage. With treatment, normal adult heights are attained. Operative correction of XX individuals and rearing as females (Prader types I–IV). Management of type V needs to be thoroughly discussed with all concerned.

Prenatal treatment with dexamethasone to prevent virilization appears possible. Begin 'blind' from the fifth or sixth week of pregnancy with a dose of 0.5 mg orally three times per day. On demonstration of a disorder, continue therapy to the end of the pregnancy.

Illustrations:
1a–d The 3-year-old sister of a boy who also has AGS.
1b The penis-like clitoris.
1c Fusion of the labia majora and urogenital sinus and clitoral hypertrophy.
1d Appearance at age 4 years and 6 months.
2 The 18-month-old sister of a boy with AGS; clitoral hypertrophy.
2b Scrotum-like hyperpigmented labia, urogenital sinus, clitoral hypertrophy.
3 A child, aged 4 years and 6 months, with masculine appearance. Salt-losing AGS; female pseudohermaphroditism (46XX) with maximal virilization (Prader type V). Gonadectomy, hysterectomy and implantation of prosthetic testes performed when the patient was 12 years old.

References:
David M, Forest M G: Prenatal treatment of congenital adrenal hyperplasia resulting from 21-hydroxylase deficiency. *J Pediatr* 1984, **105**:799–803.
Knorr, D: Das congenitale adrenogenitale Syndrom. *Monatsschr Kinderheilkd* 1985, **133**:327–335.
Miller W L, Levine L S: Molecular and clinical advances in congenital adrenal hyperplasia. *J Pediatr* 1987, **111**:1–17.
Schwab K O, Kruse K et al: Effekt einer mütterlichen Dexamethasonbehandlung... bei AGS... *Mschr Kinderheilk* 1989, **137**:293–296.
Strumberg D, Hauffa B P et al: Molecular detection of genetic defects in congenital adrenal hyperplasia due to 21-hydroxylase deficiency: a study of 27 families. *Eur J Pediatr* 1992 **151**:821–826.

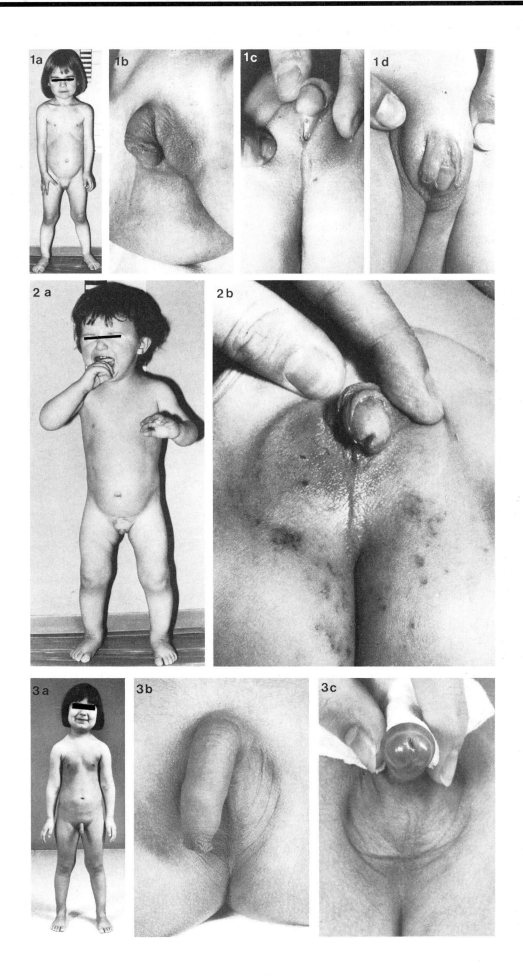

J.K.

An X-linked pseudohermaphroditism syndrome with bilateral testes, ambiguous genitalia, short, blind-ending vagina, absent uterus, and XY constitution.

Main signs:
- Inguinal or intra-abdominal testes, short blind-ending vagina, absence of uterus and fallopian tubes, clitoral hypertrophy. Male phenotype with hypospadias also possible. Only partially differentiated wolffian ducts; müllerian derivatives absent.
- Chromosomal status: 46XY.

Supplementary findings: At puberty, various degrees of masculinization and breast development. Phenotypic variability within a family. Sterility.

Manifestation: Intersex at birth.

Aetiology: X-linked recessive inheritance. Gene defect with variable expression. Unremarkable carrier mothers. Incomplete resistance to androgen: defect of the cytosol androgen receptor, which normally transports testosterone and other androgens from the cell membrane to the nucleus. Gene localization: Xq12. Diagnosis of heterozygotes by restriction fragment length polymorphism analysis.

Frequency: Including all forms of male pseudohermaphroditism, approximately 1:10 000. The ITF syndrome is correspondingly less frequent.

Course, prognosis: Various degrees of masculinization and breast development during puberty. The risk of testicular neoplasm in the first 2 decades of life is low.

Differential diagnosis: Easily differentiated from complete testicular feminization (306) (normal female external genitalia, inguinal hernias containing testes, primary amenorrhoea, absence of secondary sexual hair growth). Milder forms of androgen resistance: Lubs syndrome (female phenotype, partial labioscrotal fusion, pseudovagina); Gilbert–Dreifuss syndrome (male phenotype, small phallus, pubertal azoospermia, gynecomastia); Reifenstein syndrome (perineoscrotal hypospadias, bifid scrotum, gynaecomastia); Rosewater syndrome (male phenotype, sterility, gynaecomastia).

Treatment: Orchidectomy after puberty. Oestrogen therapy. Feminizing plastic surgery of the genitalia. In individual cases, careful differential diagnosis and psychological assessment. Prenatal diagnosis by demonstration of the androgen-cytosol-binding protein defect in cultured amniotic cells.

Illustrations:

1a and b A 13-month-old child. Clitoral hypertrophy, testes in the labioscrotal folds. Karyotype: XY.
1c and d Same child at age 5 years.
2a and b Sibling, 2 days old, ambiguous genitalia with clitoral hypertrophy; testes in the scrotum-like labia. Karyotype: 46XY.

References:
Any paediatric textbook.
Pinsky L, Kaufman M, Summitt L: Congenital androgen insensitivity due to a qualitatively abnormal androgen receptor. *Am J Med Genet* 1981 10:91–99.
Pinsky L *et al*: Human minimal androgen insensitivity with normal dihydrotestosteron-binding capacity in cultured genital skin fibroblasts: evidence for an androgen-selective qualitative abnormality of the receptor. *Am J Hum Genet* 1984, 36:965–978.
MacPhaul M J, Marcelli M, Tilley W D *et al*: Molecular basis of androgen resistance in a family with qualitative abnormality of androgen receptor and responsive to high dose androgen therapy. *J Clin Invest* 1991, 87:1413–1421.
Williams D M, Patterson M N, Hughes I A: Androgen insensitivity syndrome. *Arch Dis Child* 1993, 68:343–344.

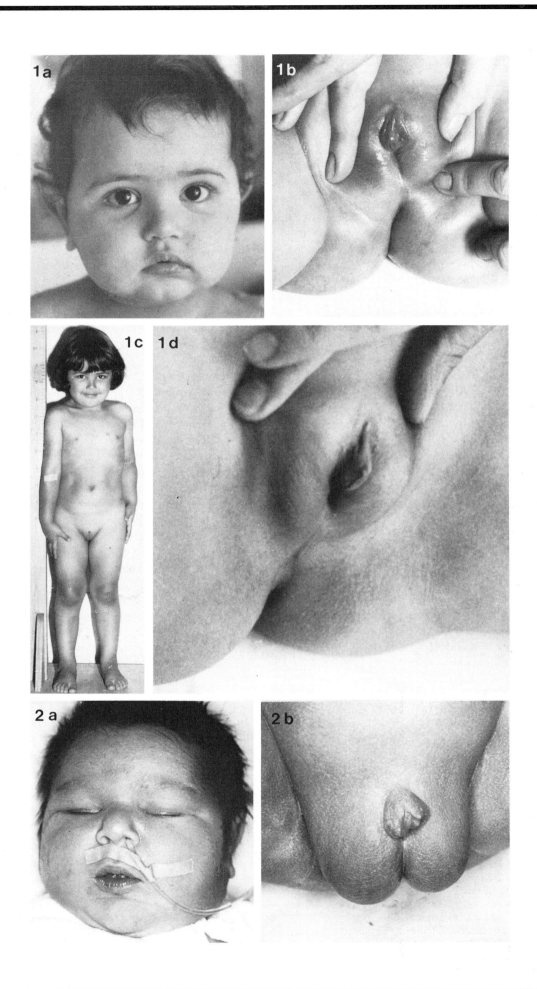

306 Complete Testicular Feminization Syndrome

('Hairless Women')

J.K.

An X-linked recessive male pseudohermaphroditism with female phenotype, primary amenorrhoea, decreased axillary and pubic hair, abdominal or inguinal testes and a male chromosome complement.

Main signs:
- Normal external female genitalia, no clitoral hypertrophy, labia majora and minora normal, separate urethral and vaginal openings.
- No differentiation of the müllerian ducts: short vagina (absence of the proximal part), no cervix, no uterus, no fallopian tubes.
- Likewise, no development of the wolffian duct: duct of epoophoron (appendix vesiculosa) and rudiments of Gartner's duct.
- The gonads are testes. They are intra-abdominal or inguinal (hernias) or in the labia.
- During puberty, normal breast development, decreased pubic and axillary hair. Primary amenorrhoea. Normal body proportions. Sterility.

Supplementary findings: Up to puberty, the testes are histologically normal. After puberty, absence of spermatogonia, infantile seminiferous tubules, no sperm formation. Leydig-cell hyperplasia. Unremarkable feminine psychosexuality.

Manifestation: At birth? However, may not be diagnosed until the menses fail to occur (primary amenorrhoea).

Aetiology: X-linked recessive inheritance.
  The genital tubercle and the foetal urogenital sinus cannot respond to induction by testicular androgens and so male genital organs do not develop. Hair follicles also do not react to androgens. Carrier mothers often show a paucity of pubic and axillary hair.
  Gene locus: Xq12. Indirect restriction fragment length polymorphism diagnosis of female carriers.

Frequency: Approximately 1:62 000 live-born male individuals.

Prognosis: In 5–20%, formation of gonadal neoplasms, such as tubular adenomas and seminomas.
  Otherwise normal life expectancy.
  Normal intelligence. Normal libido and sexual activity.

Differential diagnosis: To be differentiated from incomplete testicular feminization (305).

Treatment: Gonadal tumours do not occur before puberty. Gonadectomy after puberty is usually recommended, although some favour prepubertal removal. With prepubertal gonadectomy, oestrogen replacement therapy should be administered from the second decade of life; with postpubertal removal, correspondingly later.
  Plastic surgery to construct a deeper vagina.
Herniotomy with prior diagnostic clarification of the contents of the hernia (especially sex-chromatin diagnosis). The decision to inform the patients, who identify as females and may be married, of their male karyotype, requires very careful consideration. As a rule, patients are not told their nuclear sex.

Illustration: 1 and 2 A 17-year-old, typically affected except for relatively little breast development (primary amenorrhoea, and so on, XY constitution; androgen receptor defect demonstrated in genital-skin fibroblasts).

References:
Any textbook on gynaecology or paediatrics.
Griffin J E, Wilson I D: The syndromes of androgen resistance. *N Engl J Med* 1980, **302**:198–209.
Wieacker P, Griffin J E, Wienker T *et al*: Linkage analysis with RFLP's in families with androgen resistance syndromes: evidence for close linkage between the androgen receptor locus and the DXS1 segment. *Hum Genet* 1987, **76**:248–252.
Prior L, Bordet S *et al*: Replacement of arginen 773 cy cysteine or histidine in the human androgen receptor causes complete androgen insensitivity with different receptor phenotypes. *Am J Hum Genet* 1992, **51**:143–155.
Jakubiczka S, Werder E A, Wieacker P: Point mutation in the steroid-binding domain of the androgen receptor gene in a family with complete androgen insensitivity syndrome (CAIS). *Hum Genet* 1992, **90**:311–312.
Williams D M, Patterson M N, Hughes I A: Androgen insensitivity syndrome. *Arch Dis Child* 1993, **68**:343–344.

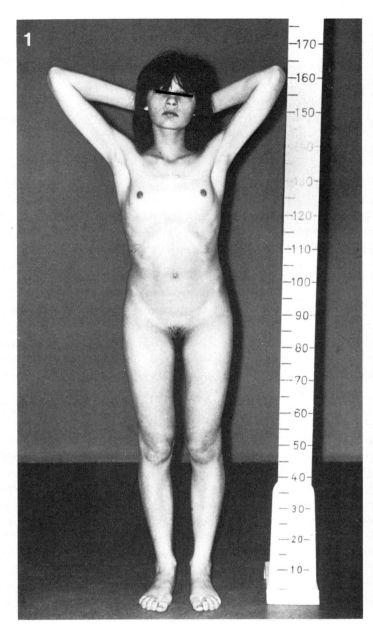

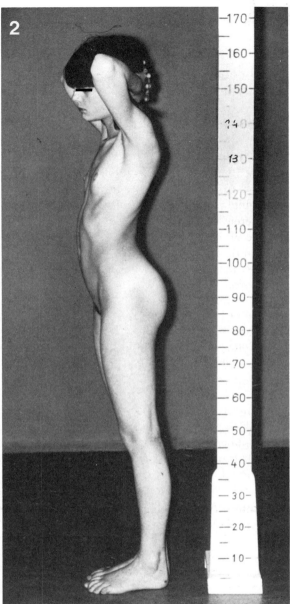

H.-R.W/
W. Sippel

Familial hypogonadotropic hypogonadism with anosmia, occurring in both sexes.

Main signs:
- Eunuchoid habitus with abnormally wide arm span and so on. Hypogonadotropic hypogonadism (1).
- Anosmia or hyposmia (seldom spontaneously reported).

Supplementary findings: Cryptorchidism and unilateral renal hypogenesis or agenesis (identified by ultrasound) may occur. Also, colour blindness, deafness; hypotelorism, cleft lip and/or palate, choanal atresia (as an expression of a mediocranial anomaly); cardiac defect, thrombocytopathy.

Manifestation: Boys with Kallmann syndrome may come to medical attention at birth because of cryptorchidism and micropenis. Parents should be carefully examined to determine whether they are affected. Early hormonal diagnosis.

Aetiology: Genetically determined neuronal migration disorder. Heterogeneity. Evidence for each of the classic modes of inheritance has been found in diverse sibships (sex-linked form localized to the region Xp22.3).
The hormonal disorder is caused by defective luteinizing hormone releasing hormone secretion by the hypothalamus; the disorder of smell, to absence of the primordial olfactory bulb and tract.

Frequency: Not so very low; estimate of one out of 10–60 000 individuals. Incidence in males appears to be approximately six times that of females. Sporadic cases (in families with isolated cases of anosmia) and also extensive observations in sibships.

Prognosis: Hormonal replacement therapy easier in girls. Prognosis for fertility less favourable in boys than in girls.

Diagnosis, differential diagnosis: Ask specifically for a history of anosmia. Test sense of smell.
Aim for early recognition, ruling out other forms of delayed puberty and hypogonadism.

Treatment: Adequate hormonal treatment to induce puberty and for maintenance therapy.
Recently, more physiological administration of luteinizing hormone releasing hormone in pulsatile form has been added to the customary method of inducing fertility by HCG/HMG treatment.

Illustrations:
1 A patient aged 13 years and 9 months; eunuchoid proportions, pubic and secondary hair, testes and penis markedly underdeveloped.
2 The same patient after 2 years of luteinizing hormone releasing hormone treatment in pulsatile form.

References:
Evain-Brion D, Gendrel D, Bozzala M *et al*: Diagnosis of Kallmann's syndrome in early infancy. *Acta Paediatr Scand* 1982 **71**:937–940.
Brämswig J H, Schellong G, König A *et al*: Familiärer Hypogonadismus mit Anosmie: Kallmann-Syndrom. *Mschr. Kinderheilk* 1983, **131**:232–234.
Hermanussen M, Sippell W G: Heterogeneity of Kallmann's syndrome. *Clin Genet* 1985, **28**:106–111.
Partsch C J, Hermanussen M, Sippell W G: Differentiation of male hypogonadotropic hypogonadism and constitutional delay of puberty by pulsatile administration of gonadotropin-releasing hormone. *J Clin Endocrin Metab* 1985, **60**:1196–1203.
Pawlowitzki I H, Diekstall P, Miny P *et al*: Abnormal platelet function in Kallmann syndrome. *Lancet* 1986, **II**:166.
Bick D, Curry, C J R *et al*: Male infant with... Kallmann syndrome... and an Xp chromosome deletion. *Am J Med Genet* 1989, **33**:100–107.
Schwanzel-Fukuda M, Pfaff D W: Origin of luteinizing hormone releasing hormone neurons. *Nature* 1989, **338**:161–164.
Meitinger T, Heye B *et al*: Definitive localization of X-linked Kallmann syndrome... to Xp22.3... *Am J Hum Genet* 1990, **47**:664–669.
Franco B, Guioli S *et al*: A gene deleted in Kallmann's syndrome... *Nature* 1991, **353**:529–536.
Bick D, Franco B *et al*: Intragenetic deletion of the Kalig-1 gene in Kallmann's syndrome. *N Engl J Med* 1992, **326**:1752–1755.
Crowley W F, Jameson J L: Gonadotropin-releasing hormone deficiency... *Endocrin Rev* 1992, **13**:635–640.
Schwanzel-Fukuda M, Jorgenson K *et al*: Biology of normal luteinizing hormone-releasing hormone neurons... *Endocrin Rev* 1992, **13**:623–634.
Birnbacher R, Wandl-Vergesslich K *et al*: Diagnosis of X-recessive Kallmann syndrome in early infancy. *Eur J Pediatr* 1994, **153**:245–247.
Mayer U: Augenbeteiligung beim Kallmann-Syndrom. *Pädiat Prax* 1994/95, **48**:479–481.
Meschede D, Behre H M *et al*: Kallmann-Syndrom. *Dtsch Med Wochenschr* 1994, **119**:1436–1442.

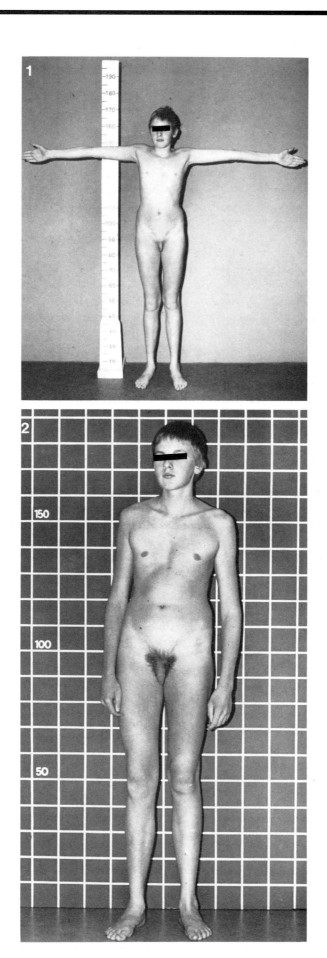

308 Klinefelter Syndrome
(XXY Syndrome)

H.-R.W/ J.K.

A hypogonadism syndrome in males with an additional X chromosome.

Main signs:

In childhood

- Frequently tall stature with mildly eunuchoid body proportions (unusually long lower extremities).
- Slightly below average intelligence, IQ 10–15 points below the average of siblings, possibly with behavioural disorders. (Relatively late onset of speech. Tendency to mild intention tremor. Increased disposition to epilepsy.)
- Possibly delayed onset of puberty, gynaecomastia.

In adolescence and adulthood

- Eunuchoid proportions with (moderate) tall stature (10 cm above average). Variable degree of gynaecomastia in approximately 40% of patients. Frequent development of obesity.
- Slightly below average intelligence (see above) with infantile tendencies, possible impulsive behaviour, or other psychological signs (anxiety, avoidance of social contact, difficulties with social adjustment).
- Normally developed penis but small firm testes of about 2.5 ml and possible poor development of secondary sexual characteristics (female distribution of pubic hair; sparse growth of beard). Plasma and urine gonadotropins elevated.

Supplementary findings: Increased disposition to varicosities of the lower legs and leg ulcers.

Below-average libido and potency; azoospermia; infertility.

X-chromatin positive on screening (buccal smear); confirmation of anomalous sex-chromosome constitution by chromosome analysis: XXY in approximately 80%; different types of mosaicism in about 20%.

Manifestation: Clinically by tall stature with relatively long legs (possibly combined with slightly below-average intelligence) in early childhood. Most patients are diagnosed after their 14th year of life.

Aetiology: The syndrome expresses a chromosomal aberration in the form of an extra X chromosome resulting from abnormal chromosome separation during oogenesis or spermatogenesis. In two-thirds of patients, both X chromosomes are of maternal origin, in one-third they are of maternal and paternal origin. Increased maternal age.

Frequency: Approximately 1:500 male newborns. Between 1:9 and 1:5 men with azoospermia are XXY.

Course, prognosis: Probably normal life expectancy. Poor social adjustment not infrequent. Infertility. (From puberty, progressive sclerosis and hyalinization of the seminiferous tubules, which in turn lead to loss of germinal tissue with subsequent secondary clumping [nodular hyperplasia] of the Leydig cells. Finally, progressive fibrosis and atrophy.)

Breast carcinoma rate as in females, that is, 3.3% of all males with breast cancer are Klinefelter patients.

Differential diagnosis: Other forms of male hypogonadism.

Treatment: If endocrinological testicular insufficiency is shown androgen therapy beginning in the 11th or 12th year of life. Surgical treatment of marked gynaecomastia may be indicated. Psychological support. Prevention of obesity.

Illustrations:

1 A proband at 8 years and 6 months: height excess, 18.5 cm; mental retardation; marked psychological signs; abnormal electroencephalogram.

4, 5, 8 The same patient at 26 years.

2, 3, 6, 7 A child aged 14 years and 3 months: 176.5 cm (above the 97th percentile); left testis 2 ml, right 3 ml, firm; moderate mental retardation.

Both patients confirmed by chromosome analysis.

References:

Any comprehensive textbook on paediatrics or internal medicine.

Netley C T: Summary overview of behavioural development in individuals with neonatally identified X and Y aneuploidy. *Birth Defects Art Ser XXII* 1986, 3:293–306.

Editorial: Klinefelter's syndrome. *Lancet* 1988, I:1316–1317.

Nielsen K J, Pelsen B, Sorensen K: Follow-up study of 30 Klinefelter males treated with testosterone. *Clin Genet* 1988, 33:262–269.

Robinson A, Bender B G, Linden M G: Summary of clinical findings in children and young adults with sex chromosome anomalies. *Birth Defects Original Article Series* 1991, 26(4):225–228.

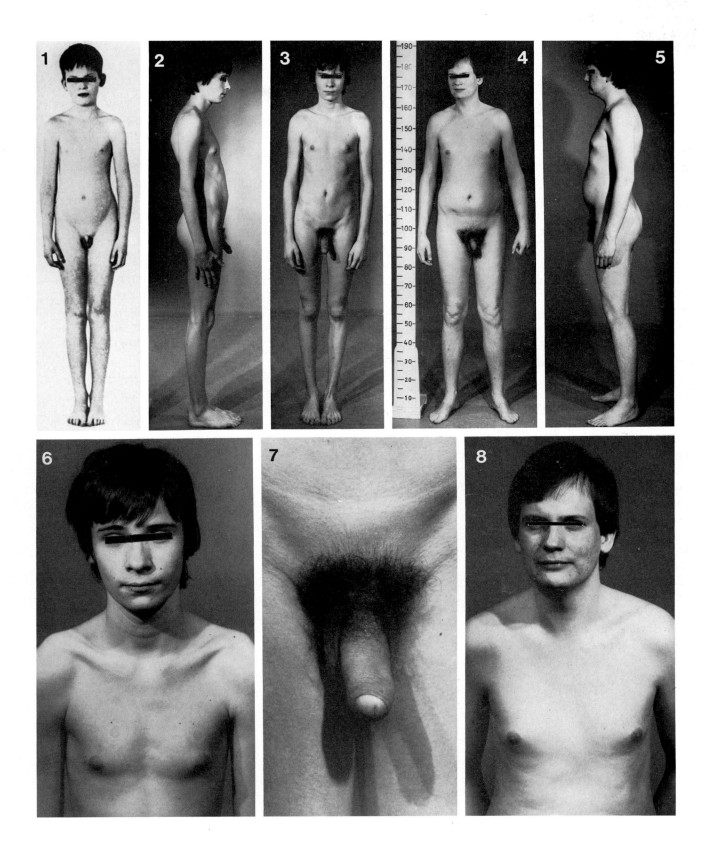

309 Idiopathic Hemihypertrophy
(Hemigigantism, Congenital Asymmetry)

J.K.

Congenital hypertrophy of unknown aetiology, which may be unilateral or partial and may occur together with involvement of the paired internal organs.

Main signs:
- Hemihypertrophy of one-half of the body or only a part thereof (face, upper and/or lower extremity, mandibles, tongue or other area); right side more frequently involved than left.
- Involvement of the internal paired organs (urogenital tract).
- Mental retardation in 10–20% of patients.
- Increased risk of Wilms' tumour (3%), adrenocortical neoplasia and hepatoblastoma; possible contralateral occurrence of these. Additionally: neuroblastoma, pheochromocytoma, testicular carcinoma.
- Radiologically, possibly accelerated bony growth on the affected side.

Supplementary findings: On the affected side: abnormal pigmentation, increased temperatures, dystrophic nails, hypertrichosis, premature dentition, enlarged pupils, heterochromia of the iris.

Manifestation: At birth; sometimes only diagnosed in the early months of life.

Aetiology: Unknown, probable heterogeneity. Different chromosomal changes described in isolated cases. Sporadic occurrence, only very isolated familial observations.
   Pathogenetically, probably a disorder of early embryogenesis; histologically, increased numbers of cells without increased size of individual cells.

Frequency: 1:14 300 in a series of children up to 6 years old; according to other authors, 1:100 000. Males are said to be more frequently affected, however, other reports speak of a 1:1 distribution.

Course, prognosis: The prognosis varies, depending on the extent of the hypertrophy; no compensatory growth of the unaffected side. Increased risk of tumours. Procedures: Up to 6 years of age, quarterly ultrasound examinations, between 6 and 10 years of age, once a year. Test catecholamines and metabolites every 1–2 years.

Differential diagnosis: Hemihypertrophy as a feature of: von Recklinghausen neurofibromatosis (*182*), hemi-3M syndrome, Klippel–Trenaunay syndrome (*198*), von Hippel-Lindau angiomatosis, Silver–Russell syndrome (*82*), Proteus syndrome (*196*), Maffucci syndrome (*233*), Wiedemann–Beckwith syndrome (*73*), McCune–Albright syndrome (*176*), Langer–Giedion syndrome (*232*), F.P. Weber syndrome (*225*), Ollier enchondromatosis (*233*).
   Distinguish from progressive hemiatrophy.
   Hemihypertrophy associated with angiomatous, lipomatous and lymphomatous malformations or tumours or with hamartomas (see also above) can be secondary.

Treatment: Dependent on the associated problems. Orthopaedic measures for different leg lengths.

Illustrations:
1a–c An 8-day-old female newborn with general left-side hemihypertrophy.
2 A 5-month-old female infant with idiopathic right-side hemihypertrophy.

References:
Ringrose R E, Jabbour J T, Keele D K: Hemihypertrophy. A review. *Pediatrics* 1965, 36:434–448.
Viljoen D, Pearn J, Beighton P: Manifestations and natural history of idiopathic hemihypertrophy: a review of eleven cases. *Clin Genet* 1984, 26:81–86.
Nudleman K, Anderman E, Anderman F *et al*: The hemi 3 syndrome: hemihypertrophy, hemihypaesthesia, hemiareflexia and scoliosis. *Brain* 1984, 107:533–546.
Mannens M, Slater R M, Heyting C *et al*: Chromosome 11, Wilms' tumor and associated congenital diseases. *Cytogenet Cell Genet* 1987, 46:655.

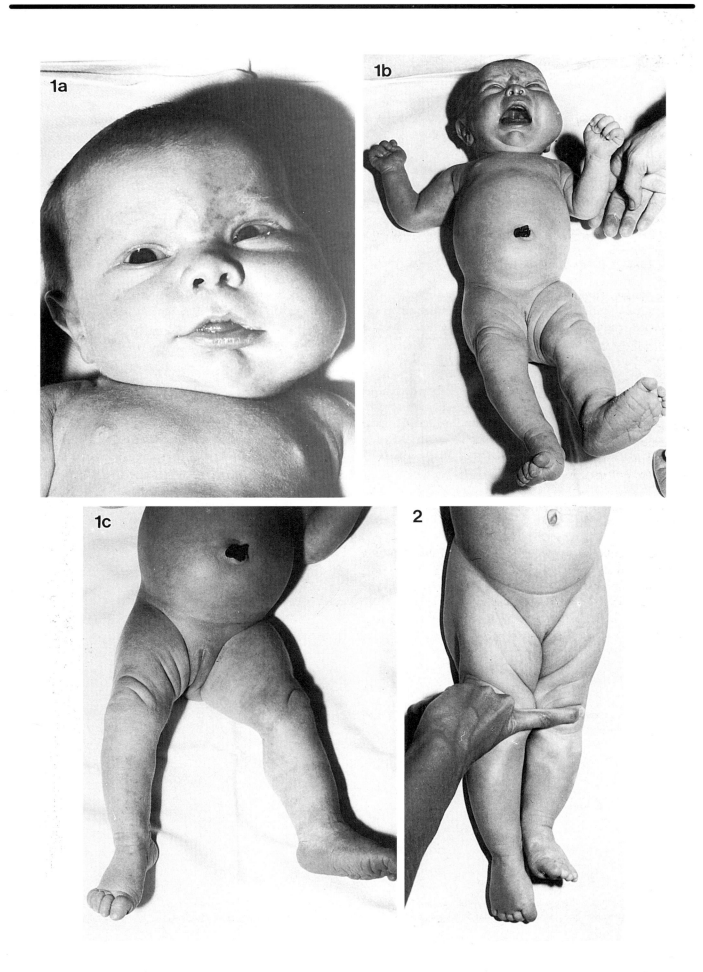

A combination of anorectal malformations, sacrococcygeal defect and presacral tumour, with familial occurrence.

Main signs:
- Anal atresia or anal stenosis and/or perineal anus.
- Sacrococcygeal defect with 'Turkish sabre' sacral deformity ('scimitar sacrum').
- Anterior meningocoele, lipoma, hamartoma, teratoma, dermoid cyst, cystic duplication of the intestines possibly with a fistula between the spinal canal and the rectum.

Supplementary findings: Chronic constipation.

Urogenital complications: urinary tract infections, vesico-ureteral reflux, neurogenic bladder; gynaecological and obstetric complications.

Meningitis.

Malignancy.

Malformations of the lower extremities, arterio-venous fistula in the knee-joint region, ambiguous genitalia, tethered cord syndrome (i.e. club feet and/or neurological defects as with manifest myelocoele, whereas only myelodysplasia, associated with an abnormally low level of the conus medullaris, is present).

Manifestation: From birth (anal obstruction) to adulthood (chronic constipation).

Aetiology: Mostly autosomal dominant inheritance; occasionally X-linked dominant inheritance and sporadic cases.

Frequency: Just under 100 patients known. Population frequency: 0.14% in children.

Prognosis: With timely diagnosis and surgical intervention, normal life expectancy. Beware: malignant degeneration.

Differential diagnosis: Caudal dysplasia 'syndrome' (*168*), diabetic embryopathy (*299*), femoral hypoplasia-unusual facies syndrome (*217*).

Treatment: Surgical.

Illustrations:

1a Patient 1: A 2-day-old female newborn with sacrococcygeal defect and 'Turkish sabre' deformity ('scimitar sacrum').

1b T2-weighted magnetic resonance imaging; patient aged 15 months; ventral meningocoele, presacral teratoma.

1c Age 15 months; anal stenosis.

2 Patient 2: A 3-month-old male infant, myelogram. Anterior sacral meningocoele and 'tethered cord' (terminal filum distinctly thickened and deeply fixed).

References:

Yates V D, Wilroy R S, Whitington G L *et al*: Anterior sacral defects: an autosomal dominantly inherited condition. *J Pediatr* 1983, **102**:239–242.
Welch J P, Atermark K: The syndrome of caudal dysplasia: a review, including etiologic considerations and evidence for heterogeneity. *Pediatr Radiol* 1984, **2**:313–327.
Janneck C, Holthusen W: Die Currarino-Trias... *Z. Kinderchir* 1988, **43**:112–116.
Chatkupt S, Speer M C *et al*: Linkage analysis of a candidate locus (HLA) in autosomal dominant sacral defect with anterior meningocele. *Am J Med Genet* 1994, **52**:1–4.

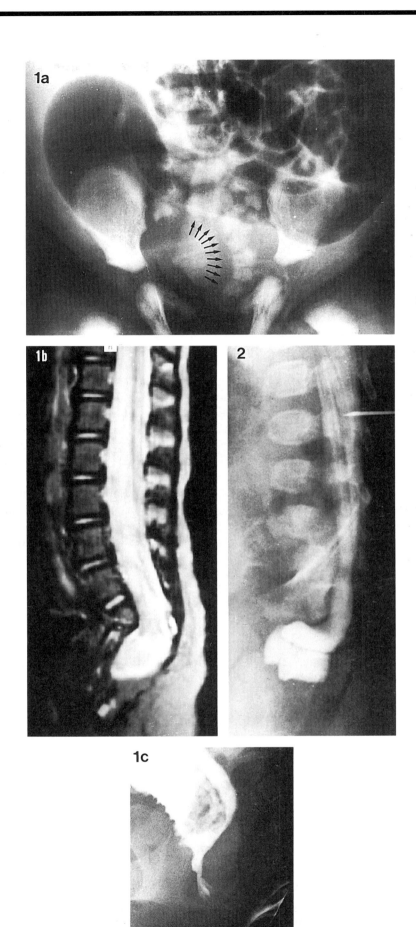

311 VATER Association

(VACTERL Syndrome: vertebral defects, anorectal atresia, cardiac anomalies, tracheo-oesophageal fistula with oesophageal atresia, renal anomalies and upper limb defects)

Main signs:
- Renal dysplasia, agenesis and other renal anomalies (73%).
- Congenital cardiac defect (73%).
- Defects of the vertebral bodies (60%).
- Tracheo-oesophageal malformations (60%).
- Anal stenosis and other anal malformations (56%)
- Radial dysplasia and other malformations of the upper extremities (44%).

Supplementary findings: Malformations of the lower extremities (43%), genital and gonadal anomalies (43.5%), rib anomalies (40%), ear anomalies (39%), ureteral anomalies (36%), single umbilical artery (33%), scoliosis, kyphosis, lordosis (32%), inguinal hernia (23.5%), anomalies of the small intestine (22%), cleft lip and palate (13%), choanal atresia (11%). Hypersegmentation with 13 or 14 ribs, several thoracic and lumbar vertebral bodies (10%). Monozygotic twins (6%). Laryngeal stenoses. Unilateral VATER association with hemihypoplasia.

Manifestation: At birth.

Aetiology: Distinct preponderance of male patients (2.6:1 in White people). Average birth weight falls to 2250 g with a gestation of about 35.5 weeks. A prolonged period of infertility before becoming pregnant is found in 10% of patients. No causative genetic factors demonstrable. Sporadic occurrence. Familial occurrence in isolated cases. Risk of recurrence 1-2%.

J.K.

Frequency: 1.6 out of 10 000 live births. Approximately 200 published patients.

Prognosis: Of those born alive, 50–85% die within the first year of life; 12% stillborn.

Differential diagnosis: Three or more components of the VATER complex occur in patients with trisomy 18 (48), trisomy 13 (47), and in the cri du chat syndrome (50). Furthermore, consider the following: Meckel–Gruber syndrome (45), Zellweger syndrome (291), sirenomelia (44), Potter sequence (43), amniotic band syndrome (219), Goldenhar 'syndrome' (30), the MURCS association (mullerian duct aplasia or hypoplasia, renal aplasia, cervicothoracic somite dysplasia), Mayer–Rokitansky–Küster–Hauser complex, Klippel-Feil syndrome (163), hereditary renal dysplasia and hemifacial microsomia (31).

Treatment: Surgery as indicated.

Illustrations:

1–5 A premature female, born in the 37th week of pregnancy, with butterfly vertebrae T4–T6, right-sided anotia, ventricular septal defect, oesophageal atresia with lower tracheal fistula, club hands with radial aplasia, nonrotation of the intestine, micrognathia, hypertelorism, 'rocker bottom' feet. Cytogenetics: 47XX, + 18.

References:

Khoury M J, Cordero J F, Greenberg, F et al: A population study of the VACTERL association: evidence for its etiologic heterogeneity. *Pediatrics* 1983, 71:815–820.

Czeizel A, Ludanyi I: An aetiologic study of the VACTERL-association. *Eur J Pediatr* 1985, 144:331–337.

Weaver D D, Mapstone C L, Yu P L: The VATER association. *AJDC* 1986, 140:225–229.

Fernbach S K, Glass R B J: The expanded spectrum of limb anomalies in the VATER association. *Pediatr Radiol* 1988, 18:215–220.

Syed S A, Onizuka K. et al: Unilateral VATER association. *Am J Med Genet* 1990, 37:60–61.

Örstavik K H, Steen-Johnsen J. et al: VACTERL or MURCS association in a girl with neurenteric cyst and identical thoracic malformations in the father: a case of gonosomal mosaicism? *Am J Med Genet* 1992, 43:1035–1038.

Corsello G, Maresi, E. et al: VATER/VACTERL association: clinical variability and expanding phenotype including laryngeal stenosis. *Am J Med Genet* 1992, 44:813–815.

Duncan P A, Shapiro L R: Interrelationships of the hemifacial microsomia-VATER, VATER, and sirenomelia phenotypes. *Am J Med Genet* 1993, 47:75–84.

Schüler L, Salzano F. M: Pattern in multimalformed babies and the question of the relationship between sirenomelia and VATERL. *Am J Med Genet* 1994, 49:29–35.

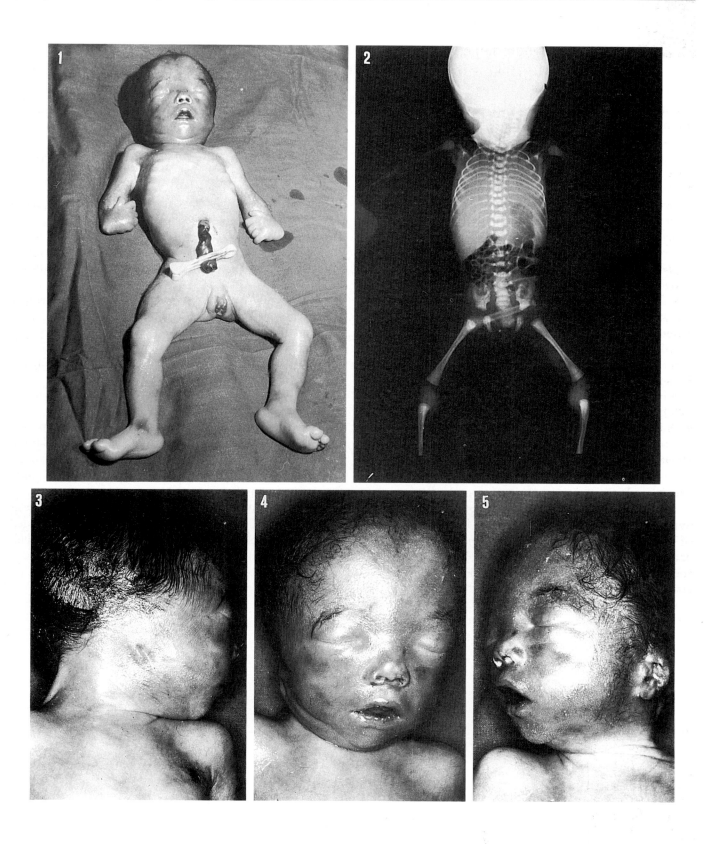

J.K.

A non-random combination of 'vertebral anomalies, anal atresia, cardiovascular anomalies, tracheo-oesophageal fistula, renal dysplasia, limb defects' and hydrocephalus.

Main signs:
- Hydrocephalus, encephalocoele, occipital meningocoele, hydranencephaly, microcephaly.
- Anal atresia, malrotation, oesophageal atresia.
- Genital anomalies: rectovaginal fistula, vaginal atresia, dorsal fusion of the labia majora, hypospadias.
- Cardiac defects: ventricular septal defect, atrial septal defect, patent ductus arteriosus, bicuspid aortic valve, endocardial fibro-elastosis, persistent superior vena cava, left.
- Renal anomalies: unilateral agenesis, bilateral hydronephrosis, renal hypoplasia, multicystic kidneys, horseshoe kidney, ectopic kidney, duplicated ureter.
- Radial anomalies: bilateral radial aplasia, aplasia of the thumbs, club hands, triphalangeal thumbs, pre-axial polydactyly, hypoplastic, bowed ulna.
- Tracheal defects: tracheal stenosis, tracheo-oesophageal fistula with esophageal stenosis, tracheal atresia.
- Vertebral anomalies: sagittal clefting of the thoracic vertebral bodies, segmentation anomalies, hemivertebrae, block vertebrae, butterfly vertebrae, sacrococcygeal defects.

Supplementary findings: Incomplete lobar development of the lungs, hypoplastic lungs, microphthalmos. Cleft lip and palate, bifid uvula. Micrognathia. Microtia, atresia of the auditory canal. Microcephaly, absent occiput, agenesis of the corpus callosum, aqueduct stenosis, agenesis and hypoplasia of the cerebellum, 'tethered cord'. Club feet. Accessory spleen, ectopic pancreas.

Manifestation: Prenatal and at birth.

Aetiology: Heterogeneity. In most cases, X-linked recessive inheritance but autosomal recessive inheritance has also been reported.

Pathogenesis: Multiple developmental fields react monogenetically like a single development unit. This supports the hypothesis put forward by *Opitz* that the development of complex embryonal structures is controlled and co-ordinated 'in an epimorphically hierarchical manner'.

Course, prognosis: In most patients, early death; maximum reported survival to date, 14 weeks.

Differential diagnosis: Hydrolethalus syndrome (*323*), Walker–Warburg syndrome (*314*), trisomy 13 (*47*), trisomy 18 (*48*).

Illustrations:
1a and b Second twin with micrognathia, macrostomia, microcephaly, occipital meningo-encephalocoele, bilateral radial aplasia, anal atresia, atrial septal defect, oesophageal atresia with tracheo-oesophageal fistula, horseshoe kidneys.
2a–d Siblings with bilateral radial aplasia, club feet, hydrocephalus, congenital cardiac defect. Right-sided renal agenesis and left-sided cystic degeneration, cerebellar hypoplasia, anal atresia.

References:
Iafolla A K, McConkie-Rosell A, Chen Y T: VATER and hydrocephalus: distinct syndrome? *Am J Med Genet* 1991, 38:46–51.
Evans J E, Stranc L C, Kaplan P, Hunter A G W: VACTERL with hydrocephalus. Further delineation of the syndromes. *Am J Med Genet* 1989, 34:177–182.
Beemer F A, Wanders R J A, Schutgens R B J: VACTERL and hydrocephalus. *Am J Med Genet* 1991, 37:425–426.
Kunze J, Huber-Schumacher S, Vogel M: VACTERL plus hydrocephalus: a monogenic lethal condition. *Eur J Pediatr* 1992, 151:467–468.
Froster-Iskenius U, Meinecke P: Encephalocele, radial defects, cardiac, gastrointestinal, anal, and renal anomalies: a new multiple congenital anomaly (MCA) syndrome? *Clin Dysmorphol* 1992, 1:37–41.
Porteous M E M, Cross I, Burn J: VACTERL with hydrocephalus: one end of the Fanconi anemia spectrum of anomalies? *Am J Med Genet* 1991, 43:1032–1034.
Genuardi M, Chiurazzi P, Capelli A, Neri G: X-linked VACTERL with hydrocephalus: the VACTERL-H syndrome. *Birth Defects: Orig Art Ser* 1993, 29(1):235–241.
Corsello G, Giuffré L: VACTERL with hydrocephalus: a further case with probable autosomal recessive inheritance. *Am.J Med Genet* 1994, 49:137–138.

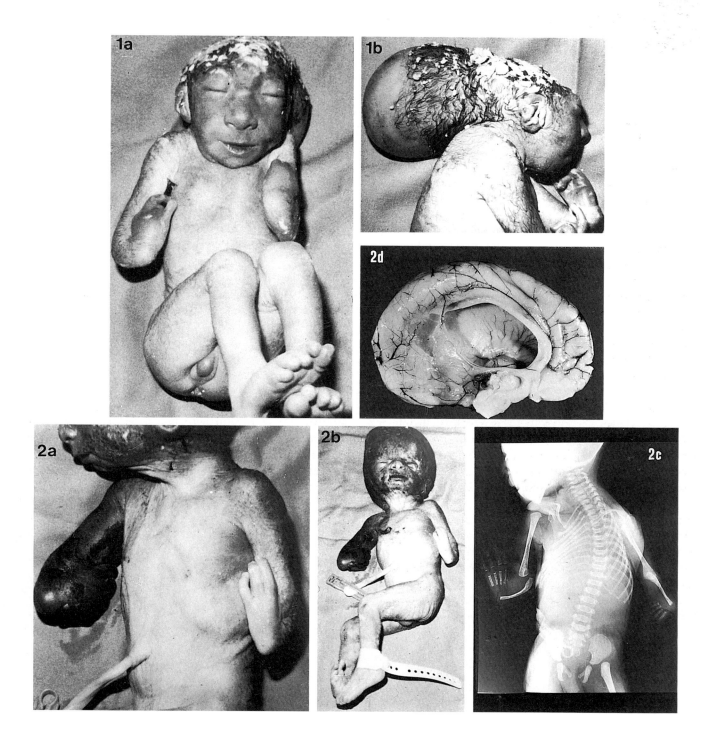

J.K.

A malformation syndrome with the characteristic triad: anal atresia, triphalangia of the thumbs and defective hearing (anus–hand–ear syndrome).

Main signs:
- Anorectal malformations: anal atresia with fistulization, ventrally positioned anus, anal stenosis.
- Malformations of the hand: pre-axial polydactyly, triphalangeal thumbs, broad thumbs, agenesis of the thumbs, arthrogryposis of the thumb joints, infrequently radius hypoplasia.
- Malformations of the ear: microtia, 'satyr ears', lop ears, pre-auricular tags and fistulas, sensorineural and conductive hearing disorders with malformations of the ossicles.

Supplementary findings:
Kidneys: unilateral renal hypoplasia, ureterostenosis, urethral valves.
Skeleton: absent/hypoplastic toes, clinodactyly of the fifth toes, pes planus, exostosis of the toes, fused metatarsals, fusion of the triquetral and hamate bones, hallux valgus, pseudo-epiphyses of the second metacarpals.
Face: mandibular hypoplasia, cleft lip and palate, widely spaced incisors, incomplete closure of the mouth.

Manifestation: At birth.

Aetiology: Autosomal dominant disorder. Over 75 patients documented.

Pathogenesis: Unknown.

Course, prognosis: With normal intelligence, dependent on the degree of accompanying malformations. Malformations of the urinary tract are always present.

Differential diagnosis: VATER association (*311*), Holt–Oram syndrome (*248*).

Treatment: Surgical correction of malformations of the hands, ears and urinary tract.

Illustrations:
1 and 2 Right-sided microtia with atresia of the auditory canal. Dysplastic left ear with pre-auricular tag.
3 and 4 Pre-axial polydactyly, triphalangeal thumb, contracture of the proximal interphalangeal joint.

1-4 from:
R König *et al.* Townes-Brocks syndrome. Eur J Pediatr 1990, **150**:100–103.

References:
Townes P L, Brocks, E: Hereditary syndrome of imperforate anus with hand, foot and ear anomalies. *J Pediatr* 1972, **81**:321–326.
Monteiro de Pina-Neto, J: Phenotypic variability in Townes-Brocks syndrome. *Am J Med Genet* 1984, **18**:147–152.
De Vries-van der Weerd M A C S, Willems P J, Mandema H M, ten Kate L P: A new family with the Townes-Brocks syndrome. *Clin Genet* 1988, **34**:195–200.
Ferraz F G, Nunes L, Ferraz M E, Sousa J P, Santos M, Carvalho C, Maroteaux P: Townes-Brocks syndrome. Report of a case and review of the literature. *Ann Génét* 1989, **32**:120–123.
O'Callaghan M, Young I D: The Townes-Brocks syndrome. *J Med Genet* 1990, **27**:457–461.
König R, Schick U, Fuchs S: Townes–Brocks syndrome. *Eur J Pediatr* 1990, **150**:100–103.
Cameron T H, Lachiewicz A M, Aylsworth A S: Townes-Brocks syndrome in two mentally retarded youngsters. *Am J Med Genet* 1991, **41**:1–4.

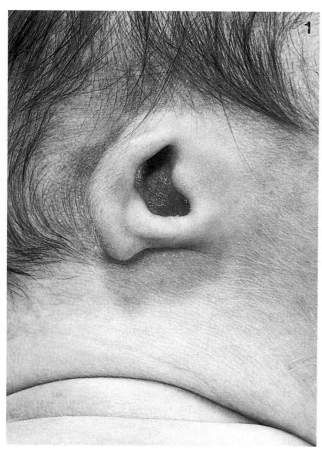

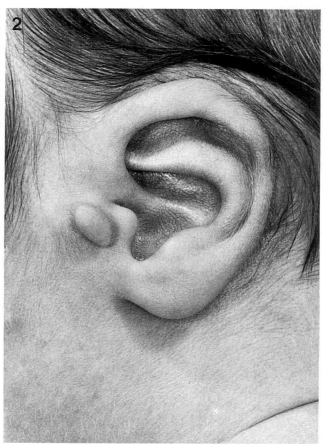

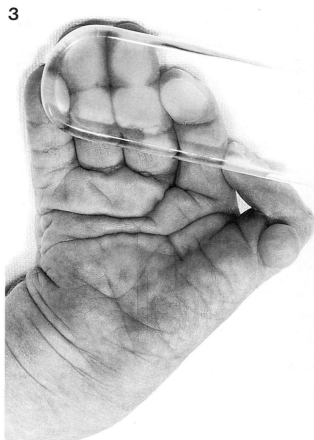

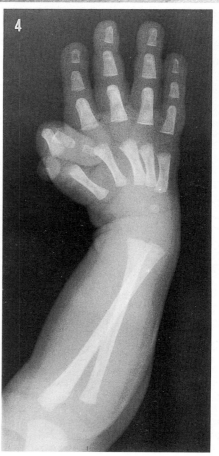

Walker–Warburg Syndrome

(Warburg Syndrome; Chemke Syndrome; Pagon Syndrome ; Cerebro-Ocular Dysplasia = COD)

J.K.

A lethal familial disorder comprising hydrocephalus, agyria, retinal dysplasia and encephalocoele (HARD + E Syndrome).

Main signs:
Hydrocephalus, usually caused by aqueduct stenosis. Dandy–Walker malformation.
Agyria (type II lissencephaly).
Retinal dysplasia, microphthalmos.
Encephalocoele.
Cerebellar malformations, hypoplasia of the cerebellar vermis. Congenital progressive muscular dystrophy, elevated creative kinase.

Supplementary findings: Cataracts, microphthalmos, hypoplasia of the iris, coloboma of the optic nerve. Cleft lip and palate. Glaucoma. Microtia and absence of the external auditory canals. Seizures. Severe developmental retardation, agenesis of the corpus callosum, hypoplasia of the white matter of the brain.

Manifestation: At birth. Hydrocephalus can be shown prenatally by ultrasound.

Aetiology: Autosomal recessive inheritance.

Frequency: Approximately 70 observations; of these, one-third are familial.

Course, prognosis: Average life expectancy 9 months. Some patients survive for a few years. Severe developmental delay.

Differential diagnosis: Lissencephaly type I (46), muscle–eye–brain disease, Fukuyama congenital muscular dystrophy.

Illustrations:
1a A 3-month-old infant. **1b** Death at age 5 months; microphthalmos left, buphthalmos right. **1c** Vitreous body histology with heterotopic retina, surrounded by older haemorrhages. **1d** Cranial magnetic resonance imaging, T^1-weighted (at 3 months), coronal section: left eye with vitreous haemorrhage. Buphthalmos right. **1e** Cranial magnetic resonance imaging, T^1-weighted, transverse section: agyria, thickening of the cortex, microphthalmos left with pathologic signals in both vitreous bodies. **1f** Iridocorneal angle histology with heterotopic retina. **1g** Superior view of the brain with agyria. **1h** Macroscopic transverse section through both cerebral hemispheres: internal hydrocephalus, agyria and fusion of the frontal cerebral fissure.
2 Patient with Miller–Dieker syndrome: coronal, T^1-weighted cranial magnetic resonance imaging: internal hydrocephalus, incomplete agyria, unremarkable cerebellum.

References:
Ayme S, Mattei J F: HARD (plus or minus) E syndrome: report of a sixth family with support for autosomal-recessive inheritance. *Am J Med Genet* 1983, **14**:759–766.
Whitley C B, Thompson T R, Mastri A R *et al*: HARD syndrome: a lethal neurodysplasia with autosomal recessive inheritance. *J Pediatr* 1983, **102**:547–552.
Williams R S, Swisher C N, Jennings M *et al*: Cerebro-ocular dysgenesis (Walker-Warburg) syndrome: neuropathologic and etiologic analysis. *Neurology* 1984, **34**:1531–1541.
Crowe C, Jassani M, Dickerman L: The prenatal diagnosis of Warburg syndrome (Abstract). *Am J Hum Genet* 1985, **37**:A214.
Crowe C, Jassani M, Dickerman L: The prenatal diagnosis of Walker-Warburg syndrome. *Prenat Diagn* 1986, **6**:177–185.
Burton B K, Dillard R G, Weaver R G: Brief clinical report: Walker-Warburg syndrome with cleft lip and cleft palate in two sibs. *Am J Med Genet* 1987, **27**:537–541.
Dobbyns W B, Pagon R A *et al*: Diagnostic criteria for Walker-Warburg syndrome. *Am J Med Genet* 1989, **32**:195–210.
Santavuori P Pihko, H *et al*: Muscle-eye-brain disease and Walker-Warburg syndrome. *Am J Med Genet* 1990, **36**:371–372.
Dobyns W B, Pagon R A *et al*: Response to Santavuori *et al*. regarding Walker-Warburg syndrome and muscle-eye-brain disease. *Am J Med Genet* 1990, **36**:373–374.
Gersoni-Baruch R, Mandel H *et al*: Walker-Warburg syndrome with microtia and absent auditory canals. *Am J Med Genet* 1990, **37**:87–91.
Wargowski D S, Chitayat D *et al*: Lethal congenital muscular dystrophy with cataracts and a minor brain anomaly: new entity or variant of Walker-Warburg syndrome? *Am J Med Genet* 1991, **39**:19–24.
Vohra N, Ghidini A *et al*: Walker-Warburg syndrome: prenatal ultrasound findings. *Prenat Diagn* 1993, **13**:575–579.
Rodgers B L, Vanner L V, Sai G S, Sens M A: Walker-Warburg syndrome: report of three affected sibs. *Am J Med Genet* 1994, **49**:198–201.

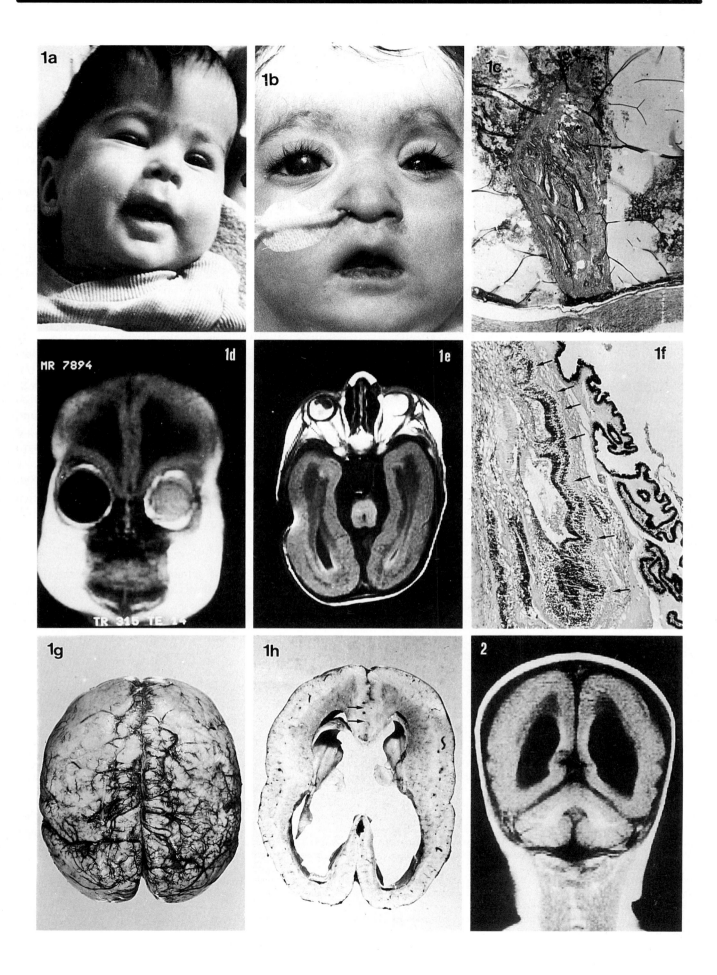

315 CHARGE Association

(CHARGE Complex, CHARGE Syndrome: coloboma, heart disease, atresia of choanae, retarded mental development, genital hypoplasia, ear anomalies and deafness)

J.K.

Main signs:
- Bilateral or unilateral coloboma of the iris, retina, and the optic nerve. Less frequently, microphthalmia or anophthalmia. Found in 80% of the patients.
- In 32% of all patients with choanal atresia, cardiac defects are found: patent ductus arteriosus, atrial septal defect, ventricular septal defect, tetralogy of Fallot, atrioventricular canal, combined defects.
- Up to two-thirds of all patients have bilateral choanal atresia. Look for further malformations.
- Mental or motor retardation in 87% and 94%, respectively, of all patients. Probably caused by hypoxic damage.
- In 74% of patients, signs of genital hypoplasia without secondary problems. Females are fertile. Males frequently show cryptorchidism and hypospadias.
- Normal or markedly dysplastic ears, may be unilateral, with sensorineural and conductive hearing impairment of various grades of severity.

Supplementary findings: One-fifth of patients show intra-uterine and postnatal growth retardation. Orofacial clefts, high palate. Oesophageal atresia, tracheo-oesophageal fistulae. Laryngomalacia, laryngeal clefts, anomalous aryepiglottic folds.
Renal malformations and dysplasia: agenesis, hypoplasia, heterotopia, hydronephrosis.
Facial dysmorphism: micrognathia, antimongoloid slant of the palpebral fissures, pug nose.
Skeletal anomalies: hemivertebrae, syndactyly, clinodactyly, scoliosis.
Neurological disorders: paresis of the facial nerve, hearing disorders, impaired pharyngeal and laryngeal co-ordination.

Manifestation: At birth.

Aetiology: Usually sporadic occurrence. Occasionally, autosomal dominant mode of inheritance (then called CHARGE syndrome). Affected siblings with healthy parents have also been observed. A similar clinical picture is seen with various chromosomal abnormalities.
Disturbance of embryological differentiation between the 35th and 38th days. Risk of recurrence in sporadic individual observations less than 1%.

Frequency: Approximately 200 patients documented.

Course, prognosis: Chances of survival poor in the case of cyanotic cardiac defects, bilateral choanal atresia or tracheo-oesophageal fistulae. Aspiration caused by impaired co-ordination of swallowing. Approximately 30% die in the first year of life; 70% reach 5 years of age. One-half show mental retardation.

Diagnosis: According to some authors, the combination of characteristic ear malformations (increased width and decreased length of the ear, 'snipped off' helix, absent ear lobe, prominent antihelix, triangular concha) with 'wedge-shaped' audiogram (loss of low frequencies of bone conduction and loss of high frequencies of air conduction) are key to the diagnosis.

Treatment: Multidisciplinary management.

Illustrations:
1 and 2 A 5-month-old female infant after surgical correction of a bilateral membranous occlusion of the posterior nares.
3 and 4 Characteristic malformation with widening of the ear, absent lobe and simply modelled helix.

References:
Koletzko B, Majewski F: Congenital anomalies in patients with choanal atresia: CHARGE-association. *Eur J Pediatr* 1984, **142**:271–275.
Davenport S L H, Hefner M A, Mitchell J A: The spectrum of clinical features in CHARGE syndrome. *Clin Genet* 1986, **29**:298–310.
Metlay L A, Smythe P S, Miller M E: Familial CHARGE syndrome: clinical report with autopsy findings. *Am J Med Genet* 1987, **26**:577–581.
Lin A E, Chin A J, Devine W. *et al*: The pattern of cardiovascular malformation in the CHARGE association. *AJDC* 1987, **141**:1010–1013.
Oley C A, Baraitser M, Grant D B: A reappraisal of the CHARGE association. *J Med Genet* 1988, **25**:147–156.
Meinecke P, Polke A, Schmiegelow, P: Limb anomalies in the CHARGE association. *J Med Genet* 1989, **26**:202–203.
Abruzzo M A, Erickson R P: Re-evaluation of new X-linked syndrome for evidence of CHARGE syndrome or association. *Am J Med Genet* 1989, **34**:397–400.
Lin A E, Siebert J R, Graham J M Jr: Central nervous malformations in the CHARGE association. *Am J Med Genet* 1990, **37**:304–310.
Blake K D, Russell-Eggitt I M *et al*: Who's in CHARGE? Multidisciplinary management of patients with CHARGE association. *Arch Dis Child* 1990, **65**:217–223.
Harvey A S, Leaper P M, Bankier A: CHARGE association: clinical manifestations and developmental outcome. *Am J Med Genet* 1991, **39**:48–55.
Clementi M, Tenconi R *et al*: Apparent CHARGE association and chromosome anomaly: chance or contiguous gene syndrome. *Am J Med Genet* 1991, **41**:246–250.
Kushnick T, Wiley J E, Oalmer S M: Agonadism in 1 patient with CHARGE association. *Am J Med Genet* 1992, **42**:9–99.
Byerley K A, Pauli R M: Cranial nerve abnormalities in CHARGE association. *Am J Med Genet* 1993, **45**:751–757.
Lubinsky M S: Properties of associations: identity, nature, and clinical criteria, with a commentary on why CHARGE and Goldenhar are not associations. *Am J Med Genet* 1994, **49**:21–25.

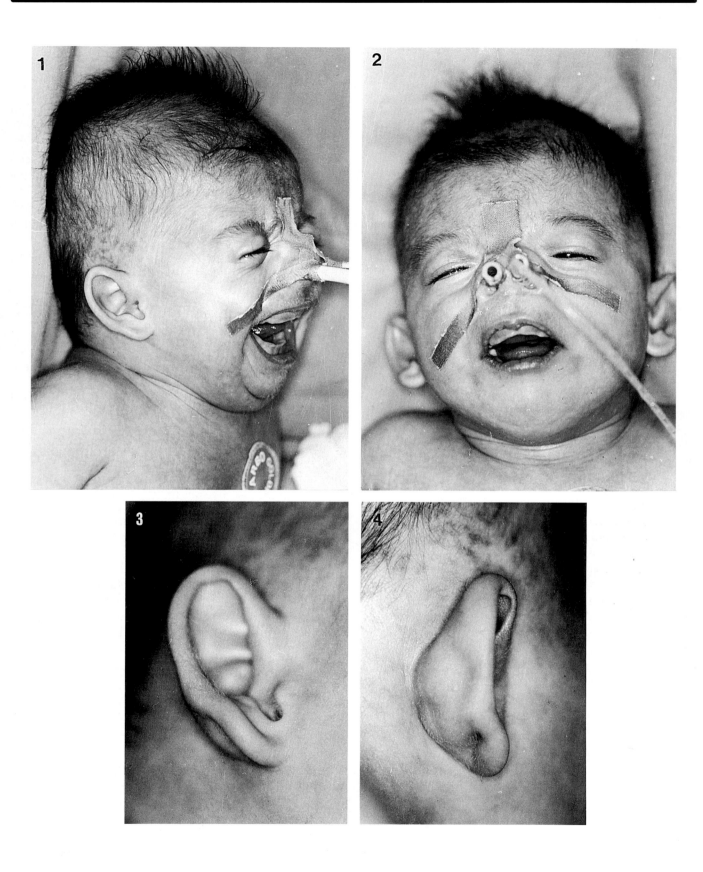

J.K.

Early embryonal developmental disorder of the cerebellum and fourth ventricle with hydrocephalus.

Main signs:
- Agenesis of the cerebellar vermis, partial or complete.
- Cystic dilation of the fourth ventricle (with atresia of the medial and lateral apertures), posterior-fossa cysts, and communication of the two cystic changes.
- Hydrocephalus.

Supplementary findings: Obstruction of the foramina of Luschka and Magendie and cystic changes of the cerebellar vermis, agenesis of the corpus callosum, hydromyelia, syringomyelia. Secondary facial deformities: prominent forehead, hypertelorism, exophthalmos.

Manifestation: Prenatal or at birth or else developing perinatally.

Aetiology: Unclear. Isolated occurrence or part of an overriding syndrome.

Pathogenesis: Primary occlusive disorders of the foramina of Luschka and Magendie.

Course, prognosis: Clinically, runs an extremely variable course, dependent also on when surgery is performed to relieve intracranial pressure and whether the Dandy–Walker malformation has occurred in isolation or as part of a syndrome.

Differential diagnosis: The Dandy–Walker malformation can be a secondary sign of the following malformation syndromes: Aase–Smith syndrome (*247*), Brachmann-de-Lange syndrome (*98*), Coffin–Siris syndrome (*94*), Ehlers-Danlos syndrome (*203*), Ellis-van-Creveld syndrome (*135*), Fraser syndrome (*42*), frontonasal dysplasia (*23*), Jones syndrome, Joubert syndrome, Meckel–Gruber syndrome (*45*), orofaciodigital syndrome, Varadi type, Walker–Warburg syndrome (*314*).
Various chromosomal disorders: Fryns syndrome (*318*), hydrolethalus syndrome (*323*).

Treatment: Shunt operation for obstruction and intracranial pressure.

Illustrations:

1a and b A 7-week-old male infant with ventriculoperitoneal shunt.

1c Cranial computerized tomography shows internal hydrocephalus and Dandy–Walker cysts.

2 Patient 2: Cranial magnetic resonance imaging, T^1-weighted, coronal section: Dandy–Walker cysts, cerebellar malformation, cerebral agyria, thickening of the cortex and hypoplasia of the medulla in the absence of myelinization. Age 5 years. In the region of the right ear, artifact because of the Rickham reservoir (child with Walker–Warburg syndrome).

References:

Murray J C, Johnson J A, Bird T D: Dandy-Walker malformation: etiologic heterogeneity and empiric recurrence risks. *Clin Genet* 1985, 28:272–283.

Stoll C, Huber C, Alembik Y, Terrade E, Maitrot D: Dandy-Walker variant malformation, spastic paraplegia, and mental retardation in two sibs. *Am J Med Genet* 1990, 37:124–127.

Nishimaki S, Yoda H, Seki K, Kawakami T, Akamatsu H, Iwasaki Y: A case of Dandy-Walker malformations associated with occipital meningocele, microphthalmos, and cleft palate. *Pediatr Radiol* 1990, 20:608–609.

Pascual-Castroviejo I, Velez A, Pascual-Pascual S I, Roche M C, Villarejo F: Dandy-Walker malformations: analysis of 38 cases. *Child Nerv Syst* 1991, 7:88–97.

Herriot R, Hallam L A, Gray E S: Dandy–Walker malformations in the Meckel syndrome. *Am J Med Genet* 1991, 39:207–210.

Cowles T, Furman P, Wilkins I: Prenatal diagnosis of Dandy-Walker malformation in a family displaying X-linked inheritance. *Prenat Diagn* 1993, 13:87–91.

Chitayat D, Moore L *et al*: Familial Dandy–Walker malformation associated with macrocephaly, facial anomalies, developmental delay, and brainstem dysgenesis. Prenatal diagnosis and postnatal outcome in brothers. A new syndrome? *Am J Med Genet* 1994, 52:406–415.

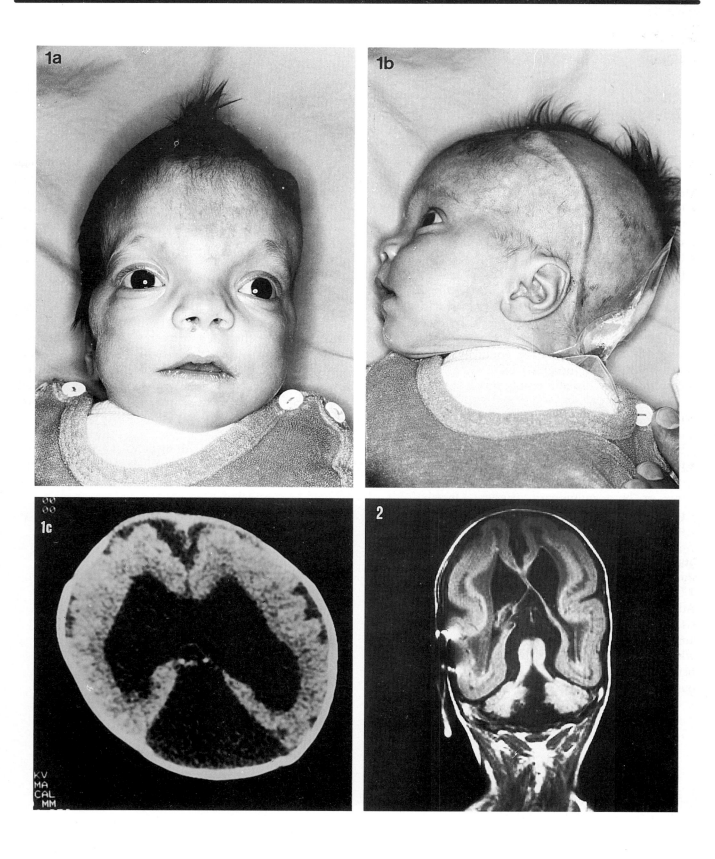

J.K.

A familial syndrome with characteristic facies, chronic cholestasis, posterior embryotoxon, butterfly-like anomalies of the vertebral arches, peripheral pulmonary stenosis and cardiac defects.

Main signs:

- Facial dysmorphism in 95%: prominent forehead; slight hypertelorism; deep-set eyes; prominent, narrow chin; saddle nose or accentuated, straight nasal bridge.
- Chronic cholestasis in 91% of patients, beginning in the first 3 months of life in 50% and between the fourth month and the third year of life in the remainder. Splenomegaly in less than one-half of the patients; one-fifth develop portal hypertension. Xanthomata on the extensor sides of the finger joints, on the back of the neck, the anal folds and the popliteal space, from the fourth year of life (progressive).
- Posterior embryotoxon: visible with a slit lamp in 89% of patients.
- Defects of the vertebral arches: in 87% of all affected individuals; failure of the arches to fuse, leading to a butterfly-like appearance.
- Cardiovascular disorders in 85%: frequently asymptomatic, isolated, nonprogressive, peripheral stenosis of one or both pulmonary arteries. One-sixth of all patients have additional cardiac defects (such as tetralogy of Fallot).

Supplementary findings: Growth retardation in 50% of the patients, increasing with age. Mesangial lipidosis in 17 out of 23 patients with only mild clinical renal signs. Additionally: infantile polycystic kidneys, nephronophthisis, stenosis of the renal artery. One patient with moyamoya disease with right-side hemiparesis. One patient with caudal dysplasia with anal stenosis, recto-urethral fistula, lumbosacral malformations. IQ below 80 in 16 out of 80 patients. Occasionally, high-pitched voice.

Manifestation: From birth to the sixth month or third year of life.

Aetiology: Autosomal dominant inheritance with high (94%) penetrance and variable expression. In 19 patients, characteristic deletions on the short arm of chromosome 20: del 20 p.11.2 and therefore gene localization presumed to be between p.11.23 and p12.2. Contiguous gene syndrome. Axial mesodermal dysplasia? Sporadic occurrence in 15%.

Frequency: Over 100 families have been reported.

Course, prognosis: Recurrent episodes of cholestasis, often associated with respiratory infections, especially in the first year of life. Malnutrition with severe cholestasis. One-quarter of all patients have died between 3 months and 23 years of age. Hepatic complications were the cause in only 5%, severe cardiac anomalies in 7.5%. Death from respiratory infections in 30%. Delayed puberty. Retarded linear growth.

Treatment: Low-fat diet with medium-chain triglycerides. Intramuscular administration of fat-soluble vitamins. Phenobarbitone to reduce pruritis. Liver transplantation should be considered.

Illustrations:

1a and b Age 21 months, broad forehead, deep-set eyes, short stature. Hepatomegaly. Caput medusae.
2a and b Age 2 years and 5 months, high forehead, prognathia with wide jaw, saddle nose.
3 Anomalies of the vertebral bodies in a newborn with Alagille syndrome.
4 Broad, high forehead, wide jaw.
5 Onset of xanthomatosis (hyperlipidemia).
6 Posterior embryotoxon.

References:

Alagille D, Estrada A, Hadchouel M *et al*: Syndromic paucity of interlobular bile ducts (Alagille syndrome or arteriohepatic dysplasia): review of 80 cases. *J Pediatr* 1987, **110**:195–200.
Rachmel A, Zeharia A *et al*: Alagille syndrome associated with moyamoya disease. *Am J Med Genet* 1989, 33:89–91.
Schnittger S, Höfers C *et al*: Molecular and cytogenic analysis of an interstitial 20p deletion associated with syndromic intrahepatic ductular hypoplasia (Alagille syndrome). *Hum Genet* 1989, 83:239–244.
Zhang F, Deleuze J F *et al*: Interstitial deletion of the short arm of chromosome 20 in arteriohepatic dysplasia (Alagille syndrome). *J Pediatr* 1990 **116**:73–77.
Anad F, Burn J *et al*: Alagille syndrome and deletion of 20p. *J Med Genet* 1990, **27**:729–737.
Legius E, Fryns J P *et al*: Alagille syndrome (arteriohepatic dysplasia) and del20p11.2. *Am J Med Genet* 1990, **35**:532–535.
Rodriguez J I, Rivera T, Palacios J: Alagille syndrome associated with caudal dysplasia sequence. *Am J Med Genet* 1991, **40**:61–64.
Teebi A S, Murthy D S K, Ismail E A R, Rehda A A: Alagille syndrome with de novo del20p11.2. *Am J Med Genet* 1992, **42**:35–38.
Dhorne-Pollet S, Deleuze J F, Hadchouel M, Bonaiti-Pellié C: Segregation analysis of Alagille syndrome. *J Med Genet* 1994 31:453–457.

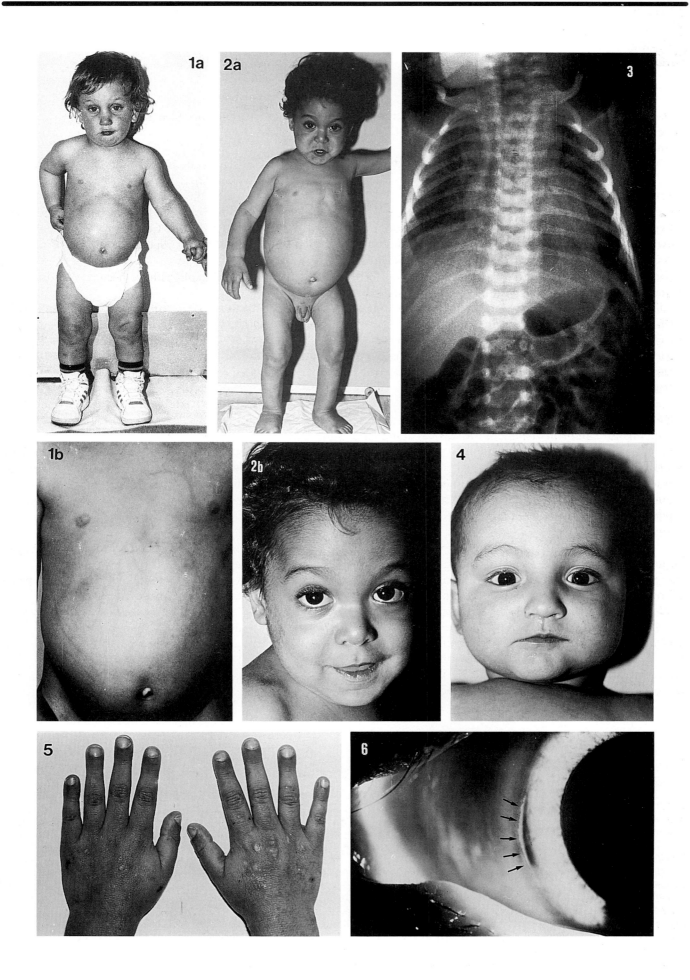

J.K.

A lethal malformation syndrome with facial dysmorphism, malformations of the distal extremities and defects of the diaphragm.

Main signs:
- Hydramnios, normal developmental data.
- Craniofacial dysmorphism: coarse facies, prominent glabella, broad flat nasal bridge, large nose with anteverted nostrils, short upper lip, macrostomia, cleft lip and palate, retrognathia, dysplastic ears.
- Brachytelephalangia (phalangeal hypoplasia in the distal region) both of the fingers and of the toes, hypoplastic nails, aplasia of the nails, camptodactyly.
- Defects of the diaphragm: aplasia of the posterolateral part continuous with hernia, secondary hypoplasia of the lungs, narrow thorax. Malrotation, multiple intestinal atresias.

Supplementary findings:
Eyes: microphthalmos, clouding of the cornea, mongoloid slant of the palpebral fissures, retinal dysplasia.
Short neck, nuchal pterygia.
Kidneys: dysplastic cystic kidneys.
Cerebrum: malformations, Dandy–Walker cysts, multiple cerebellar glioneural heterotopia.

Genitals: cryptorchidism. Bicornate uterus.
Skeleton: club feet.

Manifestation: Prenatal because 90% of patients develop a diaphragmatic hernia.

Aetiology: Autosomal recessive disorder.

Pathogenesis: Unknown.

Course, prognosis: Slim chance of survival.

Differential diagnosis: Hydrolethalus syndrome (*323*), Schinzel–Giedion syndrome, Rüdiger syndrome.

Treatment: Surgical correction of internal malformations.

Illustrations:
1–6 Craniofacial dysmorphism; hypertelorism, anteverted nostrils, broad nasal bridge, macrostomia, narrow upper lip. Short neck, diaphragmatic defect. Ventricular septal defect. Hydronephrosis, mega-ureter. Anal atresia. Deep creasing of the soles of the feet.
1–6 from:
Dix *et al.* Das Fryns-Syndrom - prä- und postnatale Diagnose. *Z Geburtshilfe Perinat* 1991, **195**:280–284.

References:
Meinecke P, Fryns J P: The Fryns syndrome: diaphragmatic defects, craniofacial dysmorphism, and distal digital hypoplasia. *Clin Genet* 1985, 28:516–520.
Fryns J P: Fryns syndrome: a variable MCA syndrome with diaphragmatic defects, coarse face, and distal limb hypoplasia. *J Med Genet* 1987, 24:271–274.
Aymé S, Julian C *et al*: Fryns syndrome: report on 8 cases. *Clin Genet* 1989, 35:191–201.
Moerman P, Fryns J P, Vandenberghe K, Devlieger H, Lauweryns J M: The syndrome of diaphragmatic hernia, abnormal face and distal limb anomalies (Fryns syndrome): report of two sibs with further delineation of this multiple congenital anomaly (MCA) syndrome. *Am J Med Genet* 1988, 31:805–814.
Bamforth J S, Leonard C O *et al*: Congenital diaphragmatic hernia, coarse facies, and acral hypoplasia: Fryns syndrome. *Am J Med Genet* 1989, 32:93–99.
Cunniff C, Jones K L, Saal H W, Stern H J: Fryns syndrome: an autosomal recessive disorder associated with craniofacial anomalies, diaphragmatic hernia, and distal digital hypoplasia. *Pediatrics* 1990, 85:499–504.
Dix U, Beudt U, Langenbeck U: Fryns-Syndrom - Prä- und postnatale Diagnose. *Z Geburtsh Perinat* 1991, **195**:280–284.
Dean J C S, Couzin D A, Gray E S, Lloyd D L, Stephen G S: Apparent Fryns' syndrome and aneuploidy: evidence for a disturbance of the midline developmental field. *Clin Genet* 1991, 40:349–352.
Stratton R F, Young R S, Heiman H S, Carter J M: Fryns syndrome. *Am J Med Genet* 1993, 45:562–564.

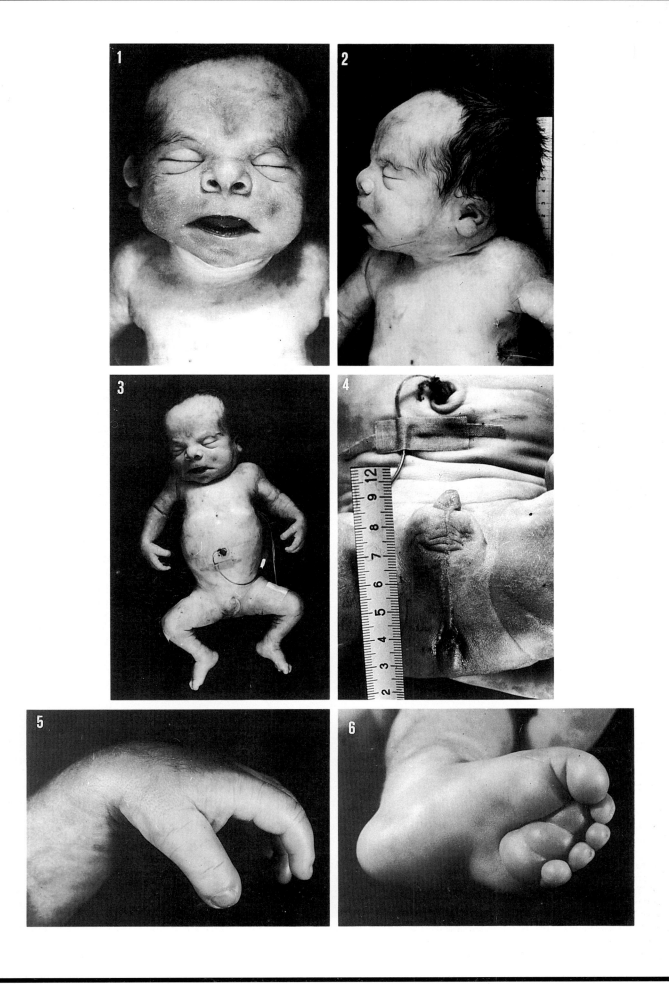

J.K.

An aetiologically heterogeneous clinical picture with a trisomy 18-like phenotype.

Main signs:
- Intra-uterine growth retardation of length and weight.
- Craniofacial anomalies: ocular hypertelorism, micrognathia, short neck, low-set and simply modelled ears, depressed tip of the nose.
- Anomalies of the extremities: retardation of growth, ankylosis of the large joints, abnormally formed fingers and toes (cylindrical), slender extremities, overlapping fingers as in trisomy 18, equinovarus positioning of the feet, 'rocker-bottom' feet, deficient calcification of the bones.
- Pulmonary hypoplasia.
- Short umbilical cord.
- Polyhydramnios (important presenting sign).
- Disorders of the central nervous system and peripheral nerves: thin cortex, dilated ventricles, polymicrogyria, neurogenic muscular atrophy.

Supplementary findings: Telecanthus, epicanthus medialis, microstomia, high palate, cleft palate, mandibular hypoplasia, camptodactyly, nuchal hygroma. Pterygia of the joints. Diverse cardiac defects. Urogenital anomalies (renal microcysts, megalo-ureter, persistent urachus, hypospadias). Choanal atresia, laryngeal stenoses. Optic atrophy. Torticollis. Hyperplasia of the thymus. Intestinal malformations, gastroschisis, malrotation, Meckel's diverticulum, anal atresia. Adrenal hypoplasia. Macrocephaly (one family).

Manifestation: At birth. Prenatal diagnosis by ultrasound is possible with a positive history.

Aetiology: Heterogeneity. Mostly autosomal recessive inheritance or sporadic patients. X-linked recessive patients also known. Even intrafamilial heterogeneity has been described. Risk of recurrence 10–15%. Maternal myasthenia. Congenital, non-neurogenic myopathy.

Frequency: Approximately 75 reports published. The syndrome is underdiagnosed: Shokeir estimates 1 out of 12 000 newborns.

Course, prognosis: One-third stillbirths; approximately 40% die within the first 14 days; demise of almost all remaining patients by the 16th week of life. Occasional survival. Weak suck, failure to thrive. Delayed motor development. Mental development normal to severely retarded. One child lived for 20 months.

Differential diagnosis: Trisomy 18 (48) can be excluded cytogenetically. Patients with the cerebro-oculo-facio-skeletal syndrome (320) (previously called Pena–Shokeir syndrome II) survive birth but then show severe, progressive psychomotor deterioration with no development of speech and death in the third year of life. Phenotypically identical to Pena–Shokeir syndrome I, suggesting different expression? Lethal congenital contracture syndrome (autosomal recessive).

Treatment: Symptomatic. Respiratory support.

Illustrations:

1a–c Foetal akinesia with hydramnios, birth in the 33rd week of pregnancy, lived for 33 h: multiple joint contractures, pulmonary hypoplasia, absent labia majora and minora, anomalies of the ears, head circumference 50th percentile, cleft palate, congenital muscular dystrophy. Spinal cord: unremarkable anterior horns.

2 Male sibling, termination of pregnancy after foetal akinesia, diagnosis in the 25th week of pregnancy by ultrasound: identical findings. Diagnosis: autosomal recessive myopathic form of the Pena–Shokeir syndrome.

References:

Shokeir M H K: Multiple ankyloses, camptodactyly, facial anomalies and pulmonary hypoplasia (Pena-Shokeir I syndrome). In: Vinken P J and Bruyn G W (eds). Handbook of clinical neurology. *Neurog dir II* 1982, **43**:437–439.

Lindhout D, Hageman G, Beemer F A *et al*: The Pena-Shokeir syndrome: report of nine Dutch cases. *Am J Med Genet* 1985, **21**:655–668.

Hunt-MacMillan R, Harbert G M, Davis W D *et al*: Prenatal diagnosis of the Pena-Shokeir syndrome type I. *Am J Med Genet* 1985, **21**:279–284.

Hall J G: Invited editorial comment: analysis of Pena Shokeir phenotype. *Am J Med Genet* 1986, **25**:99–117.

Hageman G, Willemse J, van Ketel B A *et al*: The heterogeneity of the Pena-Shokeir syndrome. *Neuropediatrics* 1987, **18**:45–50.

Ohlsson A, Fong K W, Rose T H *et al*: Prenatal diagnosis of Pena-Shokeir syndrome type I, or fetal akinesia deformation sequence. *Am J Med Genet* 1988, **29**:59–65.

Erdl R, Schmidtke K *et al*: Pena-Shokeir phenotype with major CNS-malformations: clinicopathological report of two siblings. *Clin Genet* 1989, **36**:127–135.

Lammer E J, Donnelly S, Holmes L B: Pena-Shokeir phenotypes in sibs with macrocephaly but without growth retardation. *Am J Med Genet* 1989, **32**:478–481.

Vuopala K, Herva R: Lethal congenital contracture syndrome: further delineation and genetic aspects. *J Med Genet* 1994, **31**:521–527.

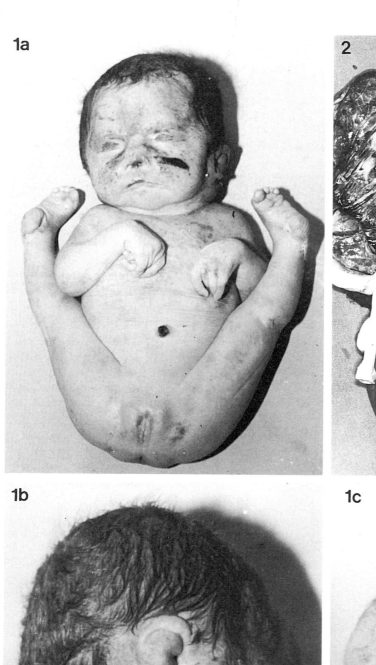

1a

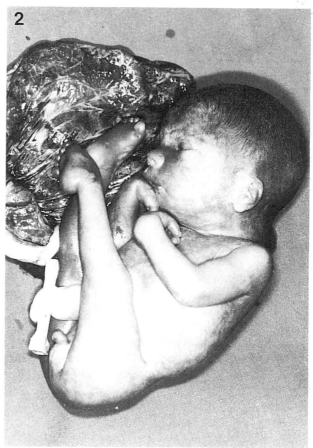

2

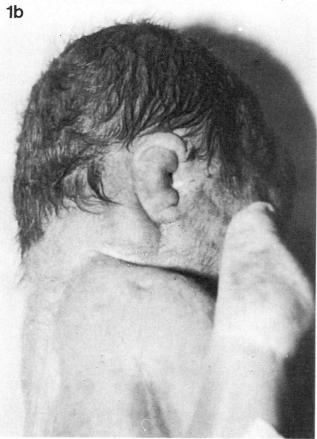

1b

1c

J.K.

An autosomal recessive clinical picture with lethal course, severe progressive psychomotor retardation, facial dysmorphism, skeletal anomalies and flexion contractures of the large joints.

Main signs:

- Microcephaly, muscular hypotonia, hyper-reflexia, areflexia, progressive psychomotor decline, no development of speech.
- Microphthalmos, anophthalmia, cataract, blepharophimosis.
- Prominent nasal bridge, micrognathia, large ears, overhanging upper lip, short neck.
- Camptodactyly, overlapping fingers, flexion contractures of the elbow and knee joints, kyphosis, dysplastic acetabula, coxa valga, 'rocker-bottom' feet, osteoporosis.

Supplementary findings: Indistinct border between the grey and white matter, lissencephaly, agenesis of the corpus callosum, reduction of neurons in the cerebrum, cerebellum, spinal cord and retina (as with neuronal destruction resulting from foetal anoxia). In older children, dilated ventricles, decrease of the white matter of the brain. Small for dates babies. Renal anomalies.

Manifestation: Birth to the sixth month of life.

Aetiology: Autosomal recessive inheritance. Parental consanguinity frequently demonstrable.

Frequency: Approximately 1 one out of 10000 newborns.

Course, prognosis: No sign of prenatal growth retardation at birth. Postnatal course of severe general developmental retardation with no development of speech. Death in the third year because of respiratory infection. Feeding difficulties.

Differential diagnosis: Pena-Shokeir syndrome I (*319*), Cockayne syndrome (*89*), trisomy 18 (*48*). Bowen–Conradi syndrome. Neu–Laxova syndrome.

Treatment: Symptomatic.

Illustrations:

1a Patient 1: a 9-day-old girl, microcephaly, small for dates, micrognathia, dysplastic ears, short neck (agenesis of the corpus callosum).
1b and c 'Trisomy 18-like' positioning of the fingers.
1d and e 'Rocker bottom' feet (as in trisomy 18).
2 Patient 2: a 5-week-old boy with characteristic prominent nasal bridge, microcephaly, hairy forehead.

References:
Shokeir M H K: Cerebro-oculo-facioskeletal (COFS) syndrome (Pena-Shokeir II syndrome). In: Vinken P J and Bruyn G W (eds.) Handbook of clinical neurology. *Neur dir II* 1982, **43**:341–343.
Silengo M C, Davi G, Bianco R *et al*: The NEU-COFS (cerebro-oculo-facio-skeletal) syndrome: report of a case. *Clin Genet* 1984, **25**:201–204.
Lerman-Sagie T, Levy Y *et al*: Syndrome of osteoporosis and muscular degeneration associated with cerebro-oculo-facio-skeletal changes. *Am J Med Genet* 1987, **28**:137–142.
Gershoni-Baruch R, Ludatscher R M *et al*: Cerebro-oculo-facio-skeletal syndrome: further delineation. *Am J Med Genet* 1991, **4**: 74–77.
Meyer R: Zerebro-okulo-fazio-skelettäres Syndrom. *Pädiat Prax* 1993/94, **46**:317–322.

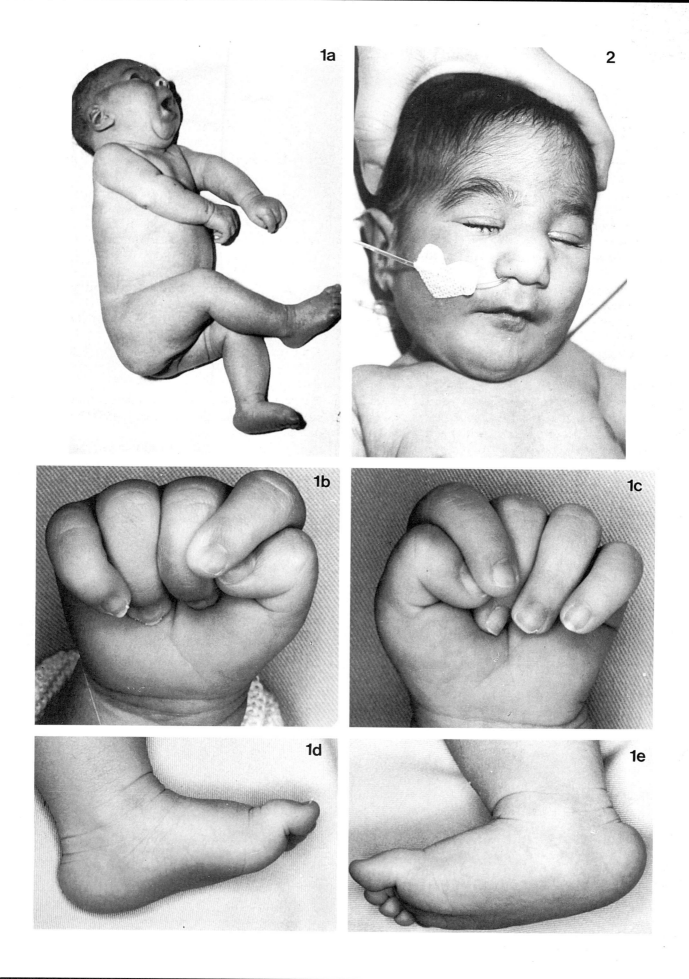

659

321 SHORT Syndrome

(Short stature, hyperextensibility of joints and hernia (inguinal), ocular depression, Rieger anomaly, delayed teething)

J.K.

Main signs:
- Short stature with intra-uterine growth retardation.
- Hyperextensibility of the joints and/or inguinal hernias.
- Deep-set eyes, megalocornea.
- Rieger anomaly (iridodental syndrome = Axenfeld syndrome).
- Delayed dentition.

Supplementary findings: Slow weight gain after birth, feeding problems in the first 2 years, recurrent infections, triangular face, telecanthus, broad nasal bridge, prominent forehead, head circumference around the 10th percentile, hypoplastic alae nasi, micrognathia, deficient subcutaneous tissue (lipo-atrophy), hearing impairment, delayed bone age, bilateral clinodactyly, delayed development of speech, normal intelligence.

Manifestation: At birth and in early childhood.

Aetiology: Autosomal recessive inheritance. Autosomal dominant inheritance has also been observed. To be differentiated from the autosomal dominant syndrome of partial lipo-atrophy with short stature and insulin-dependent diabetes.

Frequency: To date only seven observations, once in siblings, one case of vertical transmission.

Course, prognosis: Good prognosis, normal intelligence. One case of insulin-resistant diabetes mellitus has been reported.

Differential diagnosis: Silver–Russell syndrome (82), Floating Harbor syndrome (83).

Treatment: Symptomatic.

References:

Toriello H V, Wakefield S, Komar K *et al*: Report of a case and further delineation of the SHORT syndrome. *Am J Med Genet* 1985, **22**:311–314.
Lipson A H, Cowell C, Gorlin R J: The SHORT syndrome: further delineation and natural history. *J Med Genet* 1989, **26**:473–475.
Schwingshandl J, Mache C J, Rath K, Borkenstein M H: SHORT syndrome and insulin resistance. *Am J Med Genet* 1993, **47**:907–909.

GAPO Syndrome

(Growth retardation, alopecia, pseudo-anodontia, progressive optic atrophy)

J.K.

Main signs:

Severe growth retardation with retarded bone age, rhizomelic shortening.

Alopecia, severe hypotrichosis (congenital or developing during the first year), white eyelashes in isolated cases.

Pseudo-anodontia (failure of tooth eruption).

Progressive optic atrophy beginning in early childhood (not a consistent sign).

Supplementary findings: Characteristic facial appearance with high prominent forehead, midface dysplasia, prominent eyes with flat orbits, glaucoma, keratoconus. Delayed closure of the wide-open anterior fontanelle. Micrognathia. Deep-set nasal bridge. Umbilical hernias, hypogonadism: oligospermia, mammary hypoplasia, hypoplasia of the labia majora and clitoris. Skeletal anomalies: osteopenia, short metacarpals and metatarsals, exostoses, kyphosis, muscular hypertrophy, athletic habitus.

Manifestation: Usually after the first year of life. Alopecia usually at birth.

Aetiology: Autosomal recessive inheritance. Connective-tissue disorder: excessive homogeneous, amorphous hyalin material in all organs, in the interstitium and in the serosa.

Frequency: Seventeen published cases, several cases observed in siblings.

Course, prognosis: Good. Normal mental development.

Treatment: Symptomatic.

Differential diagnosis: Progeria.

References:

Tipton R E, Gorlin R J: Growth retardation, alopecia, pseudoanodontia, and optic atrophy — The GAPO syndrome: report of a patient and review of the literature. *Am J Med Genet* 1984, **19**:209–216.
Gagliardi A R T, Gonzales C H Pratesi, C.H: GAPO syndrome: report of three affected brothers. *Am J Med Genet* 1984, **19**:217–223.
Manouvrier-Hanu S, Largilliere C, Benalioua M. *et al*: Brief clinical report: the GAPO syndrome. *Am J Med Genet* 1987, **26**:683–688.
Wajntal, A, Koiffmann, C. P. et al: GAPO syndrome (McKusick 230 74) — a connective tissue disorder: report on two affected sibs and on the pathologic findings in the older. *Am J Med Genet* 1990, **37**:213–223.
Sayh B S, Gül D: GAPO syndrome in three relatives in a Turkish kindred. *Am J Med Genet* 1993, **47**:342–345.
Phadke S R, Haldhar A. *et al*: GAPO syndrome in a child without dermal hyaline deposit. *Am J Med Genet* 1994 **51**:191–193.

Hydrolethalus Syndrome
(Salonen–Herva–Norio Syndrome)

J.K.

A hereditary syndrome with severe malformations of the brain, polydactyly, pulmonary hypoplasia and facial clefts.

Main signs:
- Hydrocephalus (93%), absence of the corpus callosum and septum pellucidum, Dandy–Walker malformation, olfactory aplasia and many others.
- Polydactyly (88%): always pre-axial in the feet, occasionally additional postaxial hexadactyly of the toes. Polydactyly of the hands (when present, always postaxial. Club feet.
- Cleft lip and palate (56%).
- Micrognathia (84%), tongue small or absent.
- Malformations of the tracheobronchial tree (65%).
- Abnormal lobar development of the lungs (50%).
- Cardiac defect (58%): ventricular septal defect, atrioventricular canal.
- Polyhydramnios (100%), still birth or death immediately *post partum*.

Supplementary findings: Simply modelled nose, microphthalmos, adrenal hypoplasia in children with absent hypophysis (midline defect), no intestinal rotation, cryptorchidism, double or septate uterus. Normal kidneys. Polysplenia.

Manifestation: Prenatal and postnatal.

Aetiology: Autosomal recessive inheritance. The syndrome has been observed relatively frequently in Finland (1:20 000), but also in Arabic families and in Africans.

Frequency: Approximately 60 patients described, usually with affected siblings.

Prognosis: Always lethal. Five children lived longer: 17 days, 50 days, 4 and 8 months.

Differential diagnosis: Patients with Meckel–Gruber syndrome (*45*); also septo-optic dysplasia, the Walker–Warburg syndrome (*314*), Goldenhar 'syndrome' (*30*), Fryns syndrome (*318*), Ivemark syndrome. Patients with chromosomal disorders always have dysplastic cystic kidneys. The Smith–Lemli–Opitz syndrome (*281*) and trisomy 13 (*47*) can be clearly differentiated.

References:
Salonen R, Herva R, Norio R: The hydrolethalus syndrome: delineation of a 'new', lethal malformation syndrome based on 28 patients. *Clin Genet* 1981, 19:321–350.
Anyane-Yeboa K, Collins M, Kupsky W *et al*: Hydrolethalus (Salonen-Herva-Norio) syndrome: further clinicopathological delineation. *Am J Med Genet* 1987, 26:899–907.
Salonen R, Herva R: Hydrolethalus syndrome. *J Med Genet* 1990, 27:756–759.
Haverkamp F, Zerres K *et al*: 7 Wochen alter Säugling mit Hydroletalus-Syndrom: Fallbericht, Differentialdiagnosen und Literaturüberblick. *Klin Pädiat* 1990, 202:387–390.
Sharma A K, Phadke S *et al*: Overlap between Majewski and hydrolethalus syndromes: a report of two cases. *Am J Med Genet* 1992 43:949–953.
Pryde P G, Qureshi F *et al*: Two consecutive hydrolethalus syndromes — affected pregnancies in a non-consanguineous black couple: Discussion of problems in prenatal differential diagnosis of midline malformation syndromes. *Am J Med Genet* 1993, 46:537–541.
Seller M J, Pal K, Docherty Z, Nash T G: A fetus with an abnormal chromosome 7 and possible hydrolethalus syndrome. *Clin Dysmorphol* 1994 3:35–39.

Index

668

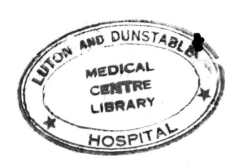